Drug Use in the Older Adult

Glenda Elaine Bilder
Patricia Brown-O'Hara

Drug Use in the Older Adult

A Guide for Nurses, Other Practicing Clinicians and Interested Older Individuals

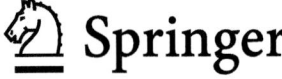

Glenda Elaine Bilder
Lederach, PA, USA

Patricia Brown-O'Hara
College of Nursing & Health Professions
Gwynedd Valley, PA, USA

ISBN 978-3-031-84830-8   ISBN 978-3-031-84831-5 (eBook)
https://doi.org/10.1007/978-3-031-84831-5

© The Editor(s) (if applicable) and The Author(s), under exclusive license to Springer Nature Switzerland AG 2025

This work is subject to copyright. All rights are solely and exclusively licensed by the Publisher, whether the whole or part of the material is concerned, specifically the rights of translation, reprinting, reuse of illustrations, recitation, broadcasting, reproduction on microfilms or in any other physical way, and transmission or information storage and retrieval, electronic adaptation, computer software, or by similar or dissimilar methodology now known or hereafter developed.

The use of general descriptive names, registered names, trademarks, service marks, etc. in this publication does not imply, even in the absence of a specific statement, that such names are exempt from the relevant protective laws and regulations and therefore free for general use.

The publisher, the authors and the editors are safe to assume that the advice and information in this book are believed to be true and accurate at the date of publication. Neither the publisher nor the authors or the editors give a warranty, expressed or implied, with respect to the material contained herein or for any errors or omissions that may have been made. The publisher remains neutral with regard to jurisdictional claims in published maps and institutional affiliations.

This Springer imprint is published by the registered company Springer Nature Switzerland AG
The registered company address is: Gewerbestrasse 11, 6330 Cham, Switzerland

If disposing of this product, please recycle the paper.

Preface

The goal of writing this book is to provide current guidance to nurses, clinicians, and older individuals on appropriate use of drugs in the treatment of age-related diseases and conditions (see back cover for details). The historic increase in life expectancy over the past century and the desire by all to spend those additional years free of disease and disability create a requisite need to better understand drug use in the older person. This book covers many topics explaining the efficacy of prescription medications, that is, what drugs can and should not do, the many ways age influences drug action, and the impact of widely used drugs obtained without a prescription (recreational drugs, Over The Counter supplements). Each chapter places a premium on discussing the scientific use of drugs in the amelioration of diseases with the view of minimizing or eliminating adverse effects. The authors have relied heavily on results from clinical trials and where available, clinical trials that included the older adult.

By way of an introduction to our book, Chap. 1 provides orientation on some important population characteristics of older adults such as size, growth rate, health status, and patterns of medication use. Additionally, it supplies essential information on the type and quality of evidence used throughout this book. Chapter 2 details the principles of pharmacokinetics and pharmacodynamics of drugs in the body and how age may influence certain aspects of pharmacokinetics and pharmacodynamics, hence requiring vigilance in prescribing. Chapter 3 continues with the most serious component of drug use, the adverse drug reaction, especially high in the older adult but mostly avoidable. Known drug combinations, polypharmacy, and potentially inappropriate drugs are discussed. Chapters 4, 5, and 6 provide essential understanding of diseases (atherosclerotic cardiovascular disease, cancer, Alzheimer's disease, Type 2 diabetes mellitus, chronic obstructive pulmonary disease, chronic kidney disease, Parkinson's disease, and many important infectious diseases), currently recommended therapies, and drug-related issues and concerns. Common geriatric syndromes (frailty, delirium, urinary incontinence, pressure injuries, falls, sarcopenia, malnutrition, cognitive impairment, unintentional weight loss, feeding/eating problems, sleeping disorders, and depression) and medications associated with geriatric syndromes that are candidates for deprescribing are presented in Chap. 7. Chapter 8 examines the use of alcohol, marijuana, and nicotine and its effects on health and interaction with other drugs. The efficacy and safety of commonly used over-the-counter drugs and dietary/herbal supplements by the older adult are reviewed in Chap. 9. Chapter 10 discusses the new field of geroscience and the search for antiaging drugs. Each chapter summarizes key points and presents them as specific guides to practice.

As authors, although with different backgrounds (PhD Pharmacology, Drug Discovery Research Career, Author of Aging Textbook, G. Bilder; PhD Nursing, Practice, Teaching, University Assistant Dean, P. Brown-O'Hara), we share an abiding interest in biological aging and appropriate drug use for the older adult. Readers will benefit from our work.

Lederach, PA, USA Glenda Elaine Bilder
Gwynedd Valley, PA, USA Patricia Brown-O'Hara

Contents

1	**Orientation: Aging, Demographics, Patterns of Medication Use**	1
	References...	8
2	**Principles of Pharmacokinetics/Pharmacodynamics**...............	13
	Pharmacokinetic Principles................................	15
	Pharmacodynamic Principles	17
	Pharmacology and Aging	18
	Pharmacokinetics and Aging...............................	19
	Pharmacodymanics and Aging	27
	Homeostatic Mechanisms.................................	32
	References...	35
3	**Adverse Drug Reactions**....................................	45
	Adverse Drug Reactions (ADRs)	46
	References...	67
4	**Medication Use in Major Age-Related Diseases: Atherosclerotic Cardiovascular Disease, Cancer, Alzheimer's Disease and Related Dementias, Type 2 Diabetes Mellitus**	77
	Atherosclerotic Cardiovascular Disease	79
	Malignancies...	88
	Alzheimer's Disease and Related Dementias	94
	Type 2 Diabetes Mellitus	100
	References...	108
5	**Medication Use in Major Age-Related Diseases: Chronic Obstructive Pulmonary Disease, Chronic Kidney Disease, and Parkinson's Disease**	123
	Chronic Obstructive Pulmonary Disease	125
	Chronic Kidney Disease	133
	Parkinson's Disease	139
	References...	151

6	**Medication Use in Infectious Diseases**	165
	Infectious Diseases	168
	COVID-19	169
	Pneumonias	175
	Influenza	178
	Tuberculosis	179
	Urinary Tract Infections	181
	Sepsis, Septic Shock	182
	Safety of Antimicrobials	184
	Vaccines	191
	References	196
7	**Geriatric Syndromes: Definition, Assessment, and Effective Therapy**	211
	References	234
8	**Recreational Drugs: Alcohol, Marijuana, Nicotine**	245
	Alcohol	246
	Marijuana	258
	Nicotine	270
	References	276
9	**Over-the-Counter Medications, Vitamins, Minerals, Biologicals, and Herbal Supplements**	289
	Over-the-Counter Drugs	292
	Vitamins and Minerals—Dietary Supplements	299
	Biologicals	306
	Botanicals (Herbal Extracts)	315
	References	322
10	**Anti-aging Drugs**	341
	Anti-aging Drugs	346
	References	356

Orientation: Aging, Demographics, Patterns of Medication Use

Abbreviations

ADRs	Adverse drug reactions
AL	Assisted living
NHANES	National Health and Nutrition Examination Survey
OTC	Over-the-counter
PD	Pharmacodynamics
PIMs	Potentially inappropriate medications
PK	Pharmacokinetics
QoL	Quality of life
RCT	Randomized clinical trial

AGING AND ITS CONSEQUENCES It seems obvious that the answer to "what is aging" should include the idea of passage of time and deteriorative changes to the body with loss of fitness. However, a recent symposium of experts in the field of biological aging could not agree on a definition of aging [1]. The greatest consensus posited that aging was a heterogeneous process, occurring unevenly across tissues, at the molecular, cellular, and higher integrative sites. There was no consensus on when aging started, whether it was reversible or as to its theoretical/evolutionary origins. As concluded from the symposium, a better understanding of aging will require integration from multiple disciplines such as demographics, epidemiology, clinical geriatrics, late-life diseases, and hallmarks of aging to name a few [1].

However, there is no escaping the convincing observation that with age, organ function progressively declines, creating a vulnerability to stress and disease and increasing the probability of death [2]. Age changes have huge ramifications, not only in permissiveness for disease/geriatric syndrome development and progression but also for the essential therapy to retard disease advancement, maintain quality of life (QoL), and reduce mortality. As part of quality therapy, it is important to understand the influence of age-related changes and associated diseases on the processing of medications in the body and equally important for the health provider to adjust to these changes so as to offer the best care to maintain QoL without unnecessary adverse drug reactions (ADRs) and hospitalizations.

DEMOGRAPHICS OF THE OLDER ADULTS Demographic data tabulates information on populations. This may include information on, for example, age, gender, race, death rate, health, disability, and education, obtained from a particular population at a particular time. With regard to aging, demographic data can provide important population insights, such as size, projected growth rate, health status, and disability of older adults, and permit comparisons across different populations and different time frames as to these characteristics. Demographic indicators of aging discussed here focus on the number of older adults globally and locally (USA), projected future numbers, and relevant attributes needed to understand drug use such as prevalence of diseases, conditions, and syndromes of aging along with prescription and nonprescription drug use.

Demographic Indicators. Influential Factors One of the most remarkable achievements of the twentieth century was the near doubling of human life expectancy from 32 years (1900) to 72 years (2020) worldwide and from 48 years to 77.5 years (2022) for Americans [3, 4] (see Table 1.1 for summary of demographic data). Life expectancy increased dramatically following the acceptance of the validity of the Germ Theory of Infectious Disease proposed by Louis Pasteur, Robert Koch, and others. This enlightenment propelled reforms in public health, hygiene, and aseptic childbirth improving chances of reaching adulthood [11]. Subsequent advances in medical technology improved management of chronic diseases, now more accessible through Medicare and Medicaid, progress that further increased the odds of surviving to older ages [11, 12]. Thus, the mortality rate declined, allowing

Table 1.1 Demographic factors defining the older adult

Demographic indicator	Global change	Local (USA) change
Life Expectancy—near doubling over the last century [3, 4]	1900—32 yrs 2020—72 yrs	1920—48 yrs 2022—77.5 yrs
Percentage of population ≥65 yrs [5–7]	2022—10% 2050—16% Females > Males	2022—17.3% 2050—23% Females > Males
Projected percentage of older adults relative to other ages [8]	Mid-2030—number of ≥80 yrs exceed number of ≤1 yr olds. 2070—number of ≥65 yrs exceeds number ≤18 yrs	2010–2020 older population increased faster than population in general [9] 2050—fastest projected growth rate of ≥85 year olds [10]

Life expectancy the projected number of years one can expect to live based on the mortality data at birth. It is a rough estimate of the health of the society, *yrs* years, ≥ equal to or greater than, ≤ equal to or less than people to live longer. The current challenge today is to expand the healthspan equal to the extended lifespan [13].

Older Adult Defined Globally *Age categories are arbitrary.* However, in most demographic studies, the older adult is considered to be 65 years and older. Data collected worldwide by the World Population Prospects 2022 [5] indicate that the population of those 65 and older is increasing more rapidly than younger age groups. As of 2022, older adults constitute 10% of the world's population and are projected to increase to 16% by 2050. By 2070, the older population is projected to be 2.2 billion and most significantly and for the first time in history, *the number of older adults will exceed the number of children under 18 years of age* [8]. Furthermore, by the mid-2030s, those 80 years and older (estimated 265 million) will exceed the number of infants of 1 year of age or less [8]. Among older adults globally, women currently outnumber men and are projected to do so representing 54% of the older population by 2050 [6].

Older Adult, USA In the United States, according to the most recent data collected by the US Census Bureau, the National Center for Health Statistics, and the Bureau of Labor Statistics [7], the number of Americans (2022), age 65 years and older is 57.8 million (31.9 million women; 25.9 million men). This age group represents 17.3% of the total US population. The change in number (15.5 million) and rate of growth (36.8%) from the decade (2010–2020) was the largest since 1880–1890 [9]. Thus, the *rate of growth of the 65 and older population was five times faster than the population itself* due to rapid increase in those 65–74 years of age followed by those 95 years and older. Older females continue to outnumber older males but a slight increase in men 100 and over occurred from 2010 to 2020 [9]. Continued growth of the 65 and older population is expected with attainment of 82 million individuals (23% of the population or nearly 1 in every 4) by 2050 [14]. The fastest rate of growth is projected to be with those 85 years and older [10] (see Table 1.1 for demographic summary).

Health Status of Older Adults In addition to defining the size of population of older adults and the projected increase over the next decade or so, knowledge of health status of older population is also essential. It provides direction for judicious use of healthcare resources and also gives encouragement for innovations in business, technology, medical science, basic research, and pharmaceutical drug/device development to improve the QoL of older adults. As shown in Table 1.2, demographic data indicate that as of 2023, approximately one-quarter of those 65 and older considered themselves to be in fair or poor health [32]. Of those 65 and older, nearly three-quarters have hypertension, and about 25% or more are living with coronary heart disease, diabetes, chronic kidney disease and the geriatric syndrome, frailty. Furthermore, 40–45% of older adults are obese and approximately a third of older adults experience one or more disabilities related to difficulties in hearing, vision, communication, concentration, mobility, and self-care [23]. Those living in nursing homes/skilled nursing facilities (24/7 medical care) constituted 2.5% of the

Table 1.2 Prevalence of disease/syndrome/disability and medication use in the population of older adults

Disease/syndrome/disability	Percentage (65–74 years of age)	Percentage (75 and more years)			
Health status—fair or poor	21.9 [15]	27.7 [15]			
Diagnosed hypertension	66.7(M), 74.4 (F) [16]	81.5(M), 86(F) [16]			
Coronary heart disease	14.3 [17]	24.2 [17]			
COPD, emphysema, chronic bronchitis	9.8 (65 years and older) [18]				
Cancer	20.3 [15]	32.6 [15]			
Type 2 Diabetes Mellitus	24.4 [19]	19.9 [19]			
Alzheimer's Disease	5.3 [20]	13.8 (75–84) 34.5 (≥85 years) [20]			
Chronic kidney disease	38% (≥65 years) [21]				
Frailty syndrome	30.4, 41(prefrailty) (≥65 years) [22]				
Obesity	41.9 (M), 45.9 (F) [16]	31.8 (M), 36.1 (F) [16]			
One or more disabilities	33 (≥65 years) [23]				
Medication use	Percentage (≥65 years)				
	One drug	≥5 drugs	≥9 drugs	≥10 drugs	OTC (drugs/supplements)
Community	90 [24]	43 [25]–65.1 [26]		6.1 [27]	37.9/63.7 [28]
Assisted living		72.2 [27]		30.2 [27]	
Nursing home		71.3 [27]	30–46 [29–31]	23.5 [27]	Supplements – 17 [29]

Diagnosed hypertension defined as systolic >130 mm Hg, diastolic >80 mm Hg or on antihypertensive medications, *disabilities* loss of vision, hearing, mobility, concentration, communication, self-care, *M* male, *F* female, *OTC* over-the-counter, *COPD* chronic obstructive pulmonary disease

older population with those 85 and older representing the largest resident age category [9].

PATTERNS OF MEDICATION USE IN THE OLDER ADULT Given the presence of diverse morbidities in the older population, it is not surprising to find high medication use. Medications encompass both prescription drugs and nonprescription drugs such as over-the-counter (OTC) drugs and dietary/herbal supplements. Several studies have determined the magnitude of medication use in older adults. The resulting general pattern of medication use in this population (discussed below) serves to emphasize the extent of drug use in each drug subcategory and, most importantly, creates an awareness of the considerable potential for drug misuse, abuse, and dependency culminating in ADRs. ADRs lead not only to poor health, hospitalizations, and death but also burden healthcare resources (discussed in Chap. 3).

Medication Use. Data Source Medication use has been evaluated by phone surveys [33], filled prescriptions [34], by in-house surveys to directly assess usage [24, 28, 35–37], and data collected from patient visits [26, 38] and from the years long National Health and Nutrition Examination Survey (NHANES) [25]. Retrospective analysis of drug use in US nursing homes has also been done [29].

Medication Use. Extent in Community-Dwellers According to the Slone Survey, a phone survey (last published survey in 2006) indicated that the use of at least one medication (prescription, OTC, vitamin/mineral, herbal) in adults was as high as 82% and that the older population consumed the most medications compared to other age groups. In-house surveys are of significance because clinicians/researchers are able to interview patients directly in their homes and ask to see both medications and prescriptions as verification. Qato et al. (2008, 2016) [28, 35] completed two studies in this fashion. Study cohorts enlisted 2351 participants in 2005–2006 and 2206 participants in 2010–2011. The authors found that "use of one prescription medication slightly increased from 84.1% in 2005–06 to 87.7% in 2010–11. Concurrent use of 5 or more medications or supplements of any type or drug obtained from multiple providers (termed polypharmacy, see fuller discussion in Chap. 3) increased substantially from 53.4% to 67.1% during this 5-year period." Thus, medication use in individuals 62–85 of age, living in communities evaluated in this manner, supports the conclusion that drug use in the older individual continues to increase. Although use of OTC drugs significantly decreased (44.4–37.9%), prescription drug use and dietary supplement use significantly increased (51.8–63.7%). Qato et al. (2016) identified the increased use of specific drugs and supplements: statins (33.8–46.2%), antiplatelet drugs (32.8–43.0%), and omega-3 fish oils (4.7–18.6%).

Analysis of NHANES (1999–2000 to 2011–2012), a larger series of in-house surveys over a 10-year period with a query of drug use in the past 30 days, found an escalation in drug use by the older adults (84–90%) and an increase in polypharmacy (24–39%) [24]. Kantor et al. (2015) additionally reported statistically significant increased drug use in 7 drug classes: antihypertensives (55–66%), antihyperlipidemic agents (21–47%), antidiabetic drugs (13–19%), antidepressants (8.4–17%), prescription proton-pump inhibitors (8.2–18%), anticoagulants (7–15%) and anticonvulsants (4.5–9%) and a significant decrease in drug use of prescription analgesics (18–14%) and antibiotics (4.4–3.5%). Use of drugs in some classes, e.g., sedatives, hypnotics, thyroid hormone, did not change over the 10 years period [24]. A recent update of NHANES (2017–2020) reported an increase in polypharmacy from 39% to 43% among the older adult population [25]. An extensive cross-sectional survey study from data collected from 2009 to 2016 in individuals 65 years and older showed an overall prevalence of polypharmacy at 65.1% with nonsteroidal antiinflammatory drugs as the most frequently prescribed medication [26]. It is clear that prescription drug use whether one drug or many is high in community-dwelling adults, 65 years and older. Of most concern is that on average 43–65.1% of the older population use multiple drugs which is a sure recipe for ADRs [28].

As noted above, the Qato study (2010–2011) reported OTC drug use at 37.9% and dietary supplement use at 63.7% among the 2000 interviewed community-dwelling older adults [28]. In a sampling of US men and women (~800 individuals, 65+), OTC drugs most frequently used were acetaminophen, aspirin, and ibuprofen [33]. Within this same sampling group, 63% used vitamins and ~26–36% consumed herbal remedies, of which the most popular was lutein (putative prevention of eye disease), followed by flaxseed oil (putative moderator of inflammation), *Ginkgo biloba* and ginseng (proposed prevention for cognitive decline) [33]. Qato et al. (2016) also found overlap with OTC drugs, aspirin, and acetaminophen noted by the Slone Survey (2006) but additionally found omeprazole (Prilosec®) and naproxen as common choices. Among dietary supplements, multivitamins/minerals, calcium, omega-3 fish oil, and vitamin D were the top four dietary supplements used by the older adult [28]. Concurrent use of prescription drugs and supplements elevated the risk of ADRs from 8.4% in 2006 to 15.1% 5 years later [28]. Similar rates of ADR (~15%) with concurrent use of dietary supplements and prescription medications were observed over a 2-year period in a geriatric clinic (survey of 400 patients) where OTC drug use and supplement use was 27.6% and 72.4%, respectively. Furthermore, combining *Ginkgo biloba*, garlic, or calcium with prescription drugs produced the majority of ADRs [39] (see Chap. 9 for OTC/herbal supplement use).

Medication Use. Extent in Assisted Living/Nursing Homes There is a scarcity of studies on drug use in settings of assisted living (AL) and nursing homes. However, one study using data from the 2015 survey of National Health and Aging Trends Study [40] on individual residences and other personal data and linking this to Medicare benefits (Part D) with permission from interviewed participants (~6000), published interesting observations [27]. The results of this study showed that 72.2% of older adults in AL used ≥5 drugs, a rate of polypharmacy slightly higher than in nursing homes (71.3%) and nearly double that of community-dwelling older adults (44.1%) [27]. Additionally, hyperpolypharmacy (use of ≥10 drugs) in AL residents was 30.2% which exceeded that in nursing homes (23.5%) and in the community (6.1%) [27]. Compared to community drug use, use of opioid analgesics, antipsychotics, benzodiazepines, gabapentinoids, and antidepressants was at least two-fold higher in AL than in nursing homes [27]. In a smaller study of 26 AL facilities (~200 participants), 51% experienced polypharmacy with an average use of 7 drugs encompassing medications to treat cardiovascular disease, gastrointestinal issues, clotting problems, high lipid levels, pain, and depression [41]. Retrospective analysis of survey data from the National Nursing Home Survey (NNHS) (2004–2005) of over 11 thousand long-term care residents of nursing homes showed that the high drug use mirrored the presence of multiple comorbidities (hypertension, vascular disease (coronary, cerebral, or peripheral), dementia, arthritis, depression, and gastro-esophageal reflux disease) [29]. The use of "health maintenance" drugs, e.g., multivitamins, laxatives, nutritional supplements, added to the polypharmacy in 17% of nursing home residents [29]. Only in the oldest residence (>85 years) except for dementia patients, was there an effort to deprescribe [29].

IMPORTANCE OF RESEARCH The discussions presented in this textbook are synthesized from many sources, namely, published science articles, reviews, textbooks, government/medical organizations, and data from clinical trials. Clinical trials are probably the least understood but of considerable value to assessing drug use. Evidenced-based data is derived from several types of clinical trials: 1) randomized clinical trials (RCTs), 2) observational studies (prospective cohort, retrospective or case-control), and 3) systematic review and meta-analysis of these studies. It is important to briefly define these study types and indicate their importance in the hierarchy of understanding drug use in the older adult.

Randomized Clinical Trial The randomized clinical trial (RCT) rests at the apex of maximum quality evidence. That is because "the RCT is the most rigorous and robust research method for determining whether a cause–effect relation exists between an intervention and an outcome" [42]. Evidence from a carefully designed and well executed RCT provides the direction for effective clinical practice that "improves patient outcomes and safety, and is generally cost-effective" [42]. It is imperative that bias, any factor that may cause the results to deviate from its true value, be eliminated from the RCT from beginning to end [42, 43]. Hence, one of many assets of the RCT is the randomization of trial participants. Randomization serves to eliminate confounding factors (known and unknown variables) between the two test groups (intervention and control). Randomization negates these variables. Another asset is allocation concealment in which the investigator's view of a prospective participant is removed and assignment (intervention or placebo) is made randomly. Additional reduction in bias occurs with a) blinding, single (participant) or double (participant, investigator), a means of blocking knowledge of assignment of the intervention or placebo and b) use of independent investigators to assess the outcome measures of the trial [42]. There are also other validated tools to determine the risk of bias in the design, conduct, and reporting of a clinical trial [44]. Absence of bias is critical to prevent erroneous conclusions [43].

Observational Studies Although the RCT is the "gold standard" for high-grade evidence, results of observational studies are also important and some consider them to be comparable in some respects [45]. However, generally, observational prospective cohort studies are placed a notch below well-designed RCTs, and retrospective case-control studies and cross-sectional studies (prevalence) are positioned even slightly lower [46]. In observational studies, the relation between the intervention (or exposure) and the disease outcome is "observed" and the investigator determines the strength of the relation between the two. Cohort studies track groups of individuals with a specified characteristic (the cohort); well-designed studies can assess cause and effect and determine disease risk. However, subject selection for the cohorts is key and because studies are long, attrition (loss of participants) creates a bias.

Case-Control Studies Observational case-control studies "are descriptive studies following one small group of subjects" [46]. Basically, an "outcome" group (e.g., response to a surgical procedure or disease diagnosis) is identified as the case and a control group with similar characteristics but without the outcome is developed. Data is collected on both groups, generally retrospectively [46]. These studies are useful for examining rare or long-term outcomes, and multiple risk factors but disadvantages of faulty recall, lack of verification of gathered information, and inability to control variables elevate the bias level for case-control studies.

Cross Sectional Studies Cross-sectional observational studies seek to define the "prevalence of disease, phenomena, or opinion in a population." Data (survey, interview, biological sampling) are collected at an indicated time point, specified period or serially over years [47]. Prevalence is displayed as a percentage of those with the designated outcome compared to the total sample size. This value gives meaning to the extent of disease burden and related "services needed, morbidity, mortality and QoL" [48]. This study design allows a wealth of data to be obtained very quickly but it cannot measure incidence of a disease or attribute (development over time) unless follow-up studies are done [47]. Similar to RCTs, observational studies are encouraged to adhere to an extensive checklist of requirements of design and reporting to improve the overall strength of such studies [49].

Systematic Reviews and Meta-Analysis Systematic reviews contribute significantly to answering a specific research question by identifying all the relevant studies on that topic and critically reviewing and analyzing them. It is a qualitative study. In contrast, a meta-analysis is a quantitative study that uses statistics to generate a pooled estimate from estimates of two or more related studies used in the systematic review, a combination that enhances the power of the final value [50]. However, the systematic review and meta-analysis are only as good as the quality of studies that are included. Inclusion follows strict criteria and if adhered to, recommendations can be valid and convincing. The network meta-analysis extends the meta-analysis. Whereas a meta-analysis assesses studies with an experimental intervention and a comparator intervention for a certain condition, the network meta-analysis can handle more than one like set of interventions and comparators [51]. This allows the comparison of multiple interventions for a specific condition and a reliable recommendation for patients who may need different options [51].

References

1. Cohen AA, Kennedy BK, Anglas U, Bronikowski AM, Deelen J, Dufour F, et al. Lack of consensus on an aging biology paradigm? A global survey reveals an agreement to disagree, and the need for an interdisciplinary framework. Mech Ageing Dev. 2020;191:111316. https://doi.org/10.1016/j.mad.2020.111316.
2. Arking R. Biology of aging: observations and principles. 3rd ed. New York: Oxford University Press; 2006. Chapter 1. p. 3–25.

References

3. https://www.statista.com/statistics/1302736/global-life-expectancy-by-region-country-historical/. National Center for Health Statistics
4. National Center for Health Statistics. https://www.cdc.gov/nchs/index.html
5. United Nations Department of Economic and Social Affairs, Population Division: (2022). World Population Prospects 2022: Summary of Results. UN DESA/POP/2022/TR/NO. 3.
6. Carey IW, Hackett C. Global population skews male, but UN projects parity between sexes by 2050. August 1, 2022. https://www.pewresearch.org/short-reads.
7. U.S. Census Bureau, the National Center for Health Statistics, and the Bureau of Labor Statistics (Administration of Aging 2024).
8. United Nations Department of Economic and Social Affairs, Population Division: (2024). World Population Prospects 2024: Summary of Results (UN DESA/POP/2024/TR/NO. 9).
9. Caplan Z, Rabe M. The Older Population: 2020, 2020 Census Briefs 2023 US Census Bureau Census.gov U.S. Census Bureau, 2023 National Population Projections Tables: Main Series.
10. Vespa J, Medina L, Armstrong DM. Demographic turning points for the United States: Population projections for 2020 to 2060. 2020. [August 3, 2021]. https://www.census.gov/content/dam/Census/library/publications/2020/demo/p25-1144.pdf.
11. Kinsella KG. Changes in life expectancy 1900–1999. Am J Clin Nutr. 1992;55(6 Suppl):1196S–202S. https://doi.org/10.1093/ajcn/55.6.1196S.
12. Population reference bureau, 2002. https://www.prb.org/resources/americans-are-living-longer-than-ever/
13. Garmany A, Yamada S, Terzic A. Longevity leap: mind the healthspan gap. NPJ Regen Med. 2021;6(1):57. https://doi.org/10.1038/s41536-021-00169-5.
14. https://www.census.gov/data/tables/2023/demo/popproj/2023-summary-tables.html
15. Interactive Summary Health Statistics for Adults, 2019–2022. https://wwwn.cdc.gov/NHISDataQueryTool/SHS_adult/index.html
16. NCHS, National Health and Nutrition Examination Survey. See Appendix I, National Health and Nutrition Examination Survey (NHANES). 2019.
17. National Center for Health Statistics, National Health Interview Survey. See Sources and Definitions, National Health Interview Survey (NHIS) and Health, United States, 2020–2021.
18. https://www.statista.com/statistics/1450851/copd-emphysema-or-chronic-bronchitis-prevalence-seniors-us/
19. https://www.cdc.gov/diabetes/php/data-research/index.html
20. Rajan KB, Weuve J, Barnes LL, McAninch EA, Wilson RS, Evans DA. Population estimate of people with clinical AD and mild cognitive impairment in the United States (2020–2060). Alzheimers Dement. 2021;17(12):1966–75. https://doi.org/10.1002/alz.12362.
21. Centers for Disease Control and Prevention. Chronic Kidney Disease in the United States, 2021. Atlanta, GA: US Department of Health and Human Services, Centers for Disease Control and Prevention; 2021.
22. Sanford AM, Morley JE, Berg-Weger M, Lundy J, Little MO, Leonard K, et al. High prevalence of geriatric syndromes in older adults. PLoS One. 2020;15(6):e0233857. https://doi.org/10.1371/journal.pone.0233857.
23. 2023 Profile of older Americans. Administration of Community Living, May, 2024.
24. Kantor ED, Rehm CD, Haas JS, Chan AT, Giovannucci EL. Trends in prescription drug use among adults in the United States from 1999–2012. JAMA. 2015;314(17):1818–31. https://doi.org/10.1001/jama.2015.13766.
25. Innes GK, Ogden CL, Crentsil V, Concato J, Fakhouri TH. Prescription medication use among older adults in the US. JAMA Intern Med. 2024;184(9):1121–3. https://doi.org/10.1001/jamainternmed.2024.2781.
26. Young EH, Pan S, Yap AG, Reveles KR, Bhakta K. Polypharmacy prevalence in older adults seen in United States physician offices from 2009 to 2016. PLoS One. 2021;16(8):e0255642. https://doi.org/10.1371/journal.pone.0255642.
27. Lei L, Samus QM, Thomas KS, Maust DT. Medication costs and use of older Americans in assisted living settings: a nationally representative cross-sectional study. J Gen Intern Med. 2023;38(2):294–301. https://doi.org/10.1007/s11606-022-07434-3.

28. Qato D, Wilder J, Gillet SLP, V, Alexander GC. Changes in prescription and over-the-counter medication and dietary supplement use among older adults in the United States, 2005 vs 2011. JAMA Intern Med. 2016;176(4):473–82. https://doi.org/10.1001/jamainternmed.2015.8581.
29. Moore KL, Patel K, Boscardin WJ, Steinman MA, Ritchie C, Schwartz JB. Medication burden attributable to chronic comorbid conditions in the very old and Vulnerable. PLoS One. 2018;13(4):e0196109. https://doi.org/10.1371/journal.pone.0196109.
30. Dwyer L, Han B, Woodwell DA, Rechtsteiner EA. Polypharmacy in nursing home residents in the United States: results of the 2004 National Nursing Home Survey. Am J Geriatr Pharmacother. 2009;8:63–72. https://doi.org/10.1016/j.amjopharm.2010.01.001.
31. Tamura BK, Bell CL, Lubimir K, Iwasaki WN, Ziegler LA, Masaki KH. Physician intervention for medication reduction in a nursing home: the polypharmacy outcomes project. J Am Med Dir Assoc. 2011;12(5):326–30. https://doi.org/10.1016/j.jamda.2010.08.013.
32. National Health Interview Survey. https://wwwn.cdc.gov/NHISDataQueryTool/SHS_adult/index.html
33. Slone Survey Patterns of medication use in the United States: A report from the Slone Survey; March 2009. http://www.bu.edu/slone/SloneSurveyWebReport2005.pdf
34. Moeller JF, Miller GE, Banthin JS. Looking inside the nation's medicine cabinet: trends in outpatient drug spending by Medicare beneficiaries, 1997 and 2001. Health Aff (Millwood). 2004;23(5):217–25. https://doi.org/10.1377/hlthaff.23.5.217.
35. Qato DM, Alexander GC, Conti RM, Johnson M, Schumm P, Lindau ST. Use of prescription and over-the-counter medications and dietary supplements among older adults in the United States. JAMA. 2008;300(24):2867–78. https://doi.org/10.1001/jama.2008.892.
36. Qato DM, Shumm LP, Johnson M, Mihai A, Lindau ST. Medication data collection and coding in a home-based survey of older adults. J Gerontol Soc Sci. 2009;64(Suppl 1):i86–93. https://doi.org/10.1093/geronb/gbp036.
37. Neves SJF, de Oliveira P, Marques A, Leal MCC, da Silva Diniz A, Medeiros TS, de Arruda IKG. Epidemiology of medication use among the elderly in an urban area of Northeastern Brazil. Rev Saude Publica. 2013;47(4):759–67; discussion 768. https://doi.org/10.1590/S0034-8910.2013047003768.
38. National Center for Health Statistics, National Ambulatory Medical Care Survey Health Center Component, January 2022–December 2023.
39. Jaqua EE, Gonzalez J, Bahjri K, Erickson S, Garcia C, Santhavachart M, et al. Analyzing potential interactions between complementary and alternative therapies, over-the-counter, and prescription medications in the older population. Perm J. 2024;28(2):70–7. https://doi.org/10.7812/TPP/23.183.
40. Kasper JD, Freedman VA. National health and aging trends study user guide: rounds 1–10 final release. Baltimore: Johns Hopkins University School of Public Health; 2021. Available from: https://nhats.org/sites/default/files/2021-07/NHATS_User_Guide_R10_Final_Release.pdf
41. Resnick B, Galik E, Boltz M, Holmes S, Fix S, Vigne E, et al. Polypharmacy in assisted living and impact on clinical outcomes. Consult Pharm. 2018;33(6):321–30. https://doi.org/10.4140/TCP.n.2018.321.
42. Bhide A, Shah PS, Achava G. A simplified guide to randomized controlled trials. Acta Obstet Gynecol Scand. 2018;97(4):380–7. https://doi.org/10.1111/aogs.13309.
43. Nair A. Quality of a randomized-controlled trial- how to assess and improve reporting? Saudi J Anaesth. 2022;16(2):257–8. https://doi.org/10.4103/sja.sja_870_21.
44. Higgins JP, Altman DG, Gøtzsche PC, Jüni P, Moher D, Oxman AD, et al. The cochrane collaboration's tool for assessing risk of bias in randomised trials. BMJ. 2011;343:d5928.
45. Concato J, Shah N, Horwitz RI. Randomized, controlled trials, observational studies, and the hierarchy of research designs. N Engl J Med. 2000;342(25):1887–92. https://doi.org/10.1056/NEJM200006223422507.
46. Song JW, Chung KC. Observational studies: Cohort and case-control studies. Plast Reconstr Surg. 2010;126(6):2234–42. https://doi.org/10.1097/PRS.0b013e3181f44abc.

47. Capili B. Overview: cross-sectional studies. Am J Nurs. 2021;121(10):59–62. https://doi.org/10.1097/01.NAJ.0000794280.73744.fe.
48. Noordzij M, Dekker FW, Zoccali C, Jager KJ. Measures of disease frequency: prevalence and incidence. Nephron Clin Pract. 2010;115(1):c17–20. https://doi.org/10.1159/000286345.
49. von Elm E, Altman DG, Egger M, Pocock SJ, Gotzsche PC, Vandenbrouche JP, et al. The strengthening the reporting of observational studies in epidemiology (STROBE) statement: guidelines for reporting observational studies. J Clin Epidemiol. 2008;61(4):344–9. https://doi.org/10.1016/j.jclinepi.2007.11.008.
50. Ahn EJ, Kang H. Introduction to systematic review and meta-analysis. Korean J Anesthesiol. 2018;71(2):103–12. https://doi.org/10.4097/kjae.2018.71.2.103.
51. Chairmani A, Caldwell DM, Li T, Higgins JPT, Salanti G. Chapter 11: Undertaking network meta-analyses. In: JPT H, Thomas J, Chandler J, Cumpston M, Li T, Page MJ, Welch VA, editors. Cochrane handbook for systematic reviews of interventions version 6.5. Cochrane; 2024. Available from: www.training.cochrane.org/handbook.

Principles of Pharmacokinetics/Pharmacodynamics

2

Abbreviations

5HT	5-hydroxytryptamine; serotonin
ACh	acetylcholine
AD	Alzheimer's Disease
ADME	absorption, distribution, metabolism, excretion
ADRs	adverse drug reactions
CNS	central nervous system
COPD	chronic obstructive pulmonary disease
CYP	cytochrome P450 enzymes
GABA	gamma-amino butyric acid
GFR	glomerular filtration rate
GI	gastrointestinal
GPCR	G-protein coupled receptor
IM	intramuscular
IV	intravenous
MAC	minimal alveolar concentration
mAChR	muscarinic acetylcholine receptors
mGluRs	metabotropic glutamate receptors
OH	orthostatic hypotension
PD	pharmacodynamics
PEPT1	human peptide transporter (1)
P-gp	P-glycoprotein
PK	pharmacokinetics
PO	oral
RCT	randomized clinical trial
SC	subcutaneous
SNS	sympathetic nervous system
SSRI	selective serotonin reuptake inhibitor

INTRODUCTION Pharmacology is the science that describes the activities of a drug in humans. It encompasses quantitative principles of pharmacokinetics (PK) and pharmacodynamics (PD) [1]. Simply and cleverly stated, "PKs describes the manner in which the body affects a drug, whereas PDs describes the manner in which the drug affects the body" [2].

Aging is one of the main risk factors for disease [3]. Hence, the older adult is more likely to develop one or more diseases. Since medication use brings amelioration or a cure to disease, the older adult with multiple comorbidities uses drugs to a greater extent than any other age group (see Chap. 1). Therefore, it is important to understand drug PK and PD and to additionally, grasp the age changes that potentially modify drug PK and PD. Clearly, the best use of medications is always required and of considerable value, both to the well-being of the older adult and to society.

It is important to stress that drug use (dosage and application) draws heavily from data generated from randomized clinical trials (RCTs). RCTs detail the pharmacology of a drug through four phases to determine PK, efficacy, and side effects to gain FDA approval. With a few exceptions, older adults (65 years and older) have been excluded from participation in clinical drug trials. This occurs despite repeated requests for inclusion from the FDA [4, 5] and a 2017 policy that "requires that clinical study applications submitted to NIH (National Institute of Health) must include a plan for enrolling individuals across the lifespan" [6]. Since the majority of pharmacological drug assessments involve individuals 18–55 years of age, prescribing clinicians are thus required to extrapolate this data in treating older adults. This approach often yields poor results (see Chap. 3, Adverse Drug Reactions). Fortunately, strategies have been proposed to encourage enrollment of healthy older adults representative of the current population in future RCTs [6]. In the interim, it is critical to understand the known effects of age on the pharmacology of each drug. This allows both the clinician and the patient insight into appropriate adjustments necessary to achieve the best efficacy with minimal side effects.

There are many factors in addition to age that influence the pharmacology of a drug. Prominent ones are gender, genetics, diseases, geriatric syndromes, environment (epigenetics, stress), and polypharmacy [7, 8]. Most of these are discussed in subsequent Chaps. 3, 4, 5, 6, and 7. The focus of this chapter is to discuss one factor, the influence of age on the pharmacology of a drug. This begins with understanding the basic principles of pharmacology and subsequently recognizing specific age changes with potential to alter these principles. The ultimate goal is to ensure that drug use is not only appropriate but also achieves the best health outcome for the older adult. The narrative is supplemented with relevant Tables 2.1 and 2.2.

PHARMACOLOGY Pharmacology consists of pharmacokinetics (PK) and pharmacodynamics (PD). PK refers to the chemical and physiological movement of a drug in the body from time of entrance to the time of exit. It entails activities of absorption, distribution, metabolism, and excretion (ADME). PD refers to the effect of a drug at its known or purported target site, to produce the desired outcome. Binding of the drug to its target site, generally a receptor or enzyme, sets in motion a cascade of cellular changes that culminate in the therapeutic effect. The essential principles of PK and PD are discussed below.

Pharmacokinetic Principles

ABSORPTION Drugs may enter the body by any number of routes: by mouth (orally, PO), sublingually/buccally (mucus membranes of the mouth), parenterally (route other than oral, e.g., injected into muscle (intramuscularly, IM) or the circulation (intravenously, IV), via the skin (topically, subcutaneously, SC), rectally, or by inhalation. Drugs that are administered IV bypass the absorption processes.

Oral Route The majority of drugs are taken by mouth, e.g., orally. These drugs are absorbed by the gastrointestinal (GI) tract in accordance with physicochemical characteristics of the drug in conjunction with biochemical factors in the GI tract. Formulation, lipid (fat) solubility, and ionization potential (degree of charge) are the main physiochemical aspects that determine drug absorption. Formulation determines drug dissolution; lipid solubility and ionization potential influence drug movement across the GI membranes. With rapid dissolution, high lipid solubility, and low ionization potential (drug in uncharged, neutral state), absorption will be rapid. Biochemical factors affecting drug absorption are: (1) GI pH (acidity or alkalinity) and fluid volume, (2) intestinal membrane permeability regulated by simple diffusion, drug transporters, and enzymes, and (3) the contribution of enzymatic activity from the microbiome (resident bacteria of the intestine) [9].

The contribution to drug absorption from enzymes and transporters on intestinal cells (enterocytes) cannot be underestimated [10, 11]. A small but important collection of metabolic enzymes, termed cytochrome P450 enzymes (CYP2C9/19, CYP2D6, CYP3A4/5, UGT1A1/3, and UGT2B7) as well as several families of transferases, have been identified [11]. The intestinal enzymes overlap with the extensive presence of cytochrome P450 metabolizing enzymes in the liver (see below). Intestinal enzymes metabolize drugs such as cyclosporine, docetaxel, midazolam, and statins to less efficacious drugs even before entering the circulation [12].

There is a wealth of intestinal transmembrane proteins that facilitate drug transport both uptake to the systemic circulation (uptake transporters, e.g., human peptide transporter 1 or return drugs to the GI lumen, e.g., permeability glycoprotein (P-gp) [10, 13]. Thus, the inhibition or stimulation at the level of intestinal transporters may dramatically influence absorption of many drugs including chemotherapeutic, steroidal, and cardiovascular drugs [14]. Adverse reactions may ensue with use of two or more drugs with opposing effects on transporters, influencing absorption of one drug in preference of another.

Parental Routes Similar to orally administered drugs, absorption of drugs by other routes, e.g., topically, SC, IM, rectally, or by inhalation is influenced by the physicochemical characteristics of a drug, membrane transport systems, and in some cases, blood flow [15, 16].

DISTRIBUTION Following drug absorption or directly with IV administration, a drug enters the cardiovascular circulation. Orally administered drugs undergo a phenomenon called first pass. First pass prevents an orally administered drug from reaching the general circulation directly from the GI tract and subjects it to potential metabolism by the liver, the main drug-metabolizing organ in the body and also as noted above, metabolism within the enterocytes. Drugs reach the liver directly from the GI tract via the hepatoportal vein. First pass produces different results for different drugs. A drug may pass through the liver/intestine unchanged or more likely, the drug will undergo biotransformation with loss of potential efficacy. Alternatively, a few drugs designed as an inactive prodrugs, experience metabolic conversion to active drugs.

Once a drug reaches the main circulation, it is distributed throughout the body. Distribution brings the drug into contact with its receptor or enzyme (site of action) enabling an effect, e.g., lower blood pressure, control of blood sugar, or anxiety relief. Distribution also delivers the drug back to the liver, site of additional metabolism and to the kidneys, site of excretion.

Factors Affecting Distribution Distribution of a drug depends on three key factors: (1) the concentration of plasma proteins, primarily albumin, (2) the lipid/water solubility characteristics of the drug, and (3) body composition (basically ratio of adipose tissue to nonadipose or lean tissue). Plasma proteins are important because all drugs bind to these proteins to some extent, some more than others. Since only the "free" or unbound drug can induce an effect, blood proteins act as reservoirs, allowing continual release of the "free" drug. Highly protein-bound drugs are slowly released and, in effect, continue to circulate to produce a longer-lasting effect compared to poorly protein-bound drugs. Lipid/water partition coefficients of drugs are important as they indicate to what extent a drug will accumulate in adipose tissue verses lean tissue (e.g., muscle). Many drugs are highly lipid soluble and hence will accumulate in adipose tissue. This too serves as a reservoir for the drug, allowing for a longer-lasting effect. Consideration of body composition (surface area, weight) is important since both adipose and lean tissue influence not only a drug's distribution but also the onset and offset of its effect. This is especially relevant to anesthetic drugs.

METABOLISM As the drug circulates, it reenters the liver. Here resides a wealth of unique proteins, cytochrome P450 enzymes, (CYP) that metabolize (biotransform) each drug to a more water-soluble entity, thereby enhancing excretion by the kidneys. Three gene families, coding for CYP1, CYP2, and CYP3, metabolically modify most drugs [17]. The specific CYPs considered of prime important to drug metabolism include CYP1A2, CYP2A6, CYP2B6, CYP2C8/9/19, CYP2D6,

CYP2E1 and CYP3A4 [18]. CYP enzymes also metabolize endogenous substances, e.g., neurotransmitters, fat-soluble vitamins, and steroid hormones.

Most drugs undergo an oxidation or reduction reaction (termed Phase I reactions). Drugs may also undergo other reactions, e.g., sulfation, glucuronidation, and acetylation (termed Phase II reactions). In addition to facilitating rapid excretion of the drug, biotransformations gradually reduce or obliterate drug efficacy. Therefore, changes in liver metabolism such as a reduction in enzyme activity, exert a major effect on the concentration of a drug. Generally, the concentration of a drug remains elevated for longer periods of time, causing a greater than expected response but also potentially inducing side effects and toxicities. It is incredibly important whenever possible to determine hepatic (liver) function prior to drug use.

EXCRETION There are many sites of drug excretion such as intestines (feces), lungs (water vapor), sweat glands (sweat), and salivary glands (saliva), but the kidneys are the main site. Excretion occurs within complex filtration units, the nephron, of which there are literally millions. Each nephron is essentially "the glomerulum (encapsulated bundle of capillaries) and the attached tubular system, consisting of different portions connected in series" [19].

Drug excretion into the urine is facilitated by prior hepatic (liver) metabolism of the drug to a more water-soluble form. A reduction in renal excretion permits the continued presence of the drug in the circulation enabling drug concentrations to rise above therapeutic values, producing side effects and toxicities. Therefore, *prior to drug use, it is critical to assess kidney function* (see more below).

Kidney Function On reaching the nephron, renal blood flow, glomerular filtration, and tubular secretion contribute to drug elimination. Glomerular filtration depends on adequate renal blood flow, and functional glomerular membranes and capillaries. Glomerular filtration removes about 20% of solutes and drugs. Although the importance of tubular secretion has been known for some time ago [20], more recent data show that tubular secretion handles about 80% of solute and drug excretion including microbiome-produced toxins bound to proteins [21]. Thus, tubular secretion becomes the main mechanism to eliminate most drugs. A family of organic anion and cation transporters residing on the basolateral side of the kidney tubule facilitates transfer of drugs from the peritubular capillaries to the proximal tubule where active transport mechanisms on the apical side (facing the lumen) move solutes and drugs into the tubules for urinary excretion [21].

Pharmacodynamic Principles

TARGET SITE ACTIVITIES Pharmacodynamic (PD) principles quantify and define the effect of a drug at its site of action. The site of action is usually a receptor or an enzyme or some component of a pathogen. Drugs act by first binding to the target site, usually with high affinity (strong attraction). This is essential for the production of the expected effect. A drug that activates its target site induces a conformational (structural/chemical) change in the target and ignites a cascade of subsequent events, collectively termed cell signaling. A drug that successfully binds to its target site and induces the appropriate cell signaling is considered efficacious and termed an agonist. Conversely, a drug that binds to the target site but prevents any subsequent cell signaling is termed an antagonist.

Most receptors are proteins and interact routinely with physiological mediators (e.g., hormones, neurotransmitters, cytokines) produced endogenously (within the organism). Therefore, drugs mimic these endogenous substances to enhance or reduce their effects. Drugs may also bind to nonreceptor proteins such as enzymes to produce an increase or decrease in enzyme activity that may affect subsequent cellular reactions.

Receptor Targets Several families of receptors have been identified and characterized. They are: cell surface receptor kinases (e.g., insulin receptor) [22]; protein kinase-associated receptors (e.g., growth hormone receptor) [23]; G-protein coupled receptors (e.g., alpha-adrenergic receptor for norepinephrine) [24]; ligand-gated ion channels (e.g., nicotinic cholinergic receptor) [25]; and transcription factors (e.g., estrogen receptor) [26]. The largest group is the guanine nucleotide-binding G-protein-coupled receptor (GPCR) that includes receptors of the sympathetic nervous system (SNS) and central nervous system (CNS).

Enzyme Targets Some of the known enzymatic targets include esterases, e.g., acetylcholinesterase of the parasympathetic nervous system and CNS [27], kinases, e.g., growth factor kinases over expressed on malignant cells [28], metabolic enzymes, e.g., HMG-CoA reductase of the cholesterol production pathway [29], protein hydrolase, e.g., angiotensin-converting enzyme, metabolizing angiotensin I to angiotensin II [30] and cyclooxygenases, e.g., conversion of arachidonic acid to prostaglandins and related lipid mediators [31].

Pharmacology and Aging

Introduction. Aging Effects on PK and PD Biological age changes are numerous and exert influence on PK and PD to different extents. The research literature supports the following biological changes progressing with age: reduced end-organ function, altered receptor/enzyme sensitivities, waning homeostatic mechanisms, and modified body composition [32], all of which affect the pharmacology of a drug. Certainly, many other factors such as the ramifications of diseases/geriatric syndromes and their associated therapies, nutritional status, and chronic stress also affect the pharmacology of a drug. These topics are covered in later chapters. It is important to emphasize that all of these factors are intertwined and are responsible for the considerable variation in drug response observed from one older individual to another. The aging process and associated factors determine the observed heterogeneity within the population of older adults. It is also important to keep in mind that many of the PK and PD studies in older adults generally were obtained from studies of approximately 20–30 healthy older adults. Drugs commonly used by an older adult are discussed in relation to age changes affecting PK/PD and hence influencing drug activity.

Pharmacokinetics and Aging

ABSORPTION As presented above, depending on the route of administration, drug absorption may occur in the GI tract (nasal and buccal mucosa, stomach, small and large intestines, rectum), skin, skeletal muscle, and lung. Age changes occur in these tissues and may influence drug absorption to different degrees.

Gastrointestinal Absorption More than half of all available drugs may be taken orally [33]. The development of "physiologically based pharmacokinetic modeling" or computer simulations is of recent interest [34, 35]. Key to the development of these predictive in vitro and in silico models is a definitive understanding of the GI physiology of the older and geriatric adults. Accordingly, the indispensable GI determinants of oral drug absorption in the older adult are: (1) gastric emptying, (2) volumes and composition of luminal fluids, and (3) intestinal permeability [35]. Although age changes are well documented, data confirming the expected change in drug absorption have been gathered mostly from small clinical studies.

Several structural/functional changes occur in the stomach with age. There is a decrease in gastric motility [36, 37] due in part to a reduction in the number and volume of the regulatory neurons, the interstitial cells of Cajal [38]. Thus, it is known that gastric emptying of noncaloric liquid and caloric solid meals is slowed in older adults [39]. Gastric emptying time following ingestion of a whey protein drink was decreased by almost half in older adults (75 years of age) compared to young adults (25 years of age) [40]. Drug gastric emptying time as measured with radioactive complexes is significantly longer in older individuals than in young [36].

Gastric volumes are generally smaller in the older adult but this may be confounded by methodology as emphasized by Stillhart et al. (2023). Also, there is "very limited understanding of the impact of advanced age on intraluminal pH, buffer capacity, and osmolality of luminal contents" [35]. In general, however, it is the disease state of atrophic gastritis, a condition of suppressed gastric acid secretion (hypochlorhydria) that hinders nutrient and drug absorption rather than aging [41]. Additionally, the chronic use of proton-pump inhibitors (e.g., omeprazole) that elevate gastric pH (decrease acid) may alter the bioavailability of some drugs that require an acid environment to attain the uncharged state. Examples of reduced drug absorption with hypochlorhydria include ketoconazole and itraconazole (antifungal), atazanavir (anti-HIV), cefpodoxime and enoxacin (antibacterial) and dipyridamole (antiplatelet) [42] and tyrosine kinase inhibitors for cancer therapy [43] or increased bioavailability of nifedipine (antihypertensive), alendronate (bisphosphonate for osteoporosis) and digoxin (heart failure treatment) [42].

A number of studies have evaluated the effect of age on intestinal permeability [44–46] and found no change except in the presence of inflammation and Type 2

Diabetes Mellitus [47] and GI symptoms of diarrhea or constipation [46]. Here again, the use of certain methodologies that alter fluid particle fluxes may have biased this data [35].

The physical presence of intestinal enzymes and transporters determined by RNA and protein analysis generally report no change with age [35, 48]. In contrast, Miki et al. [49] found a decrease in gene expression and protein level of CYP3A4 after the age of 38. Since CYP3A4 metabolizes more drugs than other CYP enzymes [50], a decrease in function would allow more unaltered drug into the circulation. "Using a validated microdose cocktail containing 5 probe substances," Rattanacheeworn et al. [51] reported that intestinal P-gp activities decreased with age (>60 years verses 20–40 years). P-gp prevents drugs from crossing the intestinal membrane. Thus, a decrease in P-gp activity would increase drug exposure.

Transdermal Delivery of drugs by transdermal systems, application of medication, or drug through the skin, (matrix-based, liquid/gel reservoirs) has many advantages including avoidance of hepatic/intestinal first pass, absence of GI upsets such as nausea, potential for more reliable steady-state drug concentrations and increased compliance [52]. Transdermal systems are helpful in the treatment of neurological diseases, e.g., Parkinson's disease [53, 54], pain management [55], and hormone therapy [56].

With time, distinct changes occur in the three layers of the skin (epidermis, dermis, hypodermis) [57]. Age changes are greatly accelerated and enhanced in unprotected skin (exposed to the environment, e.g., face, hands, arms, legs) compared to protected skin (generally covered with clothing). Therefore, the skin of the older adult is thinner with reduced physiological function in all three layers. This is attributed to (a) a reduced epithelial cell division (cell turnover), (b) senescing of fibroblasts in the dermis with production of defective matrix components such as collagen, and (c) loss of fat cells in the hypodermis [57, 58].

Results from small clinical studies on PK of transdermal drug delivery in older adults are mixed [59–61]. Several reports indicate similar transport of buprenorphine (opioid) in the young and old adults [59] while others report a significantly slower time to reach maximal drug levels for a fentanyl patch in older patients compared to young, with maximal concentration and half-life of elimination time unaffected by age [60]. More recently in a physics-based simulation to predict fentanyl delivery in the older adult, the computer simulation reported a reduction in the "maximal transdermal flux (11.4%) and maximal concentration (7%) of fentanyl in the blood" in association with a surprising 45% increase in pain relief [61]. This is an interesting virtual model that needs confirmation with large clinical trials.

Subcutaneous Subcutaneous injection or infusion into the hypodermis (bottom layer of skin) is an essential route of drug delivery for peptide/protein drugs such as insulin, parathyroid derivatives, and chemotherapeutic monoclonal antibodies or large chemical entities. There is a paucity of studies defining the effect of age on SC administration. The PK of three antibiotics (ceftriaxone, ertapenem, and teicoplanin) given SC is similar to that produced with IV administration in the older adult

[62] and SC administration of teriparatide, a smaller form of human parathyroid hormone induces serum calcium changes comparable to parathyroid hormone in postmenopausal women with osteoporosis [63]. One study determined the PK (as well as the PD) of SC administered newly formulated faster-acting insulin aspart with an earlier formulation of insulin aspart in both young and old individuals with Type 1 Diabetes [64]. Age did not influence PK or PD. Additionally, comparison of the ultra-long-acting insulin (insulin degludec) exhibited similar PK following SC administration in both young and older individuals with Type 1 Diabetes [65].

Intramuscular Gradual loss of skeletal muscle mass is a common age change [66]. Unless counteracted with a serious resistance exercise program [67], both skeletal muscle mass and to a larger extent skeletal muscle strength decline with age. Significant reduction in skeletal muscle mass, strength, and physical performance is termed sarcopenia [68].

Sadly, there is very little data assessing the effect of age on IM administration of drugs. One study reported that the PK of IM administration of the antibiotic, moxalactam in the older adult was comparable to that reported for young individuals [69]. Common sense suggests that IM administration may be quite painful in the older adult with sarcopenia. The safest of the three IM routes (ventrogluteal, dorsogluteal, and vastus lateralis) is the vastus lateralis (upper thigh) due to relatively larger muscle mass and decreased nerve and blood vessel supply.

Inhalation Pulmonary absorption accommodates inhalation drugs, e.g., volatile anesthetics and inhalation drugs for the treatment of chronic obstructive pulmonary disease (COPD), asthma, and interstitial pulmonary fibrosis [70]. Because this route offers significant advantages such as avoidance of first pass, use of this route to treat other diseases, such as with levodopa inhalation in Parkinson's disease, is proving beneficial [71].

There are significant age changes in the pulmonary system. Major changes include the gradual loss of chest cavity compliance (chest becomes stiffer), an increase in airway resistance (more energy expended to take in air), and a decrease in the amount of healthy lung tissue (reduced oxygen/carbon dioxide exchange) [72, 73]. Measurable consequences are a decrease in minute ventilation volume and a reduction of maximal ventilatory capacity with age [73].

Absorption occurs across the single epithelial cell layer of the alveolar sac. Loss of healthy lung tissue and reduced minute volume of ventilation reduces drug translocation and slows induction and emergence with anesthetic drugs [2]. The minimal alveolar concentration (MAC), defined as the anesthetic concentration (at 1 atmosphere), that prevents movement in 50% of patients exposed to a surgical incision declines significantly with age [74]. However, an explanation for the decline in MAC with age is attributed not only to an age-dependent change in absorption but also to altered distribution and receptor sensitivity plus disease-induced effects on pulmonary blood flow and cardiac output.

Intravenous The IV route (via catheter or bolus injection into a vein) is commonly used in hospital/clinic settings to administer blood products, nutrients, fluids as well as drugs [75]. IV delivery of drugs and other products goes directly into the circulatory system for immediate distribution. Frequently infused drugs fall into several classes: chemotherapeutic (doxorubicin, vincristine, cisplatin, and paclitaxel), pain-mitigating drugs (hydromorphone and morphine), antifungal drugs (fluconazole, micafungin) and antibiotics (gentamicin, vancomycin, cefazolin). Generally, drugs that are poorly bioavailable are candidates for IV administration. This route is also essential for treatment of patients with severe disease and threat of death or where oral administration is not feasible (nausea, vomiting, reduced level of consciousness). In the older adult, catheter placement/venous injection requires awareness that the skin has changed in composition, strength, and immunity. Specifically, veins are more superficial and tend to roll, skin tears readily and bruising occurs with even modest pressure of a tourniquet [76]. Additionally, aseptic procedures must be followed rigorously to prevent the induction of infections in consideration of the possible reduced immune protection due to aging and/or disease [75, 76]. Removal of the catheter/needle in patients with potentially prolonged bleeding times (anticlotting, antiplatelet drugs) requires skill to avoid excessive bleeding and bruising [76].

DISTRIBUTION Several of the essential factors influencing the circulatory distribution of a drug to organs and tissues are altered with age. First, lipid/water solubility (partition coefficient) of a drug determines distribution into the fat compartment (adipose tissue) and the water compartment (basically cellular and extracellular spaces). Therefore, body composition is critical to drug distribution and although highly variable due to diet and physical activity, body composition changes with age [77]. Total body water decreases by approximately 10–15% and body fat increases by approximately 20–40%. Two longitudinal studies: the Fels Longitudinal study [78] with data sampling twice a year for 20 years in a small group of Caucasians, 40–66 years of age, and a 6-year study in middle-aged and elderly Japanese (40–79 years of age) [79] support this general observation. A cross-sectional study also found that fat-free mass, appendicular skeletal muscle, body cell mass, and cell potassium in individuals 18–94 years of age decreased with age, especially evident after 60 years of age and fat mass increased until about 75 years of age [80]. There is no current data on the effect of age on extracellular fluid volume or plasma fluid volume.

As fat-free mass decreases in the older adult, the volume of distribution of water-soluble (polar) drugs, such as digoxin, aminoglycosides, theophylline, and ethanol, will decrease producing an increase in plasma drug concentration. If this exceeds the acceptable concentration range for efficacy (therapeutic window), adverse reactions will ensue. For lipid-soluble drugs (nonpolar drugs) such as anesthetics and hypnotic-sedative drugs, an increase in fat mass in the elderly will promote an increase in the volume of distribution. This means that the drug accumulates in the fat depots. An increase in body fat, both slows uptake and loss of the lipid-soluble drugs from the body. For example, with termination of an anesthetic drug, a slower elimination and delayed recovery is expected. In older adults, this may lead to serious consequences of respiratory and cardiovascular stress [2].

Plasma Proteins Potential determinants of drug distribution are the drug-binding plasma proteins, albumin, and alpha1-acid glycoprotein [81, 82]. Although an increase of greater than 50% in the free fraction (unbound) of certain drugs (e.g., acetazolamide, diflunisal, etomidate, naproxen, salicylate, valproate) has been reported [83] in the older adult, reduced protein binding is generally an issue that results from "physiological and pathophysiological changes or disease states" rather than to age per se [81]. Specifically, under conditions of malnutrition caused by diseases (e.g., cancer, dementia, liver disease, and some lung conditions) or frailty, the decline in plasma proteins has a serious effect on drug distribution in older adults, especially for highly bound drugs, e.g., antiepileptic phenytoin; anticoagulant warfarin. In these cases, the "free" and active drug levels will increase as the level of drug-binding proteins declines, resulting in a stronger or possibly toxic effect.

METABOLISM The steady-state concentration of a drug is determined by drug clearance. In other words, hepatic/liver metabolism is key to achieving the desired therapeutic drug concentration as well as exposing the system to drug metabolites and affecting adverse effects [84]. Both hepatic blood flow and the CYP enzymes play significant roles and are affected by age.

Flow-Dependent Drugs Hepatic/liver blood flow is important in delivering drugs to the liver. Flow-dependent drugs are highly extracted by the liver. Thus, reduction in hepatic blood flow will retard their biotransformation, extend circulatory duration, and prolong effect. Importantly, hepatic blood flow declines with age [85, 86]. Examples of flow-dependent drugs are amitriptyline, desipramine, diltiazem, fentanyl, metoprolol, and propofol.

Capacity-Dependent Drugs In contrast, capacity-dependent drugs (nonflow dependent) depend largely on intrinsic hepatic metabolism, primarily CYP enzymes of Phase I metabolism. Drug examples in this category are naproxen, valproic acid, ibuprofen, warfarin, and phenytoin. Therefore, hepatic cellular changes that may affect the functionality and/or concentration of CYP enzymes are important. In this regard, liver size (volume) as determined by ultrasound declines approximately 20–40% with age (20–91 years) [85]. Histological/cytological changes induced in the liver by aging range from minor [87] to major, thereby exhibiting all the hallmarks of aging such as genomic instability and altered intercellular communication [88].

Cytochrome P450 Enzymes The actual effect of age on CYP-dependent drug clearance is variable. On the one hand, clearance of midazolam was unaffected by age [89] as well as "most drugs with a low hepatic extraction ratio" [90]. On the other hand, drug clearance was reduced by approximately 20–60% [91] and the half-life of CYP-metabolized drugs (using hepatic biopsy samples of 226 donors) was 50–75% longer in samples from older individuals than in young individuals [92, 93]. Additional insight is predicted with development of physiological-based pharmacokinetic modeling and simulation using Simcyp®. This modeling uses data from recombinant CYP enzyme assays and liver microsomes in combination with drug probes, caffeine, S-warfarin, S-mephenytoin, desipramine, midazolam, metabolized by different CYP enzymes and exhibiting different hepatic extraction and protein binding [94]. Simulations show that from 20 to 95 years of age, drug clearance declines (20–40%) up to approximately 70 years of age. These results compared favorably with modest clinical data in 4 of 5 drugs (warfarin, [95]; midazolam, [96]; desipramine, [97] and caffeine, [98]).

Although gender differences are difficult to establish since most studies are too small and hence underpowered, Stader and Marzolini [99] pulled together over 60 clinical publications (56 drugs) on PK in men and women across the age spectrum. Applying analysis of variance, PK differences between men and women were modest with only one parameter, maximal drug concentration higher in women than men (~20%), an effect possibly due to gender differences in body weight and elimination processes.

EXCRETION Biotransformed drugs are excreted by the kidneys. Kidneys are the main site for drug elimination and a main factor in the determination of drug exposure. Thus, a reduction in kidney function will significantly increase the duration of drug activity. A persistently high drug level (above the therapeutic value) may potentially produce an adverse reaction. Therefore, prior to drug use, accurate measurement of kidney function is essential. However, there is a controversy related to the popular use of creatinine assessment of kidney function in the older adult (for details see Chap. 3). In brief review, validated methods to assess kidney function are measurement of either glomerular filtration rate (GFR) (infusion of inulin) or renal blood flow (infusion of para-aminohippurate). Since these are invasive and complicated procedures, GFR is frequently determined indirectly by blood sampling of creatinine, a metabolic product of creatine, released from skeletal muscle (estimated GFR, eGFR). Creatinine is filtered by the kidneys and only minimally altered by renal processes. However, it is affected by diet, exercise, and disease [100]. In particular, since creatinine is derived from skeletal muscles, test results from individuals with reduced muscle mass (e.g., sarcopenia) may produce a false enhancement of kidney function. This will significantly impact a variety of drugs, e.g., antibiotics (specifically aminoglycosides, vancomycin); digoxin, lithium, histamine antagonists, and diuretics.

Age Changes in Kidneys Age alters the structure of the kidneys. There is a 10% reduction in kidney mass per decade after age 40 in both healthy men and women [101] with a greater impact on the outer cortical region compared to the inner medulla [101, 102]. Nephron number [103] as well as tubular length and volume decline with age [104]. Numerous age-related changes have been reported for the glomeruli [105] that include a decrease in number of normal glomeruli, an increase in dysfunctional glomeruli, and compensatory hyper-perfusion of healthy glomeruli. The latter change eventually leads to pathological conditions, e.g., glomerulosclerosis [106].

Age-related decline in kidney function is highly variable [106]. Bolignano et al. reviewed 12 clinical studies in older adults (20–80+ years) that measured GFRs (mostly by creatinine clearance). These studies reported an average 30–46% decline in eGFR with age. In several large clinical studies, (with more than 800 older volunteers) eGFR declined 0.4 ml/min/year [107] to 2.6 ml/min/year [108]. The Baltimore Longitudinal Study of Aging collected data in healthy volunteers for 5–14 years and observed a 1.51 ml/min/year decline in GFR in individuals 40–80 years of age. Variability among participants was evident as approximately 30% exhibited no decline in kidney function and another 30% exhibited an increase in kidney function [109].

A seminal study by Davies and Shock [110] that measured renal blood flow in 70 males 24–89 years of age reported a linear decline after the age of 30 years. Others [111] confirmed an age-related decline in renal blood flow in male and female participants with average age of 26–68 years.

Tubular Secretion Renal tubular secretion, a key determinate of kidney function, has generally been assessed in diseases, e.g., chronic kidney disease [112], and infrequently in healthy older individuals. Altered cytology of outpocketing, reduced cell number, and scarring of tubules have been reported [106]. Davies and Shock (1950) [110] reported that tubular function declines with age. An in depth evaluation of the sodium/potassium ATPase and hydrogen/potassium ATPase, key enzymes in the distal tubules is lacking although use of antagonist (inhibitory) drugs binding to these enzymes, e.g., trimethoprim-sulfamethoxazole in the older adult may have severe consequences (see Chap. 3).

Kidney Transporters Renal transporters are abundant and are essential to normal kidney function [113]. "Renal transporters participate in actively secreting substances from the proximal tubular cells and reabsorbing them in the distal renal tubules" [113]. Thus, renal transporters exert a major effect on drug clearance and hence influence the duration and extent of efficacy, side effects, and toxicities. One study concluded that renal transporters in the kidney are affected by age, sex, and ethnicity [114]. Using commercially available kidney samples, the gene expression of 27 transporters was analyzed. Combining age and gender changes, significant changes (some increases, some decreases) in transporters were evident after the age of 50.

Diuretics (drugs causing increasing passing of urine) are especially troublesome in the presence of reduced kidney function since their site of action *is* the kidney and their persistence in a weakened kidney produces tissue toxicity that further worsens renal function.

Table 2.1 Effect of age on pharmacokinetics

Absorption		Distribution		Metabolism		Excretion	
Age effects	Consequences	Age effects	Consequences	Age effects	Consequences	Age effects	Consequences
↓ gastric motility	prolonged emptying time; slowed absorption	change in body composition	↑ volume of distribution slower onset & elimination for lipid-soluble drugs	↓ hepatic blood flow	↓ extraction of flow-dependent drugs — ↑ systemic exposure	↓ GFR	↑ drug exposure
↓ gastric pH (minor) atrophic gastritis & use of proton pump inhibitors (major)	hypochlorhydria that ↓ or ↑ absorption depending on drug's physical chemistry	↑ adipose tissue mass				↓ RBF	↑ drug duration of action toxicities for diuretics
		↓ lean tissue mass	↓ volume of distribution, higher drug concentration for water-soluble drugs				
↓ intestinal CYP3A enzymes	↑ availability of unchanged drug	reduction of plasma proteins	↑ amount of "free" drug → produces greater effect, possibly adverse	↓ hepatic CYP enzyme activities	variable but ↓ metabolism → longer, stronger effects	↓ tubular secretion	↑ duration and extent of effect plus possible side effects and toxicities
↓ intestinal transporter P-gp	↑ drug exposure	evident with malnutrition due to disease/frailty				↑↓ renal transporters	
skin layers thinning/dysfunctional cells	Slowed topical absorption; bruising/infection possible with IV infusions						
Muscles—loss of mass	no data; pain with injections in sarcopenia						
pulmonary ↓ lung tissue; ↓ ventilation rate	slowed induction and emergence with anesthetic drugs						

GFR glomerular filtration rate; *RBF* renal blood flow; *CYP* cytochrome P450 metabolizing enzymes; ↑ increase; ↓ decrease; → leads to; *P-gp* P-glycoprotein

Pharmacodymanics and Aging

Introduction Pharmacodynamics (PD) defines quantitatively and mechanistically the effect of a drug at its target site, generally a protein entity termed a receptor. PD characterizes the drug–receptor interaction and subsequent biochemical changes termed cell signaling that generate the expected physiological effect. Understanding the effect of age on PD is essential for best prescribing and use of drugs in the older adult. Age-dependent effects on receptors and their subsequent cell signaling can alter efficacy and lead to undesired loss of effect or adverse drug reactions (ADRs). Although not fully understood, age-related changes in several prominent receptors have been documented. It is important to note that clinical results generally are cross-sectional in design with a small sample size of older adults about 65–70 years of age.

BETA-ADRENERGIC RECEPTORS Beta(β)-adrenergic receptors, primarily of the heart, have received considerable research attention in regard to age effects. β-adrenergic receptors are members of the guanine nucleotide-binding G protein-coupled receptor (GPCR) superfamily [115]. The three receptor subclasses, β1, β2, and β3 are widely distributed in the body, specifically in the cardiovascular, pulmonary and GI systems, liver, and fat [116]. The endogenous agonists are norepinephrine, neurotransmitter of the sympathetic nervous system, and epinephrine, circulating mediator from the adrenal medulla.

Drugs classified as β1 or β2 agonists or antagonists mimic or inhibit, respectively, the actions of endogenous neurotransmitters. β1 receptors predominate in cardiac muscle, although β2 (tubular system) and β3 (nodal) receptors are also present in cardiac tissue [117]. However, β2 receptors are primarily located in the pulmonary and vascular systems and β3 receptors are expressed in fat cells [118]. Stimulation of β1-adrenergic receptors produces an increase in heart rate and enhanced contractility that together increase stroke volume, ejecting a greater quantity of blood to the rest of the body. Stimulation of β2 receptors produces relaxation of the bronchioli (smaller airways of the lungs) and vasodilatation of arterioles (small blood vessels). Stimulation of β3 receptors is involved in thermogenic activity (body heat regulation) [119].

β1-Adrenergic Receptors and Aging The extent of agonist activation of β1-adrenergic receptors is reduced with age. Specifically, cardiac function (heart rate, contractility, ejection fraction, blood pressure) is reduced following a dose response to isoproterenol (β1 agonist) in older men (60–82 years) compared to younger men (24–32 years) [120]. The cardiac response to isoproterenol in older women (60–75 years) is reduced with age but to a lesser extent than in men [121]. Nevertheless, in both men and women, this age-associated effect accounts, in large part, for exercise intolerance in the older adult [120]. Mechanistically, both receptor density and affinity decline with age, approximately 30% as observed in explanted nonfailing human hearts challenged with isoproterenol [122]. More recently, Ross et al. [123] reported that with hand grip exercise, older men (average age 67 years) "had attenuated coronary hyperemia to low-dose isoproterenol" compared to younger men (average age of 21 years).

These are significant findings. Clearly, the dose of β1 agonists required to increase heart rate or force of heart contractions is higher in older adults compared to younger adults. This is not only important in understanding exercise intolerance and loss of cardiac reserve in the older adult [124] but is critical for the treatment of heart failure [125, 126]. However, choice of an inotrope such as isoproterenol in heart failure is considered last resort and is used rarely (see Chap. 4).

β2-Adrenergic Receptors and Aging The activity of β2-adrenergic receptors also declines with age. In the vasculature, forearm vasodilation as measured by venous occlusion plethysmography to an infusion of the β2-adrenergic agonist, terbutaline, is less in postmenopausal women compared to young premenopausal women [127]. In healthy adults (24 years of age compared to 69 years of age), β2-adrenergic receptor-dependent venodilation also declines with age while response to adenosine acting through different receptors remains unchanged [128].

In the pulmonary system, activation of β2-adrenergic receptors in the bronchioles produces smooth muscle cell relaxation and widens the air passages to permit inspiration of more air [129]. Although not as well studied, β2-adrenergic receptors in the older adult are less responsive to β2-adrenergic agonists resulting in decreased bronchodilation. This was confirmed with results of reduced bronchodilation to albuterol in healthy older adults (60–76 years) compared to young adults (20–36 years) [130] and in a larger study by Banerji A et al. [131] of emergency asthmatic patients in which those 55 and older responded poorly to bronchodilators compared to young patients 18–34 years of age. Short and long-acting β2-adrenergic agonists are a significant part of the therapy for asthma [132] and chronic obstructive pulmonary disease (COPD) (see Chap. 5). Awareness of this PD age-associated change adds to the complexity of treating these diseases but assures better outcomes.

CENTRAL NERVOUS SYSTEM RECEPTORS Aging of the brain is complicated and poorly understood. However, in healthy older adults, neuronal loss is negligible and altered connectivity leading to compensation in brain function is more the norm [133]. The rate of information processing slows and there are possible reductions of other functions, e.g., executive function, reward-based behavior, and some types of memory. Many cognitive functions remain unaltered, e.g., language mastery, semantic knowledge [134]. Nevertheless, the older adult is more sensitive to central-acting drugs, e.g., anesthetics and psychotropic drugs (sedatives, hypnotics, antipsychotics, anxiolytics) than the younger adult [135]. PK may contribute in part to this enhanced sensitivity but as discussed below, major CNS receptors experience modifications with age, changes that could contribute to this age-related increase in sensitivity to CNS-acting drugs.

Gamma Amino Butyric Acid Receptors and Aging In the brain, there are two distinct gamma-amino butyric acid (GABA) receptors, $GABA_A$ and $GABA_B$, both activated by the neurotransmitter, GABA. GABA produced by GABAergic neurons binds to GABA receptors to produce an inhibitory effect that provides the counterbalance to the activity of excitatory neurons [136]. This effect is essential to learning, modulating sensory and motor activities, and optimizing neuroplasticity (growth and activation of neurons) [137].

The GABA receptors are physically dissimilar and hence respond to drugs differently. $GABA_A$ receptors are ligand-activated ion channels for chloride. $GABA_A$ receptors are considered rapidly acting receptors. $GABA_B$ receptors (also called metabotropic as they are involved in metabolic activities) is a G-protein coupled receptor (GPCR) considered a slow-acting receptor. Both are distributed throughout the brain and both have multiple components that may be drug targets and hence may enhance or diminish GABA-receptor interaction in multiple ways [138].

$GABA_A$ is of great interest since it is the target of not only the anxiolytic and antiseizure benzodiazepines, e.g., diazepam, but also "picrotoxin-like convulsants, general anesthetics including both volatile agents (like isoflurane), and intravenous agents: barbiturates, etomidate, propofol, as well as long-chain alcohols, including low potency actions of ethanol, plus neuroactive steroids" [138]. With the exception of the picrotoxin-like convulsants, these sedative and anesthetic drugs do not directly bind the $GABA_A$ receptors but instead attach elsewhere to change the structure of the receptor and hence activate indirectly (termed positive allosteric modulation) [139]. In contrast, there is only one drug, baclofen, a muscle relaxant, that is specific for the $GABA_B$ receptor [140].

Data from animal studies (rodents, nonhuman primates) and older adults with and without cognitive or motor deficiencies support the broad conclusion that the GABAergic system gradually becomes impaired with age [137]. The resulting dysregulation of GABAergic signaling in aging is difficult to pinpoint since not all brain regions change in the same way. The literature is filled with reports of increase, decrease, and no change at all in GABAergic activity [137]. Two studies in healthy older adults observed a reduction in GABAergic-dependent effects on tactile acuity [141] and hand motor activity [142].

Considering the widespread presence of the GABAergic system in the CNS and the complexities of the GABA receptors, drugs acting at these sites must be used with caution or not at all in the older adult (see Chap. 3). Specifically, the heterogeneity of the binding sites for the benzodiazepines and the varied functionality of these neurons leads to unknown potencies [143].

Metabotropic Glutamate Receptors and Aging Metabotropic glutamate receptors (MGluRs) belong to the family of GPCRs. MGluRs are distributed throughout the CNS as eight different subtypes [144]. The neurotransmitter is glutamine and "activation of mGluRs results in diverse actions on neuronal excitability and synaptic transmission by modulation of a variety of ion channels and other regulatory and signaling proteins" [145]. Thus, in contrast to GABA, glutamine is an excitatory transmitter. Unlike most GPCRs whose densities and affinities decline with age, two mGluRs subtypes, R2 and R3 increase with age [146]. MGluRs play a role in Alzheimer's Disease (AD) and Parkinson's disease possibly in part with excessive excitation that contributes to cell death and inflammation [147]. Identification of antagonists of these receptors to treat these and other neurodegenerative diseases is of considerable current interest.

Dopamine Receptors and Aging There are five dopamine receptor subtypes (D1-D5), members of the GPCR superfamily with distributions throughout the body. Subtypes D2 and D3 receptors are considered the major CNS players in "regulating mood, motivation and movement" [148]. Dopamine is the neurotransmitter produced by the dopaminergic neurons. Striking changes in the dopamine system occur in Parkinson's disease and AD that affect motor and cognitive/memory functions (see Chapters 4 and 5 for details). However, the age-related changes evident in healthy older adults differ from the pathology of Parkison's disease and AD [149].

In human aging, dopaminergic transmission is reduced due to loss of neurons and dysfunction of receptors and transporters [149]. Autopsy analysis of individuals across the lifespan shows loss of dopaminergic neurons with age [150]. The density and affinity of D2 and D3 receptors decline in the striatum and substantia nigra [146]; the decline of D2 receptors is estimated at "9% pre decade from early childhood" [149]. The ability of the dopamine transporter that removes dopamine from the synapse back into the nerve terminal for reuse also declines with age, slowing neurotransmitter turnover and subsequent CNS activities [151, 152]. These age-associated changes result in functional deficits such as reduced control of olfaction [153] and balance [154]. Also, simple reaction time and motor speed [151, 152] and gait [154] are affected by impaired dopaminergic activity.

It is important to appreciate the dysfunction of the dopaminergic system in the older adult. The class of drugs called typical antipsychotics, e.g., haloperidol, used in the treatment of psychotic disorders, e.g., schizophrenia and bipolar as well as affective (mood) disorders, act in large part by inhibiting the D2 receptors [155]. If typical antipsychotics are used in the older adult, extreme caution is required because these drugs will add to and exacerbate the age-related changes in the dopaminergic system. This will enable an additional reduction in reaction time, balance, and/or gait that promotes errors, accidents, falls, and hospitalizations.

Muscarinic Acetylcholine Receptors and Aging The muscarinic acetylcholine receptors (mAChR) of which there five subtypes (M1–5) belong to the GPCR family [156]). Cortical and hippocampal cholinergic neurons release the neurotransmitter, acetylcholine (ACh). ACh activates the mAChRs to affect a multiplicity of downstream cell signaling events, e.g., potassium and calcium fluxes inducing excitatory nerve functions. As revealed from extensive studies using knock-out mice, the cholinergic system is complex [157]. Cholinergic neurons interact negatively with dopaminergic neurons in the striatum to influence motor function, assist with learning and memory in the hippocampus, and influence brain plasticity throughout the brain.

A great deal is known about the changes in structure/function of the cholinergic neurons in AD. Progressive loss of cholinergic responses results in continuous memory loss [158] (see Chap. 4). Less is known about the effect of normal aging on this system. Decrements in the cholinergic neurons are thought to account for age-related decline in some cognitive functions especially serious attention-demanding tasks [159]. Supporting data indicate that indeed, the density and affinity of the mAChR-M2 declines with age in the (pre)frontal, hippocampus, and striatum [146]. Additionally, the success on memory tests, e.g., delayed word recall is correlated with optimal cholinergic function as determined by PET scans and radiolabeled ligands for cholinergic enzyme marker, acetylcholinesterase in the brain [160].

"At least 600 drugs/medicinal products are recognized to have anticholinergic activity" [161]. Hence, inhibition of cholinergic activity as a main effect needed in the treatment of overactive bladder or arising as a side effect [162] is likely to occur in the older adult. The limited evidence for age-associated changes in the cholinergic system suggests that it is best to avoid drugs that would further dampen this system and lead to perturbations in cognition and increased risk of dementia [163].

Serotonin Receptors and Aging Serotonin is the neurotransmitter that stimulates anyone of 15 different serotonin (5HT) GPCR receptors distributed throughout the CNS and periphery [164]. Cellular responses are diverse due not only to the many subtypes but also the multitude of proteins that modulate these receptors, placing the serotonin system in high regard [164]. The serotonin system is key in regulating normal physiology of sleep, food intake, mood, and libido. Consequently, disruption of the system underlies CNS disorders of depression, schizophrenia, anxiety/panic, eating, and migraines as well as peripheral disorders of hypertension and irritable bowel syndrome [165].

Numerous studies reviewed by de Oliveira et al. [146] using PET and a specific radioligand, found that the 5HT1A and 5HTB receptors in the cortex decline with age [166, 167]. Similar findings were noted in cortical membranes from postmortem samples (1–88 years of age) [168].

Drugs that affect the serotonin system are numerous. Several selective antagonists, ondansetron, granisetron, and palonosetron are approved to treat nausea and vomiting. Additionally, the atypical antipsychotics, e.g., risperidone, act by antagonizing either 5HT2A, 5HT1A, or 5HT1C receptors in addition to D2 antagonism [155]. Serotonin agonists, e.g., buspirone are useful in the treatment of anxiety and migraines. Another class of drugs acting on the serotonin system and primarily used to treat depression is the selective serotonin reuptake inhibitors (SSRIs) that prevent the reuptake of serotonin in the presynaptic terminal and hence increase its availability at the postsynaptic receptors, in effect acting as indirect 5HT receptor agonists [169]. Well-known SSRIs include escitalopram, fluoxetine, and paroxetine.

Considering the complexity of the serotonin system in the CNS and the evolving understanding of how 5HT agonists, antagonists and SSRIs actually exert their effects, use of these drugs should proceed with caution and if necessary, for short-term use only.

Other Receptors and Aging The comprehensive review by de Oliveir et al. [146] also reported that in addition to those mentioned above, the density and affinity of other members of the GPCR family either decreased with age, e.g., alpha2-adrenergic, opioid (kappa), somatostatin, cannabinoid receptor1, and oxytocin or increased with age, e.g., angiotensin1 receptors.

Table 2.2 Effect of age on pharmacodynamics

Receptors, location	Age effects	Consequences
β1-adrenergic receptors, heart	↓ density, sensitivity	↓ cardiac function→ ↓ heart rate, contractility, ejection fraction; exercise intolerance; reduced response to isoproterenol; implications for treatment of heart failure
β2-adrenergic receptors, blood vessels	↓ receptor responsiveness	↓ vasodilation to agonists
β2-adrenergic receptors, airways	↓ receptor responsiveness	↓ bronchodilation to agonists (albuterol); implications for treatment of respiratory diseases
GABA$_A$ receptors, CNS	Variable	↑ sensitivity to many classes of drugs (anxiolytics, anesthetics, hypnotics, sedative)
metabotropic glutamate receptors, CNS	↑ activity of mGluR2, 3; other subtypes ↓	Postulated pathological role in AD
dopamine receptors, CNS	↓ dopaminergic transmission due to neuronal loss, ↓D2 and D3 receptors and dopamine transporters	↓ in reaction time, balance, and/or gait; effects of typical antipsychotic drugs (D2 antagonists) are additive to age changes
muscarinic acetylcholine receptors, CNS	↓ density and affinity of the mAChR M2; decline in some cholinergic-dependent CNS functions	drugs with anticholinergic activity block cholinergic influence on memory/cognition and additive with age changes; also affects functions of the dopaminergic system; use of anticholinergic drugs is to be avoided (Chap. 3)
serotonin receptors	↓ density/affinity of 5HT1A and 5HT1B	Widespread serotonergic actions perturbed with mood and neurological disorders. Many drugs modulate the serotonergic activity, e.g., atypical antipsychotics and antidepressants (SSRIs)

GABA gamma-amino butyric acid; *mGluR* metabotropic glutamate receptor; *D2, D3* dopamine receptor subtypes; *mAChR M2* muscarinic acetylcholine receptor subtype; *5HT1A and 5HT1B* serotonin receptor subtypes; *AD* Alzheimer's Disease; *SSRIs* selective serotonin reuptake inhibitors; ↑ increase; ↓ decrease, CNS central nervous system

Homeostatic Mechanisms

Homeostatic mechanisms seek to restore the organism to its normal balanced state. Those likely to be affected negatively by age and drug use include orthostatic hypotension prevention reflex, cough reflex, laryngeal reflexes, thermoregulation, response to dehydration, and prevention of hemorrhage. These mechanisms weaken with age and hence create a serious vulnerability. The presence of drugs further inhibits these mechanisms. Orthostatic hypotension prevention reflex, cough reflex, and the laryngeal reflex will be discussed here.

Orthostatic Hypotension and Aging Orthostatic hypotension (OH) is defined as a "drop in blood pressure of at least 20 mmHg for systolic blood pressure and at least 10 mmHg for diastolic blood pressure within 3 minutes of standing up" [170]. The older adult is likely to experience OH as it is one of several homeostatic mechanisms diminished by age and exacerbated by medications.

The homeostatic mechanism preventing OH is a reflex initiated by mechanoreceptors (pressure sensors) and chemoreceptors (gas sensors) in the carotid sinus and aortic arch, respectively. These sensors relay information to the vasomotor center in the brain stem to increase the sympathetic nervous system outflow to increase heart rate, contractility, and vasoconstriction in skin and muscle. This reflex serves to maintain blood flow to the brain in cases where it is likely to fall abruptly as in positional change from supine or sitting to standing. Slowing of this reflex leads to light-headedness and loss of consciousness with serious consequences such as falls and fractures [170].

Saedon et al. [171] reported that 22.2% of community-dwelling older adults and 23.9% of older individuals in long-term care experience a reduction in the adequacy of the OH reflex. Others have reported similar degrees of loss [172, 173]. Use of certain medications adds to this age change. Vasodilator and alpha1-adrenergic antagonists, diuretics, mixed beta and alpha blockers, and tricyclic antidepressants facilitate OH in the older adult [174]. OH is an adverse drug reaction that can be minimized or avoided with identification of OH-inducing drugs (see Chap. 3). Also, other strategies to counteract OH include patient education, medical review, avoidance of large carbohydrate-dense meals, counseling on diet and hydration, and physical counter-pressure maneuvers [175].

> *Alert*: Since 46.1% of older adults experience reduction in the adequacy of the orthostatic hypotension reflex, safety/falls are a big concern.

Cough Reflex and Age The cough reflex is another protective reflex that serves to expel foreign debris from entering the airways. It involves numerous afferent fibers from all parts of the respiratory system and elicits rapid efferent responses to respiratory, laryngeal, and abdominal muscles to generate a forceful air pressure to rid the bronchial tree of potentially harmful debris [176]. Neurological diseases, e.g., Parkinson's Disease, lung disorders, e.g., COPD and age-related diminished mass and strength of skeletal muscles reduce the efficacy of the cough reflex. Cough reflex reduction is undesirable because it elevates the risk of respiratory infections and aspiration pneumonia [177]. Furthermore, in the frail older adult, there is some data to support the proposal that pneumonia may arise from "repeated microaspiration" that establishes chronic airway inflammation in the absence of pathogens. This "silent pneumonia" compromises respiratory function and increases mortality [177].

Assessment of lung function essential in the older adult is worthwhile so that appropriate treatment can be advised. Beta2-agonists or muscarinic antagonists in COPD (see Chap. 5) improve airway flow and improve the cough reflex [176]. Mechanical devices termed Manual Insufflator/Exsufflator that provide some cough reflex improvement in neurological and muscular deficiencies are considered valuable aids [178].

Laryngeal Reflex The laryngeal reflex, a component of the cough reflex, is a protective airway response that closes the glottis and prevents aspiration (intake of oropharyngeal and gastric substances into the airways). A 3–six fold age-related decrease in responsiveness was demonstrated in two studies with volunteers (17–96 years of age) [179, 180]. The lower fold change was attributed to exclusion of smokers and methodological improvements [180]. Nevertheless, this depressed reflex sensitivity is sufficient to raise concerns for aspiration during anesthesia recovery facilitating aspiration pneumonia and for the use of sedatives in the older adult [180].

Guidance
1. Knowledge of pharmacokinetics (PK) and pharmacodynamics (PD) is essential to appropriate drug use. Since aging and disease influence these principles, reasonable modifications in drug use must be implemented.
2. Aging affects PK of a drug in multiple ways. Awareness of age-related decline in organ function, especially of the liver and kidneys and age-related changes in body composition alerts the prescriber to potentially major changes in systemic drug exposure and duration of action. Age-related changes in absorption are incompletely understood but at present considered minor.
3. As receptors decrease or increase in abundance and activity, so does the PD of a drug. Familiarity with age-related loss of receptors and associated functional decline allows for choice of the appropriate dose and avoidance of adverse reactions.
4. Age-related reduction in homeostatic reflexes contributes to orthostatic hypotension, increased risk of respiratory infections, and aspiration pneumonia. Drugs that add to these changes are to be used with caution.
5. Since the rate of biological aging is specific to each person, age-dependent changes in receptors, blood flow, reflexes, and end-organ function vary with the individual. Use of drugs in the older adult requires an individualized approach based on accurate measurement of function.

References

1. Pharmacokinetics & pharmacodynamics. In: Ernstmeyer K, Christman E, editors Nursing Pharmacology, 2nd ed. Open Resources for Nursing (Open RN). Eau Claire: Chippewa Valley Technical College; 2023. Sections 1.1–1.11. https://www.ncbi.nlm.nih.gov/books/NBK595000/
2. Andres TM, McEvoy MD, Allen BFS. Geriatric Pharmacology: An Update. Anesthesiol Clin. 2019;37(3):475–92. https://doi.org/10.1016/j.anclin.2019.04.007.
3. Niccoli T, Partridge L. Ageing as a risk factor for disease. Curr Biol. 2012;22(17):R741–52. https://doi.org/10.1016/j.cub.2012.07.024.
4. GAO-07-47R: Elderly persons in clinical drug trials. 2007. Available online at: http://www.gao.gov/products/GAO-07-47R
5. Grimsrud KN, Sherwin CMT, Constance JE, Tak C, Zuppa AF, Sigarelli MG, et al. Special population considerations and regulatory affairs for clinical research. Clin Res Regul Aff. 2015;32(2):47–56. https://doi.org/10.3109/10601333.2015.1001900.
6. National Academies of Sciences, Engineering, and Medicine. 2021. Drug research and development for adults across the older age span: Proceedings of a workshop. Washington, DC: Tational Academies Press. https://doi.org/10.17226/25998.
7. Pazan F, Wehling M. Polypharmacy in older adults: a narrative review of definitions, epidemiology and consequences. Eur Geriatr Med. 2021;12(3):443–52. https://doi.org/10.1007/s41999-021-00479-3.
8. Ramos-Lopez O, Milagro FI, Riezu-Boj JI, Martinez JA. Epigenetic signatures underlying inflammation: an interplay of nutrition, physical activity, metabolic diseases, and environmental factors for personalized nutrition. Inflamm Res. 2021;70(1):29–49. https://doi.org/10.1007/s00011-020-01425-y.
9. Salazar N, Gonzalez S, Nogacka AM, Rios-Covian D, Arboleya S, Gueimonde M, et al. Microbiome: Effects of ageing and diet. Curr Issues Mol Biol. 2020;36:33–62. https://doi.org/10.21775/cimb.036.033.
10. Müller J, Keiser M, Drozdzik M, Oswald S. Expression, regulation and function of intestinal drug transporters: an update. Biol Chem. 2017;398(2):175–92. https://doi.org/10.1515/hsz-2016-0259.
11. Drozdzik M, Busch D, Lapczuk J, Muller J, Ostrowski M, Kurzawski M, et al. Protein abundance of clinically relevant drug-metabolizing enzymes in the human liver and intestine: a comparative analysis in paired tissue specimens. Clin Pharmacol Ther. 2018;104(3):515–24. https://doi.org/10.1002/cpt.967.
12. Peters SA, Jones CR, Ungell A-L, Hatley OJD. Predicting drug extraction in the human gut wall: assessing contributions from drug metabolizing enzymes and transporter proteins using preclinical models. Clin Pharmacokinet. 2016;55(6):673–96. https://doi.org/10.1007/s40262-015-0351-6.
13. Kiela PR, Ghishan FK. Physiology of Intestinal Absorption and Secretion. Best Pract Res Clin Gastroenterol. 2016;30(2):145–59. https://doi.org/10.1016/j.bpg.2016.02.007.
14. Wessler JD, Grip LT, Mendell J, Giugliano RP. The P-glycoprotein transport system and cardiovascular drugs. J Am Coll Cardiol. 2013;61(25):2495–502. https://doi.org/10.1016/j.jacc.2013.02.058.
15. Freckmann G, Pleus S, Haug C, Bitton G, Nagar R. Increasing local blood flow by warming the application site: beneficial effects on postprandial glycemic excursions. Diabetes Sci Technol. 2012;6(4):780–5. https://doi.org/10.1177/193229681200600407.
16. Saeed S, Irfan M, Naz S, Liaquat M, Jahan S, Hayat S. Routes and barriers associated with protein and peptide drug delivery system. Med Assoc. 2021;71(8):2032–9. https://doi.org/10.47391/JPMA.759.
17. Zhao Y, Yang Y, Li Q, Li J. Understanding the unique microenvironment in the aging liver. Front Med (Lausanne). 2022;9:842024. https://doi.org/10.3389/fmed.2022.842024.

18. Zanger UM, Schwab M. Cytochrome P450 enzymes in drug metabolism: regulation of gene expression, enzyme activities, and impact of genetic variation. Pharmacol Ther. 2013 Apr;138(1):103–41. https://doi.org/10.1016/j.pharmthera.2012.12.007.
19. Gekle M. Kidney and aging - A narrative review. Exp Gerontol. 2017;87(Pt B):153–5. https://doi.org/10.1016/j.exger.2016.03.013.
20. Smith HW, Goldring W, Chasis H. The measurement of the tubular excretory mass, effective blood flow, and filtration rate in the normal human kidney. J Clin Invest. 1938;17(3):263–78. https://doi.org/10.1172/JCI100950.
21. Wang K, Kestenbaum B. Proximal tubular secretory clearance: a neglected partner of kidney function. Clin J Am Soc Nephrol. 2018;13(8):1291–1296. https://doi.org/10.2215/CJN.12001017.
22. Clerk A, Sugden PH. The insulin receptor family in the heart: new light on old insights. Biosci Rep 2022;42(7):BSR20221212. doi: https://doi.org/10.1042/BSR20221212.
23. Waters MJ. The growth hormone receptor. Growth Hormon IGF Res. 2016;28:6–10. https://doi.org/10.1016/j.ghir.2015.06.001.
24. Perez DM. Current developments on the role of alpha(1)-adrenergic receptors in cognition, cardioprotection, and metabolism. Front Cell Dev Biol. 2021;9:652152. https://doi.org/10.3389/fcell.2021.652152.
25. Yakel JL. Cholinergic receptors: functional role of nicotinic ACh receptors in brain circuits and disease. Pflugers Arch. 2013;465(4):441–50. https://doi.org/10.1007/s00424-012-1200-1.
26. Fuentes N, Silveyra P. Estrogen receptor signaling mechanisms. Adv Protein Chem Struct Biol. 2019;116:135–70. https://doi.org/10.1016/bs.apcsb.2019.01.001.
27. Trang A, Khandhar PB. Physiology, acetylcholinesterase. In: StatPearls [Internet]. Treasure Island: StatPearls Publishing; 2024 Jan. 2023 Jan 19. PMID: 30969557.
28. Voldborg BR, Damstrup L, Spang-Thomsen M, Poulsen HS. Epidermal growth factor receptor (EGFR) and EGFR mutations, function and possible role in clinical trials. Ann Oncol. 1997;8(12):1197–206. https://doi.org/10.1023/a:1008209720526.
29. Friesen JA, Rodwell VW. The 3-hydroxy-3-methylglutaryl coenzyme-A (HMG-CoA) reductases. Genome Biol. 2004;5(11):248. https://doi.org/10.1186/gb-2004-5-11-248.
30. Bernstein KE, Giani JF, Shen XZ, Gonzalez-Villalobos RA. Renal angiotensin-converting enzyme and blood pressure control. Curr Opin Nephrol Hypertens. 2014;23(2):106–12. https://doi.org/10.1097/01.mnh.0000441047.13912.56.
31. Fitzpatrick FA. Cyclooxygenase enzymes: regulation and function. Pharm Des. 2004;10(6):577–88. https://doi.org/10.2174/1381612043453144.
32. Bilder GE. Human biological aging: From macromolecules to organ systems. Hoboken: John Wiley & Sons Publishers; 2016. pp. 168–82, 19–201, 228–40, 312–7.
33. Algahtani MS, Kazi M, Alsenaidy MA, Ahmad MZ. Advances in oral drug delivery. Front Pharmacol. 2021;12:618411. https://doi.org/10.3389/fphar.2021.618411.
34. Demeester C, Robins D, Edwina AE, TournoyJ AP, Ince I, et al. Physiologically based pharmacokinetic (PBPK) modeling of oral drug absorption in older adults—an AGePOP review. Eur J Pharm Sci. 2023;188:106496. https://doi.org/10.1016/j.ejps.2023.106496.
35. Stillhart C, Asteriadis A, Bocharova E, Eksteen G, Harder F, Kusch J, et al. The impact of advanced age on gastrointestinal characteristics that are relevant to oral drug absorption: An AGePOP review. Eur J Pharm Sci. 2023;187:106452. https://doi.org/10.1016/j.ejps.2023.106452.
36. Evans MA, Triggs EJ, Cheung M, Broe GA, Creasey H. Gastric emptying rate in the elderly: implications for drug therapy. J Am Geriatr Soc. 1981;29(5):201–5. https://doi.org/10.1111/j.1532-5415.1981.tb01766.x.
37. Dumic I, Nordin T, Jecmenica M, Lalosevic MS, Milosavlievic T, Milovanovic T, et al. Gastrointestinal tract disorders in older age. Can J Gastroenterol Hepatol. 2019;2019:6757524. https://doi.org/10.1155/2019/6757524.
38. Gomez-Pinilla PJ, Gibbons SJ, Sarr MG, Kendrick ML, Shen KR, Cima RR, et al. Changes in interstitial cells of cajal with age in the human stomach and colon. Neurogastroenterol Motil. 2011;23(1):36–44. https://doi.org/10.1111/j.1365-2982.2010.01590.x.

39. Soenen S, Rayner CK, Jones KL, Horowitz M. The ageing gastrointestinal tract. Curr Opin Clin Nutr Metab Care. 2016;19(1):12–8. https://doi.org/10.1097/MCO.0000000000000238.
40. Giezenaar C, Trahair LG, Rigda R, Hutchison AT, Feinle-Bisset C, Luscombe-Marsh ND, et al. Lesser suppression of energy intake by orally ingested whey protein in healthy older men compared with young controls. Am J Physiol Regul Integr Comp Physiol. 2015;309(8):R845–54. https://doi.org/10.1152/ajpregu.00213.2015.
41. Porter KM, Hoey L, Hughes CF, Ward M, Clements M, Strain J, et al. Associations of atrophic gastritis and proton-pump inhibitor drug use with vitamin B-12 status, and the impact of fortified foods, in older adults. Am J Clin Nutr. 2021;114(4):1286–94. https://doi.org/10.1093/ajcn/nqab193.
42. Lahner E, Annibale B, Fave GD. Systematic review: impaired drug absorption related to the co-administration of antisecretory therapy. Aliment Pharmacol Ther. 2009;29(12):1219–29. https://doi.org/10.1111/j.1365-2036.2009.03993.x.
43. Sharma M, Holmes HM, Mehta HB, Chen H, Aparasu RR, Shih Y-CT, et al. The concomitant use of tyrosine kinase inhibitors and proton pump inhibitors: Prevalence, predictors, and impact on survival and discontinuation of therapy in older adults with cancer. Cancer. 2019;125(7):1155–62. https://doi.org/10.1002/cncr.31917.
44. Saweirs WM, Andrews DJ, Low-Beer TS. The double sugar test of intestinal permeability in the elderly. Age Ageing. 1985;14(5):312–5. https://doi.org/10.1093/ageing/14.5.312.
45. Saltzman JR, Kowdley KV, Perrone G, Russell RM. Changes in small-intestine permeability with aging. J Am Geriatr Soc. 1995;43(2):160–4. https://doi.org/10.1111/j.1532-5415.1995.tb06382.x.
46. Mall JPG, Lofvendahl L, Lindqvist CM, Brummer RJ, Keita AV, Schoultz I. Differential effects of dietary fibres on colonic barrier function in elderly individuals with gastrointestinal symptoms. Sci Rep. 2018;8(1):13404. https://doi.org/10.1038/s41598-018-31492-5.
47. Valentini L, Ramminger S, Haas V, Postrach E, Werich M, Fischer A, et al. Small intestinal permeability in older adults. Physiol Rep. 2014;2(4):e00281. https://doi.org/10.14814/phy2.281.
48. Lindell M, Karlsson MO, Lennernas H, Pahlman L, Lang MA. Variable expression of CYP and Pgp genes in the human small intestine. Eur J Clin Investig. 2003;33(6):493–9. https://doi.org/10.1046/j.1365-2362.2003.01154.x.
49. Miki Y, Suzuki T, Tazawa C, Blumberg B, Sasano H. Steroid and xenobiotic receptor (SXR), cytochrome P450 3A4 and multidrug resistance gene 1 in human adult and fetal tissues. Mol Cell Endocrinol. 2005;231(1–2):75–85. https://doi.org/10.1016/j.mce.2004.12.005.
50. Werk AN, Cascorbi I. Functional gene variants of CYP3A4. Clin Pharmacol Ther. 2014;96(3):340–8. https://doi.org/10.1038/clpt.2014.129.
51. Rattanacheeworn P, Kerr SJ, Kittanamongkolchai W, Townamchai N, Udomkarnjananun S, Praditpornsilpa K, et al. Quantification of CYP3A and drug transporters activity in healthy young, healthy elderly and chronic kidney disease elderly patients by a microdose cocktail approach. Front Pharmacol. 2021;12:726669. https://doi.org/10.3389/fphar.2021.726669.
52. Sabbagh F, Kim BS. Recent advances in polymeric transdermal drug delivery systems. J Control Release. 2022;341:132–46. https://doi.org/10.1016/j.jconrel.2021.11.025.
53. Priano L, Gasco MR, Mauro A. Transdermal treatment options for neurological disorders: impact on the elderly. Drugs Aging. 2006;23(5):357–75. https://doi.org/10.2165/00002512-200623050-00001.
54. Ibrahim H, Woodward Z, Pooley J, Richfield EW. Rotigotine patch prescription in inpatients with Parkinson's disease: evaluating prescription accuracy, delirium and end-of-life use. Age Ageing. 2021;50(4):1397–401. https://doi.org/10.1093/ageing/afaa256.
55. Vadivelu N, Hines RL. Management of chronic pain in the elderly: focus on transdermal buprenorphine. Clin Interv Aging. 2008;3(3):421–30. https://doi.org/10.2147/cia.s1880.
56. Muensterman ET, Jaynes HA, Sowinski KM, Overholser BR, Shen C, Kovacs RJ, et al. Effect of transdermal testosterone and oral progesterone on drug-induced qt interval lengthening in older men: a randomized, double-blind, placebo-controlled

crossover-design study. Circulation. 2019;140(13):1127–9. https://doi.org/10.1161/CIRCULATIONAHA.119.041395.
57. Zhang J, Yu H, Man M-Q, Hu L. Aging in the dermis: Fibroblast senescence and its significance. Aging Cell. 2023;00:e14054. https://doi.org/10.1111/acel.14054.
58. Zouboulis CC, Makrantonaki E, Nikolakis G. When the skin is in the center of interest: An aging issue. Clin Dermatol. 2019;37(4):296–305. https://doi.org/10.1016/j.clindermatol.2019.04.004.
59. Al-Tawil N, Odar-Cederlof I, Berggren A-C, Johnson HE, Persson J. Pharmacokinetics of transdermal buprenorphine patch in the elderly. Eur J Clin Pharmacol. 2013;69(2):143–9. https://doi.org/10.1007/s00228-012-1320-8.
60. Thompson JP, Bower S, Liddle AM, Rowbotham DJ. Perioperative pharmacokinetics of transdermal fentanyl in elderly and young adult patients. Br J Anaesth. 1998;81(2):152–4. https://doi.org/10.1093/bja/81.2.152.
61. Bahrami F, Rossi RM, Defraeye T. Predicting transdermal fentanyl delivery using physics-based simulations for tailored therapy based on the age. Drug Deliv. 2022;29(1):950–69. https://doi.org/10.1080/10717544.2022.2050846.
62. Colin E, Baldolli A, Verdon R, Saint-Lorant G. Subcutaneously administered antibiotics. Med Mal Infect. 2020;50(3):231–42. https://doi.org/10.1016/j.medmal.2019.06.007.
63. Satterwhite J, Heathman M, Miller PD, Marín F, Glass EV, Dobnig H. Pharmacokinetics of teriparatide (rhPTH[1-34]) and calcium pharmacodynamics in postmenopausal women with osteoporosis. Calcif Tissue Int. 2010;87(6):485–92. https://doi.org/10.1007/s00223-010-9424-6.
64. Heise T, Hovelmann U, Zijlstra E, Stender-Petersen K, Bonde J, Haahr H. A comparison of pharmacokinetic and pharmacodynamic properties between faster-acting insulin aspart and insulin aspart in elderly subjects with type 1 diabetes mellitus. Drugs Aging. 2017;34(1):29–38. https://doi.org/10.1007/s40266-016-0418-6.
65. Korsatko S, Deller S, Mader JK, Glettler K, Koehler G, Treiber G, et al. Ultra-long pharmacokinetic properties of insulin degludec are comparable in elderly subjects and younger adults with type 1 diabetes mellitus. Drugs Aging. 2014;31(1):47–53. https://doi.org/10.1007/s40266-013-0138-0.
66. Wilkinson DJ, Piasecki M, Atherton PJ. The age-related loss of skeletal muscle mass and function: Measurement and physiology of muscle fibre atrophy and muscle fibre loss in humans. Ageing Res Rev. 2018;47:123–32. https://doi.org/10.1016/j.arr.2018.07.005.
67. Zhao H, Cheng R, Song G, Teng J, Shen S, Xuancheng F, et al. Effect of resistance training on the rehabilitation of elderly patients with sarcopenia: a meta-Analysis. Int J Environ Res Public Health. 2022;19(23):15491. https://doi.org/10.3390/ijerph192315491.
68. Cruz-Jentoft AJ, Bahat G, Bauer J, Boirie Y, Bruyere O, Cederholm T, et al. Sarcopenia: revised European consensus on definition and diagnosis. Age Ageing. 2019;48(1):16–31. https://doi.org/10.1093/ageing/afy169.
69. Andritz MH, Smith RP, Baltch AL, Griffin PE, Conroy JV, Sutphen N, et al. Pharmacokinetics of moxalactam in elderly subjects. Antimicrob Agents Chemother. 1984;25(1):33–6. https://doi.org/10.1128/AAC.25.1.33.
70. Cho SJ, Stout-Delgado HW. Aging and lung disease. Annu Rev Physiol. 2020;82:433–59. https://doi.org/10.1146/annurev-physiol-021119-034610.
71. Paik J. Levodopa inhalation powder: A review in Parkinson's disease. Drugs. 2020;80(8):821–8. https://doi.org/10.1007/s40265-020-01307-x.
72. Lowery EM, Brubaker AL, Kuhlmann E, Kovacs EJ. The aging lung. Clin Interv Aging. 2013;8:1489–96. https://doi.org/10.2147/CIA.S51152.
73. Schneider JL, Rowe JH, Garcia-De-Alba C, Kim CF, Sharpe AH, Haigis MC. The aging lung: Physiology, disease, and immunity. Cell. 2021;184(8):1990–2019. https://doi.org/10.1016/j.cell.2021.03.005.
74. Nickalls RWD, Mapleson WW. Age-related iso-MAC charts for isofurane, sevofurane and desfurane in man. Br J Anaesth. 2003;91(2):170–4. https://doi.org/10.1093/bja/aeg132.

75. Waitt C, Waitt P, Pirmohamed M. Intravenous therapy. Postgrad Med J. 2004;80(939):1–6. https://doi.org/10.1136/pmj.2003.010421.
76. Moureau NL. Tips for inserting an i.v. in an older patient. Nursing. 2004;34(7):18. https://doi.org/10.1097/00152193-200407000-00017.
77. St-Onge MP, Gallagher D. Body composition changes with aging: the cause or the result of alterations in metabolic rate and macronutrient oxidation? Nutrition. 2010;26(2):152–5. https://doi.org/10.1016/j.nut.2009.07.004.
78. Guo SS, Zeller C, Chumlea WC, Siervogel RM. Aging, body composition, and lifestyle: the Fels Longitudinal Study. Am J Clin Nutr. 1999;70(3):405–11. https://doi.org/10.1093/ajcn/70.3.405.
79. Kitamura I, Koda M, Otsuka R, Ando F, Shimokata H. Six-year longitudinal changes in body composition of middle-aged and elderly Japanese: age and sex differences in appendicular skeletal muscle mass. Geriatr Gerontol Int. 2014;14(2):354–61. https://doi.org/10.1111/ggi.12109.
80. Kyle UG, Gremion G, Genton L, Slosman DO, Golay A, Pichard C. Physical activity and fat-free and fat mass by bioelectrical impedance in 3853 adults. Med Sci Sports Exerc. 2001;33(4):576–84. https://doi.org/10.1097/00005768-200104000-00011.
81. Grandison MK, Boudinot FD. Age-related changes in protein binding of drugs: implications for therapy. Clin Pharmacokinet. 2000;38(3):271–90. https://doi.org/10.2165/00003088-200038030-00005.
82. Cabrerizo S, Cuadras D, Gomez-Busto F, Artaza-Artabe I, Marin-Ciancas F, Malafarina V. Serum albumin and health in older people: Review and meta analysis. Maturitas. 2015;81(1):17–27. https://doi.org/10.1016/j.maturitas.2015.02.009.
83. Wallace SM, Verbeeck RK. Plasma protein binding of drugs in the elderly. Clin Pharmacokinet. 1987;12(1):41–72. https://doi.org/10.2165/00003088-198712010-00004.
84. McLachlan AJ, Pont LG. Drug metabolism in older people--a key consideration in achieving optimal outcomes with medicines. J Gerontol A Biol Sci Med Sci. 2012;67(2):175–80. https://doi.org/10.1093/gerona/glr118.
85. Wynne HA, Cope LH, Mutch E, Rawlins MD, Woodhouse KW, James OF. The effect of age upon liver volume and apparent liver blood flow in healthy man. Hepatology. 1989;9(2):297–301. https://doi.org/10.1002/hep.1840090222.
86. Wynne HA, Goudeveos J, Rawlins MD, James OF, Adams PC, Woodhouse KW. Hepatic drug clearance: the effect of age using indocyanine green as a model compound. Br J Clin Pharmacol. 1990;30(4):634–7. https://doi.org/10.1111/j.1365-2125.1990.tb03826.x.
87. Morsiani C, Bacalini MG, Santoro A, Garagnani P, Collura S, D'Errico A, et al. The peculiar aging of human liver: A geroscience perspective within transplant context. Ageing Res Rev. 2019;51:24–34. https://doi.org/10.1016/j.arr.2019.02.002.
88. Hunt NJ, Kang SWS, Lockwood GP, LeCouteur DG, Cogger VC. Hallmarks of aging in the liver. Comput Struct Biotechnol J. 2019;17:1151–61. https://doi.org/10.1016/j.csbj.2019.07.021.
89. Klotz U. Pharmacokinetics and drug metabolism in the elderly. Drug Metab Rev. 2009;41(2):67–76. https://doi.org/10.1080/03602530902722679.
90. Shi S, Klotz U. Age-related changes in pharmacokinetics. Curr Drug Metab. 2011;12(7):601–10. https://doi.org/10.2174/138920011796504527.
91. Butler JM, Begg EJ. Free drug metabolic clearance in elderly people. Clin Pharmacokinet. 2008;47(5):297–321. https://doi.org/10.2165/00003088-200847050-00002.
92. Sotaniemi EA, Arranto AJ, Pelkonen O, Pasanen M. Age and cytochrome P450-linked drug metabolism in humans: an analysis of 226 subjects with equal histopathologic conditions. Clin Pharmacol Ther. 1997;61(3):331–9. https://doi.org/10.1016/S0009-9236(97)90166-1.
93. Ginsberg G, Hattis D, Russ A, Sonawane B. Pharmacokinetic and pharmacodynamic factors that can affect sensitivity to neurotoxic sequelae in elderly individuals. Environ Health Perspect. 2005;113(9):1243–9. https://doi.org/10.1289/ehp.7568.

94. Polasek TM, Patel F, Jensen BP, Sorich MJ, Wiese MD, Doogue MP. Predicted metabolic drug clearance with increasing adult age. Br J Clin Pharmacol. 2013;75(4):1019–28. https://doi.org/10.1111/j.1365-2125.2012.04446.x.
95. Jensen BP, Chin PKL, Roberts RL, Begg EJ. Influence of adult age on the total and free clearance and protein binding of (R)- and (S)-warfarin. Br J Clin Pharmacol. 2012;74(5):797–805. https://doi.org/10.1111/j.1365-2125.2012.04259.x.
96. Greenblatt DJ, Abernethy DR, Locniskar A, Harmatz JS, Limjuco RA, Shader RI. Effect of age, gender, and obesity on midazolam kinetics. Anesthesiology. 1984;61(1):27–35. PMID: 6742481.
97. Abernethy DR, Greenblatt DJ, Shader RI. Imipramine and desipramine disposition in the elderly. J Pharmacol Exp Ther. 1985;232(1):183–8. PMID: 3965690.
98. Blanchard J, Sawers SJ. Comparative pharmacokinetics of caffeine in young and elderly men. J Pharmacokinet Biopharm. 1983;11(2):109–26. https://doi.org/10.1007/BF01061844.
99. Stader F, Marzolini C. Sex-related pharmacokinetic differences with aging. Eur Geriatr Med. 2022;13(3):559–65. https://doi.org/10.1007/s41999-021-00587-0.
100. Alikhani R, Pai MP. Reconsideration of the current models of estimated kidney function-based drug dose adjustment in older adults: The role of biological age. Clin Transl Sci. 2023;16:2095–105. https://doi.org/10.1111/cts.13643.
101. Gourtsoyiannis N, Prassopoulos P, Cavouras D, Pantelidis N. The thickness of the renal parenchyma decreases with age: a CT study of 360 patients AJR. Am J Roentgenol. 1990;155(3):541–4. https://doi.org/10.2214/ajr.155.3.2117353.
102. Griffiths GJ, Robinson KB, Cartwright GO, Mclachlan MS. Loss of renal tissue in the elderly. Br J Radiol. 1976;49(578):111–7. https://doi.org/10.1259/0007-1285-49-578-111.
103. Denic A, Glassock RJ, Rule AD. Structural and functional changes with the aging kidney. Adv Chronic Kidney Dis. 2016;23(1):19–28. https://doi.org/10.1053/j.ackd.2015.08.004.
104. Kaplan C, Pasternack B, Shah H, Gallo G. Age-related incidence of sclerotic glomeruli in human kidneys. Am J Pathol. 1975;80(2):227–34. PMID: 51591.
105. Roseman DA, Hwang S-J, Oyama-Manabe N, Chuang ML, O'Donnell CJ, Manning WJ, et al. Clinical associations of total kidney volume: the Framingham Heart Study. Nephrol Dial Transplant. 2017;32:1344–50. https://doi.org/10.1093/ndt/gfw237.
106. Bolignano D, Mattace-Raso F, Sijbrands EJG, Zoccali C. The aging kidney revisited: A systematic review. Ageing Res Rev. 2014;14:65–80. https://doi.org/10.1016/j.arr.2014.02.003.
107. Wetzels JFM, Kiemeney LALM, Swinkels DW, Willems HL, den Heijer M. Age- and gender-specific reference values of estimated GFR in Caucasians: the Nijmegen Biomedical Study. Kidney Int. 2007;72(5):632–7. https://doi.org/10.1038/sj.ki.5002374.
108. Lauretani F, Semba RD, Bandinelli S, Miller ER 3rd, Ruggiero C, Cherubini A, et al. Plasma polyunsaturated fatty acids and the decline of renal function. Clin Chem. 2008;54:475–81. https://doi.org/10.1373/clinchem.2007.095521.
109. Lindeman RD, Tobin J, Shock NW. Longitudinal studies on the rate of decline in renal function with age. J Am Geriatr Soc. 1985;33(4):278–85. https://doi.org/10.1111/j.1532-5415.1985.tb07117.x.
110. Davies DF, Shock NW. Age changes in glomerular filtration rate, effective renal plasma flow, and tubular excretory capacity in adult males. J Clin Invest. 1950;29(5):496–507. https://doi.org/10.1172/JCI102286.
111. Fliser D, Franek E, Joest M, Block S, Mutschler E, Ritz E. Renal function in the elderly: Impact of hypertension and cardiac function. Kidney Int. 1997;51(4):1196–204. https://doi.org/10.1038/ki.1997.163.
112. Suchy-Dicey AM, Laha T, Hoofnagle A, Newitt R, Sirich TL, Meyer TW, et al. Tubular secretion in CKD. J Am Soc Nephrol. 2016;27(7):2148–55. https://doi.org/10.1681/ASN.2014121193.
113. Lin K, Kong X, Tao X, Zhai X, Lv L, Dong D. Research methods and new advances in drug-drug interactions mediated by renal transporters. Molecules. 2023;28(13):5252. https://doi.org/10.3390/molecules28135252.

114. Joseph S, Nicolson TJ, Hammons G, Word B, Green-Knox B, Lyn-Cook B, et al. Expression of drug transporters in human kidney: impact of sex, age, and ethnicity. Biol Sex Differ. 2015;6:4. https://doi.org/10.1186/s13293-015-0020-3.
115. Syrovatkina V, Alegre KO, Dey R, Huang X-Y. Regulation, signaling, and physiological functions of G-proteins. J Mol Biol. 2016;428(19):3850–68. https://doi.org/10.1016/j.jmb.2016.08.002.
116. Fu Q, Xiang YK. Trafficking of β-adrenergic receptors: Implications in intracellular receptor signaling. Prog Mol Biol Transl Sci. 2015;132:151–88. https://doi.org/10.1016/bs.pmbts.2015.03.008.
117. Nakao S, Yanagisawa K, Ueyama T, Hasegawa K, Kawamura T. Eur Cardiol. 2021;16:e58. https://doi.org/10.15420/ecr.2021.16.PO2.
118. Lymperopoulos A, Rengo G, Koch WJ. Adrenergic nervous system in heart failure: pathophysiology and therapy. Circ Res. 2013;113(6):739–53. https://doi.org/10.1161/CIRCRESAHA.113.300308.
119. Pan R, Zhu X, Maretich P, Chen Y. Combating obesity with thermogenic fat: Current challenges and advancements. Front Endocrinol (Lausanne). 2020;11:185. https://doi.org/10.3389/fendo.2020.00185.
120. Stratton JR, Cerqueira MD, Schwartz RS, Levy WC, Veith RC, Kahn SE, et al. Differences in cardiovascular responses to isoproterenol in relation to age and exercise training in healthy men. Circulation. 1992;86(2):504–12. https://doi.org/10.1161/01.cir.86.2.504.
121. Turner MJ, Mier CM, Spina RJ, Schechtman KB, Ehsani AA. Effects of age and gender on the cardiovascular responses to isoproterenol. J Gerontol A Biol Sci Med Sci. 1999;54(9):B393–400. https://doi.org/10.1093/gerona/54.9.b393.
122. White M, Roden R, Minobe W, Khan MF, Larrabee P, Wollmering M, et al. Age-related changes in beta-adrenergic neuroeffector systems in the human heart. Circulation. 1994;90(3):1225–38. https://doi.org/10.1161/01.cir.90.3.1225.
123. Ross AJ, Gao Z, Pollck JP, Leuenberger UA, Sinoway LI, Muller D. β-Adrenergic receptor blockade impairs coronary exercise hyperemia in young men but not older men. Am J Physiol Heart Circ Physiol. 2014;307(10):H1497–503. https://doi.org/10.1152/ajpheart.00584.2014.
124. Howlett LA, Lancaster MK. Reduced cardiac response to the adrenergic system is a key limiting factor for physical capacity in old age. Exp Gerontol. 2021;150:111339. https://doi.org/10.1016/j.exger.2021.111339.
125. Santulli G, Iaccarino G. Adrenergic signaling in heart failure and cardiovascular aging. Maturitas. 2016;93:65–72. https://doi.org/10.1016/j.maturitas.2016.03.022.
126. Mahmood A, Ahmed K, Zhang Y. β-adrenergic receptor desensitization/down-regulation in heart failure: A friend or foe? Front Cardiovasc Med. 2022;9:925692. https://doi.org/10.3389/fcvm.2022.925692.
127. Harvey RE, Ranadive SM, Limberg JK, Baker SE, Nicholson WT, Curry B, et al. Forearm vasodilatation to a β2-adrenergic receptor agonist in premenopausal and postmenopausal women. Exp Physiol. 2020;105(5):886–92. https://doi.org/10.1113/EP088452.
128. Ford GA, Hoffman BB, Vestal RE, Blaschke TF. Age-related changes in adenosine and -adrenoceptor responsiveness of vascular smooth muscle in man. Br J Clin Pharmacol. 1992;33(1):83–7. https://doi.org/10.1111/j.1365-2125.1992.tb04004.x.
129. Matera MG, Rinaldi B, Calzetta L, Rogliani P, Cazzola M. Advances in adrenergic receptors for the treatment of chronic obstructive pulmonary disease: 2023 update. Expert Opin Pharmacother. 2023;13:1–10. https://doi.org/10.1080/14656566.2023.2282673.
130. Connolly MJ, Crowley JJ, Charan NB, Nielson CP, Vestal RE. Impaired bronchodilator response to albuterol in healthy elderly men and women. Chest. 1995;108(2):401–6. https://doi.org/10.1378/chest.108.2.401.
131. Banerji A, Clark S, Afilalo M, Blanda MP, Cydulka RK, Camargo CA Jr. Prospective multicenter study of acute asthma in younger versus older adults presenting to the emergency department. J Am Geriatr Soc. 2006;54(1):48–55. https://doi.org/10.1111/j.1532-5415.2005.00563.x.

132. Reed CE. Asthma in the elderly: diagnosis and management. J Allergy Clin Immunol. 2010;126(4):681–7; quiz 688–9. https://doi.org/10.1016/j.jaci.2010.05.035.
133. Stern Y, Barnes CA, Grady C, Jones RN, Raz N. Brain reserve, cognitive reserve, compensation, and maintenance: operationalization, validity, and mechanisms of cognitive resilience. Neurobiol Aging. 2019;83:124–9. https://doi.org/10.1016/j.neurobiolaging.2019.03.022.
134. Nyberg L, Lovden M, Riklund K, Lindenberger U, Blackman L. Memory aging and brain maintenance. Trends Cogn Sci. 2012;16(5):292–305. https://doi.org/10.1016/j.tics.2012.04.005.
135. Trifiro G, Spina E. Age-related changes in pharmacodynamics: focus on drugs acting on central nervous and cardiovascular systems. Curr Drug Metab. 2011;12(7):611–20. https://doi.org/10.2174/138920011796504473.
136. Terunuma M. Diversity of structure and function of $GABA_B$ receptors: a complexity of $GABA_B$-mediated signaling. Proc Jpn Acad Ser B Phys Biol Sci. 2018;94(10):390–411. https://doi.org/10.2183/pjab.94.026.
137. Rozycka A, Liguz-Lecznar M. The space where aging acts: focus on the GABAergic synapse. Aging Cell. 2017;16(4):634–43. https://doi.org/10.1111/acel.12605.
138. Olsen RW. $GABA_A$ receptor: Positive and negative allosteric modulators. Neuropharmacology. 2018;136(Pt A):10–22. https://doi.org/10.1016/j.neuropharm.2018.01.036.
139. Goldschen-Ohm MP. Benzodiazepine modulation of $GABA_A$ receptors: a mechanistic perspective. Biomolecules. 2022;12(12):1784. https://doi.org/10.3390/biom12121784.
140. Evenseth LSM, Gabrielsen M, Sylte I. The $GABA_B$ receptor-structure, ligand binding and drug development. Molecules. 2020;25(13):3093. https://doi.org/10.3390/molecules25133093.
141. Lenz M, Tegenthoff M, Kohlhaas K, Stude P, Hoffken O, Tossi MAG, et al. Increased excitability of somatosensory cortex in aged humans is associated with impaired tactile acuity. J Neurosci. 2012;32:1811–6. https://doi.org/10.1523/JNEUROSCI.2722-11.2012.
142. Heise K-F, Zimerman M, Hoppe J, Gerloff C, Wegscheider K, Hummel FC. The aging motor system as a model for plastic changes of GABA-mediated intracortical inhibition and their behavioral relevance. J Neurosci. 2013;33(21):9039–49. https://doi.org/10.1523/JNEUROSCI.4094-12.2013.
143. Shen W, Nan C, Nelson PT, Ripps H, Slaughter MM. $GABA_B$ receptor attenuation of $GABA_A$ currents in neurons of the mammalian central nervous system. Physiol Rep. 2017;5(6):e13129. https://doi.org/10.14814/phy2.13129.
144. Habrian C, Latorraca N, Fu Z, Isacoff EY. Homo- and hetero-dimeric subunit interactions set affinity and efficacy in metabotropic glutamate receptors. Nat Commun. 2023;14(1):8288. https://doi.org/10.1038/s41467-023-44013-4.
145. Niswender CM, Conn PJ. Metabotropic glutamate receptors: Physiology, pharmacology, and disease. Annu Rev Pharmacol Toxicol. 2010;50:295–322. https://doi.org/10.1146/annurev.pharmtox.011008.145533.
146. de Oliveira PG, Ramos MLS, Amaro AJ, Dias RA, Vieira SI. Gi/o-protein coupled receptors in the aging brain. Front Aging Neurosci. 2019;11:89. https://doi.org/10.3389/fnagi.2019.00089.
147. Gautam D, Naik UP, Naik MU, Yadav SK, Chauasia RN, Dash D. Glutamate receptor dysregulation and platelet glutamate dynamics in Alzheimer's and Parkinson's diseases: Insights into current medications. Biomolecules. 2023;13(11):1609. https://doi.org/10.3390/biom13111609.
148. Kim KM. Unveiling the differences in signaling and regulatory mechanisms between Dopamine D(2) and D(3) receptors and their impact on behavioral sensitization. Int J Mol Sci. 2023;24(7):6742. https://doi.org/10.3390/ijms24076742.
149. Taylor WD, Zald DH, Felger JC, Christman S, Claassen DO, Horga G, et al. Influences of dopaminergic system dysfunction on late-life depression. Mol Psychiatry. 2022;27(1):180–91. https://doi.org/10.1038/s41380-021-01265-0.
150. Rudow G, O'Brian R, Savonenko AV, Resnick SM, Zonderman AB, Pletnikova O, et al. Morphometry of the human substantia nigra in ageing and Parkinson's disease. Acta Neuropathol. 2008;115(4):461–70. https://doi.org/10.1007/s00401-008-0352-8.

151. Yang YK, Chiu NT, Chen CC, Chen M, Yeh TL, Lee IH. Correlation between fine motor activity and striatal dopamine D2 receptor density in patients with schizophrenia and healthy controls. Psychiatry Res. 2003;123(3):191–7. https://doi.org/10.1016/s0925-4927(03)00066-0.
152. Van Dyck CH, Avery RA, MacAvoy MG, Marek KL, Quinlaan DM. Baldwin RM et al Striatal dopamine transporters correlate with simple reaction time in elderly subjects. Neurobiol Aging. 2008;29(8):1237–46. https://doi.org/10.1016/j.neurobiolaging.2007.02.012.
153. Wong KK, Muller MLTM, Kuwabara H, Studenski SA, Bohen NI. Olfactory loss and nigrostriatal dopaminergic denervation in the elderly. Neurosci Lett. 2010;484(3):163–7. https://doi.org/10.1016/j.neulet.2010.08.037.
154. Cham R, Perera S, Studenski SA, Bohnen HI. Striatal dopamine denervation and sensory integration for balance in middle-aged and older adults. Gait Posture. 2007;26(4):516–25. https://doi.org/10.1016/j.gaitpost.2006.11.204.
155. Siafis S, Wu H, Wang D, Burschinski A, Nomura N, Takeuchi H, et al. Antipsychotic dose, dopamine D2 receptor occupancy and extrapyramidal side-effects: a systematic review and dose-response meta-analysis. Mol Psychiatry. 2023;28(8):3267–3277. https://doi.org/10.1038/s41380-023-02203-y.
156. Brown DA. Acetylcholine and cholinergic receptors. Brain Neurosci Adv. 2019;3:2398212818820506. https://doi.org/10.1177/2398212818820506.
157. Thomsen M, Sorensen G, Dencker D. Physiological roles of CNS muscarinic receptors gained from knockout mice. Neuropharmacology. 2018;136(Pt C):411–20. https://doi.org/10.1016/j.neuropharm.2017.09.011.
158. Davis SE, Cirincione AB, Jimenez-Torres AC, Chu J. The impact of neurotransmitters on the neurobiology of neurodegenerative diseases. Int J Mol Sci. 2023;24(20):15340. https://doi.org/10.3390/ijms242015340.
159. Dumas JA, Newhouse PA. The cholinergic hypothesis of cognitive aging revisited again: cholinergic functional compensation. Pharmacol Biochem Behav. 2011;99(2):254–61. https://doi.org/10.1016/j.pbb.2011.02.022.
160. Richter N, Allendorf I, Onur OA, Kract L, Dietlein M, Tittgemeyer M, et al. The integrity of the cholinergic system determines memory performance in healthy elderly. NeuroImage. 2014;100:481–8. https://doi.org/10.1016/j.neuroimage.2014.06.031.
161. Migirov A, Datta AR. Physiology, anticholinergic reaction. In: StatPearls [Internet]. Treasure Island: StatPearls Publishing; 2023.
162. Khastgir J. Antimuscarinic drug therapy for overactive bladder syndrome in the elderly - are the concerns justified? Expert Opin Pharmacother. 2019;20(7):813–20. https://doi.org/10.1080/14656566.2019.1574749.
163. Gray SL, Hanlon JT. Anticholinergic medication use and dementia: latest evidence and clinical implications. Ther Adv Drug Saf. 2016;7(5):217–24. https://doi.org/10.1177/2042098616658399.
164. Mitroshina EV, Marasanova EA, Vedunova MV. Functional dimerization of serotonin receptors: Role in health and depressive disorders. Int J Mol Sci. 2023;24(22):16416. https://doi.org/10.3390/ijms242216416.
165. Pytliak M, Vargova V, Mechirova V, Felsoci M. Serotonin receptors - from molecular biology to clinical applications. Physiol Res. 2011;60(1):15–25. https://doi.org/10.33549/physiolres.931903.
166. Meltzer CC, Drevets WC, Price JC, Mathis CA, Lopresti B, Greer PJ, et al. Gender-specific aging effects on the serotonin 1A receptor. Brain Res. 2001;895(1–2):9–17. https://doi.org/10.1016/s0006-8993(00)03211-x.
167. Matuskey D, Pittman B, Planeta-Wilson B, Walderhaug E, Henry S, et al. Age effects on serotonin receptor 1B as assessed by PET. J Nucl Med. 2012;53:1411–4. https://doi.org/10.2967/jnumed.112.103598.

168. Gonzalez-Maeso J, Torre I, Rodríguez-Puertas R, García-Sevilla JA, Guimón J, Meana JJ. Effects of age, postmortem delay and storage time on receptor-mediated activation of G-proteins in human brain. Neuropsychopharmacology. 26:468–78. https://doi.org/10.1016/S0893-133X(01)00342-6.
169. Edinoff AN, Akuly HA, Hanna TA, Ochoa CO, Patti SJ, Ghaffar YA, et al. Selective serotonin reuptake inhibitors and adverse effects: A narrative review. Neurol Int. 2021;13(3):387–401. https://doi.org/10.3390/neurolint13030038.
170. Joseph A, Wanono R, Flamant M, Vidal-Petiot E. Orthostatic hypotension: A review. Nephrol Ther. 2017;13(Suppl 1):S55–67. https://doi.org/10.1016/j.nephro.2017.01.003.
171. Saedon NI, Tan MP, Frith J. The prevalence of orthostatic hypotension: A systematic review and meta-analysis. J Gerontol A Biol Sci Med Sci. 2020;75(1):117–22. https://doi.org/10.1093/gerona/gly188.
172. Shin C, Abbott RD, Lee H, Kim J, Kimm K. Prevalence and correlates of orthostatic hypotension in middle-aged men and women in Korea: the Korean Health and Genome Study. Hypertension. 2004;18(10):717–23. https://doi.org/10.1038/sj.jhh.1001732.
173. Low PA, Tomalia VA. Othrostatic hypotension: mechanisms, causes, management. J Clin Neurol. 2015;11(3):220–6. https://doi.org/10.3988/jcn.2015.11.3.220.
174. Rivasi G, Ungar A. Orthostatic hypotension in older adults: the role of medications. Monaldi Arch Chest Dis. 2020;90(4) https://doi.org/10.4081/monaldi.2020.1254.
175. Dani M, Dirksen A, Taraborrelli P, Panagopolous D, Torocastro M, Sutton R, et al. Orthostatic hypotension in older people: considerations, diagnosis and management. Clin Med (Lond). 2021;21(3):e275–82. https://doi.org/10.7861/clinmed.2020-1044.
176. Francesco A, Marina A, Ciuseppina B, Ernesto C, Alfredo C. Cough, a vital reflex. Mechanisms, determinants and measurements. Acta Biomed. 2018;89(4):477–80. https://doi.org/10.23750/abm.v89i4.6182.
177. Ebihara S, Sekiya H, Miyagi M, Ebihara T, Okazaki T. Dysphagia, dystussia, and aspiration pneumonia in elderly people. J Thorac Dis. 2016;8(3):632–9. https://doi.org/10.21037/jtd.2016.02.60.
178. Belli S, Prince I, Savio G, Paracchini E, Cattaneo D, Bianchi M, et al. Airway clearance techniques: the right choice for the right patient. Front Med (Lausanne). 2021;s:544826. https://doi.org/10.3389/fmed.2021.544826.
179. Pontoppidan H, Beecher HK. Progressive loss of protective reflexes in the airway with the advance of age. JAMA. 1960;174:2209–13. https://doi.org/10.1001/jama.1960.03030180029007.
180. Erskine RJ, Murphy PJ, Langton JA, Smith G. Effect of age on the sensitivity of upper airway reflexes. Br J Anaesth. 1993;70(5):574–5. https://doi.org/10.1093/bja/70.5.574.

Adverse Drug Reactions 3

Abbreviations

ACEI	angiotensin-converting enzyme inhibitor
ADEs	adverse drug events
ADRs	adverse drug reactions
ARB	angiotensin receptor blocker
ARNI	angiotensin receptor neprilysin inhibitor
BCRP	breast cancer resistance protein
CNS	central nervous system
CVD	cardiovascular disease
CYP	cytochrome P450 enzymes
DAAs	direct acting antiviral drugs
DDIs	drug–drug interactions
DOACs	direct oral anticoagulants
GFR	glomerular filtration rate
GI	gastrointestinal
HRT	hormone replacement therapy
MATE1, MATE2	multidrug and toxic compound extrusion transporters
MRP2	multidrug resistance protein 2
NSAIDs	nonsteroidal anti-inflammatory drugs
OAT1, OAT2	organic anion transporters
OCT2	organic cation transporters
OTC	over-the-counter
PD	pharmacodynamics

P-gp	P-glycoprotein
PIMs	potential inappropriate medications
PK	pharmacokinetics
PXR	pregnane X receptor
QoL	quality of life
RXR	retinoid X receptor
SNRIs	selective serotonin/norepinephrine reuptake inhibitors
SSRIs	selective serotonin reuptake inhibitors
TCAs	tricyclic antidepressants
TKIs	tyrosine kinase inhibitors

INTRODUCTION *The prime goal of pharmacological therapy is the amelioration of the destructive effect(s) of a disease or geriatric syndrome without unnecessary harm to the patient.* When prescribed judiciously, most drugs achieve this goal, and the use of medications continues as a successful approach to disease management. However, for the older adult, many factors converge on the pharmacology of a drug to produce less-than-optimal outcomes. Significant factors are (1) age-dependent changes in pharmacokinetics (PK)/pharmacodynamics (PD), (2) multimorbidities, (3) polypharmacy, (4) frailty, (5) genetics, and (6) environmental influences [1]. These factors produce undesired, unnecessary, and potentially avoidable reactions, termed adverse drug reactions (ADRs) [1–3].

This chapter will discuss the many facets of ADRs: what constitutes an ADR, major causes of ADRs such as polypharmacy/potentially inappropriate medications (PIMs), the path to avoidance for prescribers (Beers Criteria®), and deprescribing strategies. The goal is to describe the key reasons that create susceptibility to ADRs and to provide understanding to facilitate prevention in the future. The narrative is supplemented in Tables 3.1, 3.2, 3.3, and 3.4.

Adverse Drug Reactions (ADRs)

Adverse Drug Reactions. Definitions ADRs are unwanted drug reactions ranging in degree from unpleasant to harmful to lethal [4]. ADRs are unintentional outcomes to a therapeutic medication [5]. ADRs "may be expected or unexpected, and may occur at dosages used for the prophylaxis, diagnosis, or therapy of disease, or for modifying physiological function" [3]. Deliberate poisonings or overdosing are not considered ADRs. ADRs require special attention and treatment and necessitate a clear indication of future drug avoidance or reduction in dose or change in treatment [6]. ADRs range from minor to fatal reactions. ADRs are costly both with regard to financial health care expenses and quality of life (QoL) of the older adult [7]. Table 3.1 displays common ADRs from mild to severe.

Table 3.1 Examples of reported adverse drug reactions

Mild
Cutaneous hypersensitivity—skin rash, pruritus
GI disturbances—upsets, dyspepsia, nausea, altered taste, diarrhea
Abnormal liver function tests
Dizziness, mild headache, palpitations
Moderate
Anticholinergic effects—dry mouth, urinary retention, constipation
GI gastric/duodenal ulcers—increased risk of bleeding
Orthostatic hypotension
Skeletal muscle pain
Infections—Urinary, pulmonary
Hypoglycemia
Sedation
Sexual dysfunction
Thrombophlebitis—Superficial
Ototoxicity—Reversible
Fatigue
Severe
Life-threatening anaphylaxis
Cutaneous hypersensitivity—Stevens Johnson syndrome/toxic epidermal necrolysis[a]
Extrapyramidal side effects such as akathisia, dyskinesias, and parkinsonian-like syndromes[b]
Increased risk of a major bleeding episode
Thrombophlebitis—Deep vein
Liver, lung, or kidney toxicities
Decreased cognition, enhanced dementia/delirium
Hyponatremia, hyperkalemia
Adverse cardiovascular events—Stroke, myocardial ischemia, hypotension, angina
GI, prostate, breast malignancies
Seizures
Death

[a]Line et al. [152]
[b]Messiha [153]

Side effects "refer to pharmacological effects of drugs beyond the purpose of treatment that occur after the standard dose of the drug is taken" [8]. Unacceptable side effects of drugs are essentially ADRs and may result from super-pharmacological doses, therapeutic effects but off-target, nontherapeutic effects but off-target, and multiple effects of all aforementioned [9]. However, since no drug has a single action, all drugs can be expected to have side effects, albeit over a range of minor and acceptable to major and unacceptable effects.

Another important term is adverse drug events (ADEs), loosely defined as "harmful and unintended consequences of medications" [10]. In one sense, ADE is the umbrella term, whereas ADR is a subset member. However, ADE is often used interchangeably with ADR because a specific consensus definition for ADE does not exist. A systematic review of pharmacovigilance international reporting systems uncovered an extensive number of definitions varying in scope from classification and severity of ADE to timelines and management [10]. There was a "lack of standardization between systems" that hinders advancement in pharmacovigilance [10]. Hence, ADR is the better term for this chapter.

Adverse Drug Reactions. Classifications Over the years, attempts to organize ADRs have resulted in several classification schemes. The division of ADRs into two subcategories, "augmented-bizarre" or Type A and Type B, was one of the first [11]. Type A included reactions that occurred due to dose (quantitatively)-enhanced effect of a drug's basic effect (qualitatively) where a high dose produces toxicities. Type A ADRs are influenced by changes in pharmacokinetics, especially reduced kidney function that decreases drug elimination, causing an elevation in the drug level, and pharmacodynamic changes that affect end-organ responsiveness. An example of Type A ADRs is the expected side effect of a drug as evident at higher doses with many drugs (e.g., antihistamines, antipsychotics, antidepressants, antispasmodics, antimuscarinics) that produce anticholinergic activity (dry mouth, skin flushing, constipation, urinary retention, blurred vision, tachycardia, sedation, confusion). See Table 3.4 for drugs with anticholinergic effects [12].

The majority of ADRs (~80%) are dose- and time-related [3]. The remainder are dose-independent, unpredictable, and immune-related [13, 14]. These "Type B reactions," also called drug hypersensitivity reactions, are costly worldwide in terms of morbidity, mortality, and health care costs [15]. Common examples are (a) Immunoglobulin E-mediated, rapid onset of "urticaria (hives), anaphylaxis, and bronchospasm" and (b) delayed hypersensitivity due to activated T-lymphocytes combined with human leukocyte antigen alleles [15]. Immune-mediated ADRs may arise by direct stimulation of a drug at the T-cell receptor or by a drug or its metabolite binding to a protein to induce immunogenicity in a traditional manner. However, where known, prior screening for susceptible alleles is a path to prevention of hypersensitivity and other ADR reactions [16].

Adverse Drug Reactions. Prevalence It is important to assess the prevalence (frequency) of ADRs because ADRs cause a significant number of unscheduled hospital admissions as well as additional problems during the hospital stay and after discharge [6]. Although many ADRs are not serious systemic events, they, nevertheless, impact health care costs, associated morbidity/mortality, and the prescriber–patient relationship [6].

It is difficult, if not impossible, to assign a prevalence or percentage of occurrence for ADRs. This is because many factors influence the rate of ADRs. The main ones are (a) just how an ADR is defined, detected, and reported, (b) the nature of the population under review, and (c) location of the study [3]. Thus, the frequency of occurrence depends on the method of ADR identification, population, and study location. The majority of available studies relate to hospitalized patients rather than to primary care patients because of the constant monitoring and clear evidence of drug use present in a hospital setting. The frequency of ADRs is the highest in long-term care facilities (18.5–82.6%) [17, 18], followed by hospital-related ADRs (4.6–30%) [19–24], then primary care at 4–25% [25–27]. The class of drugs most commonly responsible for ADRs varied with the population under study but drugs classified as cardiovascular (cardiac glycosides, warfarin, diuretics) and antianxiety drugs (benzodiazepines) were most commonly responsible for ADRs in these studies [17, 23, 27, 28].

Of all the confounding issues influencing the frequency of ADRs, assessment of causality is of prime importance. Many methods have been proposed to validate causality with the goal of optimizing pharmacovigilance. There are basically three assessment measures [29]. They are (a) global introspection exemplified by the World Health Organization-Uppsala Monitoring Center (WHO-UMC) [30] method that seeks the likely relation in a clinical setting, i.e., expert judgment, (b) algorithms exemplified by the Naranjo algorithm [31] that is question-based and score-enhanced to reduce bias, and c) probabilistic methods that rely on principles of statistics and probability [32]. Generally, agreement between and among these methods is poor [33, 34].

Adverse Drug Reactions. Initiating Factors There are numerous reasons why the older adult experiences an unacceptably high occurrence of ADRs (see Fig. 3.1). ADRs result from age changes that` affect pharmacokinetics (PK) and pharmacodynamics (PD), various chronic diseases requiring individualized pharmacological therapies, inappropriate therapies for frailty syndromes, polypharmacy (generally defined as the use of more than five medications) (see below), the use of potentially inappropriate medications (PIMs), patient noncompliance, and lack of clinician/patient education and other factors, e.g., drug abuse and over-the-counter (OTC) drug and herbal remedy use (see Fig. 3.1).

PK and PD changes significantly influenced by age are discussed in Chap. 2 and will be briefly reviewed here. Interactions of disease/geriatric syndromes and drug PK and PD to produce ADRs are described in Chaps. 4, 5, 6, and 7 devoted to drug use in specific age-related diseases/syndromes. Drug abuse and OTC drug/dietary

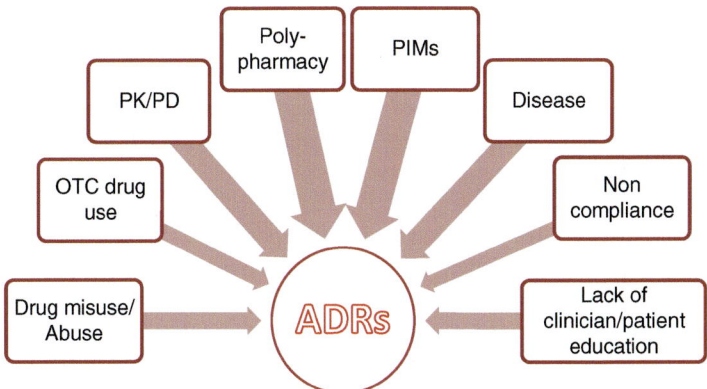

Fig. 3.1 Causes of Adverse Drug Reactions (ADRs) in the older adult
PIMs potentially inapprorpriate medications; *PK/PD* Pharmacokinetics/Pharmacodynamics; *OTC* over-the-counter

supplement use are featured in Chaps. 8 and 9, respectively. Polypharmacy, PIMs (Beers' criteria), and clinician/patient-related issues are discussed below.

Adverse Drug Reactions. Pharmacokinetics/Pharmacodynamics/Aging Age-related changes affect all aspects of PK (absorption, distribution, metabolism, and excretion) and PD. However, the most clinically relevant age change that contributes in a major way to ADRs is a reduction in kidney function, also emphasized in Beers Criteria® [12]. The kidneys handle drugs via processes of glomerular filtration, tubular secretion, and tubular reabsorption. It is, therefore, essential that kidney function in the older adult be assessed prior to drug and dose prescribing. This remains a challenge since standard biomarkers of kidney function, serum creatinine and cystatin C, are incompatible with accurate determination of kidney function in the older adult [35]. Creatinine, a metabolic by-product produced by active skeletal muscles, is filtered unchanged by the kidneys, and hence serum values of creatinine are used to determine estimated glomerular filtration rate (eGFR). It is an estimate to be used cautiously. In the older adult, due to age-associated loss of muscle mass, reduced physical activity, and frailty, creatinine output declines and hence no longer accurately reflects eGFR. Furthermore, renal tubules also actively secrete a portion of the creatinine concentration and a variety of drugs, e.g., fenofibrate, tyrosine kinase inhibitors (TKIs), antiviral drugs, block tubular secretion, and when present, negate the validity of serum creatinine as a biomarker of kidney function [36].

Serum cystatin C, a protein biomarker of kidney function, is a substitute for serum creatinine since it is less affected by age and muscle mass. However, cystatin C assay suffers from other issues, e.g., standardization, cost, interference from steroids, systemic inflammation, and thyroid dysfunction [36].

Serum creatinine is still widely used despite serious issues discussed above. "The most widely used kidney function equation for drug dosing is the Cockcroft-Gault (CG) equation" [35]. It calculates creatinine clearance taking chronological age, weight, and sex into account. Whereas it has successfully measured the decline in kidney function from 40 to 80 years of age in diverse populations, accuracy of kidney function on an individual basis is achievable only with substitution of biological age for chronological age [35].

Adverse Drug Reactions. Effects of Diseases/Geriatric Syndrome The effects of disease and geriatric syndromes on the development of ADRs are discussed in Chaps. 4, 5, 6, and 7.

Adverse Drug Reactions. Polypharmacy Polypharmacy, a major cause of ADRs, sadly has no consensus definition. In fact, there are over 143 different definitions of polypharmacy [37]. A reasonable definition of polypharmacy is an "increase in the number of medications or the use of more medications than are medically necessary" [38]. Another reasonable definition is having multiple health providers prescribing medications, regardless of the number of medications [39]. Frequently, a quantitative, albeit arbitrary, definition of five or more medications daily is used [37]. Medications include not only prescription drugs but also OTC drugs and dietary supplements (including herbal remedies). Often, information on OTC drugs and dietary supplements is absent, compounding understanding of ADRs.

Polypharmacy. Prevalence Lack of agreement on a definition of polypharmacy impedes comparison of different studies on the prevalence of polypharmacy among older adults. Accordingly, "prevalence ranges from 4% among community-dwelling older people to over 96.5% in hospitalized patients" [37]. Thus, polypharmacy differs in different settings [38]. Specifically, approximately 30% of community-dwelling elderly (75–85 years) used five or more drugs, and nearly half took one or more OTC or dietary supplements [40]. More recent data found that the prevalence of polypharmacy (five or more drugs) (NHANES survey) in 60–79-year-olds to be 34.5% [41]. However, the avoidance of polypharmacy in ambulatory care is often unrealistic, especially in the presence of two or more diseases [38].

In hospital settings described in different studies, polypharmacy is between 40 and 50% on discharge and admissions, respectively [38]. In a British 8-month retrospective study, patients (mean age of 77 years) were discharged from the hospital with 9.3 prescriptions, and polypharmacy was significantly associated with potential inappropriate medications (PIMs) and omissions [42]. Additionally, in an analysis of patients with heart failure (Medicare beneficiaries 2003–2014), polypharmacy was the norm with 84% on admission and 95% on discharge taking five or more medications [43].

In long-term care facilities/nursing homes across the United States, findings from a retrospective, cross-sectional study of over 13,000 residents found the prevalence of polypharmacy (≥ 9 drugs) to be 40% in 2004 [44]. A National Nurses Home Survey (on-site record review by experts) of 1000 facilities (2004–2005, mean age 85) indicated that half of residents received six or more drugs and 30% received nine or more drugs. Polypharmacy was positively related to the number of diagnoses [45]. Prevalence of polypharmacy in a smaller review study of nursing home residents taking nine or more drugs was 46.2% [46].

Polypharmacy is the foremost risk factor for ADRs [47]. The reason for this is largely twofold: drug–drug interactions (DDIs) and potential inappropriate medications (PIMs). These issues are discussed in the following sections.

Trends in rising polypharmacy among older adults have been reported [48–50] and are expected as the population ages [51]. As polypharmacy increases, so do ADRs, but this relationship is complex and frequently inconsistent, except in certain settings, e.g., hospitals and inappropriate prescribing [52]. In those situations, according to Davies et al. (2020) [52], a reduction of polypharmacy would clearly reduce ADRs.

Alert: There are numerous reasons why the older adult experiences an unacceptably high occurrence of adverse drug reactions. Polypharmacy is the highest risk factor.

Adverse Drug Reactions. Drug–Drug Interactions The potential for two or more drugs to interact beneficially or adversely within the realm of PK and/or PD is high and inevitable [53]. The interaction of the active chemical entity of one drug with another may result in a response ranging from a stronger effect (potentiation), no effect, or loss of efficacy [54]. A stronger effect is sometimes needed, for example, when two chemotherapeutic drugs are combined to produce additive effects culminating in tumor cell death, hindrance of future metastases, and prevention of drug resistance [55]. This is a desired outcome. Alternatively, a stronger-than-expected effect may produce an undesired outcome, hence an ADR as detailed below. A loss of efficacy is equally problematic, allowing the persistence of a worsening medical issue. For every five drugs, one drug–drug interaction (DDI) can be expected as determined by a mathematical study that cross-referenced electronic medical records with databases of DDIs [56]. Furthermore, DDIs increase in proportion to the number of drugs used [56]. DDIs also arise when the same drug with different brand names is consumed. This is a frequent occurrence when a patient is cared for by multiple specialty physicians, unaware of medications prescribed by the other.

DDIs may be PK-dependent or PD-dependent or both. Unfavorable drug interactions can occur during any process of PK—absorption, distribution, metabolism (biotransformation), and excretion—as well as during PD at receptors and downstream events. Drug interactions at either the PK or PD level generally take the form of (1) antagonism (inhibition), (2) additive effects (sum of two drug effects), or (3) synergy (enhancement of expected efficacy) [54]. In the majority of cases, the outcome is undesirable.

Adverse Drug Reactions. Pharmacokinetic-Dependent Drug–Drug Interactions The underpinnings of PK-DDIs begin with the nuclear receptor, pregnane X receptor (PXR). Many chemical entities, whether medications (xenobiotics) or environmental chemicals (endobiotics), bind to PXR [57]. The ligand-bound PXR combines with the second nuclear receptor (retinoid X receptor, RXR) to induce transcription of a plethora of genes involved in drug PK [58]. Gene products are the numerous transporters that regulate the absorption, distribution, and excretion of drugs and the cytochrome P450 enzymes (CYP) that metabolize drugs. Therefore, one important mechanism of DDIs results from the translational increase or decrease of transporters and metabolic enzymes by one drug, thereby affecting the transport or metabolism of another drug.

Drug–Drug Interactions and Transporters Beginning with absorption following oral consumption, PK-dependent DDIs occur at the level of the intestinal efflux transports, ATP-binding cassette transporters, e.g., P-glycoprotein (P-gp, ABCB1), the multidrug resistance protein 2 (MRP2), and the breast cancer resistance protein (BCRP) [59]. Most is known about the former. Intestinal efflux transporters restrict drug absorption by directing the drug back into the intestine. Some drugs act as PXR ligands to increase (inducers) or reduce (inhibitors) P-gp function. Also, many drugs are substrates of P-gp.

Adverse Drug Reactions (ADRs)

Reduction of P-gp, for example, by one drug will permit unhindered absorption of a second drug normally a substrate transported by P-gp. This DDI results in a higher drug concentration and hence greater exposure of the second drug. If this concentration exceeds the therapeutic level, unwanted effects can be expected. Alternatively, drug-induced enhancement of P-gp decreases the exposure of a second transport-dependent drug and produces a less-than-optimal effect or no effect at all. Thus, it is essential to know which drugs are substrates, inducers, or inhibitors of transporters to avoid DDIs (see Table 3.2 [60]).

Interactions of drugs at intestinal transporters are numerous. Specifically, the combination of digoxin with the macrolide clarithromycin produces greater exposure of digoxin [61] and intoxication [62] due to the inhibition of P-gp by clarithromycin in the gastrointestinal (GI) tract. Similarly, the coadministration of dronedarone, an anti-arrhythmic drug, and strong P-gp inhibitor, coadministered with dabigatran, a direct oral anticoagulant (DOAC) increases blood levels of dabigatran and elevates the risk of a major bleeding episode [63]. Other P-gp inhibitors of moderate strength (amiodarone, quinidine, and verapamil) may also increase the risk of bleeding when combined with dabigatran and other DOACs (rivaroxaban,

Table 3.2 Drugs interacting with intestinal P-gp transporter[a]

Substrates
Opioids—loperamide, morphine
Antihypertensives—aliskiren, carvedilol
Anticoagulants—dabigatran, **rivaroxaban, apixaban, and edoxaban**
Cardiac glycosides—digoxin
Immunosuppressants—cyclosporin, tacrolimus, sirolimus
Protease inhibitors—indinavir, saquinavir
Statins—atorvastatin, lovastatin, simvastatin
Antineoplastic agents—paclitaxel, anthracyclines, vinca alkaloids, etoposide, imatinib
Inducers
Anticonvulsants—carbamazepine (oxcarbazepine less so), phenytoin, phenobarbital, primidone
Tuberculostatics—rifampin (e.g., rifampin decreases exposure of DOACs → risks of clots)
Antiretroviral—efavirenz
St. John's wort extract—hyperforin
Inhibitors
Antimycotics—itraconazole, ketoconazole
Calcium channel blockers—diltiazem, felodipine, nicardipine, nifedipine, verapamil
Macrolide antibiotics—erythromycin, clarithromycin, not azithromycin (e.g., clarithromycin increases digoxin exposure → toxicities)
HIV protease inhibitors—indinavir, nelfinavir, ritonavir, saquinavir
Immunosuppressants—cyclosporin
Anti-arrhythmic drugs—amiodarone, quinidine, propafenone, **dronedarone** (e.g., dronedarone increases exposure **of** dabigatran→↑ bleeding risk)
DOACs—direct oral anticoagulants, → leads to, ↑ increases

Drug in bold are new additions
[a]Revised with permission from Cascorbi (2012) [60]

apixaban, and edoxaban) [63]. On the other hand, coadministration of the antimicrobial, rifampin, with DOAC decreases exposure of DOACs since rifampin is a strong inducer of P-gp, potentially permissive for clot formation [63]. Concomitant use of St. John's Wort (SJW), a dietary supplement in the United States used for depression, lowered the concentration of the immunosuppressant, cyclosporine, resulting in several reports of liver and heart transplant rejections [64]. The active component of SJW is hyperforin, a strong inducer of P-gp (and additionally cytochrome P450 enzymes) (see below) accounting for the reduced absorption and subsequent increased metabolism of cyclosporine [64]. Ritonavir, an antiviral drug combined with nirmatrelvir, a protease inhibitor, has been successful in the therapy of COVID-19 in high-risk patients [65]. Since many patients with COVID-19 are taking other drugs such as DOACs for atrial fibrillation or venous thromboembolism, there exists potential for excess bleeding with concomitant use of ritonavir and DOACs [63]. Thus, PK-dependent DDI effects can dramatically transform efficacy to a serious outcome or negate efficacy altogether.

The kidneys are the site of drug elimination. This process requires contribution from glomerular filtration, tubular secretion, and tubular reabsorption. Among these, tubular secretion is the main process perturbed by multiple drugs that cause unwanted DDIs [66]. Tubular activities are regulated by charge-selective transporters: organic cation transporters (OCT2) and organic anion transporters (OAT1, OAT3) located on the basolateral membrane (outward-facing the blood vessels) and multidrug and toxic compound extrusion transporters (MATE1 and MATE2) on the brush border membrane (inward) [66]. Drugs that affect renal tubular secretory transporters have a major impact on the PK of a second drug and, additionally, have the potential to cause nephrotoxicity [66].

Inhibitors of OCT2, MATE1, and MATE2 transporters are cimetidine (H_2 antagonist for acid reduction), pyrimethamine (antiparasitic), and dolutegravir (HIV integrase inhibitor). Consequently, renal elimination of substrates by these transporters, such as metformin, is reduced and drug levels remain elevated [67–69]. Additionally, serum creatinine (biomarker for kidney function, see above) is a substrate of these transporters. Thus, creatinine will be elevated in the presence of inhibitors, providing an inaccurate value of kidney function [70].

Probenecid (increases uric acid excretion) is a potent inhibitor of the organic anion transporters OAT1/3, and as such, coadministration with furosemide (diuretic), cidofovir (antiviral), or fexofenadine (antihistamine) reduces their elimination and increases their exposure [70]. One positive effect of combining probenecid with, for example, antibiotics such as penicillin, is to prolong the effect of the latter, a rapidly secreted drug. Probenecid is currently of interest to increase the bioavailability of drugs used to treat central nervous system diseases [71].

Drug–Drug Interactions. Liver Enzyme Metabolism DDIs may occur during drug metabolism, primarily in the liver but also elsewhere, as in the intestine [54]. The cytochrome P450 enzymes (CYPs) are responsible for metabolizing drugs to a more water-soluble metabolite that is readily excreted by the kidneys. DDIs occur in several ways: (1) translational-induction, that is, drugs act as ligands for the PXR to increase/decrease the concentration of a CYP enzyme and/or (2) more commonly, competition at the CYP enzyme itself [72]. Although the CYP family of enzymes is large, three families, CYP1, 2, and 3, are responsible for metabolism of more than three quarters of all drugs [72]. Among these three families, the isoforms CYP3A4 and CYP2D6 handle half of all drug metabolism [72] as shown in Table 3.3.

Table 3.3 Prominent cytochrome P450 enzymes and their substrates, inhibitors, and inducers[a]

CYP1A2	CYP2C9	CYP2C19	CYP2D6	CYP3A4/5		CYP2C8
Antidepressants	*NSAIDs*	*Proton pump inhibitors*	*Beta-blockers*	*Macrolide antibiotics*	*Miscellaneous*	*Anticancer*
Imipramine	Celecoxib	Omeprazole	Metoprolol	Clarithromycin	Aripiprazole	Imatinib
Duloxetine	Diclofenac	Lansoprazole	Propafenone	Erythromycin	Buspirone	Paclitaxel
Fluvoxamine	Ibuprofen	Pantoprazole	Timolol	Telithromycin	Quinidine	Dasabuvir
Mirtazapine.	Naproxen[b]	Rabeprazole	*Anti-arrhythmics*	*Benzodiazepines*	Quinine	Enzalutamide
Atypical antipsychotic	Piroxicam	*Antidepressants*	Encainide	Alprazolam	Ethinylestradiol	*Antidiabetic*
Olanzapine	*Antidiabetics*	Amitriptyline	Flecainide	Diazepam	Imatinib	Pioglitazone
Clozapine	Glipizide	Clomipramine	Perhexiline	Midazolam	Sildenafil	Repaglinide,
Anti-arrhythmic	Tolbutamide	Citalopram	Propafenone	Triazolam	Tamoxifen	Rosiglitazone
Mexiletine	*Angiotensin receptor blockers*	Escitalopram	Sparteine	Brotizolam	Vincristine	*Miscellaneous*
Miscellaneous	Irbesartan	Imipramine	*Antidepressants*	Partially quazepam,	ivacaftor	Loperamide
Naproxen	Losartan	Moclobemide	Amitriptyline	diazepam,	*Tyrosine kinase inhibitors*[c]	Montelukast
Phenacetin	*Miscellaneous*	Sertraline	Clomipramine	flunitrazepam		Amodiaquine
Tacrine	Cyclophosphamide	*Anti-seizure*	Desipramine	*Calcium channel blockers*	*Inhibitors*	Cerivastatin
Ciprofloxacin	Fluvastatin	Phenytoin	Duloxetine	Amlodipine	Ketoconazole	*Inhibitors*
Theophylline	Phenytoin	Phenobarbitone	Imipramine	Diltiazem	Itraconazole	Clopidogrel
Caffeine,	Sulfamethoxazole	S-mephenytoin	Paroxetine	Felodipine	*Inducers*	Gemfibrozil
Propranolol	Torasemide	hexobarbital	Venlafaxine	Nifedipine	Phenobarbital	Trimethoprim
R-warfarin	S-Warfarin	*Miscellaneous*	Fluvoxamine	Nisoldipine	Phenytoin	*Inducer*
Inhibitor	Fluoxetine	Proguanil	Nortriptyline	Nitrendipine	Rifampicin	Rifampicin
Simeprevir	Torsemide	Clopidogrel	Mianserin	Verapamil	St. John's Wort	
Inducers	*Inducers*	Cyclophosphamide	*Antipsychotics*	*Immunosuppressants*	Glucocorticoids.	
Rifampicin	Rifampicin	*Antianxiety*	Aripiprazole	Ciclosporin	Enzalutamide	
Omeprazole	Enzalutamide	Diazepam	Haloperidol	Tacrolimus	Lumacaftor	
		Carisoprodol	Risperidone	Sirolimus		
		Inducer	Thioridazine	*HIV protease inhibitors*		
		Rifampicin	Perphenazine	Indinavir		
			Thioridazine	Ritonavir		
			Zuclopenthixol	Saquinavir		
			Opioids	*Statins*		
			Codeine	Atorvastatin		
			Dextromethorphan	Lovastatin		
			Tramadol	Simvastatin		
			Miscellaneous	*Anticoagulants*		
			Ondansetron	Apixaban		
			Tamoxifen	Rivaroxaban		
			Phenformin	Phenprocoumon		
			Debrisoquine			
			Tolterodine			
			Debrisoquine			

[a]modified from Cascorbi (2012) [60]; [b]major metabolic pathway; [c]Pathway for 41/43 tyrosine kinase inhibitors; Additional references: Backman et al. [154], Bolleddula et al. [83], FDA drug interactions [155]

Information is available for most drugs as to the requisite metabolizing CYP enzyme isoform [73]. Metabolism of two drugs by the same CYP isoform leads to metabolism of one drug and increased exposure (no or little metabolism) of the second drug. For example, the combination of glyburide (a sulfonylurea antidiabetic drug) used with co-trimoxazole (broad-spectrum antibiotic of trimethoprim and sulfamethoxazole) results in hypoglycemia and hospitalization. This is because the antibiotics inhibit CYP2C9, the same isoform used to metabolize sulfonylureas, thereby increasing drug levels of glyburide and enhancing its glucose-lowering effect [74]. Similarly, as noted by Beers Criteria® (2023 update) [12], phenytoin (antiseizure) toxicity occurs in the presence of co-trimoxazole that results from competition between phenytoin and sulfamethoxazole at CYP2C9 [75]. This combination should be avoided. Others to avoid are coadministration of theophylline, an antiasthma drug with cimetidine, antacid, or ciprofloxacin, an antibiotic, due to CYP competition resulting in increased exposure of theophylline and subsequent toxicity [12]. This also applies to avoidable DDIs with warfarin, an anticoagulant, and amiodarone, an anti-arrhythmic, due to amiodarone's inhibition of CYP2C9, an enzyme needed to metabolize warfarin. Coadministration results in the potential for excessive bleeding [12].

Exposure of direct-acting antiviral drugs (DAA), e.g., dasabuvir, developed for the treatment of hepatitis C virus is greatly increased with strong inhibitors of CYP2C8 (clopidogrel, gemfibrozil), the enzymes that metabolize dasabuvir [76]. Clopidogrel, an antiplatelet drug, strongly inhibits CYP2C8, and hence its coadministration with dasabuvir is contraindicated [76, 77]. Generally, DAAs are given in combination, and since they are both substrates and inhibitors of several CYPs as well as transporters, numerous DDIs (with proton pump inhibitors, antidepressants, benzodiazepines, and statins) have been reported [78, 79].

The antiviral protease inhibitor, ritonavir, is the most potent inhibitor of CYP3A4 [80]. It is frequently used at a low dose to boost the bioavailability of other drugs that are rapidly metabolized by CYP3A4. This is the case with the combination of lopinavir-ritonavir, to treat HIV and more recently used successfully for the treatment of SARS-CoV-2 infections [81, 82]. However, "Ritonavir-boosted therapy leads to several important DDIs with cardiac medications" and should not be used with "ranolazine, dronedarone, colchicine, simvastatin, and sildenafil" [82]. This is because of ritonavir inhibition of CYP3A4 in addition to inhibition of CYP2D6 and induction of CYP2B6, CYP2C19, CYP2C9, and CYP1A2 [82]. One study, in particular, showed that coadministration of ritonavir with clopidogrel significantly decreases the efficacy of clopidogrel, creating a clotting risk [77]. The metabolic enzyme, CYP3A4, that converts clopidogrel (a prodrug) to its active metabolite is inhibited by ritonavir [77].

Rifampin, an antibiotic mainly used for tuberculosis, if coadministered with other drugs, should be done so with caution. Rifampin is a potent translational inducer of CYP3A4 and CYP2C19 and a moderate inducer of CYP1A2, CYP2B6, CYP2C8, and CYP2C9 [83], a potent inducer of intestinal/hepatic P-gp transporters

[84] and an inhibitor of the hepatic uptake transporters, organic anion-transporting polypeptides (OATP1B1/3) [85]. The multitude of PK affected by rifampin complicates the predictability of DDIs when coadministered with other drugs such as anticancer drugs that are metabolized by CYP 3A4 enzymes [86] and substrates of OATP-1B1/3 [87].

A review of studies assessing coadministration of anticancer tyrosine kinase inhibitors (TKIs) with other drugs emphasized the potential for serious consequences of hepatotoxicity and anticoagulation irregularities [86]. Regarding metabolism, most TKIs are metabolized by CYP3A4 enzymes, such that strong inducers (rifampin, carbamazepine, ritonavir) and inhibitors (ketoconazole, itraconazole) affect TKI exposure and efficacy [86].

Adverse Drug Reactions. Pharmacodynamic-Dependent Drug–Drug Interactions Similar to PK-dependent DDIs, PD-dependent DDIs are classified as additive, synergistic, or antagonistic and may occur at the same target site, or unlike PK-DDIs, through different downstream pathways yielding similar biological endpoints [88]. Additionally, DDIs may arise as side effects or target effects in nonspecific tissues. An additive effect is generated when two or more drugs given simultaneously produce an effect that equals the sum of each when given alone. For example, if drug 1 reduces blood pressure by 5 mm Hg and drug 2 reduces blood pressure by the same amount, given together an additive effect would be a fall of 10 mm Hg. A synergistic effect of several drugs, sometimes termed potentiation, exceeds that expected by adding the effects of each drug individually. In the example above, if blood pressure fell 15 mm Hg with coadministration of drugs 1 and 2, this would be a synergistic effect. Synergism is of considerable interest in the treatment of microbial diseases (e.g., tuberculosis) since synergism allows for dose reduction of individual drugs, thereby decreasing unwanted side effects and the potential risk of resistance [89]. Antagonism is the reduction or inhibition of the effect of one drug by another. However, these terms are more precisely applied to defined drug-receptor effects observed in vitro and ex vivo [88]. Unlike PK, these effects occur in the presence of unaltered plasma levels of each drug.

The Beers Criteria®: Guide to Potential Inappropriate Medication (PIM) The Beers Criteria® [12], a proven and comprehensive guide to PIMs for the older adult (see details below), emphasizes specific additive effects that should be avoided. In particular, according to the Beers Criteria®, combining an opioid with a non-opioid, e.g., gabapentin, produces dangerous sedation, possible respiratory depression and death; use of opioids and benzodiazepines is a recipe for sedation and death. Other examples of additive effects that should be avoided are the use of two anticholinergic drugs (see Table 3.4) that add together to diminish cognition, enhance delirium, and promote falls, fractures, and hospitalizations. Other additive combinations that result in increased risk of falls and fractures are the use of three or more drugs characterized as antiseizure, antipsychotics, antidepressants, opioids, skeletal muscle relaxants, benzodiazepines, and non-benzodiazepines [12]. Additionally, two drugs, each with the same potential for an adverse effect, when combined, elevate the risk for that effect. An example is the coadministration of a nonspecific peripheral alpha 1 inhibitor with oral or transdermal estrogen use, each alone causing some degree of urinary incontinence and combined producing a significantly elevated risk of urinary incontinence in women [90]. Antimicrobial drugs, such as the fluoroquinolones and macrolides, have the potential to produce abnormal heart rhythms, primarily QT interval prolongation (time between ventricular contraction and relaxation), but also torsades de pointes (TdP), ventricular tachycardia, and sudden cardiac death [91]. Coadministration of drugs from these two classes is to be avoided [60].

Assessing downstream adverse events, e.g., anticoagulation, hyperkalemia (elevation in potassium in the blood), and hypotension, is challenging, and PD-DDIs are actually infrequently assessed in clinical situations [88]. One commonly reported PD-DDI is the combination of an angiotensin-converting enzyme inhibitor (ACEI), e.g., enalapril, and a potassium-sparing diuretic, e.g., spironolactone, that results in hyperkalemia especially manifest in the presence of reduced kidney function, heart failure, diabetes, and risk of dehydration [92, 93]. The potassium-sparing diuretics interfere with sodium/potassium exchange in the renal tubule, such that sodium is excreted and potassium is reabsorbed. An ACEI exacerbates this because it increases potassium levels by blocking the effect of aldosterone on sodium/potassium exchange [94]. Similarly, the antibiotic combination, trimethoprim–sulfamethoxazole, is potassium-sparing and should not be used with an ACEI [75]. Also, the combination of lithium, an antimanic drug, and any one of the numerous renin-angiotensin-aldosterone (RAAS) inhibitors, e.g., ACEI, angiotensin receptor blocker (ARB), and angiotensin receptor neprilysin inhibitor (ARNI), produces lithium toxicity due to the alteration of lithium excretion by RAAS inhibitors [12].

More recently, a noted example of PD-DDI is the combination of monoclonal antibodies with DOACs. Monoclonal antibodies increase the risk of bleeding especially alemtuzumab (anti-CD52, used to treat multiple sclerosis). If coadministered with DOCAs, there is an increased risk of bleeding [63]. Other anticancer monoclonals, e.g., bevacizumab (anti-VEGF), caplacizumab (anti-vWF), ipilimumab (anti-CTLA4), and ramucirumab (anti-VEGFR2), are to be used with caution as they too can influence anticoagulation [63].

The nonsteroidal anti-inflammatory drugs (NSAIDs), although beneficial as anti-inflammatory and analgesic/antipyretic drugs, present a risk when used with many other drugs. Some NSAIDs such as ibuprofen and naproxen are available at low doses (OTC) and higher doses (prescription). Diclofenac, ketorolac, and celecoxib (COX-2 inhibitor) are prescription only NSAIDs. DDIs are largely dependent on dose and duration [95]. A case series analysis of over 100,000 patients with upper gastrointestinal (GI) bleeding reported that coadministration of NSAIDs or low-dose aspirin with selective serotonin reuptake inhibitor (SSRIs), corticosteroids, aldosterone antagonists, or anticoagulants significantly elevated the risk of GI bleeding [96].

The GI bleeding propensity of NSAIDs is related to their mechanism of action, in which NSAIDs inhibit the enzymatic activity of constitutive (always present) and inducible cyclooxygenases (COX) [97, 98]. Cyclooxygenases produce lipid mediators, prostaglandins such as thromboxane A2, and prostacyclin that generally prevent platelet aggregation [97, 98]. Drugs that also produce anticoagulation effects such as DOACs, warfarin, aspirin, and SSRIs produce an additive effect on GI bleeding when combined with NSAIDS [98]. Alternatively, the risk of possible bleeding with warfarin is greatly enhanced in the presence of other drugs that affect platelet aggregation (SSRIs) or kill vitamin K-producing bacteria (macrolides, trimethoprim-sulfamethoxazole) [12].

A small elevation of blood pressure has been noted with simultaneous use of NSAIDs and thiazide diuretics and antihypertensive drugs (ACEI ARB), explained by an additive effect on renal fluid retention [99]. Greater use of NSAIDs is predicted in the future [100]. NSAIDs are now considered important suppressors of inflammation. NSAIDs inhibit mediators of inflammation, e.g., nuclear factor-κB and activate anti-inflammatory mediators, e.g., peroxisome proliferator-activated receptor gamma, and are positioned to enhance anticancer therapies and treat CNS disorders [100]. As the use of NSAIDs increases, previous understanding of NSAID-dependent DDIs should help to prevent future DDIs.

GENERAL ISSUES FOR DRUG–DRUG INTERACTIONS Prior to prescribing, it is reasonable for physicians to ascertain the potential interaction(s) between or among drugs. DDIs are avoidable, yet they continue to occur. In the assessment of DDIs, many investigators lament the lack of methods to standardize DDIs [93, 101]. Better agreement among the available evidence-based databases, e.g., Micromedex, Lexicomp, and others, is needed [102]. A call for "appropriate mechanistic, pathophysiological system models" to assist with understanding and preventing DDI, especially PD-dependent DDI, has been proposed [101]. One such system model is the quantitative systems pharmacology model (QSPM) that with the help of mathematical modeling, "can integrate and recapitulate the fundamental interactions in biological systems, simulate drug activity as perturbations of those systems, and evaluate drug effects within the context of the properties of the system" [101]. Unlike PD, information on PK-DDIs with regard to metabolism and transporters is required by the FDA for drug approval [103]. Additionally, although hurdles remain, pharmacogenetics offers the opportunity to identify genetic variants of metabolic enzymes and transporters, thereby assisting in the selection of appropriate drugs and avoidance of ADRs [104].

Potential Inappropriate Medications (PIMs) Although reduction of polypharmacy reduces ADRs, decreasing polypharmacy may not be feasible in cases where drugs have benefits that outweigh the risks. A successful means to reduce polypharmacy, DDIs, ADRs and improve clinical outcomes for patients is deprescribing [105]. Part of this strategy requires identification of potentially inappropriate medications (PIMs) [106, 107].

The Beers Criteria® and Its Guidance The Beers Criteria® is one of the best guides to identify PIMs [12]. Beers Criteria® is derived from rigorous scientific analyses to identify PIMs for the older adult (≥65 years of age) in "ambulatory, acute, institutionalize settings of care but not hospice or end of life" [12]. Beers Criteria® (2023) is the seventh update of PIMs, originated in 1991 by Dr. Mark Beers to identify those medications used in nursing homes that were injurious and hence inappropriate. Subsequent Beers Criteria® expanded beyond nursing homes, as noted above. The goal of Beers Criteria® is to provide an "explicit list of potentially inappropriate medications" to be avoided in most circumstances [12]. As emphasized repeatedly by Beers' panel of experts, the list of PIMs is to be used as important supportive and insightful information for clinicians and patients in the "clinical decision-making" process [12]. The ultimate outcome is a reduction in ADRs, improved quality of life, and better use of health care expenditures for the older adult.

To develop the most recent PIM list, the expert panel performed a systematic review (2017–2022) on drugs, drug classes, ADRs, and ADE and assessed the data using the American College Physician approach [108] and a grade-based approach [109]. The former designated evidence as high (well-designed/implemented randomized clinical trials, RCT), moderate (RCTs with limitations), or low-quality (observational study) evidence. The grade-based assessment reviewed the data according to five factors that included risk of bias, inconsistency, indirectness, imprecision, and publication bias. Recommendations for each criterion were strong or weak based on several factors: quality of evidence, frequency and severity of ADR, and its relation to possible benefit.

Beers Criteria® is expansive and covers medications identified as PIMs to be avoided, PIMs relevant in diseases, PIMs to be used with caution, PIM as DDIs, and PIMs requiring dosage change [12].

Drugs with Anticholinergic Effects According to the Beers Criteria®, important PIMs are the antihistamines, e.g., brompheniramine; chlorpheniramine, cyproheptadine, triprolidine, hydroxyzine, and others considered first generation, due to their strong anticholinergic effects. Anticholinergic effects (blockade of the acetylcholine cholinergic receptors) are undesirable in older adults because their effects are widespread and adverse, as noted above. To repeat, anticholinergic effects are dry mouth, constipation, urinary retention, bowel obstruction, dilated pupils, blurred vision, increased heart rate, and decreased sweating. Concomitant use of multiple drugs with anticholinergic effects (see Table 3.4) leads to confusion, delirium, and severe cognitive decline, creating an elevated risk for accidents and falls [110–113]. Some drugs with anticholinergic effects are prescribed for potentially beneficial antimuscarinic activity (as in overactive bladder), but a wider range of drugs are prescribed for other reasons (depression, psychosis) but come with anticholinergic side effects. Only in acute allergic reactions, however, is the antihistamine, diphenhydramine considered a reasonable choice [12].

Table 3.4 Drugs with strong anticholinergic effects[a]

Antidepressants	Amitriptyline Amoxapine Clomipramine Desipramine Doxepin	Imipramine Nortriptyline Paroxetine Protriptyline Trimipramine
Antiemetics	Prochlorperazine Promethazine	
Antihistamines (first generation)	Brompheniramine Chlorpheniramine Clemastine Cyproheptadine Dexchlorpheniramine Diphenhydramine	Doxylamine Dimenhydrinate Hydroxyzine Meclizine Phenindamine Triprolidine
Antimuscarinic	Darifenacin Fesoterodine Flavoxate Oxybutynin	Solifenacin Tolterodine Trospium
Antiparkinsonian agents	Benztropine Trihexyphenidyl	
Antipsychotics	Chlorpromazine Clozapine Loxapine Olanzapine	Perphenazine Thioridazine Trifluoperazine
Antispasmodics	Atropine Clidinium-chlordiazepoxide Dicyclomine Homatropine Hyoscyamine Scopolamine	
Skeletal muscle relaxants	Cyclobenzaprine Methocarbamol Orphenadrine	
Anti-arrhythmics	Disopyramide	

[a]Revised from AGS 2023 Beers' Criteria® update, with permission

Anticoagulant Drugs Regarding anticoagulants, Beers Criteria® recommends prescribing direct oral anticoagulants (DOAC) rather than warfarin for prevention of clots in non-valvular atrial fibrillation and venous thromboembolism. The latter carries a greater risk of cranial bleeding. The exception to this recommendation applies to patients who have successful long-term experience with warfarin without adverse effects and with expected international normalized ratio (INR) clotting time 70% of the time. Although DOACs are safer than warfarin, not all DOACs provide the same benefit/risk profile. Rivaroxaban should be avoided due to its high potential for major bleeding; among the other DOAC, apixaban is a better choice than dabigatran. The latter should be used with caution due to the potential for major bleeding. In all cases, dose consideration and kidney function assessment are essential prior to treatment [12].

Inhibition of P2Y12 ADP receptors on platelets is a novel means to block activation/aggregation of platelets. However, members of this class, prasugrel (irreversible inhibitor) and ticagrelor (reversible inhibitor), are to be used with caution as they promote bleeding.

> *Alert*: The Beers Criteria® recommends prescribing direct oral anticoagulants rather than warfarin due to the risk of cranial bleeding.

Low-Dose Aspirin Low-dose aspirin has been used for years as a primary and secondary prevention of cardiovascular disease (CVD) [114]. However, a reassessment of aspirin's benefit/risk profile revised this former view. According to conclusions from an extensive systemic review and micro-simulation modeling by the US Preventive Services Task Force, the use of low-dose aspirin for primary prevention of adverse events stemming from cardiovascular disease (myocardial infarction, stroke, mortality) offers no benefit [115]. The Beers Criteria® suggests that due to the risk of GI bleeding and lack of CVD prevention benefit, deprescribing is reasonable, although use of low-dose aspirin for secondary prevention in patients with CVD remains a beneficial addition [116].

Antihypertensive Drugs In the antihypertensive class, dipyridamole (phosphodiesterase inhibitor), doxazosin (nonselective alpha 1 blocker), clonidine (centrally acting agonist), and nifedipine (calcium channel blocker) are to be avoided as these drugs promote orthostatic hypotension, adverse CNS effects (clonidine) and hypotension (nifedipine). Orthostatic hypotension is a major cause of dizziness and subsequent falls [117]. Better antihypertensive drugs are available.

Anti-arrhythmic Drugs The Beers Criteria® recommends that there are better choices for therapy of atrial fibrillation than amiodarone, dronedarone, and digoxin. Amiodarone is a potential inducer of serious pulmonary toxicities [118] and its use is only recommended for rhythm control in heart failure and ventricular hypertrophy. Dronedarone, a derivative of amiodarone, is to be avoided in cases of permanent atrial fibrillation or severe decompensated heart failure since it is associated with increased mortality and hospitalizations [119]. Digoxin has a narrow therapeutic window requiring careful dosing and kidney function assessment. It is not the best drug for heart failure with reduced ejection fraction.

Centrally Acting Drugs Among the centrally acting drugs, Beers Criteria® recommends avoidance of antidepressants with strong anticholinergic activity (e.g., amitriptyline; desipramine and antiparkinson disease drug, benztropine) (also see Table 3.4). Amitriptyline and desipramine are also sedating and produce orthostatic hypotension; benztropine is inappropriate for treatment of Parkinson's Disease as well as the extrapyramidal side effects (abnormal muscle contractions) of antipsychotics.

The antipsychotic drugs, whether typical or atypical, pose serious harm of increased risk of stroke and accelerated decline in dementia [120]. They are to be avoided in psychotic episodes in delirium and dementia and only used in conditions of defined schizophrenia, bipolar, Parkinson's Disease psychosis, and as an adjunct to major depression. Furthermore, the first line of treatment for neuropsychiatric symptoms of dementia should be non-pharmacological [121].

Select sedatives/hypnotics should be avoided since they produce dependence (phenobarbital) and addiction (benzodiazepines, e.g., midazolam, diazepam, and non-benzodiazepine z-drugs, e.g., zolpidem and similar acting, meprobamate). These drugs also have potential for misuse and abuse. Exceptions for benzodiazepine use include as treatment for seizures, severe anxiety, and perioperative procedures.

Antidepressants of major classes, e.g., selective serotonin reuptake inhibitors (SSRIs), selective serotonin/norepinephrine reuptake inhibitors (SNRIs), and tricyclic antidepressants (TCAs) should be used with caution because they cause water retention-induced hyponatremia (low level of sodium in blood). Similar effects may occur with antiseizure drugs, oxcarbazepine and carbamazepine, thiazide diuretics, and antipsychotics [122].

Hormone Therapies PIMs among specific hormone therapies include testosterone, estrogen (with and without progesterone), insulin, desiccated thyroid, and progestin (megestrol). Hormone replacement therapy (HRT) to restore in part of the age-related loss of testosterone (in men) and estrogen (in women) is controversial [123–126]. Testosterone is the drug of choice for validated hypogonadism but long-term use raises the risk of cardiovascular adverse events [127, 128] and possibly prostate cancer, which remains unsubstantiated [129].

Results of three large clinical trials (Estrogen replacement and atherosclerosis study, Heart and estrogen/progestin replacement study, Women's health initiative) showed that HRT of estrogen (with and without progesterone) did not prevent CVD and increased the incidence of thromboembolic events, coronary heart disease, stroke, and pulmonary embolism [123, 130, 131]. However, administration of estrogen 12 years postmenopause is considered a flaw in the design of these clinical trials and HRT to women in the perimenopausal and early menopause phase produces no adverse effects [126]. On the other hand, long-term use of estrogen is associated with an increased risk of breast cancer [132, 133]. The Beers Criteria® suggests the use of vaginal estrogens for treatment of atrophy-related symptoms or genitourinary syndrome of menopause, e.g., dryness, painful urination, painful intercourse, recurrent urinary tract infections [134].

Other hormones of concern are short- or rapid-acting insulins, which produce a high risk of hypoglycemia; desiccated thyroid with potential cardiac effects and for which better drugs are available; megestrol with potential for clotting and little efficacy to treat weight loss and growth hormone with minimal positive effects on body composition but many negative effects (increase in fasting glucose level, headache, tinnitus (ringing in the ears), and benign intracranial hypertension) [135–137].

Anti-Inflammatory Drugs As discussed above, NSAIDs, and non-NSAIDs, e.g., aspirin, interfere with clotting mechanisms, thereby increasing the risk of bleeding. Coadministration enhances this risk as does combination with corticosteroids (glucocorticoid) and is significantly associated with the induction of peptic ulcer bleeding [138].

Proton Pump Inhibitors Several adverse effects have been associated with long-term use of proton pump inhibitors. These ADRs are the risk of osteoporosis-related fractures, intestinal *Clostridium difficile* infection, poor absorption of vitamins and minerals, pneumonia, kidney disease, and gastric cancer [139]. The Beers Criteria® recommends avoidance. Another GI-related drug, metoclopramide (antiemetic), may cause tardive dyskinesia (involuntary muscle movements) and should be used only for one indication, gastroparesis (chronic disease with impaired gastric emptying and reduced intestinal motility) [140].

Other Drugs Other drugs, desmopressin (antidiuretic associated with hyponatremia), atropine (antispasmodic with anticholinergic effects), and meperidine (narcotic analgesic), have little efficacy and should be avoided. Adverse effects of hypoglycemia, cardiac events, and all-cause mortality are associated with sulfonylureas and should be avoided, especially long-acting sulfonylureas, e.g., glyburide. The sodium-glucose co-transporter 2 inhibitor, canagliflozin, used in the treatment of diabetes, is associated with the risk of urinary tract infections and diabetic ketoacidosis [141] and should be used with caution.

Antibiotics Nitrofurantoin, an antibiotic used to treat urinary tract infections, has the potential to cause toxicity involving liver, lungs, and kidneys in the older adult with reduced kidney function (creatinine clearance <30 ml/min). It should be avoided. Trimethoprim–sulfamethoxazole combination also used to treat urinary tract infections poses a risk of hyperkalemia when used with drugs blocking the renin-angiotensin system, e.g., ACEI as noted above. Beers Criteria® recommends this antibiotic combo to be used with caution by dose reduction or avoidance with creatinine clearance <15 ml/min. Ciprofloxacin carries the risks of central nervous system toxicities and requires care in dosage with reduced kidney function.

Reduced Kidney Function. Issues Several antithrombotic drugs, enoxaparin (low molecular weight heparin), fondaparinux (synthetic heparin/factor Xa inhibitor), edoxaban (direct oral anticoagulant), and rivaroxaban (factor Xa inhibitor) are to be avoided in the presence of reduced kidney function. These drugs are either not efficacious (edoxaban) or cause bleeding. Similarly, depressed kidney function increases the risk of hyperkalemia with diuretics, amiloride, triamterene, and spironolactone and should be avoided. Other drugs to avoid with diminished kidney function include baclofen (skeletal muscle relaxant), duloxetine (antidepressant), gabapentin/pregabalin (anti-seizure), cimetidine and histamine H_2 receptor blockers, colchicine and probenecid (antigout), tramadol (opioid), NSAIDS, and dofetilide (anti-arrhythmic). If not, CNS adverse effects (baclofen, gabapentin/pregabalin, tramadol), QTc prolongation (rate of ventricular contraction and relaxation corrected for heart rate) and torsades de pointes (dofetilide), or other toxicities, GI, kidney (NSAIDs, colchicine) are to be expected.

Beers Criteria® has also identified PIMs of drugs interacting with disease. These will be discussed in related chapters on drug use in disease.

OTHER GUIDES TO APPROPRIATE MEDICATION PRESCRIBING A European guide designated STOPP (Screening Tool of Older Persons' potentially inappropriate Prescriptions)/START (Screening Tool to Alert doctors to Right Treatment) was developed in 2008 after the earlier acceptance of the Beers Criteria® in 1991. The aim of STOPP/START is to provide an "explicit list of potentially inappropriate medications and potential prescribing omissions aimed at optimizing medication and minimizing adverse drug reactions and events during medication review in older people, particularly those with multi-morbidity and polypharmacy" [142]. The STOPP criteria relate to deprescribing PIMs, and the START criteria relate to potentially prescribing omissions, something not addressed in the Beers Criteria®.

Deprescribing/prescribing tools may be explicit or implicit. The Beers Criteria® and STOPP/START are explicit lists of PIMs because they are developed with rigorous standards to facilitate rapid decision-making yet without consideration of patient issues [2]. Explicit lists emphasize errors of commission or omission in prescribing and focus on frequently used drugs that should be avoided. In contrast, two other tools, Medication Appropriate Index (MAI) [143, 144] and Fit For The Ages (FORTA) [145], are implicit tools, which, in the case of MAI, is based on physician's knowledge and judgment (answering/rating ten drug-related questions per drug see https://globalrph.com/medcalcs/medication-appropriateness-index-calculator/) rather than a set of defined criteria; in the case of FORTA, 190 drugs in 20 groups are rated in four categories of A (indispensable), B (drugs with proven or obvious efficacy but limited), C (questionable efficacy, use with caution), and D (avoid) [145]. Ratings by an expert panel consider "factors such as adherence issues, age-dependent tolerance and frequency of relative contraindications" [145]. According to the Cochrane review [146], no one tool is all encompassing in its assessing PIMs or polypharmacy and similarly no one tool is significantly better than another. The Cochrane review also was skeptical as to whether these tools yielded improved patient health outcomes.

DEPRESCRIBING "Deprescribing is the process of tapering or stopping drugs, aimed at minimizing polypharmacy and improving patient outcomes" [147]. Although there is considerable disagreement on a definition of "patient outcomes" [148], in a meta-analysis of over 100 select randomized clinical trials on deprescribing, an individualized-patient intervention reduced mortality [149]. Deprescribing is a reasonable strategy to reduce inappropriate polypharmacy albeit a challenge to implement [148].

"Deprescribing is a complex and nuanced process in a heterogeneous group of patients" [149]. Consequently, there are significant barriers to deprescribing [148, 150]. Specifically, there exists a lack of education relating specific guidelines to deprescribing and their application to individual patients. This generates concerns for prescriber–patient relations and possible medico-legal issues [148, 150]. Another barrier is factors associated with the health system, e.g., lack of time to review medications for deprescribing and lack of coordination among clinicians in different specialties. Patient-related factors create additional barriers. These include resistance from patients to change medications arising from misconceptions on potential outcomes or due to lack of education about age changes, diseases, and therapeutic benefits and risks or poor communication between prescriber and patient.

Deprescribing Strategies There are a number of strategies to overcome these barriers [148]. Suggestions are to take advantage of (1) "triggers," i.e., situations that prompt the possibility of deprescribing, such as the presence of ADRs, decline in cognitive function, patient's age and comorbidities; (2) "opportunities," i.e., situation that requires a medical review and hence possible deprescribing such as transition in care or patient's questions about medications; and (3) "facilitating influences and strategies," e.g., situations favorable to reviewing medication, such as on hospital admissions or coordinating with specialists, and strategies of creating a team approach, educating of patient and family on the concept of deprescribing and risks of inappropriate polypharmacy, and educating of the clinician on deprescribing and use of evidence-based guidelines, e.g., Beers' Criteria® [148].

Another strategy is the use of a "drug holiday," which is an agreed cessation of medication for a period of time. The drug holiday is "framed as a longitudinal structured 'pause and monitor' process, with a patient-focused approach" [151]. The drug is stopped and the patient's response is followed closely. If restarting the medication is necessary, the patient needs to be advised that their body may be more sensitive and thus may require a lower starting dose. Sometimes, a drug holiday is recommended before tolerance develops to maintain sensitivity to the drug.

Guidance
1. Adverse drug reactions (ADRs) are unintended and undesired outcomes of medical therapy. ADRs may cause serious harm, negatively absorb health care resources, and reduce quality of life. ADRs are avoidable.
2. ADR avoidance strategies
   (a) Recognize the relation between polypharmacy and the potential for drug–drug interactions (DDIs); 2 or more drugs may produce additive, synergistic or antagonistic effects that are unwanted
   (b) Consider the wealth of information of PK-dependent DDIs—presented in this chapter on transporter/hepatic enzyme DDIs
   (c) Understand known PD-DDIs—especially the adverse additive effects of drugs with anticholinergic, sedative, or anticoagulation effects
   (d) Adhere to Beers Criteria® of explicit list of potentially inappropriate medications (PIMs); always determine kidney function prior to prescribing; know concerns of renal biomarkers of serum creatinine/cystatin C
3. Acknowledge that deprescribing to reduce polypharmacy and PIMs is difficult, but it has the potential to reduce ADRs and improve patient care. It requires education and communication between prescriber, team care givers, patient, and family.

References

1. Aronson JK, Ferner RE. Joining the DoTS: new approach to classifying adverse drug reactions. BMJ. 2003;327(7425):1222–5. https://doi.org/10.1136/bmj.327.7425.1222.
2. Halli-Tierney AD, Scarbrough C, Carroll D. Polypharmacy: evaluating risks and Deprescribing. Am Fam Physician. 2019;100(1):32–8. PMID: 31259501.
3. Zazzara MB, Palmer K, Vetrano DL, Carfi A, Onder G. Adverse drug reactions in older adults: a narrative review of the literature. Eur Geriatr Med. 2021;12(3):463–73. https://doi.org/10.1007/s41999-021-00481-9.
4. Aronson JK, Ferner RE. Clarification of terminology in drug safety. Drug Safety. 2005;28(10):851–70. https://doi.org/10.2165/00002018-200528100-00003.
5. Montané E, Santesmases J. Adverse drug reactions. Med Clin (Barc). 2020;154(5):178–84. https://doi.org/10.1016/j.medcli.2019.08.007.
6. Coleman JJ, Pontefract SK. Adverse drug reactions. Clin Med J R Coll Physicians (Lond). 2016;16(5):481–5. https://doi.org/10.7861/clinmedicine.16-5-481.
7. Robinson EG, Hedna K, Hakkarainen KM, Gyllensten H. Healthcare costs of adverse drug reactions and potentially inappropriate prescribing in older adults: a population-based study. BMJ Open. 2022;12(9):e062589. https://doi.org/10.1136/bmjopen-2022-062589.
8. Jiang M, Zhou B, Chen L. Identification of drug side effects with a path-based method. Math Biosci Eng. 2022;19(6):5754–71. https://doi.org/10.3934/mbe.2022269.
9. Berger SI, Iyengar R. Role of systems pharmacology in understanding drug adverse events. Wiley Interdiscip Rev Syst Biol Med. 2011;3(2):129–35. https://doi.org/10.1002/wsbm.114.
10. Bailey C, Peddie D, Wickham ME, Badke K, Small SS, Doyle-Waters MM, et al. Adverse drug event reporting systems: a systematic review. Br J Clin Pharmacol. 2016;82(1):17–29. https://doi.org/10.1111/bcp.12944.
11. Rawlins MD. Adverse reactions to drugs. Br Med J (Clin Res Ed). 1981;282(6268):974–6. https://doi.org/10.1136/bmj.282.6268.974.
12. By the 2023 American Geriatrics Society Beers Criteria® Update Expert Panel. American Geriatrics Society 2023 updated AGS Beers Criteria® for potentially inappropriate medication use in older adults. J Am Geriatr Soc. 2023;71(7):2052–81. https://doi.org/10.1111/jgs.18372.
13. Karnes JH, Miller MA, White KD, Konvinse KC, Pavlos K, Redwood AJ, et al. Applications of immunopharmacogenomics: predicting, preventing, and understanding immune-mediated adverse drug reactions. Annu Rev Pharmacol Toxicol. 2019;59:463–86. https://doi.org/10.1146/annurev-pharmtox-010818-021818.
14. Lee AY. Immunological mechanisms in cutaneous adverse drug reactions. Biomol Ther (Seoul). 2024;32(1):1–12. https://doi.org/10.4062/biomolther.2023.170.
15. Pavlos R, Mallal S, Ostrov D, Buus S, Metushi I, Peters B, et al. T cell-mediated hypersensitivity reactions to drugs. Annu Rev Med. 2015;66:439–54. https://doi.org/10.1146/annurev-med-050913-022745.
16. Rollinson V, Turner R, Pirmohamed M. Pharmacogenomics for primary care: an overview. Genes (Basel). 2020;11(11):1337. https://doi.org/10.3390/genes11111337.
17. Storms H, Marquet K, Aertgeerts B, Claes N. Prevalence of inappropriate medication use in residential long-term care facilities for the elderly: a systematic review. Eur J Gen Pract. 2017;23(1):69–77. https://doi.org/10.1080/13814788.2017.1288211.
18. Lexow M, Wernece K, Schmid GL, Sultzer R, Bertsche T, Schiek S. Considering additive effects of polypharmacy : analysis of adverse events in geriatric patients in long-term care facilities. Wien Klin Wochenschr. 2021;133(15–16):816–82. https://doi.org/10.1007/s00508-020-01750-6.
19. Chan M, Nicklason F, Vial JH. Adverse drug events as a cause of hospital admission in the elderly. Intern Med J. 2001;31(4):199–205. https://doi.org/10.1046/j.1445-5994.2001.00044.x.

20. Shehab N, Patel PR, Srinivasan A, Budnitz DS. Emergency department visits for antibiotic-associated adverse events. Clin Infect Dis. 2008;47(6):735–43. https://doi.org/10.1086/591126.
21. Kongkaew C, Noyce PR, Ashcroft DM. Hospital admissions associated with adverse drug reactions: a systematic review of prospective observational studies. Ann Pharmacother. 2008;42(7):1017–25. https://doi.org/10.1345/aph.1L037.
22. Marcum ZA, Amuan ME, Hanlon JT, Aspinall SL, Handler SM, Ruby CM, et al. Prevalence of unplanned hospitalizations caused by adverse drug reactions in older veterans. J Am Geriatr Soc. 2012;60(1):34–41. https://doi.org/10.1111/j.1532-5415.2011.03772.x.
23. Al Hamid A, Ghaleb M, Aljadhey H, Aslanpour Z. A systematic review of hospitalization resulting from medicine-related problems in adult patients. Br J Clin Pharmacol. 2013;78(2):202–17. https://doi.org/10.1111/bcp.12293.
24. Parameswaran Nair N, Chalmers L, Peterson GM, Bereznicki BJ, Castelino L, Bereznicki LR. Hospitalization in older patients due to adverse drug reactions -the need for a prediction tool. Clin Interv Aging. 2016;11:497–505. https://doi.org/10.2147/CIA.S99097.
25. Gurwitz JH, Field TS, Harrold LR, Rothschild J, Debellis K, Seger AC, et al. Incidence and preventability of adverse drug events among older persons in the ambulatory setting. JAMA. 2003;289(9):1107–16. https://doi.org/10.1001/jama.289.9.1107.
26. Placido AI, Herdeiro MT, Morgado M, Figueiras A, Roque F. Drug-related problems in home-dwelling older adults: A systematic review. Clin Ther. 2020;42(4):559–572.e14. https://doi.org/10.1016/j.clinthera.2020.02.005.
27. Khalil H, Huang C. Adverse drug reactions in primary care: a scoping review. BMC Health Serv Res. 2020;20(1):5. https://doi.org/10.1186/s12913-019-4651-7.
28. Jennings E, Murphy K, Gallagher P, O'Mahony D. In-hospital adverse drug reactions in hospitalized older adults—a systematic review. Age Ageing. 2020;49(6):948–58. https://doi.org/10.1093/ageing/afaa188.
29. Shukla AK, Jhaj R, Misra S, Ahmed SN, Nanda M, Chaudhary D. Agreement between WHO-UMC causality scale and the Naranjo algorithm for causality assessment of adverse drug reactions. Family Med Prim Care. 2021;10(9):3303–8. https://doi.org/10.4103/jfmpc.jfmpc_831_21.
30. http://www.who-umc.org/Graphics/24734.pdf
31. Naranjo CA, Busto U, Sellers EM, Sandor P, Ruiz I, Roberts EA, et al. A method for estimating the probability of adverse drug reactions. Clin Pharmacol Ther. 1981;30(2):239–45. https://doi.org/10.1038/clpt.1981.154.
32. Théophile H, André M, Miremont-Salamé G, Arimone Y, Bégaud B. Comparison of three methods (an updated logistic probabilistic method, the Naranjo and Liverpool algorithms) for the evaluation of routine pharmacovigilance case reports using consensual expert judgement as reference. Drug Saf. 2013;36(10):1033–44. https://doi.org/10.1007/s40264-013-0083-1.
33. Belhekar M, Taur S, Munshi R. A study of agreement between the Naranjo algorithm and WHO-UMC criteria for causality assessment of adverse drug reactions. Indian J Pharmacol. 2014;46(1):117–20. https://doi.org/10.4103/0253-7613.125192.
34. Theophile H, Arimone Y, Miremont SG, Moore N, Fourrier RA, Haramburu B, et al. Comparison of three methods (consensual expert judgment, algorithmic and probabilistic approaches) of causality assessment of adverse drug reactions: an assessment using reports made to a French Pharmacovigilance center. Drug Saf. 2010;33(11):1045–54. https://doi.org/10.2165/11537780-000000000-00000.
35. Alikhani R, Pai MP. Reconsideration of the current models of estimated kidney function-based drug dose adjustment in older adults: the role of biological age. Clin Transl Sci. 2023;16(11):2095–105. https://doi.org/10.1111/cts.13643.
36. Chen DC, Potok OA, Rifkin D, Estrella MM. Advantages, limitations, and clinical considerations in using cystatin C to estimate GFR. Kidney360. 2022;3(10):1807–14. https://doi.org/10.34067/KID.0003202022.

37. Pazan F, Wehling M. Polypharmacy in older adults: a narrative review of definitions, epidemiology and consequences. Eur Geriatr Med. 2021;12(3):443–52. https://doi.org/10.1007/s41999-021-00479-3.
38. Masnoon N, Shakib S, Kalisch-Elett L, Caughey GE. What is polypharmacy? A systemic review of definitions. BMC Geriatr. 2017;17(1):230. https://doi.org/10.1186/s12877-017-0621-2.
39. Linsky A, Simon SR, Marcello TB, Bokhour B. Clinical provider perceptions of proactive medication discontinuation. Am J Manag Care. 2015;21(4):277–83. PMID: 26014466.
40. Qato DM, Alexander GC, Conti R, Johnson M, Schumm P, Lindau ST, et al. Use of prescription and over-the-counter medications and dietary supplements among older adults in the United States. JAMA. 2008;300(24):2867–78. https://doi.org/10.1001/jama.2008.892.
41. Hales CM, Servais J, Martin CB, Kohen D. Prescription drug use among adults aged 40-79 in the United States and Canada. NCHS Data Brief. 2019;347:1–8. PMID: 31442200.
42. Counter D, Millar JWT, McLay JS. Hospital readmissions, mortality and potentially inappropriate prescribing: a retrospective study of older adults discharged from hospital. Br J Clin Pharmacol. 2018;84(8):1757–63. https://doi.org/10.1111/bcp.13607.
43. Unlu O, Levitan EB, Reshetnyak E, Kneifati-Hayek J, Diaz I, Archambault A, et al. Polypharmacy in older adults hospitalized for heart failure. Circ Heart Fail. 2020;13(11):e00697. https://doi.org/10.1161/CIRCHEARTFAILURE.120.006977.
44. Dwyer L, Han B, Woodwell DA, Rechtsteiner EA. Polypharmacy in nursing home residents in the United States: results of the 2004 National Nursing Home Survey. Am J Geriatr Pharmacother. 2010;8(1):63–72. https://doi.org/10.1016/j.amjopharm.2010.01.001.
45. Moore KL, Patel K, Boscardin WJ, Steinman MA, Ritchie C, Schwartz JB. Medication burden attributable to chronic co-morbid conditions in the very old and vulnerable. PLoS One. 2018;13(4):e0196109. https://doi.org/10.1371/journal.pone.0196109.
46. Tamura BK, Bell CL, Lubimir K, Iwasaki WN, Ziegler LA, Masaki KH. Physician intervention for medication reduction in a nursing home: the polypharmacy outcomes project. J Am Med Dir Assoc. 2011;12(5):326–30. https://doi.org/10.1016/j.jamda.2010.08.013.
47. Rodrigues MC, de Oliveira C. Drug-drug interactions and adverse drug reactions in polypharmacy among older adults: an integrative review. Rev Lat Am Enfermagem. 2016;24:e2800. https://doi.org/10.1590/1518-8345.1316.2800.
48. Kantor ED, Rehm CD, Haas JS, Chan AT, Giovannucci EL. Trends in prescription drug use among adults in the United States from 1999–2012. JAMA. 2015;314:1818–31. https://doi.org/10.1001/jama.2015.13766.
49. Qato DM, Wilder J, Schumm LP, Gillet V, Alexander GC. Changes in prescription and over-the-counter medication and dietary supplement use among older adults in the United States, 2005 vs 2011. JAMA Intern Med. 2016;176(4):473–82. https://doi.org/10.1001/jamainternmed.2015.8581.
50. Martin CB, Hales CM, Gu Q. Ogden CL prescription drug use in the United States, 2015-2016. NCHS Data Brief. 2019;334:1–8. PMID: 31112126.
51. WHO Medication Safety in Polypharmacy, 2019 WHO/UHC/SDS/2019.11. https://apps.who.int/iris/bitstream/handle/10665/325454/WHO-UHC-SDS-2019.11-engpdf?ua=1.
52. Davies LE, Spiers G, Kingston A, Todd A, Adamson J, Hanratty B. Adverse outcomes of polypharmacy in older people: systematic review of reviews. J Am Med Dir Assoc. 2020;21(2):181–7. https://doi.org/10.1016/j.jamda.2019.10.022.
53. Bettonte S, Berton M, Marzolini C. Magnitude of drug-drug interactions in special populations. Pharmaceutics. 2022;14(4):789. https://doi.org/10.3390/pharmaceutics14040789.
54. Buxton ILO. General principles. In: Brunton LL, Lazo JS, Parker KL, editors. Goodman and Gilman's the pharmacological basis of therapeutics. 11th ed. New York: McGraw-Hill Medical Publishing Division; 2006. p. 1–39.
55. Mokhtari RB, Homayouni TS, Baluch N, Morgatskaya E, Kumar S, Das B, et al. Combination therapy in combating cancer. Oncotarget. 2017;8(23):38022–43. https://doi.org/10.18632/oncotarget.16723.

56. Butkiewicz M, Restrepo NA, Haines JL, Crawford DC. Drug-drug interaction profiles of medication regimens extracted from a de-identified electronic medical records system. AMIA Summits Transl Sci Proc. 2016;2016:33–40. PMCID: PMC5001747
57. Gee RRF, Huber AD, Chen T. Regulation of PXR in drug metabolism: chemical and structural perspectives. Expert Opin Drug Metab Toxicol. 2024:1–15. https://doi.org/10.1080/17425255.2024.2309212.
58. Ma X, Idles JR, Gonzalez FJ. The Pregnane X receptor: from bench to bedside. Expert Opin Drug Metab Toxicol. 2008;4(7):895–908. https://doi.org/10.1517/17425255.4.7.895.
59. Dominguez CJ, Tocchetti GN, Rigalli JP, Mottino AD. Acute regulation of apical ABC transporters in the gut. Potential influence on drug bioavailability. Pharmacol Res. 2021;163:105251. https://doi.org/10.1016/j.phrs.2020.105251.
60. Cascorbi I. Drug interactions-principles, examples and clinical consequences. Dtsch Arztebl Int. 2012;109:546–56. https://doi.org/10.3238/arztebl.2012.0546.
61. Gurley GJ, Swain AS, Williams DK, Barone G, Battu SK. Gauging the clinical significance of P-glycoprotein-mediated herb-drug interactions: comparative effects of St. John's wort, Echinacea, clarithromycin, and rifampin on digoxin pharmacokinetics. Mol Nutr Food Res. 2008;52(7):772–9. https://doi.org/10.1002/mnfr.200700081.
62. Chan ALF, Wang M-T, Su C-Y, Tsai F-H. Risk of digoxin intoxication caused by clarithromycin-digoxin interactions in heart failure patients: a population-based study. Eur J Clin Pharmacol. 2009;65(12):1237–43. https://doi.org/10.1007/s00228-009-0698-4.
63. Ferri N, Colombo E, Tenconi M, Baldessin L, Corsini A. Drug-drug interactions of direct oral anticoagulants (DOACs): from pharmacological to clinical practice. Pharmaceutics. 2022;14(6):1120. https://doi.org/10.3390/pharmaceutics14061120s.
64. Nicolussi S, Drewe J, Butterweck V, Meyer Zu Schwabedissen HE. Clinical relevance of St. John's wort drug interactions revisited. Br J Pharmacol. 2020;177(6):1212–26. https://doi.org/10.1111/bph.14936.
65. Reis S, Metzendorf M-I, Kuehn R, Popp M, Gagyor I, Kranke P, et al. Nirmatrelvir combined with ritonavir for preventing and treating COVID-19. Cochrane Database Syst Rev. 2022;2022(9):CD015395. https://doi.org/10.1002/14651858.CD015395.pub2.
66. Yin J, Wang J. Renal drug transporters and their significance in drug-drug interactions. Acta Pharm Sin B. 2016;6(5):363–73. https://doi.org/10.1016/j.apsb.2016.07.013.
67. Matsushima S, Maeda K, Inoue K, Ohta K-y, Yuasa H, Kondo T, et al. The inhibition of human multidrug and toxin extrusion 1 is involved in the drug-drug interaction caused by cimetidine. Drug Metab Dispos. 2009;37(3):555–9. https://doi.org/10.1124/dmd.108.023911.
68. Kusuhara H, Ito S, Kumagai Y, Jiang M, Shiroshita T, Moriyama Y, et al. Effects of a MATE protein inhibitor, pyrimethamine, on the renal elimination of metformin at oral microdose and at therapeutic dose in healthy subjects. Clin Pharmacol Ther. 2011;89(6):837–44. https://doi.org/10.1038/clpt.2011.36.
69. Song IH, Zong J, Borland J, Jerva F, Wynne V, Zamek-Gliszczynski MJ, et al. The effect of Dolutegravir on the pharmacokinetics of metformin in healthy subjects. J Acquir Immune Defic Syndr. 2016;72(4):400–7. https://doi.org/10.1097/QAI.0000000000000983.
70. Nakada T, Kudo T, Ito K. Quantitative consideration of clinical increases in serum creatinine caused by renal transporter inhibition. Drug Metab Dispos. 2023;51(9):1114–26. https://doi.org/10.1124/dmd.122.000969.
71. Garcia-Rodriguez C, Mujica P, Illanes-Gonzalez J, Lopez A, Vargas C, Saez JC, et al. Probenecid, an old drug with potential new uses for central nervous system disorders and neuroinflammation. Biomedicines. 2023;11(6):1516. https://doi.org/10.3390/biomedicines11061516.
72. Zhao M, Ma J, Li M, Zhang Y, Jiang B, Zhao X, et al. Cytochrome P450 enzymes and drug metabolism in humans. Int J Mol Sci. 2021;22(23):12808. https://doi.org/10.3390/ijms222312808.
73. https://www.fda.gov/drugs/drug-interactions

74. Tan A, Holmes HM, Kuo Y-F, Raji MA, Goodwin JS. Coadministration of co-trimoxazole with sulfonylureas: hypoglycemia events and pattern of use. J Gerontol A Biol Sci Med Sci. 2015;70(2):247–54. https://doi.org/10.1093/gerona/glu072.
75. Antoniou T, Gomes T, Juurlink DN, Loutfy MR, Glazier RH, Mamdani MM. Trimethoprim-sulfamethoxazole-induced hyperkalemia in patients receiving inhibitors of the renin-angiotensin system: a population-based study. Arch Intern Med. 2010;170(12):1045–9. https://doi.org/10.1001/archinternmed.2010.142.
76. King JR, Zha J, Khartri A, Dutta S, Menon RM. Clinical pharmacokinetics of dasabuvir. Clin Pharmacokinet. 2017;56(10):1115–24. https://doi.org/10.1007/s40262-017-0519-3.
77. Itkonen MK, Tornio A, Lapatto-Reiniluoto O, Neuvonen M, Neuvonen PJ, Niemi M, et al. Clopidogrel increases dasabuvir exposure with or without ritonavir, and ritonavir inhibits the bioactivation of clopidogrel. Clin Pharmacol Ther. 2019;105(1):219–28. https://doi.org/10.1002/cpt.1099.
78. Smolders EJ, Berden FAC, de Kanter CTMM, Kievit W, Drenth JPH, Burger DM. The majority of hepatitis C patients treated with direct acting antivirals are at risk for relevant drug-drug interactions. United European Gastroenterol J. 2017;5(5):648–57. https://doi.org/10.1177/2050640616678151.
79. Kuo MH, Tseng CW, Lee CH, Tseng KC. Drug-drug interactions between direct-acting antivirals and statins in the treatment of chronic hepatitis C. Tzu Chi Med J. 2020;32(4):331–8. https://doi.org/10.4103/tcmj.tcmj_247_19.
80. Loos NHC, Beijnen JH, Schinkel AH. The mechanism-based inactivation of CYP3A4 by ritonavir: what mechanism? Int J Mol Sci. 2022;23(17):9866. https://doi.org/10.3390/ijms23179866.
81. Macias J, Pinilla A, Lao-Dominguez FA, Corma A, Macias EC, Gonzalez-Serna A, et al. High rate of major drug-drug interactions of lopinavir-ritonavir for COVID-19 treatment. Sci Rep. 2020;10(1):20958. https://doi.org/10.1038/s41598-020-78029-3.
82. Agarwal S, Agarwal SK. Lopinavir-ritonavir in SARS-CoV-2 infection and drug-drug interactions with cardioactive medications. Cardiovasc Drugs Ther. 2021;35(3):427–40. https://doi.org/10.1007/s10557-020-07070-1.
83. Bolleddula J, Gopalakrishnan S, Hu P, Dong J, Venkatakrishnan K. Alternatives to rifampicin: a review and perspectives on the choice of strong CYP3A inducers for clinical drug-drug interaction studies. Clin Transl Sci. 2022;15(9):2075–95. https://doi.org/10.1111/cts.13357.
84. Elmeliegy M, Vourvahis M, Guo C, Wang DD. Effect of P-glycoprotein (P-gp) inducers on exposure of P-gp substrates: review of clinical drug-drug interaction studies. Clin Pharmacokinet. 2020;59(6):699–714. https://doi.org/10.1007/s40262-020-00867-1.
85. Shitara Y. Clinical importance of OATP1B1 and OATP1B3 in drug-drug interactions. Drug Metab Pharmacokinet. 2011;26(3):220–7. https://doi.org/10.2133/dmpk.DMPK-10-RV-094.
86. Teo YL, Ho HK, Chan A. Metabolism-related pharmacokinetic drug-drug interactions with tyrosine kinase inhibitors: current understanding, challenges and recommendations. Br J Clin Pharmacol. 2015;79(2):241–53. https://doi.org/10.1111/bcp.12496.
87. Khurana V, Minocha M, Pal D, Mitra AK. Inhibition of OATP-1B1 and OATP-1B3 by tyrosine kinase inhibitors. Drug Metabol Drug Interact. 2014;29(4):249–59. https://doi.org/10.1515/dmdi-2014-0014.
88. Niu J, Straubinger RM, Mager DE. Pharmacodynamic drug-drug interactions. Clin Pharmacol Ther. 2019;105(6):1395–406. https://doi.org/10.1002/cpt.1434.
89. Yadav R, Bulitta JB, Schneider EK, Shin BS, Velkov T, Nation RL, et al. Aminoglycoside concentrations required for synergy with carbapenems against Pseudomonas aeruginosa determined via mechanistic studies and modeling. Antimicrob Agents Chemother. 2017;61(12):e00722–17. https://doi.org/10.1128/AAC.00722-17.
90. Ruby CM, Hanlon JT, Boudreau RM, Newman AB, Simonsick EM, Shorr RI, et al. The effect of medication use on urinary incontinence in community-dwelling elderly women. Health, Aging and Body Composition Study. J Am Geriatr Soc. 2010;58(9):1715–20. https://doi.org/10.1111/j.1532-5415.2010.03006.x.

91. Cubeddu LX. QT prolongation and fatal arrhythmias: a review of clinical implications and effects of drugs. Am J Ther. 2003;10(6):452–7. https://doi.org/10.1097/00045391-200311000-00013.
92. Schepkens H, Vanholder R, Billiouw JM, Lameire N. Life-threatening hyperkalemia during combined therapy with angiotensin-converting enzyme inhibitors and spironolactone: an analysis of 25 cases. Am J Med. 2001;110(6):438–41. https://doi.org/10.1016/s0002-9343(01)00642-8.
93. Hughes JE, Waldron C, Bennett KE, Cahir C. Prevalence of drug- drug interactions in older community-dwelling individuals: a systematic review and meta-analysis. Drugs Aging. 2023;40(2):117–34. https://doi.org/10.1007/s40266-022-01001-5.
94. Juurlink DN, Mamdani M, Kopp A, Laupacis A, Redelmeier DA. Drug-drug interactions among elderly patients hospitalized for drug toxicity. JAMA. 2003;289(13):1652–8. https://doi.org/10.1001/jama.289.13.1652.
95. Dugowson CE, Gnanashanmugam P. Nonsteroidal anti-inflammatory drugs. Phys Med Rehabil Clin N Am. 2006;17(2):347–54, vi. https://doi.org/10.1016/j.pmr.2005.12.012.
96. Masclee GMC, Valkhoff VE, Coloma PM, de Ridder M, Romio S, Schuemie MJ, et al. Risk of upper gastrointestinal bleeding from different drug combinations. Gastroenterology. 2014;147(4):784–92.e9. https://doi.org/10.1053/j.gastro.2014.06.007.
97. Rao P, Knaus EE. Evolution of nonsteroidal anti-inflammatory drugs (NSAIDs): cyclooxygenase (COX) inhibition and beyond. J Pharm Pharm Sci. 2008;11(2):81s–110s. https://doi.org/10.18433/j3t886.
98. Moore N, Scheiman JM. Gastrointestinal safety and tolerability of oral non-aspirin over-the-counter analgesics. Postgrad Med. 2018;130(2):188–99. https://doi.org/10.1080/00325481.2018.1429793.
99. Moore N, Pollack C, Butkerait P. Adverse drug reactions and drug-drug interactions with over-the-counter NSAIDs. Ther Clin Risk Manag. 2015;11:1061–75. https://doi.org/10.2147/TCRM.S79135.
100. Sokołowska P, Bleibel L, Owczarek J, Wiktorowska-Owczarek A. PPARγ, NF-κB and the UPR pathway as new molecular targets in the anti-inflammatory actions of NSAIDs: novel applications in cancers and central nervous system diseases? Adv Clin Exp Med. 2024; https://doi.org/10.17219/acem/174243.
101. Peterson MC, Riggs MM. FDA advisory meeting clinical pharmacology review utilizes a Quantitative Systems Pharmacology (QSP) model: a watershed moment? CPT Pharmacometrics Syst Pharmacol. 2015;4(3):e00020. https://doi.org/10.1002/psp4.20.
102. Bories M, Bouzillé G, Cuggia M, Le Corre P. Drug-drug interactions in elderly patients with potentially inappropriate medications in primary care, nursing home and hospital settings: a systematic review and a preliminary study. Pharmaceutics. 2021;13(2):266. https://doi.org/10.3390/pharmaceutics13020266.
103. https://www.fda.gov/files/drugs/published/In-Vitro-Metabolism%2D%2Dand-Transporter%2D%2DMediated-Drug-Drug-Interaction-Studies-Guidance-for-Industry.pdf
104. Jing L, Legeay S, Gagnon A-L, Frigon M-P, Tessier L, Tremblay K. Moving towards the implementation of pharmacogenetic testing in Quebec. Front Genet. 2024;14:1295963. https://doi.org/10.3389/fgene.2023.1295963.
105. Zhou D, Chen Z, Tian F. Deprescribing interventions for older patients: a systematic review and meta-analysis. J Am Med Dir Assoc. 2023;24(11):1718–25. https://doi.org/10.1016/j.jamda.2023.07.016.
106. Bloomfield HE, Greer N, Linsky AM, Bolduc J, Naidl T, Vardeny O, et al. Deprescribing for community-dwelling older adults: a systematic review and meta-analysis. J Gen Intern Med. 2020;35(11):3323–32. https://doi.org/10.1007/s11606-020-06089-2.
107. Rochon PA, Petrovic M, Cherubini A, Onder G, O'Mahony D, Sternberg SA, et al. Polypharmacy, inappropriate prescribing, and deprescribing in older people: through a sex and gender lens. Lancet Healthy Longev. 2021;2(5):e290–300. https://doi.org/10.1016/S2666-7568(21)00054-4.

108. Qaseem A, Snow V, Owens DK, Shekelle P. Clinical Guidelines Committee of the American College of Physicians The development of clinical practice guidelines and guidance statements of the American College of Physicians: summary of methods. Ann Intern Med. 2010;153(3):194–9. https://doi.org/10.7326/0003-4819-153-3-201008030-00010.
109. Guyatt GH, Oxman AD, Montori V, Vist G, Kunz R, Brozek J, et al. GRADE guidelines: 5. Rating the quality of evidence--publication bias. J Clin Epidemiol. 2011;64(12):1277–82. https://doi.org/10.1016/j.jclinepi.2011.01.011.
110. Tune LE. Anticholinergic effects of medication in elderly patients. Clin Psychiatry. 2001;62(Suppl 21):11–4. PMID: 11584981.
111. Araklitis G, Robinson D, Cardozo L. Cognitive effects of anticholinergic load in women with overactive bladder. Clin Interv Aging. 2020;15:1493–503. https://doi.org/10.2147/CIA.S252852.
112. Egberts A, Moreno-Gonzalez R, Alan H, Ziere G, Mattace-Raso FUS. Anticholinergic Drug Burden and Delirium: A Systematic Review. J Am Med Dir Assoc. 2021;22(1):65–73.e4. https://doi.org/10.1016/j.jamda.2020.04.019.
113. Naseri A, Sadigh-Eteghad S, Seyedi-Sahebari S, Hosseini M-S, Hajebrahimi S, Salehi-Pourmehr H. Cognitive effects of individual anticholinergic drugs: a systematic review and meta-analysis. Neuropsychology. 2023;17:e20220053. https://doi.org/10.1590/1980-5764-DN-2022-0053.
114. Dasa O, Pepine CJ, Pearson TA. Aspirin in primary prevention: what changed? A critical appraisal of current evidence. Am J Cardiol. 2021;141:38–48. https://doi.org/10.1016/j.amjcard.2020.11.014.
115. Davidson KW, Barry MJ, Mangione CM, Cabana M, Chelmow D, Coker TR, et al. Aspirin use to prevent cardiovascular disease: US preventive services task force recommendation statement. JAMA. 2022;327(16):1577–84. https://doi.org/10.1001/jama.2022.4983.
116. Ittaman SV, VanWormer JJ, Rezkalla SH. The role of aspirin in the prevention of cardiovascular disease. Clin Med Res. 2014;12(3–4):147–54. https://doi.org/10.3121/cmr.2013.1197.
117. Dani M, Dirksen A, Taraborrelli P, Panagopolous D, Toroastro M, Sutton R, et al. Orthostatic hypotension in older people: considerations, diagnosis and management. Clin Med (Lond). 2021;21(3):e275–82. https://doi.org/10.7861/clinmed.2020-1044.
118. Feduska ET, Thoma BN, Torjman MC. Goldhammer JE acute amiodarone pulmonary toxicity. J Cardiothorac Vasc Anesth. 2021;35(5):1485–94. https://doi.org/10.1053/j.jvca.2020.10.060.
119. Naccarelli GV. Kowey PR the role of dronedarone in the treatment of atrial fibrillation/flutter in the aftermath of PALLAS. Curr Cardiol Rev. 2014;10(4):303–8. https://doi.org/10.2174/1573403x10666140513110247.
120. Li ZP, You YS, Wang JD, He LP. Underlying disease may increase mortality risk in users of atypical antipsychotics. World J Psychiatry. 2022;12(8):1112–4. https://doi.org/10.5498/wjp.v12.i8.1112.
121. Rogowska M, Thornton M, Creese B, Velayudhan L, Aarsland D, Ballard C, et al. Implications of adverse outcomes associated with antipsychotics in older patients with dementia: a 2011-2022 update. Drugs Aging. 2023;40(1):21–32. https://doi.org/10.1007/s40266-022-00992-5.
122. Kim G-H. Pathophysiology of drug-induced hyponatremia. J Clin Med. 2022;11(19):5810. https://doi.org/10.3390/jcm11195810.
123. Rossouw JE, Anderson GL, Prentice RL, LaCroix AZ, Kooperberg C, Stefanick ML, et al. JAMA. 2002;288(3):321–33. https://doi.org/10.1001/jama.288.3.321.
124. Yabluchanskiy A, Tsitouras PD. Is testosterone replacement therapy in older men effective and safe? Drugs Aging. 2019;36(11):981–9. https://doi.org/10.1007/s40266-019-00716-2.
125. Gersh F, O'Keefe JH, Elagizi A, Lavie CJ, Laukkanen JA. Estrogen and cardiovascular disease. Prog Cardiovasc Dis. 2024:S0033-0620(24)00015-X. https://doi.org/10.1016/j.pcad.2024.01.015.

126. The NAMS 2017 Hormone Therapy Position Statement Advisory Panel. The 2017 hormone therapy position statement of the North American Menopause Society. Menopause. 2017;(24):728–53. https://doi.org/10.1097/GME.0000000000000921.
127. Basaria S, Coviello AD, Travison TG, Storer TW, Farwell WR, Jette AM, et al. Adverse events associated with testosterone administration. N Engl J Med. 2010;363(2):109–22. https://doi.org/10.1056/NEJMoa1000485.
128. Finkle WD, Greenland S, Ridgeway GK, Adams JL, Frasco MA, Cook MB, et al. Increased risk of non-fatal myocardial infarction following testosterone therapy prescription in men. PLoS One. 2014;9(1):e85805. https://doi.org/10.1371/journal.pone.0085805.
129. Barone B, Napolitano L, Abate M, Cirillo L, Reccia P, Passaro F, et al. The role of testosterone in the elderly: what do we know? Int J Mol Sci. 2022;23(7):3535. https://doi.org/10.3390/ijms23073535.
130. Hodis HN, Mack WJ, Lobo RA, Shoupe D, Sevanian A, Mahrer PR, et al. Estrogen in the prevention of atherosclerosis. A randomized, double-blind, placebo-controlled trial. Ann Intern Med. 2001;135(11):939–53. https://doi.org/10.7326/0003-4819-135-11-200112040-00005.
131. Grady D, Herrington D, Bittner V, Blumenthal R, Davidson M, Hlatky M, et al. Cardiovascular disease outcomes during 6.8 years of hormone therapy: heart and estrogen/progestin replacement study follow-up (HERS II). JAMA. 2002;288(1):49–57. https://doi.org/10.1001/jama.288.1.49.
132. Beral V. Breast cancer and hormone-replacement therapy in the Million Women Study Million Women Study Collaborators. Lancet. 2003;362(9382):419–27. https://doi.org/10.1016/s0140-6736(03)14065-2.
133. Vinogradova Y, Coupland C, Hippisley-Cox J. Use of hormone replacement therapy and risk of breast cancer: nested case-control studies using the QResearch and CPRD databases. BMJ. 2020;371:m3873. https://doi.org/10.1136/bmj.m3873.
134. Rahn DD, Carberry C, Sanses TV, Mamik MM, Ward RM, Meriwether KV, et al. Vaginal estrogen for genitourinary syndrome of menopause: a systematic review. Obstet Gynecol. 2014;124(6):1147–56. https://doi.org/10.1097/AOG.0000000000000526.
135. Price DA, Clayton PE, Lloyd IC. Benign intracranial hypertension induced by growth hormone treatment. Lancet. 1995;345(8947):458–9. https://doi.org/10.1016/s0140-6736(95)90444-1.
136. Harman SM, Blackman MR. The effects of growth hormone and sex steroid on lean body mass, fat mass, muscle strength, cardiovascular endurance and adverse events in healthy elderly women and men. Horm Res. 2003;60(Suppl 1):121–4. https://doi.org/10.1159/000071236.
137. Forrest L, Sedmak C, Sikder S, Grewal S, Harman SM, Blackman MR, et al. Effects of growth hormone on hepatic insulin sensitivity and glucose effectiveness in healthy older adults. Endocrine. 2019;63(3):497–506. https://doi.org/10.1007/s12020-018-01834-4.
138. Tseng CL, Chen YT, Huang CJ, Luo J-C, Peng Y-L, Huang D-F, et al. Short-term use of glucocorticoids and risk of peptic ulcer bleeding: a nationwide population-based case-crossover study. Aliment Pharmacol Ther. 2015;42(5):599–606. https://doi.org/10.1111/apt.13298.
139. Chinzon D, Domingues G, Tosetto N, Perrotti M. Safety of long-term proton pump inhibitors: facts and myths. Arq Gastroenterol. 2022;59(2):219–25. https://doi.org/10.1590/S0004-2803.202202000-40.
140. Rao AS, Camilleri M. Review article: metoclopramide and tardive dyskinesia. Aliment Pharmacol Ther. 2010;31(1):11–9. https://doi.org/10.1111/j.1365-2036.2009.04189.x.
141. Juneja D, Nasa P, Jain R, Singh O. Sodium-glucose Cotransporter-2 inhibitors induced euglycemic diabetic ketoacidosis: a meta summary of case reports. World J Diabetes. 2023;14(8):1314–22. https://doi.org/10.4239/wjd.v14.i8.1314.
142. O'Mahony D, Cherubini A, Guiteras AR, Denkinger M, Beuscart J-B, Onder G, et al. STOPP/START criteria for potentially inappropriate prescribing in older people: version 3. Eur Geriatr Med. 2023;14(4):625–32. https://doi.org/10.1007/s41999-023-00777-y.
143. Hanlon JT, Schmader KE, Samsa GP, Weinberger M, Uttech KM, Lewis IK, et al. A method for assessing drug therapy appropriateness. J Clin Epidemiol. 1992;45(10):1045–51. https://doi.org/10.1016/0895-4356(92)90144-c.

144. Hanlon JT, Schmader KE. The medication appropriateness index: a clinimetric measure. Psychother Psychosom. 2022;91(2):78–83. https://doi.org/10.1159/000521699.
145. Kuhn-Thiel AM, Weiß C, Wehling M. FORTA authors/expert panel members consensus validation of the FORTA (Fit fOR The Aged) list: a clinical tool for increasing the appropriateness of pharmacotherapy in the elderly. Drugs Aging. 2014;31(2):131–40. https://doi.org/10.1007/s40266-013-0146-0.
146. Rankin A, Cadogan CA, Patterson SM, Kerse N, Cardwell CR, Bradley MC, et al. Interventions to improve the appropriate use of polypharmacy for older people. Cochrane Database Syst Rev. 2018;9:CD008165. https://doi.org/10.1002/14651858.CD008165.pub4.
147. Scott IA, Hilmer SN, Reeve E, Potter K, Le Couteur D, Rigby D, et al. Reducing inappropriate polypharmacy: the process of deprescribing. JAMA Intern Med. 2015;175(5):827–34. https://doi.org/10.1001/jamainternmed.2015.0324.
148. Robinson M, Mokrzecki S, Mallett AJ. Attitudes and barriers towards deprescribing in older patients experiencing polypharmacy: a narrative review. NPJ Aging. 2024;10(1):6. https://doi.org/10.1038/s41514-023-00132-2.
149. Page AT, Clifford R, Potter K, Schwartz D, Etherton-Beer CD, et al. The feasibility and effect of deprescribing in older adults on mortality and health: a systematic review and meta-analysis. Br J Clin Pharmacol. 2016;82(3):583–623. https://doi.org/10.1111/bcp.12975.
150. Ailabouni NJ, Weir KF, Reeve E, Turner JT, Norton JW, Gray SL. Barriers and enablers of older adults initiating a deprescribing conversation. Patient Educ Couns. 2022;105(3):615–24. https://doi.org/10.1016/j.pec.2021.06.021.
151. Mangin D, Lamarche L, Agarwal G, Ali A, Cassels A, et al. Team approach to polypharmacy evaluation and reduction: feasibility randomized trial of a structured clinical pathway to reduce polypharmacy. Pilot Feasibil Stud. 2023;9(1):84. https://doi.org/10.1186/s40814-023-01315-0.
152. Line J, Saville E, Meng X, Naisbitt D. Why drug exposure is frequently associated with T-cell mediated cutaneous hypersensitivity reactions. Front Toxicol. 2023;5:1268107. https://doi.org/10.3389/ftox.2023.1268107.
153. Messiha FS. Fluoxetine: adverse effects and drug-drug interactions. J Toxicol Clin Toxicol. 1993;31(4):603–30. https://doi.org/10.3109/15563659309025765.
154. Backman JT, Filppula AM, Niemi M, Neuvonen PJ. Role of cytochrome P450 2C8 in drug metabolism and interactions. Pharmacol Rev. 2016;68(1):168–241. https://doi.org/10.1124/pr.115.011411.
155. https://www.fda.gov/drugs/drug-interactions-labeling/drug-development-and-drug-interactions-table-substrates-inhibitors-and-inducers

4. Medication Use in Major Age-Related Diseases: Atherosclerotic Cardiovascular Disease, Cancer, Alzheimer's Disease and Related Dementias, Type 2 Diabetes Mellitus

Abbreviations

ACC	American College of Cardiology
AD	Alzheimer's disease
ADA	American Diabetic Association
ADRD	AD and related dementia
AHA	American Heart Association
ASCVD	atherosclerotic cardiovascular disease
CGA	comprehensive geriatric assessment
CRC	colorectal cancer
CSVD	cerebral small vessel disease
CV	cardiovascular
DAPT	dual antiplatelet therapy
DM	diabetes mellitus
HF	heart failure
IDF	International Diabetes Federation
LDL-C	low-density lipoprotein cholesterol
mAbs	monoclonal antibodies
MDR	multidrug resistance
MI	myocardial infarction
QoL	quality of life
RCT	randomized clinical trial
SGLT2	sodium-glucose co-transporter-2
T2DM	type 2 diabetes mellitus
TG	triglycerides
TIA	transient ischemic attack
TK	tyrosine kinase
TKIs	tyrosine kinase inhibitors
WHO	World Health Organization

INTRODUCTION. Relation Between Aging and Disease Aging is one of the main risk factors for disease. It took dramatic changes in life expectancy (discussed in Chap. 1) to understand that aging and disease were distinct but intertwined entities. The longer lifespan of humans encouraged scientific inquiry into the distinction between aging and disease. It became apparent that the characteristics of aging common across all species differ markedly from the pathological changes of disease [1]. Additionally, if medical science developed cures for all the known diseases, life expectancy would increase, but the rate of aging would be unaffected. Thus, there is an interdependence between aging and disease in that *aging creates a vulnerability to disease*. The medical community treats the consequences of disease but more realistically should be treating the underlying age changes [2], an approach that has launched the discovery of anti-aging drugs (see Chap. 10).

There are a number of age changes, termed the hallmarks of aging, that create the milieu for age-related diseases [3, 4]. These are discussed in detail in Chap. 10. However, one hallmark, cell senescence, will be presented here since it is intricately involved in the diseases of this chapter [5–7]. The hallmark is termed cell senescence.

Cell Senescence Cell senescence is the process, possible in all cell types but especially evident in fibroblasts, endothelial cells and immune cells, whereby normal cells change their phenotype (appearance and function) and gene expression over time. Senescent cells are characterized by (1) irreversible growth arrest (no cell renewal and tissues cannot improve), (2) enlargement and production/secretion of pro-inflammatory mediators and harmful enzymes in place of cell-specific normal factors (resulting from "turning on" of silent genes), and (3) resistance to cell death (apoptosis) [5, 6]. Hence, senescent cells persist as abnormal cells and chronically damage neighboring cells by continuous production of harmful compounds [8].

Cell senescence contributes to disease in the following ways: senescent endothelial cells (cell lining blood vessels) promote vascular pathology by permitting uptake of lipids, decreasing synthesis of anticlotting molecules, and limiting production of factors that ensure vascular relaxation, all of which create a vulnerability to atherosclerosis [9]. In malignancies, senescent immune cells shift the positive balance of T and B cells in favor of highly aggressive proinflammatory immune cells. Also, senescent cells are postulated to initiate tumorigenesis (initiate tumor production) in neighboring cells [10]. In the brains of patients with Alzheimer's disease (AD) senescent brain cells, e.g., astrocytes, microglia, endothelial cells, and neurons, have been identified as players in AD development and progression [11]. In type 2 diabetes mellitus (T2DM), there is a relation between senescent adipocytes, the presence of which is increased in obesity. The aberrant effects of senescent adipocytes lead to reduced fat metabolism, inflammation, and insulin resistance, changes that significantly influence the progression of T2DM [12].

This chapter will discuss drug use in four major disease categories that affect the older adult. For orientation, some pathophysiology, disease prevalence/incidence, and risk factors will be presented. The narrative is supported by Tables 4.1, 4.2, 4.3, and 4.4 and Fig. 4.1.

DISEASE RANK ON MORTALITY As reported by the National Vital Statistics (data 2021), the cause of death (ages 65 and older) from various diseases (most frequent to least frequent) is attributed to diseases of the heart, malignancies, COVID-19, cerebrovascular diseases such as stroke, chronic lower respiratory diseases, AD, diabetes mellitus, accidents (unintentional injuries), kidney disorders, e.g., nephritis (inflammation), and kidney dysfunction, Parkinson's disease, essential hypertension and hypertensive renal disease, influenza and pneumonia, septicemia, chronic liver disease, and cirrhosis and pneumonitis (lung inflammation) [26].

Atherosclerotic Cardiovascular Disease

ATHEROSCLEROTIC CARDIOVASCULAR DISEASE. Overview and Prevalence Atherosclerotic cardiovascular disease (ASCVD) constitutes the major cause of morbidity and mortality in the older adult, both globally and in the United States [27]. The prevalence of ASCVD (2017–2020, those >20 years of age) in both sexes was 48.8% [28]. ASCVD increases with age in both sexes [28].

Atherosclerosis is the pathological process underlying cardiovascular (CV) diseases that affects medium- and large-sized blood arteries, such as the coronary, carotid, renal, femoral arteries, and the aorta. The clinical manifestations of atherosclerosis depend on the affected blood vessel. In coronary arteries, atherosclerosis causes coronary heart disease with complications of angina (chronic chest pain), heart attack (myocardial infarction, MI), and congestive heart failure (HF) after repeat MIs. As of 2021, coronary heart disease was the most common type of ASCVD [28]. In carotid and cerebral arteries, atherosclerosis causes cerebrovascular diseases with outcomes of transient ischemic attacks (TIAs), stroke, dementia, cognitive decline, and possibly cerebral small vessel disease (CSVD affecting smaller vessels in the brain). Prevalence of stroke (2017–2020, >20 years) was 3.3% (>20 years of age). Stroke prevalence increases with age [28]. Atherosclerosis of the femoral arteries causes peripheral vascular disease that results in chronic leg pain (intermittent claudication) with potential for gangrene in the presence of diabetes. Atherosclerosis of renal arteries leads to chronic kidney disease and hypertension, and atherosclerosis in the aorta creates the potential for an aneurysm, a perforation in the artery wall producing fatal hemorrhage. ASCVDs may be silent or subclinical for years, but clinical manifestations will eventually ensue if risk factors (see Table 4.1) are not reduced [29].

Table 4.1 Risk factors for cardiovascular disease; primary prevention [13–15]

Risk factor	Prevention
Age (50 and older)	Choose a healthy lifestyle throughout life
Hypertension: systolic BP 130 mm Hg or higher; Diastolic BP 80 mm Hg or higher	Non-pharmacological: weight loss, sodium reduction, physical activity program, healthy diets, ↓ alcohol intake Pharmacological: antihypertensive/diuretic drugs
Persistently elevated blood cholesterol LDL-C > 160 mg/dl; Total cholesterol >200 mg/dl; HDL-C < 40 mg/dl	Statin therapy—intensity based on degree of LDL-C elevation
Triglycerides ≥175 mg/dL; generally associated with elevated LDL-C	Diet—Mediterranean-style + weight loss, ↓ simple CHO intake, ↑ dietary fiber, ↓ fructose and saturated fatty acids, consuming marine-derived omega-3 PUFAs
Body mass index (BMI) 25–29.9 kg/m^2—overweight ≥30 kg/m^2—obese	Weight reduction
T2DM—to improve glycemic control	Non-pharmacological—nutrition and dietary change, physical exercise (150 min/wk. moderate intensity or 75 min/wk. vigorous intensity), weight loss Pharmacological—metformin, see Table 4.4
Smoking	Cessation—behavioral and pharmacotherapy assistance
Behavioral—poor diet, sedentary lifestyle	Physical exercise (as above), diet of fruits, vegetables, legumes, nuts, whole grains, fish and ↓ intake of sodium, processed meats, refined carbohydrates, and sweetened beverages
Family history of premature atherosclerotic cardiovascular disease, inflammatory diseases, e.g., HIV, rheumatoid arthritis, psoriasis	Awareness and treatment if possible
Other measurable factors: high sensitivity C-reactive protein >2.0 mg/dL; Lipoprotein(a) (Lp[a]) levels ≥50 mg/dL Apolipoprotein B ≥130 mg/dL Ankle-brachial index <0.9	

BP blood pressure, ↓ decrease, *LDL-C* low-density lipoprotein cholesterol, *HDL-C* high density lipoprotein cholesterol, *T2DM* type 2 diabetes mellitus, *CHO* carbohydrates, *omega-3 PUFAs* omega-3 polyunsaturated fatty acids

Atherosclerotic Cardiovascular Disease. Pathophysiology Atherosclerosis is a chronic progressive autoimmune inflammatory disease of the artery wall [30]. The resulting pathological wall remodeling may appear as fatty streaks, intimal and medial thickenings, and/or complex atherosclerotic plaques. Wall thickenings and atherosclerotic plaques slowly reduce the size of the artery lumen, a change that decreases blood flow and produces chronic ischemic tissue damage. Complex plaques have the potential to rupture, an event that completely occludes the artery lumen, deprives distal tissue of oxygen, and produces widespread organ damage that is life-threatening. Plaque rupture is the cause of most MIs [31].

It takes decades for the artery wall to develop a complex plaque that compromises blood flow and/or has the potential to rupture and generate an MI. The main driving force for these changes is the intricate activities of innate and adaptive immune cells that are chronically stimulated by various lipids and toxins, especially low-density lipoprotein cholesterol (LDL-C) [32, 33]. Uptake of lipids and toxins, e.g., smoking components and pollutants into the arterial wall, sets up a cascade of oxidation, macrophage and immune cell participation, generating continuous inflammatory damage that leads to increased wall thickness, growth of the plaque toward the lumen, loss of endothelial antithrombotic properties, creation of a plaque cap, and necrosis of the artery area underneath the plaque cap [34–38].

It is well established that cell senescence is a key factor in the pathophysiology of CVD [39, 40], not only for its role in aberrantly modifying endothelial cells but other cells, e.g., myocardial cells as well [41]. Age-related changes in the mitochondria contribute to the pathology of heart disease [42]. Mitochondria are cellular organelles that are abundant in myocardial cells since they produce the energy molecule, ATP. Mitochondria are involved in nutrient metabolism, calcium metabolism, and regulation of cell death. As they become dysfunctional, ATP production decreases, and oxidative stress and cell death increase [43]. Both cell senescence and mitochondrial dysfunction promote inflammation initiating and advancing ASCVD [42].

Atherosclerotic Cardiovascular Disease. Risk Factors Primary prevention necessitates the reduction of modifiable risk factors. Many of these risk factors were identified over the past 65 years through the research of the Framingham Heart Study, a multigenerational longitudinal study of the epidemiology of cardiovascular disease [44]. The primary risk factor for ASCVD is age [42]. Modifiable risk factors are hypertension (elevated systolic pressure) [45, 46], elevated LDL-C [47], obesity [48], and diabetes [49]. Additional research by others has identified supplementary risk factors: smoking [50], family history of premature ASCVD, persistently elevated triglycerides (TGs), metabolic syndrome (a cluster of symptoms that include abdominal obesity, insulin resistance, hypertension, hyperlipidemia), chronic inflammatory diseases, elevated "high sensitive" c-reactive protein (CRP) (inflammatory marker detected at low levels with newer tests), elevated lipoprotein(a) (rare but harmful lipid) [13, 14] (see Table 4.1).

Alert: The primary risk factor of ASCVD is age; modifiable risk factors are hypertension, obesity, and diabetes.

Primary Prevention. Non-pharmacological "The most important way to prevent ASCVD, heart failure, and atrial fibrillation is to promote a healthy lifestyle throughout life" [13]. Results of numerous clinical trials confirm lifestyle interventions of routine physical activity, weight loss, and a healthy diet, e.g., Mediterranean-style diet, are effective primary preventions against ASCVD [51–54] (see Table 4.1).

Primary Prevention. Pharmacotherapy. Statins For the older adult between 65 and 75 years of age, "statin therapy represents a substantial potential for safe, effective, and inexpensive primary prevention of ASCVD" [55] especially primary prevention of a nonfatal MI [56]. Statins (atorvastatin, fluvastatin, lovastatin, pitavastatin, pravastatin, rosuvastatin, simvastatin) inhibit the activity of HMG-CoA reductase, the rate-limiting enzyme in the synthesis of cholesterol. Inhibition lowers hepatic cholesterol concentration, upregulates liver LDL receptors (more receptors to bind and internalize LDL), and enhances clearance of circulating LDL-C [57], thereby reducing elevated plasma LDL-C, now considered the causative agent of ASCVD [58]. A recent systematic review by the US Preventive Services Task Force of 22 clinical trials with 6 months to 6 years of follow-up comparing statins with placebo or no placebo or another statin observed that statin therapy for primary prevention reduced all-cause mortality and cardiovascular events but not cardiovascular deaths [59]. (See Table 4.2 for ASCVD pharmacotherapy).

Table 4.2 Age-related diseases and treatment strategies

ASCVD	Cancers	Dementias	Diabetes Mellitus
Prevention of CV events: MI, ischemic stroke, need for Revascularization, PAD, and CV death	**All types of malignancies**	**Alzheimer's disease (AD)**	**Type 2 diabetes mellitus (T2DM)**
Primary prevention: 1. Lower LDL-C: statins, ezetimibe. Bile acid sequesterants, PCSK9 inhibitors (e.g., evolocumab) 2. Treat hypertension—beta blocker, ACEI, ARB, chlorthalidone 3. Encourage lifestyle changes Secondary prevention: 4. Prevent vascular thrombosis: aspirin; P2Y12 inhibitors (e.g., clopidogrel): DOACs (e.g., dabigatran) 5. Lower TGs: icosapent ethyl	1. CGA—if possible surgery, radiation, chemotherapy 2. Chemotherapy: (a) Cytotoxic drugs; (b) Hormones/hormone antagonists; (c) Tyrosine kinase inhibitors (TKIs); (d) Immune check point inhibitors (ICIs)	1. Mild/moderate AD: Anticholinesterase inhibitors (e.g., donepezil) 2. Moderate/severe AD: add-on -NMDA receptor inhibitor (memantine) 3. Plaque-removers- β-amyloid-antibodies (e.g., lecanemab)	1. Weight loss, physical activity, healthy diet 2. CGA 3. Biguanide (metformin), DPP-4 inhibitor (e.g., sitagliptin), GLP-1 agonists (oral/SC) (e.g., semaglutide), Sulfonylureas (e.g., glyburide), SGLT2 inhibitors (e.g., dapagliflozin)

(continued)

Table 4.2 (continued)

ASCVD	Cancers	Dementias	Diabetes Mellitus
Prevention of HF	**First line treatments**	**Cerebrovascular dementias**	**First- and second-line treatments**
Stage A—treat risk factors of hypertension, T2DM, encourage lifestyle changes **Stage B**—RAS inhibitors, beta-blockers, exercise training **Stage C/D**—RAS inhibitors, β-blockers, loop diuretics, SGLT-2 inhibitors, inotrope rarely	1. Hematological cancer, breast cancers and sarcomas—cytotoxic anthracyclines 2. Early stage/advanced prostate/breast cancers—hormone/hormone antagonists 3. Non-small cell lung cancer (EGFR-mutations), chronic myelogenous leukemia (Bcr-Abl)—TKIs, 4. Non-Hodgkin lymphoma, CRC, HER2 breast cancer—mAb TKI Advanced melanoma—ICI	1. Reduce CV risk factors—smoking cessation, ↑ PA, treat T2DM, and hypertension 2. Antiplatelet drugs for stroke prevention 3. Rehabilitation?	First line—metformin Second line—sulfonylureas; SGLT2 inhibitors Unmet HbA1c target basal insulin—short-acting, long-acting, rapid-acting analogues for meals avoid hypoglycemia

ASCVD atherosclerotic cardiovascular disease, *CV* cardiovascular, *MI* myocardial infarction, *PAD* peripheral artery disease, *LDL-C* low-density lipoprotein-cholesterol, *DOAC* direct oral anticoagulant, *TG* triglyceride, *HF* heart failure, *T2DM* type 2 Diabetes Mellitus, *RAS* renin-angiotensin system, *SGLT2* sodium glucose co-transporter 2, *CGA* comprehensive geriatric assessment, *PA* physical activity, *HbA1c* hemoglobin A1c, *PCSK9* proprotein convertase subtilisin/kexin type 9, *P2Y12* platelet receptor, *ACEI* angiotensin-converting enzyme inhibitor, *ARB* angiotensin receptor blocker, *EGFR* epithelial growth factor receptor, *CRC* colorectal cancer, *ICI* immune checkpoint inhibitors, *mAb* monoclonal antibody, *TKI* tyrosine kinase inhibitor, *SC* subcutaneous↑ increase

Whether statin therapy is appropriate as primary prevention of ASCVD for individuals older than 75 years of age is controversial. This is due to the paucity of randomized clinical trials (RCTs) with predominant enrollment of older adults and concern that extrapolation of data from RCTs with mainly younger adults is risky [60]. Furthermore, American College of Cardiology (ACC)/American Heart Association (AHA) risk assessment protocol has a cutoff of 79 years of age [61]. On the one hand, an ad hoc secondary analysis of the Antihypertensive and Lipid-Lowering Treatment to Prevent Heart Attack Trial–Lipid-Lowering Trial (ALLHAT-LLT) of approximately 1400 patients on pravastatin and an equal number on usual care found no significant benefit of pravastatin on all-cause mortality or cardiovascular heart events [62]. Another RCT (PROspective study of pravastatin in the elderly at risk, PROSPER) of over 2000 patients 70–82 years in the pravastatin and placebo groups showed a significant reduction in risk of coronary heart disease death or risk of nonfatal MI but no decrease of stroke risk over a 3-year follow-up [63, 64]. With meager data, unanswered questions remain, such as the potential for increased risk of adverse reactions, likely with multiple morbidities and polypharmacy, and equally important is how to achieve the best balance between benefit and harm.

Furthermore, the criteria used to determine the initiation of statin therapy for primary prevention of ASCVD differ significantly, depending on the use of (a) ACC and AHA guidelines [65, 66], (b) RCT results, or (c) combination of risk and trial results [67]. Risk assessment is determined by rigorously developed cohort equations of evidence-based risk factors [66]. For the ACC/AHA guidelines, initiation of statin therapy depends on a $\geq 7\%$ risk in 10 years of ASCVD event and LDL-C of 70–189 mg/dl. In a test comparison of these three approaches, "the clinical performance of the ACC/AHA risk-based approach for primary prevention of ASCVD with statins was superior to the trial-based and hybrid approaches" [67].

Statins Cautions In the use of statin therapy, it is important to advise the patient of the following: (a) consumption of grapefruit juice is to be avoided since grapefruit juice contains compounds that inhibit intestinal CYP3A4, the enzyme metabolizing statins, especially atorvastatin, lovastatin, and simvastatin, resulting in higher-than-expected levels of statins in the blood, (b) routine monitoring of liver enzymes is important since statins tend to increase certain liver enzymes requiring a change to another statin, (c) a statin should be taken at night when cholesterol synthesis is highest, and (d) muscle/leg weakness, memory loss, and confusion should be reported immediately to the health care provider [68].

Primary Prevention. Pharmacotherapy. Antihypertensive Drugs To minimize the risk factor of elevated blood pressure, several antihypertensive drugs are considered successful primary preventatives. In a systematic review and meta-analysis of 58 RCTs with an average follow-up of 3 years, antihypertensive drug use was associated with reduced cardiovascular death and all-cause mortality [69]. Antihypertensive drugs include beta blockers (propranolol, metoprolol, timolol), angiotensin-converting enzyme inhibitors, ACEIs (trandolapril, enalapril, lisinopril), ARBs (losartan, valsartan, telmisartan, candesartan), and thiazide diuretic chlorthalidone [69]. Although antihypertensive drugs have been associated with an increase in the incidence of falls and fractures [70, 71], this analysis found no evidence of this independent of drug class. There was an association with antihypertensive medications and syncope (fainting), which is a serious life-threatening effect [69]. However, antihypertensive drug use is associated with acute kidney injury, hyperkalemia, hypotension, and syncope [69] related to drugs blocking the renin-angiotensin system (RAS). These potentially adverse effects of RAS inhibitors in the presence of reduced kidney function are discussed in Chap. 3.

Atherosclerotic Cardiovascular Disease. Secondary Prevention In the presence of established ASCVD, such as with a diagnosis of coronary artery disease (CAD), secondary prevention is implemented to thwart future serious cardiovascular events of MI, ischemic stroke, need for revascularization, peripheral artery disease (PAD), and cardiovascular death [72]. As with primary prevention, lifestyle choices, especially the addition of a physical rehabilitation program (or doctor-approved exercise program), are not only beneficial but cost-effective [73].

Secondary Prevention. Lipid-Lowering Drugs The principal pharmacological strategies of secondary prevention of ASCVD focus on marked lowering of circulating LDL-C and clot prevention [74, 75]. Key drug classes are the statins/other cholesterol-lowering non-statin drugs and the antiplatelet/anticoagulant drugs (see Table 4.2). Guidelines for the management of high cholesterol [74, 75] propose that LDL-C should be reduced "by at least 50% with a high intensity statins; and if necessary, to achieve LDL-C <55–70 mg/dL" [75]. Results of RCTs indicate that the greater the reduction in LDL-C, the greater the benefit in secondary prevention [75] to include a life-threatening ischemic stroke [76, 77].

Although monotherapy with statins remains the main therapy for many, adjunct therapy with other lipid-lowering drugs is needed for high-risk patients (e.g., familial hypercholesterolemia, an inherited disorder of extremely high LDL-C, or statin intolerance). Other lipid-lowering drugs that lower the risk of ASCVD and are now used in clinical practice are ezetimibe (cholesterol absorption inhibitor), bile acid sequestrants, and proprotein convertase subtilisin/kexin type 9 (PCSK9 inhibitor) [78]. All lipid-lowering drugs increase the clearance of LDL-C but by different mechanisms. Ezetimibe inhibits intestinal uptake of cholesterol by blocking the transmembrane protein (Niemann-Pick C1-Like1) [79]; bile acid sequestrants (cholestyramine, colestipol, and colesevelam) increase LDL receptor number by reduction of the enterohepatic pool of cholesterol [75, 80]; PCSK9 inhibitors (monoclonal antibodies, evolocumab, and alirocumab) prevent PCSK9 from masking LDL receptors, thereby improving LDL-C clearance [81].

Hypertriglyceridemia, the elevation of triglycerides (TGs) (neutral fats), represents an important risk factor [82]. TGs are packaged with cholesterol and found as components of very low-density lipoproteins and ultralow-density lipoproteins called chylomicrons. Lipid-lowering guidelines in the United States propose lowering hypertriglyceridemia of moderate extent (triglyceride levels 2.0–5.6 mmol/L[175–499 mg/dL]) and severe (triglyceride levels ≥5.6 mmol/L [≥500 mg/dL]) [75]. Icosapent ethyl, an omega-3 fatty acid, is a recommended adjunct to statin therapy [75].

Secondary Prevention. Lipoprotein (a) Reduction Another lipid that has received scrutiny is lipoprotein(a) (Lp(a)) because elevated levels, >125 nmol/L (50 mg/dL), are associated with ASCVD, aortic stenosis, and possibly venous thrombosis [83]. The result of the FOURIER trial (Further Cardiovascular Outcomes Research with PCSK9 Inhibition in Subjects with Elevated Risk) with a 2-year follow-up showed that evolocumab treatment lowered Lp(a) and reduced risks of coronary artery disease [83]. Several drugs to lower Lp(a) are currently in clinical trial [84].

Secondary Prevention. Antiplatelet and Anticoagulant Drugs Based on the pathophysiology of a dysfunctional endothelial layer as essential for the development and progression of ASCVD, atherothrombotic events are inevitable [85]. They include "clinical scenarios such as stable and unstable angina, acute myocardial infarction, ischemic stroke and peripheral arterial occlusive disease" [86]. Use of antiplatelet and anticoagulant drugs has reduced the risk of these major CV events [87, 88]. Antiplatelet drugs encompass aspirin and the P2Y12 inhibitors (clopidogrel, prasugrel, ticagrelor, cilostazol, and dipyridamole). P2Y12 drugs inhibit platelet aggregation by inhibition of the adenosine diphosphate platelet receptor [89]. Aspirin is an irreversible inhibitor of cyclooxygenase (COX-1) that eventually leads to a decrease in the production of thromboxane A2, a promoter of platelet activation/aggregation (early step in clotting). "Aspirin therapy is associated with reductions in serious vascular events, including stroke and coronary events, and a 10% reduction in total mortality" [90]. However, *aspirin is no longer recommended for primary prevention as a prophylactic because efficacy is poor and bleeding potential is high* (see Chap. 3). Dual antiplatelet therapy (DAPT) is successful in the avoidance of thrombotic events of ASCVD such as percutaneous coronary intervention (PCI) or surgical revascularization [88, 90]. DAPT is available for the older adult with the recommendation choice of clopidogrel rather than prasugrel or ticagrelor [91].

The direct oral anticoagulants (DOAC) (dabigatran, apixaban, rivaroxaban, and edoxaban) have generally replaced warfarin, as demonstrated by their greater efficacy in randomized clinical trials (RCTs) for the prevention and treatment of various thrombotic events, e.g., venous thromboembolism (VTE), pulmonary embolism, and cardioembolic stroke in nonvalvular atrial fibrillation [92]. DOACs disrupt the clotting cascade by blocking key factors such as factor Xa (apixaban, rivaroxaban, edoxaban) or thrombin (dabigatran) in contrast to warfarin, which antagonizes the vitamin K epoxide reductase complex [93]. Results of several RCTs observed reduced risk of bleeding with DOAC compared to warfarin [94]. Beers Criteria® proposes selection of DOAC over warfarin [95]. As with DAPT, results of the COMPASS trial showed that low-dose aspirin (100 mg) in combination with rivaroxaban (2.5 mg twice daily) reduces the risk of major cardiovascular events, such as MI, stroke, and death [96], and is approved for patients with coronary artery disease or peripheral artery disease [97].

HEART FAILURE Heart failure (HF) results from the inability to supply adequate amounts of oxygenated blood to peripheral tissues, either due to inadequate ventricular filling or reduced ejection of blood by the ventricles [98]. This is the progressive outcome of heart muscle, structurally or functionally damaged by any number of factors such as ASCVD, hypertension, T2DM, resulting in reduced cardiac output and pulmonary vascular congestion that eventually defies therapy [99].

"Heart failure is a major cause of mortality, hospitalizations, and reduced quality of life and a major burden for the healthcare system" [100]. The ACC/AHA/Heart Failure Society of America (HFSA) guidelines separate HF into four stages: *Stage A*, at risk for HF; *Stage B*, preheart HF; *Stage C*, symptomatic HF; and *Stage D*, advanced HF [98].

Heart Failure. Pharmacotherapy Pharmacological management (see Table 4.2) for *Stage A* is directed at HF risk factor reduction that includes antihypertensive drugs for hypertension and SGLT2 inhibitors for treatment of T2DM. Management of normal weight, healthy diet, adequate physical exercise [101], and smoking cessation are encouraged in *Stage A*.

Stage B identifies structural changes that may accelerate asymptomatic HF to symptomatic Stage C/D. Drugs of value in this stage are the RAS inhibitors and the β-blockers (carvedilol). Both ACEI (e.g., enalapril) and beta-blockers (e.g., carvedilol) are recommended for asymptomatic left ventricular (LV) dysfunction after an MI where LV ejection fraction is $\leq 40\%$. The success of these two classes of drugs is attributed to their ability to prevent abnormal cardiac remodeling and reduce hospitalizations. Avoidance of antidiabetic thiazolidinediones (TZD; e.g., rosiglitazone) and calcium channel blockers (e.g., diltiazem) is recommended as these drugs offer no benefit.

Exercise training is strongly recommended in HF *Stage C* because results of numerous randomized clinical trials (RCTs) show clear benefit in decreasing cardiovascular (CV) mortality and hospitalizations and improving QoL. Drugs of value are loop diuretics (bumetanide, furosemide, and torsemide) in relieving congestion or fluid retention. RAS inhibitors (ACEI, ARB, and angiotensin receptor neprilysin inhibitor, ARNI) are recommended with a preference for ARNI (sacubitril-valsartan, a combination of ARB and ARNI) that achieves inhibition of angiotensin and numerous other vasoactive peptides. The outcome is improvement in survivability and reduction in hospitalizations in symptomatic HF with reduced ejection fraction compared to enalapril alone. Beta-blockers, specifically bisoprolol, sustained-release metoprolol (succinate), and carvedilol are also recommended as is the SGLT2 inhibitor (dapagliflozin) with or without diabetes since it reduces hospitalizations, CV deaths, and all-cause mortality.

In *Stage D*, advanced HF with hypotension or hypoperfusion, inotropes (drugs to enhance cardiac contractility) are used cautiously [102] and as a bridge to other therapies (assist circulatory devices or heart transplant) in those with end organ hypoperfusion and refractory to other therapies.

Atherosclerotic Cardiovascular Disease. Adverse Drug Reactions Statins, first approved by the FDA in 1987, remain the most effective drugs to lower LDL-C [103, 104]. Potentially adverse myotoxicities, e.g., myopathy (muscle weakness), myalgia (muscle pain), myositis (muscle inflammation), or the rare but life-threatening rhabdomyolysis (breakdown of muscle tissue, huge increase in creatine kinase), are largely related to higher-than-expected concentrations of statins [105]. Statins are also associated with a modest diabetogenic effect observed in patients with prediabetes or metabolic syndrome [106]. However, the cardiovascular benefits of statins outweigh this adverse effect [106]. Drugs such as protease inhibitors, cyclosporine (immunosuppressant), amiodarone (anti-arrhythmic), and some fibrates, known to interfere with the metabolism and transport of statins, should be avoided.

Although antiplatelet and anticoagulant therapy is essential for secondary prevention of ASCVD, the concern for a major bleeding event is real. Additive or synergistic effects are likely when two drugs in these classes are used concurrently. Importantly, in the presence of reduced kidney function, factor Xa inhibitors (edoxaban, rivaroxaban) and direct thrombin inhibitors (dabigatran) should be avoided [95].

In guideline-directed medical therapy for HF, drugs from several drug classes have been shown in RCTs to reduce hospitalizations and CV deaths [100]. Nevertheless, the resulting polypharmacy is of concern. Beers Criteria® recommends that drugs that promote water retention should be avoided. These are non-dihydropyridine calcium channel blockers (diltiazem, verapamil), COX-2 inhibitor (celecoxib), and nonsteroidal anti-inflammatory drugs (e.g., ibuprofen, naproxen). Other drugs to be avoided in HF are the anti-arrhythmic drug dronedarone, which worsens HF with Q-T prolongation, the antiplatelet drug cilostazol, and the combination of dextromethorphan-quinidine, both of which increase HF mortality. Additionally, the thiazolidinediones, e.g., pioglitazone, rosiglitazone offer no benefit in HF [95, 98]. Renin-angiotensin system (RAS) inhibitors are important in therapy of HF because they prevent cardiac remodeling. However, they should not be combined with potassium-sparing diuretics (amiloride, spironolactone) due to the risk of hyperkalemia highly associated with arrhythmias and death [95]. RAS inhibitors can produce angioedema (edema of skin and mucous membranes due to increased vascular permeability) that may be life-threatening [107].

Malignancies

CANCERS. Prevalence and Incidence "Cancer is the second-leading cause of death in the United States overall" [108]. Assessing literature data from 2011 to 2016, the prevalence and incidence of cancer increase with age up to 85–89 years with a declining rate thereafter [109]. Incidence varies among cancer types, gender, and ethnicities [110]. More than half of all newly diagnosed cancers in developed countries are in the older adult ≥65 years of age [111]. Despite age as the major risk factor for cancer, and a growing older population, new diagnosis in those ≥65 years decreased from 61% (1995) to 58% (2019–2020), possibly due to a reduced incidence of prostate and smoking-related cancers in older men [108]. Cancers producing the most deaths in the older population, ≥65 years of age, are lung, prostate, colorectal (CRC), and pancreas for men and lung, breast, CRC, and pancreas for women [108].

Cancers. Pathophysiology The words "malignancies" and "cancers" are used interchangeably, as are cancer and neoplastic cells. They define a disease characterized by loss of cell cycle control mechanisms [112]. Cell cycle refers to stages of cell division that are tightly regulated to assure a final product of two identical daughter cells. In contrast, cancer cells divide continuously, uncontrollably, and spread throughout tissues because they express "core hallmark capabilities" [113] identified as capabilities to (1) produce ongoing proliferative signals that encourage cell division, (2) evade growth suppressors exerted by tumor suppressors such as P53 [114], (3) defy cell death signals generally called apoptosis, (4) divide indefinitely, (5) penetrate the vasculature via cell migration to create metastases, (6) alter cell metabolism to benefit the cancer cell survival, and (7) avoid immunological surveillance and potential obliteration [113].

Cancers. Risk Factors Based on findings from data-driven analytical approaches and theory-driven models for carcinogenesis, risk factors may be viewed as intrinsic (due to mutations in DNA replication) and non-intrinsic factors (both endogenous occurring within the body and exogenous or external) [25]. Figure 4.1 provides specifics that show cancer risk is multifactorial, encompassing both modifiable (fully or partially) and non-modifiable factors [25].

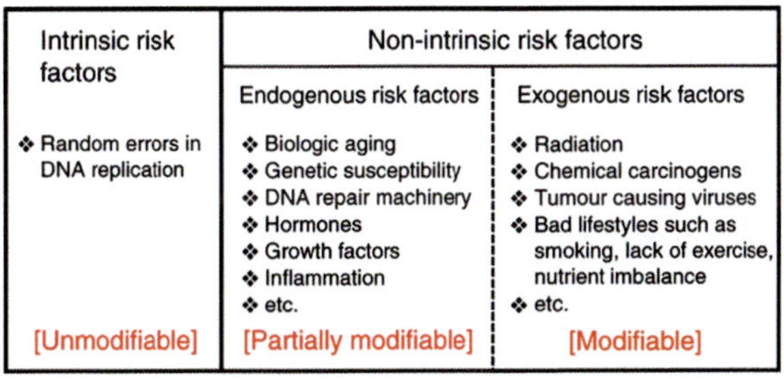

Intrinsic risk factors	Non-intrinsic risk factors	
	Endogenous risk factors	Exogenous risk factors
❖ Random errors in DNA replication	❖ Biologic aging ❖ Genetic susceptibility ❖ DNA repair machinery ❖ Hormones ❖ Growth factors ❖ Inflammation ❖ etc.	❖ Radiation ❖ Chemical carcinogens ❖ Tumour causing viruses ❖ Bad lifestyles such as smoking, lack of exercise, nutrient imbalance ❖ etc.
[Unmodifiable]	[Partially modifiable]	[Modifiable]

Fig. 4.1 Three types of cancer risk factors. The overall cancer risk factors are divided into two mutually exclusive components: the unmodifiable intrinsic and the modifiable, at least partially, non-intrinsic risk factors. The intrinsic risk factors refer to random errors resulting from DNA replication. The non-intrinsic risk factors further consist of endogenous and exogenous risk factors depending on whether such factors are more internal or external to an individual. (Ref. [25] licensed under Commons Attribution 4.0 International License)

Clearly, the major risk factor for cancer is age [115]. One explanation for this is the overlap between the hallmarks of cancer and the hallmarks of aging (see Chap. 10), e.g., changes such as genomic instability, deregulated nutrient sensing [3] and the continuous production of senescent cells that secrete pro-tumor factors [115–117]. Additionally, a key cell function, termed autophagy, associated with tumor suppression, declines with age [118]. Autophagy is the efficient recycling of damaged proteins and organelles by other organelles termed lysosomes, to prevent further harm to healthy cell components [119, 120]. Another age-related change that creates a vulnerability to malignancies is immunosenescence. Complex changes occur over time in both natural (innate) and adaptive (T and B-cell dependent) immunity that decrease important activities of immunological surveillance (chronic tumor cell detection) and cytotoxicity (immediate killing) of an aberrant cell [121]. The loss of these functions permits tumor cell proliferation and the onset of a malignancy [121, 122].

Modifiable factors causally linked to cancers include "smoking and lung cancer, sun exposure and skin cancer, human papillomavirus (HPV) and cervical cancer, Helicobacter pylori (H. pylori) and gastric cancer, and viral hepatitis and hepatocellular cancer" [25]. Modifiable risk factors noted by the CDC include active and passive smoking, overweight and obesity, high alcohol consumption, and infectious diseases. All of these significantly increase the risk of cancer. Specifically, active smoking accounts for 80–90% of lung cancer deaths, and overweight and obesity are linked to 13 types of cancer including uterine, breast, and CRC cancers [123, 124]. Risk factors do not act alone [25, 124]. Risk factors are influenced by epigenetic changes (changes in DNA expression via alteration in the protein milieu around DNA) [125], tumor suppressor genes, e.g., p53 [114], and the role of stem cells in modulating risk factors [126].

> *Alert*: The modifiable risk factors for cancer are active and passive smoking, obesity, high alcohol consumption, and infectious diseases.

Cancers. Pharmacological Treatments Treatment for malignancies in young individuals is aggressive surgery, chemotherapy, and radiation [127]. However, these approaches represent significant hurdles for the older adult who might not have the physiological reserve to handle this approach [128, 129]. Therefore, cancer therapy for the older adult is challenging. Unfortunately, because older adults have been largely excluded from clinical cancer trials (especially those >75 years of age), validated treatment therapies are sparse.

Cancers. Comprehensive Geriatric Assessment An inclusive systematic review concluded that a *Comprehensive Geriatric Assessment (CGA) is the most successful approach to achieve the best outcomes for the older patient with cancer* [129]. Successes of a CGA include improved communications and discussion of goals-of-care, lower toxicity and complication rates, enhanced likelihood of treatment completion, and improved physical functioning and quality of life (QoL) [129].

The CGA is a rigorous assessment of physical health, functional status, psychological well-being, and socioeconomic factors [128, 130]. The following domains are evaluated: comorbidities and assessment of risk factors; functional status using activities of daily living (ADL, e.g., independent feeding, bathing, toileting, dressing) and instrumental activities of daily living (IADL, e.g., shopping, preparing food, handling finances); physical status (battery of physical activities, [131]; cognitive performance (validated screening tests, [132]); psychological and socioeconomic support; nutritional status; and medications. If a patient has no or few ADL issues, full aggressive drug therapy is considered possible. Clinical assessment needs to be repeated frequently, and special attention needs to be paid to areas of cognition, pain/thermal sensitivity, and cardiac function. Dose reduction is reasonable, and therapies including the use of growth factors for hematopoietic depression, cytoprotective drugs, and prophylactic antibiotics in association with cytotoxic drugs are acceptable. For patients with reduced functional reserve or frail individuals (see Chap. 7 geriatric syndromes), the possibility of therapy-induced toxicity must be considered, and the alternative of palliative therapy and maintenance would be an option [128, 130].

Cancers. Pharmacotherapy Cancer treatment for the older adult (see Table 4.2) should be based on an assessment of the physiology, psychology, and social environment of the individual and not on chronological age [128, 130]. The best outcomes occur when this is matched with complete understanding of the malignancy, its characteristics related to growth, invasiveness, and drug resistance in the context of the older environment. Where possible, genomics (profiles) of patient, tumors, and healthy tissue assist with the determination of the correct drug, the correct dose, and better safety [133].

There are four major groups of anticancer drugs: (1) cytotoxic drugs (alkylating agents, antimetabolites, antitumor antibiotics, plant extracts, and miscellaneous cytotoxic drugs), (2) hormones and hormone antagonists (estrogen/androgen antagonists), (3) target-based agents (tyrosine kinase (TK) receptor/non-receptor inhibitors), and (4) immuno-modulators (enabling T-cell anticancer functions) (see Table 4.2).

Cytotoxic Drugs Cytotoxic drugs were the early anticancer drugs. Cytotoxic drugs inhibit rapidly dividing cells, both neoplastic and normal. Toxicity is high and generally dose-related. Cytotoxic drugs exert diverse actions on DNA, RNA, and metabolic cell function to prevent cell division and enhance cell death [134]. Examples are alkylating compounds with reactive nitrogen and sulfur, e.g., busulfan, cyclophosphamide. Alkylating drugs combine chemically with DNA and proteins to cause cell death. Other important alkylating agents are the platinum analogs, e.g., carboplatin, cisplatin, oxaliplatin, that are highly successful in treating a range of solid tumors. Additional cytotoxic drugs are the antimetabolites, e.g., methotrexate (folic acid antagonist), 5-fluorouracil (prodrug with multiple activities blocking RNA/DNA synthesis/function), gemcitabine (blocks nucleotide and nucleic acid synthesis). The anthracyclines or antitumor antibiotics, e.g., doxorubicin, epirubicin, mitomycin, dactinomycin, bleomycin, idarubicin, exert multiple actions to inhibit cell division but also generate damaging reactive radicals. Anthracyclines remain highly effective and are first-line treatment options for hematological cancers (leukemias, lymphomas), breast cancers and sarcomas (tumors in bone and soft tissue) in patients of all ages [135]. The cytotoxic plant derivatives consist of taxanes, e.g., paclitaxel, docetaxel, that perturb mitotic spindle formation needed for cell division, vinblastine and vincristine that disrupt microtubule formation essential for cell division, and epipodophyllotoxins, e.g., etoposide, teniposide, that block the enzyme, topoisomerase II, late in cell division causing DNA damage and cell death [134].

Hormones and Hormone Antagonists Another class of anticancer drugs is the hormones and hormone antagonists [134]. Examples of hormones are leuprolide and goserelin, the synthetic peptide analogs of endogenous gonadotropin-releasing hormone. By effectively manipulating levels of pituitary hormones, follicle-stimulating hormone (FSH) and luteinizing hormone (LH), these hormones dramatically lower testosterone levels and are used in the treatment of advanced prostate cancer. Hormone antagonists include the antiestrogen drug, tamoxifen, that inhibits the estrogen receptor and is beneficial in the treatment of early stage and metastatic breast cancer. The aromatase inhibitors, e.g., aminoglutethimide, anastrozole, and letrozole block the first step in the conversion of cholesterol to pregnenolone resulting in complete inhibition of estrone and estradiol synthesis. Aromatase inhibitors are of benefit in estrogen receptor-positive metastatic breast cancer in postmenopausal women. Antiandrogens, flutamide, and bicalutamide inhibit androgenic effects and are used in the treatment of early stage and metastatic prostate cancer.

Targeted Therapies Targeted therapies are of more recent vintage. In this category are the small molecules that inhibit tyrosine kinases (TKs), both receptor or non-receptor tyrosine kinases. From 2001 to 2019, the FDA approved 43 tyrosine kinase inhibitors (TKIs) [136]. TKs are important targets because they are key regulators of normal and abnormal cell function [136]. Inhibition of TKs leads to the cessation of cell division and other related activities such as angiogenesis (initiation of blood vessel formation) [136]. TKIs are effective therapies in cancers where TKs are overexpressed or aberrant and hence abnormally controlling cell function. TKIs (erlotinib, gefitinib, and afatinib or osimertinib) are first-line therapy for non-small cell lung cancers (NSCLC) with epidermal growth factor receptor (EGFR)-activating mutations [136]. A long-term success is the treatment of chronic myelogenous leukemia (a hematopoietic stem cell cancer) (CML) inhibited with the first generation of TKIs (ibrutinib). Ibrutinib blocks the oncoprotein, Bcr-Abl kinase in CML [136].

Inhibition of TKs with infusion of humanized monoclonal antibodies (mAbs) is another approach of targeted therapy. This therapy is successful because it offers greater specificity for the target and has the potential to exert additional anticancer effects [137]. Antibodies are unique proteins produced by immune B cells following activation on binding to a specific antigen. The normal function of antibodies is to enhance the destruction of pathogens as well as tumors [137]. Anticancer mAbs (although made commercially) act in the same fashion, and so the FDA has approved a number for anticancer mAb therapies (see list in [137]). Rituximab successfully treats non-Hodgkin's lymphoma by blocking CD20 kinase, panitumumab is used in CRC by blocking the EGFR and trastuzumab and pertuzumab are of value in the treatment of human epidermal growth factor 2 (HER2) kinase-dependent breast cancer [137]. Although the aforementioned mAbs act as cytotoxic effectors, most mAbs are weak anticancer drugs and are used conjugated to toxic compounds([137].

Immune Checkpoint Inhibitors The fourth class of anticancer drugs is the immune checkpoint inhibitors (ICIs). ICIs are antibodies designed to interrupt specific immune mechanisms that serve to control immune cell activity and hence preserve self-tolerance and prevent secondary tissue damage [138]. ICIs liberate immune cells in multiple ways to aggressively destroy cancer cells. Checkpoints targeted with ICIs are cytotoxic T lymphocyte antigen 4 (CTLA-4) (ipilimumab, tremelimumab), used successfully for advanced melanoma, and programmed death receptor-1 (PD-1) (pembrolizumab, nivolumab, cemiplimab) and its ligand (PDL-1) (atezolizumab, avelumab, durvalumab) used to treat advanced melanoma and other solid cancers [139].

CANCERS. ADVERSE DRUG REACTIONS All anticancer therapies, whether targeted or non-targeted, produce toxicities, acute and delayed, some appearing years after completing therapy [140, 141]. Toxicities of conventional chemotherapy are well known and are inevitable due to the intrinsic biological toxicity of inhibiting and killing rapidly dividing cells, normal and neoplastic. Expected toxicities are gastrointestinal toxicity, e.g., mucositis (inflammation of the GI tract), nausea, vomiting, diarrhea, and constipation contributed in part by a perturbed microbiota [142], neuropathies, e.g., neuropathic pain, numbness, motor dysfunction [143], cardiovascular toxicities, e.g., QT prolongation, heart failure [144], dermatological toxicities of skin, hair, and nails [145], hormone impairment/infertility, nephrotoxicity [146], and myelosuppression, e.g., anemia (decreased red blood cell production), neutropenia or granulocytopenia (decreased white cell production) and thrombocytopenia (decreased platelet production) [147]. These toxicities are managed with dose reduction/delays and supportive care where possible such as hematopoietic growth factors/blood transfusions for myelosuppression [148].

TKIs are associated with a number of serious cardiopulmonary toxicities to include QT prolongation, torsade de pointes (rare ventricular arrhythmia), cardiac arrhythmias, heart failure, pleural effusion (fluid around lungs), and pulmonary hypertension [149]. Compared to other anticancer drugs, "cardiovascular events were more frequent with TKIs" [149]. The mechanism of this toxicity is not fully understood but it may be related to on-target effects, off-target actions affecting a range of other TKs, genetic predisposition, and the presence of cardiovascular risk factors. The latter two issues should be assessed prior to the use of TKIs.

Cancers. Multidrug Resistance A major barrier to successful chemotherapy is multidrug resistance (MDR). MDR is "a kind of acquired resistance of microorganisms and cancer cells to chemotherapeutic drugs that are characterized by different chemical structures and different mechanisms of action" [150]. MDR is responsible for 90% of deaths in advanced cancers [151]. MDR is associated with metastases and reoccurrence of tumors with long-term therapy [150]. MDR develops in tumors in several ways: by overexpression of membrane transporters, e.g., P-glycoprotein (MDR1, ABCB1) and multidrug resistance-associated protein (MRP) that transport drugs out of cells preventing efficacy; by blocking drug uptake into tumor cells; and/or by metabolism of the drug with enhancement of P450 enzymes within the tumor cell [150].

Different resistance mechanisms limit the efficacy of TKIs and mAbs. Tumor cells innately have mutations that circumvent targeted therapy or readily produce mutations within the antibody target. Resistance may occur when tumor cells acquire new signal pathways or become migratory (metastasize) by changing from epithelial to mesenchymal cells [137]. Targeted mAbs also produce immune-related adverse events (AE)—some life-threatening, e.g., encephalopathy, pneumonia, nephritis (inflammation of the kidneys), hepatitis (liver inflammation), myocarditis (heart inflammation), and colitis (inflammation of the colon). Other reported AEs include fatigue, musculoskeletal pain, decreased appetite, pruritus (itchy skin), diarrhea, nausea, rash, pyrexia (elevated body temperature), cough, dyspnea (shortness of breath), constipation, pain, and abdominal pain [139].

In consideration of drug-induced toxicities and resistance, treatment trends are favoring combinations of two mAbs or combinations of mAbs with TKI, ICIs, cytotoxic agents, and radiation [137]. Currently, a retrospective meta-analysis of clinical trials concluded that the combination of cetuximab (mAb) and a PD-1 inhibitor is more effective compared with PD-1 inhibitor monotherapy in patients with human papillomavirus-negative head and neck squamous cell carcinoma [114]. Future improvements in chemotherapy are expected to benefit from research on the role of the microbiota in chemotherapy from efficacy to toxicity [152] and development of nanoparticles to deliver drugs without eliciting resistance while reducing toxicity [150].

Alzheimer's Disease and Related Dementias

ALZHEIMER'S DISEASE AND RELATED DEMENTIAS. Introduction De mentia is the umbrella term for the brain disease in which there is a progressive and eventual global loss of brain function. Cognitive functions of memory, intellect, judgment, and executive function gradually diminish. Alzheimer's disease (AD) is the most common type of dementia with a defined set of symptoms and biomarkers. It comprises slightly over half of all irreversible dementias. Other irreversible dementias are cerebrovascular-dependent (20–30%) due to multiple infarctions, atherosclerosis, or cerebral small vessel disease (CSVD), frontotemporal degeneration (FTD) (3%) due to nerve death and temporal (side lobes) shrinkage, hippocampal sclerosis (3–13%) due to scarring/shrinkage of the hippocampal region, and Lewy body dementia (LBD) (5%) due to the accumulation of aberrant protein deposits in nerves [20]. The majority of AD patients have mixed neuropathologies, presenting with more than one type of dementia [153].

Alzheimer's Disease. Prevalence and Incidence As of 2023, about 6.7 million older adults in the United States are living with AD dementia. This number is expected to double by the year 2060 [20]. Using several sources (Chicago Health and Aging Project, a population-based health conditions project and US census demographic projection data 2020–2060), the prevalence of AD was estimated at 5.3% (65–74 years), 13.8% (75–84 years), and 34.5% ($\geq$85 years) [154]. AD prevalence increases with age. Estimates relative to race/ethnicity show that the prevalence of AD is highest in African Americans, followed by Hispanics and Non-Hispanic whites with the lowest estimate [154]. The prevalence of AD from 2020 to 2060 is expected to double or nearly double in all age groups $\geq$65 years [154]. All prevalence estimates are based on clinical symptoms and not on AD validated pathological brain changes [20].

The number of newly diagnosed AD cases estimated per year as of 2011 and 2015 is 0.4% ($\geq$65–74 years), 3.2% ($\geq$75–84 years), and 7.6% ($\geq$ 85 years) [154, 155]. By 2050, AD incidence is expected to double [156]. There is controversy surrounding the trends in falling AD prevalence and incidence over the past 25 years [20]. These changes are attributed to greater awareness and reduction in AD risk factors, especially cardiovascular risk factors [20].

Alzheimer's Disease. Pathophysiology The brain is comprised of billions of interconnected neurons and supporting cells, microglia, astrocytes, and oligodendrocytes. Information is relayed through a multiplicity of nerve impulses, generating the basis of cognition. Nerves communicate with one another through small molecules, i.e., neurotransmitters, released from the terminus of one neuron, diffuse across a small space (synapse), and interact with the dendrites (extensions with receptors) of another neuron. AD and related dementias (ADRD) interfere with this complex network.

The exact etiology of AD is not known. However, three prominent changes in the brain are considered hallmarks of the disease [21]. They are beta-amyloid (Aβ) plaques, phosphorylated tau fibrillar tangles, and neurodegeneration. These are considered biomarkers of AD and are used in conjunction with clinical symptoms of cognitive loss to determine a diagnosis. Among the biomarkers, Aβ plaques provide the most definitive diagnosis of AD [21]. Aβ plaques arise outside the nerve from normal synaptic production and secretion of the amyloid precursor protein that is subsequently cleaved into Aβ peptides [157]. Why Aβ peptides aggregate to form plaques that eventually induce inflammation [158] and neuronal death [159] is not clear. Therapeutic strategies to prevent Aβ formation, aggregation, and inflammation have been generally unsuccessful [157].

The presence of extracellular Aβ plaques is necessary for the formation of intracellular phosphorylated tau fibrillar tangles [160]. In contrast to Aβ aggregation, the progression of tau pathology correlates well with the clinical progression of AD, suggesting that tau pathology is the requisite driver of neurodegeneration [160–162]. Tau is a soluble protein produced within neurons. Once produced, it is modified in many ways, one of which is by phosphorylation. Its function is unknown, although it has binding sites for neuronal microtubules, and when highly phosphorylated, tau aggregates to disrupt microtubules [160]. Aggregates are mobile and prion-like and hence migrate to the neocortex to accelerate cognitive decline [163].

One significant contribution to the pathology of AD comes from apolipoprotein E (ApoE). Many studies of different types verified that ApoE is the strongest risk factor for late-onset AD [164]. ApoE is a lipoprotein produced in the liver and brain (astrocytes, microglia) to assist with the transport of lipids and cholesterol. There are three variants: ApoE e2, ApoE e3, and ApoE e4. The highest risk of AD occurs with the inheritance of two copies of ApoE e4 (12-fold increase) while inheritance of ApoE e2 is protective [165].

Alzheimer's Disease. Assessment. Brain Imaging Many of the pathological changes of AD are observed with imaging technology. Positron emission tomography (PET) is used to identify amyloid deposits in the brain; 18-fluorodeoxyglucose (18F-FDG-PET) follows the extent of change in brain metabolism associated with AD; the magnetic resonance imaging (MRI) is used to measure medial temporal lobe atrophy associated with AD; and Tau-PET uses tau binding ligands to track the development of tau pathology [21]. Another validated test is the measurement of secreted Aβ42 in the cerebrospinal fluid. Patients with AD, mild cognitive impairment (MCI), and preclinical AD diagnosis exhibit reduced amounts of Aβ42 peptides correlated with increased amounts remaining in brain plaques [166].

Alzheimer's Disease. Assessment. Clinical Signs The clinical signs of AD are progressive, beginning with preclinical AD [20]. Preclinical AD is characterized by the presence of biomarkers, e.g., Aβ deposits in PET scans, but no evidence of memory loss attributed to neuronal compensation. MCI is characterized by the presence of biomarkers in addition to very modest loss of memory and thinking ability. Progression to dementia is variable with about 15% and 30% advancing to dementia in 2 and 5 years, respectively. Dementia is characterized by the presence of biomarkers as discussed above and progressively worsening degrees of cognitive impairment. In mild dementia, patients are fairly independent but may require some help on complicated tasks but generally keep daily routines. Patients with moderate dementia struggle with instrumental activities of daily living (IADLs), e.g., shopping, preparing food, handling finances, have worsening memory and language, may experience emotional and behavioral changes, and may not recognize loved ones. Patients with severe dementia require constant care, verbalize little, are less mobile (more bed-bound), and eventually have difficulty swallowing, creating the potential of aspiration pneumonia [20]. Patients may be successfully cared for at home during the early and intermediate stages of AD, but later stages with the occurrence of behavior disorders and major organ system changes require nursing care [20].

Alzheimer's Disease. Risk Factors A key risk factor for AD is advanced age [21]. It is noted that AD changes differ from normal aging in several respects. In normal aging, the variable changes in cognition, e.g., decrease in processing speed, changes in semantic and short-term memory, and reduced focus, may be minimized with positive neuroplasticity (engagement in serious activities that stimulate the brain) [167]. However, as with all diseases, the hallmarks of aging create the vulnerability to disease [3, 4]. Measurable age changes are the conversion of normal brain cells to senescent ones [168] resulting in a decrease in neurogenesis (development of new neurons), loss of dendrites (neuronal extensions accepting incoming information), decrease in synaptic plasticity (reduced connectivity among neurons), and increased apoptosis (cell death) [169].

Another age change relates to the functional decline in the brain's lymphatic drainage system primarily failing to remove waste products (Aβ peptides and other metabolic toxins) from the brain to the peripheral lymphatic system [170]. This drainage system includes meningeal (membranes surrounding the brain), the glymphatics (a glia-dependent system connecting the blood, interstitial fluid around cells and the cerebrospinal fluid) and drainage sites in other spaces such as the basement membrane of cerebral arteries [170, 171]. The lymphatic outflow rate of this system declines with age [171, 172]. Since the brain filtration system works mostly during sleep, a causal relation between sleep disturbances and neurodegenerative diseases exists via impact on eventual buildup of metabolic toxins [22]. Thus, sleep impairments are positioned as a risk factor for AD. Based on studies in normal volunteers and animals, sleep reduction (slow-wave decrease or sleep deprivation in animals) results in decreases in cerebral spinal fluid Aβ peptides (reduction in brain clearance of toxins) [21, 173].

Specific genetic changes elevate the risk of AD. As referenced above, a key risk factor for AD is the expression of ApoE e4 variant (discussed above) and a family history of AD [20]. Depending on the study type, 56–65% of patients with diagnosed AD expressed at least one copy of ApoE e4 [20]. Down syndrome (trisomy 21) is associated with an increased risk of AD, explained by the presence of an extra chromosome 21 on which the gene producing amyloid proteins is located [174]. A family history of one or more close relatives with AD confers a high risk of AD [175].

Approximately one-third of AD and related dementia (ADRD) are statistically associated with modifiable risk factors. In data collected from a self-reported survey (US Behavioral Risk Factor Surveillance Survey) over one year (2018), eight modifiable risk factors were identified [23]. The three factors of highest risk were midlife obesity, physical inactivity, and low education. Other modifiable risk factors were depression, diabetes, hearing loss, midlife hypertension, and smoking [23] (see Table 4.3 Risk Factors).

Table 4.3 Risk factors and Interventions for Alzheimer's disease and related dementias

Risk factors	Interventions
Non-modifiable [20, 21] Age APOE e4 gene presence Family history of dementias	Awareness; genetic testing
Modifiable [22–24] Hearing Loss Inadequate sleep Midlife obesity Physical inactivity Low education Depression Diabetes Hypertension Smoking	Lifestyle choices Hearing aids 7–9 hours continuous sleep per night Weight loss Exercise program Intellectually stimulating activities Counseling Above plus healthy diet or drug therapy Lifestyle changes or drug therapy Smoking cessation

Self-reported data tends to underestimate the contribution of hearing loss to ADRD, which elevates it as the most important modifiable risk factor [24]. Data from observational studies, e.g., the National Health and Aging Trends Study (annual in-home interviews of community-dwelling older adult over 5-year period) [24] and meta-analysis of nine prospective cohort studies over a 10-year period [176], found that the prevalence of dementia was significantly associated with the severity of the hearing loss and that the use of hearing aids reduced prevalence, hence reducing the risk of dementia [24]. Furthermore, hearing loss accelerated the rate of cognitive decline [176]. At present, the mechanism for this is speculative but it essentially points to a loss of cognitive reserve with hearing loss that increases a vulnerability to "to functional impairment secondary to existing neuropathological damage" [177].

> *Alert*: Four of the highest modifiable risk factors of Alzheimer's Disease are midlife obesity, physical inactivity, low education and uncorrected hearing loss.

Alzheimer's Disease. Pharmacotherapy *There is no cure for AD*. At best, cognitive decline is slowed by treatment with drugs that promote the survival of the neurotransmitter, acetylcholine (see Table 4.2). Cholinergic neurons (those making acetylcholine) are essential for memory and related cognitive activities and these neurons, identified on autopsy, are the ones damaged by amyloid plaques and neurofibrillary tangles [178].

Alzheimer's Disease. Anticholinesterase Inhibitors The most frequently prescribed drug for AD is donepezil (Aricept). Donepezil is an anticholinesterase inhibitor and acts by blocking the enzyme that degrades acetylcholine [179]. In addition to donepezil, there are galantamine and rivastigmine with the latter also blocking butyrylcholinesterase [179]. Donepezil, a short-acting reversible inhibitor, is used for mild to moderate AD and has benefit in ameliorating the pathological progression of AD [180] but produces a range of adverse effects (insomnia, nausea, loss of appetite, diarrhea, muscle cramps, and muscle weakness) [181]. Galantamine (short-acting, reversible) and rivastigmine (longer-acting, somewhat irreversible) have side effects similar to donepezil, e.g., nausea, stomach cramps, muscle weakness but may also cause convulsions, confusion, and watering eyes [182, 183]. The overall efficacy of these compounds is considered modest at best [184].

Memantine Another drug used to treat AD is memantine. Memantine inhibits the N-methyl-D-aspartate (NMDA) receptor and is used in moderate/severe AD to reduce the neurodegenerative effects of the neurotransmitter, glutamate [185]. A meta-analysis of 54 clinical trials (Asia, Europe, North America) combining memantine with donepezil found the combination produced "superior outcomes in cognition, global assessment, daily activities and neuropsychiatric symptoms" compared to monotherapy or placebo [186]. Although the outcomes were better for the combination therapy and adverse effects were similar, patient preference was for monotherapy with memantine [186]. Remaining therapy entails addressing the development of new behavioral and physiological changes as they appear.

Monoclonal Antibodies Two drugs, lecanemab (2023) and donanemab (2024), recently FDA and Medicare approved, are the first to target the reduction of the proposed cause of AD, the amyloid plaques [187, 188]. Both drugs are monoclonal antibodies directed at Aβ protein deposits. They were evaluated in numerous randomized clinical trials, in patients with early MCI or dementia (average age 70 years, some difference in races/ethnicities). Cognition was assessed at baseline and 18 months later with the clinical dementia rating scale that incorporates evaluations of cognitive domains of memory, orientation, judgment/problem-solving, in conjunction with functional domains of community affairs, home/hobbies, personal care. Both drugs dose-dependently decreased Aβ plaques and slowed cognitive decline by 27% (lecanemab) and 22% (donanemab) over 1.5 years. Approximately 20–30% of patients experience serious adverse effects that include amyloid-related image abnormalities (ARIA) of brain swelling, effusions, and spotty bleeding [188]. Other similar drugs are in development that may offer greater slowing of cognitive loss and a reduction in adverse effects.

CEREBROVASCULAR DEMENTIA Cerebrovascular dementia (VaD) is the second most common type of dementia ([189]. VaD is vascular brain damage caused by ischemia, infarction, or hemorrhage [190]. These are insults induced by atherosclerosis (affecting large arteries), arteriosclerosis (affecting medium-sized arteries), cerebral amyloid angiography (Aβ plaques around pia mater membrane and cortical arteries and capillaries), and microvascular disease (affecting capillaries) [190].

Results of structural and functional neuroimaging reveal the heterogeneity of VaD and its overlap with AD as well as the complexity of cognitive loss based on variations in VaD-induced brain network disruptions [190]. Neuroimaging defines the affected brain regions and explains the cognitive impairments. This information plus the reduction of cardiovascular risk factors is the essence of successful therapy. The main risk factors for VaD are smoking, hypertension, diabetes, and physical inactivity. Additionally, possession of the APOE e4 gene is another important risk factor contributing to cerebral amyloid angiography.

Cerebrovascular Dementia. Assessment The type and degree of cognitive loss vary with the affected brain region. Assessment into one of four phenotypic categories seems helpful. They are subcortical ischemic vascular dementia with marked reduction in executive function, post-stroke dementia affecting language/memory with immediate (or within 6 months) onset and no recovery, multi-infarct dementia causing apraxia (inability to response with movements), aphasia (difficulty understanding language), and visual field cut (normal visual field reduced) and mixed dementia with the co-existence of AD and VaD [190].

Cerebrovascular Dementia. Pharmacotherapy Therapy is focused on identification and reduction of cardiovascular risk factors. Secondary prevention of stroke with antiplatelet therapy is important but the use of anticholinesterase drugs or memantine is controversial, with none to modest efficacy [190]. Rehabilitation cognitive strategies may improve some aspects of cognitive loss [191].

Type 2 Diabetes Mellitus

Type 2 Diabetes Mellitus. Introduction The World Health Organization (WHO) defines diabetes as a "chronic, metabolic disease characterized by elevated levels of blood glucose (or blood sugar), which leads over time to serious damage to the heart, blood vessels, eyes, kidneys and nerves" [192]. There are many forms of DM but the most common, as noted by the WHO and estimated at 90%, is type 2 diabetes mellitus (T2DM). The WHO's definition of T2DM is general but touches on the three main aspects of the diseases: its metabolic nature that disrupts regulation of key nutrients of sugar, fats, and proteins; the unacceptable elevation in blood glucose both in the fasted and fed state which is both diagnostic and pathological; and the long-term consequences of vascular damage that cause morbidity and death [193].

Type 2 Diabetes Mellitus. Prevalence and Incidence T2DM has reached epidemic proportions globally [194]. The International Diabetes Federation (IDF) explains the increase prevalence in T2DM as a composite of socioeconomic, genetic, and environmental factors that "include urbanization, an ageing population, decreasing levels of physical activity and increasing prevalence of overweight and obesity" [194]. Locally, as of 2021, according to the National Diabetes Statistics Report, 2021, an estimated 29.2% of older adults have diabetes [195]. This is the highest of any age category. The incidence of diabetic cases in those ≥65 years of age is estimated at 6.8%. The age-adjusted (18 and older) incidence trend appears to be drifting downward but it is still too high for a disease that is preventable.

Type 2 Diabetes Mellitus. Pathophysiology The etiology of T2DM is complex and involves the actions of two hormones, insulin and glucagon, and the pancreatic cells that produce them, the β and α cells, respectively. External factors as well as genetics influence these hormones in their production, secretion, and activities [196]. In the healthy liver, insulin stimulates, via activation of the insulin receptor, the storage of glucose into glycogen and transcriptionally inactivates genes that promote synthesis of glucose. Insulin also acutely blocks lipolysis (breakdown of fats) in white adipose tissue (predominate fat type in the body) which supplies the liver with products of lipolysis, e.g., nonesterified or free fatty acids and glycerol, that stimulate synthesis of glucose (gluconeogenesis) [197]. Insulin also facilitates the transport of glucose into muscles and adipocytes (fat cells) and additionally supports proteins and triglycerides (fatty acid) storage in these tissues. Insulin's actions are mediated directly (activation of the insulin receptor) and indirectly via effects of metabolic products [197]. Glucagon, also through receptor-mediated and indirect effects, opposes the actions of insulin [198].

The underlying etiology of T2DM is the dysregulation of glucose [197]. T2DM is characterized by a decreased ability of insulin to exert its normal metabolic regulatory functions. The effects of insulin (e.g., transport of glucose, amino acids, and fats into muscle and liver, and promotion of biosynthesis of storage molecules, glycogen, proteins, and triglycerides) and opposition to other antagonistic hormones (e.g., glucagon) are reduced. This blunted physiological response of insulin, regardless of the concentration of circulating insulin, is called insulin resistance (or reduced insulin sensitivity) [196].

Type 2 Diabetes Mellitus. Risk Factors Based on results of observational, epidemiological, and clinical trial results, an extensive list of risk factors has been amassed [16, 17]. The major modifiable risk factors, or those with validated interventions that prevent or forestall T2DM are adiposity (obesity), physically inactivity, unhealthy dietary patterns, metabolic syndrome, and smoking [16]. Age and genetics are two main non-modifiable risk factors [17–19] (see Table 4.4).

Table 4.4 Risk factors and interventions for type 2 diabetes mellitus [16–19]

Risk factors	Interventions
Non-modifiable	
Age Genetics— ~ 400 T2DM-related gene variants	Awareness, genetic testing in future
Modifiable	
Obesity—BMI ≥30 kg/m^2; Waist circumference (≥36.2 in) Physical inactivity Unhealthy dietary patterns Metabolic syndrome	Weight loss Routine exercise (aerobics/resistance) Healthy diet, e.g., Mediterranean diet Improve lipid profile with statins, reduce BP with antihypertensive drug
Smoking	Quit smoking

BMI Body mass index, *BP* Blood pressure, *in* inches, *kg/m^2* kilogram per meter squared, *T2DM* Type 2 diabetes mellitus

Results of an 8-year-long study (Nurses' Health Study) observed that obesity (body mass index (BMI) ≥ 30 kg/m^2), waist-hip ratio (3.1), and waist circumference (36.2 inches) were strong risk factors for women in T2DM [199]. Weight loss either with time-restricted eating [200] or personalized weight loss strategies [201] decreased the risk for T2DM. Mechanistically, enlargement of visceral fat in obesity attracts macrophages primed to produce inflammatory mediators that reduce insulin sensitivity and induce the vicious cycle of lipolysis, fatty acid release and continued insulin resistance [202, 203].

Physical inactivity determined by sedentary time and TV watching time is another significant risk factor for T2DM as confirmed in an extensive meta-analysis [204]. Risk significantly increased with total sitting time greater than 6–8 h/day and 3–4 h/day of TV viewing [204]. Exactly how physical inactivity creates a risk for T2DM is unknown but postulated to be linked to abnormal glucose and fatty acid metabolism in large muscles on chronic sitting [205] and to poor diet with increased consumption of calories in watching TV [204]. On the other hand, results of numerous randomized controlled trials have shown the ability of physical exercise programs to decrease the risk of T2DM [206]. Short-term lack of exercise impairs postprandial (after meal intake) glycemia regardless of age [207]. In contrast, an intensive 1-year lifestyle intervention that included a healthy diet (with calorie reduction) and program of exercise, three times weekly, 30-min aerobics (75–85% maximal heart rate), and 30-min resistance exercises plus stretches and balance exercises in the older adult with diabetes lowered hemoglobin A1c (HbA1c, a measure of blood sugar over past 2–3 months), improved insulin sensitivity, reduced fat mass and body weight, improved physical performance and QoL [208]. The benefits of chronic moderate intensity exercise to normalize glucose regulation make it the main management strategy for newly diagnosed diabetics [209].

A systematic review and meta-analysis of clinical trials and prospective studies concluded that adherence to the Mediterranean diet decreased T2DM risk [210]. Additionally, it was observed that in the prevention of T2DM, common components of a healthy diet were table oils (olive oil) and whole grains, fruits, nuts, vegetables, legumes and protein-rich foods (white meat, seafood), moderate alcohol consumption, and reduced intake of red/processed meat and sweetened beverages [210, 211]. The positive effect of the Mediterranean diet on T2DM is attributed to its ability to raise the blood level of diet-derived antioxidants, to influence the oxidative potential of iron, to lower C-reactive protein, and to prevent the detrimental oxidative effects of hyperglycemia throughout the body [210].

The mechanism by which chronic smoking elevates the risk of T2DM is incompletely understood. Results from human and animal studies suggest the central and peripheral activation of the nicotinic cholinergic receptors by nicotine leads to dysregulation of glucose and insulin resistance [212].

Two non-modifiable risk factors for T2DM are age and genetics or genetic predisposition. As with all diseases, age is a major risk factor. The contribution of the senescent cell cannot be underestimated [213]. Senescent cells in visceral fat enhance lipolysis that increase insulin resistance and senescent cells in muscle and liver reduce the effects of insulin [213]. Additionally, senescent cells prevent β-cell proliferation, reducing insulin production [214, 215]. Furthermore, age-dependent changes in body composition with fat accumulation and loss of skeletal muscle mass (sarcopenia) exacerbated by physical inactivity and poor dietary choices elevate T2DM risk [216].

T2DM is considered a heterogeneous polygenic disease. Hence, genetic predisposition is under serious investigation [217]. Approximately 400 gene variants have been identified as associated with T2DM risk. These variants were further analyzed and linked to several pathophysiological changes evident in T2DM, e.g., β-cell abnormalities of insulin secretion, and adiposity [18]. The goal is to precisely define the etiology of T2DM, which would enable identification of those at high risk and assure development of the best treatment strategy [217].

Alert: Modifiable risk factors for T2DM are obesity, physical inactivity, unhealthy diet, smoking, and metabolic syndrome.

Type 2 Diabetes Mellitus. Diagnosis 8–12 h fasting glucose levels of 100–125 mg/dL (5.6–6.9 mmol/L) and HbA1c of 5.7–6.4% are the most frequently used tests to support a diagnosis of prediabetes. Screening should be initiated at age 45 unless other risk factors, e.g., BMI $\geq$25 kg/m^2, hypertension, and family history of diabetes are present. A diagnosis of T2DM is supported by results from several tests: fasting glucose of $\geq$126 mg/dL or 7.0 mmol/L, results of $\geq$200 mg/dL or 11.1 mmol/L glucose after an ingestion of 75 g of glucose/water solution (oral glucose tolerance test) and HbA1c of $\geq$6.5% [218].

Type 2 Diabetes Mellitus. Non-pharmacological Therapy As with all of the diseases discussed in this chapter, T2DM can be prevented or delayed with lifestyle choices that include a physical exercise program, and a healthy diet. Years of study by the Diabetes Prevention Program Research Group (DPPRG) reported a nearly 60% reduction in diabetic risk in 3 years with exercise that followed a protocol of a minimum of 150 min/week of moderate-intensity exercise (e.g., 15–20-min/mile walking) or 75 min/week of vigorous physical activity (e.g., running) performed over at least 3 days [219–221]. Additional beneficial changes were weight loss of a minimum of 7% and dietary changes that included a reduction of dietary fats and saturated fats, an increase in fiber, and reduction in alcohol consumption [222, 223]. These lifestyle choices are beneficial for prediabetics, diabetics, and healthy older adults.

Type 2 Diabetes Mellitus. Pharmacotherapy Drugs used to treat T2DM are oral antidiabetic drugs that serve to achieve good glycemic control by targeting the pathological changes that characterize T2DM [224]. Classes of drugs used to treat

T2DM are the biguanides, sulfonylureas, thiazolidinediones (TZD), alpha-glucosidase inhibitors, dipeptidyl peptidase 4 (DPP-4) inhibitors, meglitinide, and sodium-glucose co-transporter-2 (SGLT2) inhibitors [225].

Metformin The first-line oral drug choice, regardless of age, is metformin, a biguanide. Metformin enhances the uptake of glucose by the liver and reduces gluconeogenesis primarily by its effect on the mitochondrial respiratory complex I (oxidative phosphorylation) and secondarily on suppression of a metabolic sensor (AMP-activated protein kinase), although other actions of enhanced insulin receptor expression and function have been reported [226]. Metformin therapy retards T2DM progression and reduces the risk of complications and mortality [226]. Although GI disturbances occur in 30% of patients, overall metformin has an excellent safety record. Because renal excretion is the main route of elimination, metformin is used at reduced doses in patients with GFR <30 mL/min/1.73 m^2. It is essential to monitor levels of vitamin B_{12} and folic acid since metformin can induce deficiencies. This is frequently overlooked in the older adult [227].

Dipeptidyl Peptidase 4 Inhibitors The dipeptidyl peptidase 4 (DPP-4) inhibitors (sitagliptin, saxagliptin, linagliptin, and alogliptin) are termed incretin mimetics because they preserve the presence of the hormone, glucose-dependent insulinotropic polypeptide (GIP, or incretin). GIP and a second hormone, glucagon-like peptide (GLP-1), regulate orally ingested sugars by enhancing insulin secretion. Both are rapidly destroyed by DPP-4, hence their preservation, especially GIP with DPP-4 inhibitors. Most common adverse effects reported in clinical trials were nasopharyngitis (irritation of nose and throat), upper respiratory tract infection, and headache. Low doses are considered safe in moderate and severe renal disease [225].

GLP-1 Agonists GLP-1 agonist (liraglutide, exenatide, dulaglutide) are resistant to enzymatic breakdown by DPP-4. These drugs activate the GLP-1 receptor to increase insulin secretion, increase satiety, and decrease glucagon production [224]. GLP-1 agonist (semaglutide) and dual GLP-1 and GIP agonist (tirzepatide) injected subcutaneously, exert multiple actions: lower blood sugar, promote weight loss, improve blood lipid profile and exert beneficial effects on the cardiovascular system [228]. Mild-moderate GI distress has been reported and hypoglycemia is of concern when used with other antidiabetic drugs. Both have been approved for weight loss in obese patients [228].

Sulfonylureas The sulfonylureas (chlorpropamide, tolazamide, glyburide, glimepiride, glipizide) achieve normal glycemic control by increasing insulin secretion and reducing clearance, reducing hepatic gluconeogenesis, and decreasing lipolysis [229]. These effects result from the ability of sulfonylureas to block the ATP-sensitive potassium channels in the β-cells [230]. Sulfonylureas are second-line medications. Their major side effect is hypoglycemia, especially evident with glyburide [95]; the best choice is glimepiride. The risk of hypoglycemia is enhanced when used with other drugs: β-blockers, aspirin, sulfonamides, fibrates, and allopurinol [224]. Sulfonylureas should be avoided in patients with liver or kidney diseases.

Meglitinides The meglitinides (repaglinide and nateglinide) although not sulfonylureas act as insulin secretagogues similar to sulfonylureas but with a shorter half-life [224]. Basically, these drugs are used in patients with irregular feeding schedules or those experiencing hypoglycemia with sulfonylureas.

Sodium-Glucose Co-Transporter Inhibitors Sodium-glucose co-transporter inhibitors (SGLT2 inhibitors) (bexagliflozin, canagliflozin, dapagliflozin, empagliflozin, ertugliflozin) act on the kidney to block reabsorption of glucose [231]. Filtered glucose is reabsorbed entirely back into the blood by the kidney tubules. SGLT2 inhibitors bind to SGLT transporters on the luminal membrane of the renal tubules and block glucose reabsorption by 50–60% [231]. Because of this unique mechanism of action, they are valid add-on drugs in severe T2DM [224]. Most common side effects are female genital mycotic (fungal) infections, urinary tract infections, and increased urination; use is restricted in kidney disease [232]. Although a systematic network meta-analysis of 36 clinical trials showed that the risk for diabetic ketoacidosis (increase in ketone acids in blood) was no higher with SGLT2 inhibitors than other antidiabetic drugs [233], for the older adult, the Beers Criteria® suggests SGLT2 inhibitors, especially canagliflozin be used with caution [95].

Pioglitazone The TZD class currently contains one drug, pioglitazone. Pioglitazone activates the PPARγ-receptor to modify gene expression that culminates in enhancement of insulin's effects on glucose uptake and hepatic inhibition of gluconeogenesis [234]. The use of TZD has diminished over the years due to the initiation of heart failure. Therefore, this drug is to be avoided [95].

Insulin Insulin therapy is useful when HbA1c target values are unmet despite more than 3 months of combination therapy. Specifically, when biomarkers show HbA1c at ≥ 10–12%, and hyperglycemia at ≥ 300–350 mg/dL, and additionally, there are other symptoms, e.g., weight loss, ketosis (ketone bodies from hepatic fat metabolism), and persistent thirst and urination [235]. In conjunction with metformin, insulin therapy is commenced, starting with basal insulins such as the short-acting neutral protamine Hagedorn (NPH) insulin (isophane insulin) with 10 U or 0.1–0.2 U/kg), gradually increased 2 U every 4–7 days until glycemic control is achieved. Longer-acting basal insulins are U-100 regular (Humulin R), U-300 glargine, and U-200 degludec. The latter two (second-generation basal insulin) produce comparable metabolic control with lower rates of hypoglycemia and no weight gain [236]. If glycemic control is lacking, rapidly acting insulin analogues (lispro, aspart, or glulisine) may be added before meals [224]. Additional drugs such as

SGLT2 inhibitors may be added if glycemic control is unreliable with dosage changes in insulin. Inhalation insulin available only as the Technosphere insulin-inhalation system (Afrezza) has a low risk of hypoglycemia due to its rapid glucose-lowering action. Adequate pulmonary function is required; a cough develops in 9% of individuals [237].

The benefits of intensive glucose management on microvascular complications, such as retinopathy, nephropathy, and neuropathy, have been shown in several large randomized clinical trials (RCTs) [238]. Study results show that for risk reduction, glucose control must be initiated early in the T2DM disease course. In long-standing T2DM, addressing all cardiovascular risk factors is especially important. One concern of rigorous glucose control is the possibility of hypoglycemic episodes that may precipitate serious consequences such as increased incidence of falls, exacerbation of comorbidities and worse, coma [239].

Type 2 Diabetes Mellitus. Assessment For the older adult, lack of definitive guidance from RCT results that exclude the older adult, aggressive glycemic control should be individualized and supervised in consideration of comorbidities, functional and cognitive status, polypharmacy, kidney function, age-related changes in body composition and handling of drugs, frailty syndromes, and risk of hypoglycemia plus relevant social and psychological issues including cost-effectiveness of glycemic control [240–242]. In other words, a *Comprehensive Geriatric Assessment* is essential in the treatment of T2DM in the older adult.

Specifically, the objective is to achieve the best glycemic control that both slows disease progression, reduces the advent of adverse complications, and avoids episodes of hypoglycemia. A comprehensive geriatric assessment should be the starting point. Additionally, providers need to incorporate into their health care objectives for the older patient with diabetes, the following considerations [243]: (1) individual patient analysis of overall health status (remembering that chronological age does not equal biological age), presence of comorbidities and associated drug use, characteristics of the diabetes (onset, duration, complications), and the patient's personal views, financial and social assistance sphere; (2) geriatric syndromes (see Chap. 7) should be identified and appropriately treated. Many of these such as cognitive decline indicate that the patient may require additional aid with self-care to achieve treatment goals; (3) education for both the patient, family, and caregivers must be on point, easy to understand, and implemented and reinforced as needed; (4) selection of insulin-delivering devices and blood glucose meters should be optimized for the patient. Insulin pens are easier to use than syringes and meters with large print or audio capabilities are available for those with visual disabilities; (5) adjust glucose monitoring to the patient's ability, advise on symptoms of hypoglycemia (confusion, weakness), and develop a plan to counter-act such an episode; (6) provide appropriate nutritional advice regarding healthy eating, advising consistency in carbohydrate intake to keep glucose level constant, engage family in simplifying meals and changing lifestyle choices; (7) weight loss is not advised in the older adult as it may lead to malnutrition, compounding diabetes; (8) physical activity of all types (with safety advice from a physical/

occupational therapist) is recommended as it not only assures independence but provides numerous ameliorating benefit to diabetes; and (9) as with all medications prescribed to the older adult, initial dose should be the lowest dose possible, with constant monitoring of efficacy and adverse effects and dose increase only if necessary. Select drugs with least risk of hypoglycemia, measure kidney function with actual glomerular filtration rate rather than serum creatinine, measure kidney and liver enzymes periodically and consider financial situation of patient if prescribing recently approved expensive antidiabetic drugs [243].

Guidance
1. Although age is a primary risk factor for diseases, atherosclerotic cardiovascular disease, cancers, Alzheimer's disease/other dementias and type 2 diabetes mellitus, the older adult should be counseled on the main *modifiable* risk factors for age-related diseases, and effective validated interventions. This non-pharmacological strategy applied over a lifetime involves maintenance of a normal weight (avoid overweight/obesity), healthy dietary selections (similar to the Mediterranean diet), chronic participation in aerobic and resistance exercises, and no smoking. These are key interventions (although there are others, e.g., adequate sleep, hearing loss correction) that significantly reduce the risk of major age-related diseases.
2. Pharmacological therapies should be initiated only after a Comprehensive Geriatric Assessment in which the totality (physical, mental, social, psychological, comorbidities, polypharmacy) of the older adult is assessed. This determines the degree of therapeutic aggressiveness as well as drug selection and dose.
3. Drug selection is disease specific:
    (a) Atherosclerotic Cardiovascular Disease (ASCVD)—the statins are the drugs of choice for primary and secondary prevention of ASCVD; addition of antihypertensive drugs for primary prevention and antiplatelet/anticoagulant drugs for secondary prevention are highly effective; treatment of heart failure depends on the stage of failure and requires inhibitors of the renin-angiotensin system, beta-blockers, loop diuretics, and possibly others.
    (b) Cancers—the four classes of drugs (cytotoxic, hormones/antagonists, tyrosine kinase inhibitors, immune checkpoint inhibitors) have success in suppressing specific types of cancers. However, generally the cytotoxic drugs are more efficacious but produce more adverse reactions. All anticancer drugs produce some type of drug resistance. Combinations of drugs with smaller doses of each are beneficial with fewer side effects.

(continued)

(c) Alzheimer's disease (AD)—anticholinesterase inhibitors are helpful therapy in early to moderate AD and the NMDA receptor inhibitor (memantine) is useful in moderate/severe AD. β-amyloid antibodies that remove brain plaques modestly retard cognitive loss. Better pharmacological therapies are needed. Cerebrovascular dementias benefit from CV risk reduction and antiplatelet therapy.

(d) Type 2 diabetes mellitus—the goal of therapy is glycemic control and normal HbA1c values to avoid long-term damage to major organs. Metformin is the mainstay with, if necessary, add-ons of sulfonylureas and SGLT2 inhibitors. Worsening episodes of hyperglycemia may require the use of basal insulins. Drugs should be used at doses that do not produce hypoglycemia, which can lead to falls and fractures.

References

1. Hayflick L. The not-so-close relationship between biological aging and age-associated pathologies in humans. J Gerontol A Biol Sci Med Sci. 2004;59(6):B547–50; discussion 551–3. https://doi.org/10.1093/gerona/59.6.b547.
2. Kirkland JL. Translating advances from the basic biology of aging into clinical application. Exp Gerontol. 2013;48(1):1–5. https://doi.org/10.1016/j.exger.2012.11.014.
3. López-Otín C, Blasco MA, Partridge L, Serrano M, Kroemer G. The hallmarks of aging. Cell. 2013;153(6):1194–217. https://doi.org/10.1016/j.cell.2013.05.039.
4. López-Otín C, Blasco MA, Partridge L, Serrano M, Kroemer G. Hallmarks of aging: an expanding universe. Cell. 2023;186(2):243–78. https://doi.org/10.1016/j.cell.2022.11.001.
5. Campisi J. Senescent cells, tumor suppression, and organismal aging: good citizens, bad neighbors. Cell. 2005;120(4):513–22. https://doi.org/10.1016/j.cell.2005.02.003.
6. Campisi J. Aging, cellular senescence, and cancer. Annu Rev Physiol. 2013;75:685–705. https://doi.org/10.1146/annurev-physiol-030212-183653.
7. Freund A, Orjalo AV, Desprez PY, Campisi J. Inflammatory networks during cellular senescence: causes and consequences. Trends Mol Med. 2010;16(5):238–46. https://doi.org/10.1016/j.molmed.2010.03.003.
8. Gorgoulis V, Adams PD, Alimonti A, Bennett DC, Bischof O, Bishop C, et al. Cellular senescence: defining a path forward. Cell. 2019;179(4):813–27. https://doi.org/10.1016/j.cell.2019.10.005.
9. Childs BG, Durik M, Baker DJ, van Deursen JM. Cellular senescence in aging and age-related disease: from mechanisms to therapy. Nat Med. 2015;21(12):1424–35. https://doi.org/10.1038/nm.4000.
10. Laberge R-M, Awad P, Campisi J, Desprez P-Y. Epithelial-mesenchymal transition induced by senescent fibroblasts. Cancer Microenviron. 2012;5(1):39–44. https://doi.org/10.1007/s12307-011-0069-4.
11. Liu RM. Aging, Cellular Senescence, and Alzheimer's Disease. Int J Mol Sci. 2022 Feb 11;23(4):1989. https://doi.org/10.3390/ijms23041989.
12. Spinelli R, Parrillo L, Longo M, Florese P, Desiderio A, Zatterale F, et al. Molecular basis of ageing in chronic metabolic diseases. J Endocrinol Investig. 2020;43(10):1373–89. https://doi.org/10.1007/s40618-020-01255-z.

References

13. Arnett DK, Blumenthal RS, Albert MA, Buroker AB, Goldberger ZD, Hahn EJ. 2019 ACC/AHA guideline on the primary prevention of cardiovascular disease: executive summary: a report of the American College of Cardiology/American Heart Association Task Force on Clinical Practice Guidelines. Circulation. 2019;140(11):e563–95. https://doi.org/10.1161/CIR.0000000000000677.
14. Hariri EH, Hammoud MMA, Nissen SE, Hammer DF. Primary and secondary prevention of atherosclerotic cardiovascular disease: a case-based approach. Cleve Clin J Med. 2022;89(9):513–22. https://doi.org/10.3949/ccjm.89a.21103.
15. Miller M, Stone NJ, Ballantyne C, Bittner V, Criqui MH, Ginsberg HN. Triglycerides and cardiovascular disease: a scientific statement from the American Heart Association. Circulation. 2011;123(20):2292–333. https://doi.org/10.1161/CIR.0b013e3182160726.
16. Bellou V, Belbasis L, Tzoulaki I, Evangelou E. Risk factors for type 2 diabetes mellitus: an exposure-wide umbrella review of meta-analyses. PLoS One. 2018;13(3):e0194127. https://doi.org/10.1371/journal.pone.0194127.
17. Laakso M. Biomarkers for type 2 diabetes. Mol Metab. 2019;27S(Suppl):S139–46. https://doi.org/10.1016/j.molmet.2019.06.016.
18. Mahajan A, Taliun D, Thurner M, et al. Fine-mapping type 2 diabetes loci to single-variant resolution using high-density imputation and islet-specific epigenome maps. Nat Genet. 2018;50(11):1505–13. https://doi.org/10.1038/s41588-018-0241-6.
19. Al-sofiani ME, Ganji SS, Kalyani RR. Body composition changes in diabetes and aging. J Diabetes Complicat. 2019;33(6):451–9. https://doi.org/10.1016/j.jdiacomp.2019.03.007.
20. Alzheimer's Association. Alzheimer's disease facts and figures. Alzheimers Dement. 2023;2023, 19(4) https://doi.org/10.1002/alz.13016.
21. Scheltens P, De Strooper B, Kivipelto M, Holstege H, Chételat G, Teunissen CE, et al. Lancet. 2021;397(10284):1577–90. https://doi.org/10.1016/S0140-6736(20)32205-4.
22. Nedergaard M, Goldman SA. Glymphatic failure as a final common pathway to dementia. Science. 2020;370(6512):50–6. https://doi.org/10.1126/science.abb8739.
23. Nianogo RA, Rosenwohl-Mack A, Yaffe K, Carrasco A, Hoffmann CM, Barnes DE. Risk factors associated with Alzheimer disease and related dementias by sex and race and ethnicity in the US. JAMA Neurol. 2022;79(6):584–91. https://doi.org/10.1001/jamaneurol.2022.0976.
24. Huang AR, Jiang K, Lin FR, Deal JA, Reed NS. Hearing loss and dementia prevalence in older adults in the US. JAMA. 2023;329(2):171–3. https://doi.org/10.1001/jama.2022.20954.
25. Wu S, Zhu W, Thompson P, Hannun YA. Evaluating intrinsic and non-intrinsic cancer risk factors. Nat Commun. 2018;9(1):3490. https://doi.org/10.1038/s41467-018-05467-z.
26. Centers for Disease Control and Prevention, National Center for Health Statistics. National Vital Statistics System, Mortality 2018–2021 on CDC WONDER Online Database, released in 2021 http://wonder.cdc.gov/ucd-icd10-expanded.
27. Virani SS, Alonso A, Benjamin EJ, Bittencourt MS, Callaway CW, Carson AP, et al. American Heart Association Council on Epidemiology and Prevention Statistics Committee and Stroke Statistics Subcommittee. Heart Disease and stroke statistics-2020 update: a report from the American Heart Association. Circulation. 2020;141(9):e139–596. https://doi.org/10.1161/CIR.0000000000000757.
28. Tsao CW, Aday AW, Almarzooq ZI, Anderson CAM, Arora P, Avery CL, et al. Heart Disease and Stroke Statistics-2023 update: a report from the American Heart Association. American Heart Association Council on Epidemiology and Prevention Statistics Committee and Stroke Statistics Subcommittee. Circulation. 2023;147(8):e93–e621. https://doi.org/10.1161/CIR.0000000000001123.
29. https://www.nhlbi.nih.gov/health/atherosclerosis, 2022.
30. Wolf D, Ley K. Immunity and Inflammation in Atherosclerosis. Circ Res. 2019;124(2):315–27. https://doi.org/10.1161/CIRCRESAHA.118.313591.

31. Ambrose JA, Tannenbaum MA, Alexopoulos D, Hjemdahl-Monsen CE, Leavy J, Weiss M, et al. Angiographic progression of coronary artery disease and the development of myocardial infarction. J Am Coll Cardiol. 1988;12(1):56–62. https://doi.org/10.1016/0735-1097(88)90356-7.
32. Ait-Oufella H, Taleb S, Mallat Z, Tedgui A. Recent advances on the role of cytokines in atherosclerosis. Arterioscler Thromb Vasc Biol. 2011;31(5):969–79. https://doi.org/10.1161/ATVBAHA.110.207415.
33. Roy P, Orecchioni M, Ley K. How the immune system shapes atherosclerosis: roles of innate and adaptive immunity. Nat Rev Immunol. 2022;22(4):251–65. https://doi.org/10.1038/s41577-021-00584-1.
34. Ley K, Miller YI, Hedrick CC. Monocyte and macrophage dynamics during atherogenesis. Arterioscler Thromb Vasc Biol. 2011;31(7):1506–16. https://doi.org/10.1161/ATVBAHA.110.221127.
35. Moutachakkir M, Lamrani Hanchi A, Baraou A, Boukhira A, Chellak S. Immunoanalytical characteristics of C-reactive protein and high sensitivity C-reactive protein. Ann Biol Clin (Paris). 2017;75(2):225–9. https://doi.org/10.1684/abc.2017.1232.
36. Nahrendort M. Myeloid cell contributions to cardiovascular health and disease. Nat Med. 2018;24(6):711–20. https://doi.org/10.1038/s41591-018-0064-0.
37. Kelly P, Meade KG, O'Farrelly C. Non-canonical inflammasome-mediated IL-1beta production by primary endometrial epithelial and stromal fibroblast cells is NLRP3 and Caspase-4 dependent. Front Immunol. 2019;10:102. https://doi.org/10.3389/fimmu.2019.00102.
38. Winkels H, Wolf D. Heterogeneity of T cells in atherosclerosis defined by single-cell RNA-sequencing and cytometry by time of flight. Arterioscler Thromb Vasc Biol. 2021 Feb;41(2):549–63. https://doi.org/10.1161/ATVBAHA.120.312137.
39. Booth LK, Redgrave RE, Tual-Chalot S, Spyridopoulos I, Phillips HM, Richardson GD. Heart disease and ageing: the roles of senescence, mitochondria, and telomerase in cardiovascular disease. Subcell Biochem. 2023;103:45–78. https://doi.org/10.1007/978-3-031-26576-1_4.
40. Witham MD, Granic A, Miwa S, Passos JF, Richardson GD, Sayer AA. New horizons in cellular senescence for clinicians. Age Ageing. 2023;52:afad127. https://doi.org/10.1093/ageing/afad127.
41. Redgrave R, Dookun E, Booth L, Folaranm O, Tual-Chalot S, Gill J, et al. Senescent cardiomyocytes contribute to cardiac dysfunction following myocardial infarction. NPJ Aging. 2023;9:15. https://doi.org/10.1038/s41514-023-00113-5.
42. Camacho-Encina M, Booth LK, Redgrave RE, Folaranmi O, Spyridopoulos I. Richardson GD cellular senescence, mitochondrial dysfunction, and their link to cardiovascular disease. Cells. 2024;13(4):353. https://doi.org/10.3390/cells13040353.
43. Chistiakov DA, Shkurat TP, Melnichenko AA, Grechko AV, Orekhov AN. The role of mitochondrial dysfunction in cardiovascular disease: a brief review. Ann Med. 2018;50:121–7. https://doi.org/10.1080/07853890.2017.1417631.
44. Mahmood SS, Levy D, Vasan RS, Wang TJ. The framingham heart study and the epidemiology of cardiovascular disease: a historical perspective. Lancet. 2014;383(9921):999–1008. https://doi.org/10.1016/S0140-6736(13)61752-3.
45. Kannel WB, Dawber TR, Kagan A, Revotskie N, Stokes J 3rd. Factors of risk in the development of coronary heart disease–six year follow-up experience. The Framingham Study. Ann Intern Med. 1961;55:33–50. https://doi.org/10.7326/0003-4819-55-1-33.
46. Kannel WB, Gordon T, Schwartz MJ. Systolic versus diastolic blood pressure and risk of coronary heart disease: the Framingham study. Am J Cardiol. 1971;27:335–46. https://doi.org/10.1016/0002-9149(71)90428-0.
47. Gordon T, Castelli WP, Hjortland MC, Kannel WB, Dawber TR. High density lipoprotein as a protective factor against coronary heart disease: the Framingham study. Am J Med. 1977;62:707–14. https://doi.org/10.1016/0002-9343(77)90874-9.
48. Hubert HB, Feinleib M, McNamara PM, Castelli WP. Obesity as an independent risk factor for cardiovascular disease: a 26-year follow-up of participants in the Framingham Heart Study. Circulation. 1983;67:968–77. https://doi.org/10.1161/01.cir.67.5.968.

49. Garcia MJ, McNamara PM, Gordon T, Kannell WB. Morbidity and mortality in diabetics in the Framingham population: sixteen year follow-up study. Diabetes. 1974;23:105–11. https://doi.org/10.2337/diab.23.2.105.
50. Ambrose JA, Barua RS. The pathophysiology of cigarette smoking and cardiovascular disease: an update. J Am Coll Cardiol. 2004;43:1731–7. https://doi.org/10.1016/j.jacc.2003.12.047.
51. Kuller LH, Kriska AM, Kinzel LS, Simkin-Silverman LR, Sutton-Tyrrell K, Johnson BD, et al. The clinical trial of women on the move through activity and nutrition (WOMAN) study. Contemp Clin Trials. 2007;28(4):370–81. https://doi.org/10.1016/j.cct.2006.10.009.
52. McDermott MM, Guralnik JM, Criqui MH, Ferrucci L, Zhao L, Liu K, et al. Home-based walking exercise in peripheral artery disease: 12-month follow-up of the GOALS randomized trial. J Am Heart Assoc. 2014;3(3):e000711. https://doi.org/10.1161/JAHA.113.000711.
53. Salas-Salvadó J, Díaz-López A, Ruiz-Canela M, Basora J, Fitó M, Corella D, et al. Effect of a lifestyle intervention program with energy-restricted mediterranean diet and exercise on weight loss and cardiovascular risk factors: one-year results of the PREDIMED-Plus trial. PREDIMED-Plus investigators. Diabetes Care. 2019;42(5):777–88. https://doi.org/10.2337/dc18-0836.
54. Garcia-Lunar I, van der Ploeg HP, Fernández Alvira JM, van Nassau F, Castellano Vázquez JM, van der Beek AJ, et al. Effects of a comprehensive lifestyle intervention on cardiovascular health: the TANSNIP-PESA trial. Eur Heart J. 2022;43(38):3732–45. https://doi.org/10.1093/eurheartj/ehac378.
55. Collins R, Reith C, Emberson J, Armitage J, Baigent C, Blackwell L, et al. Interpretation of the evidence for the efficacy and safety of statin therapy. Lancet. 2016;388:2532–61. https://doi.org/10.1016/S0140-6736(16)31357-5.
56. Mortensen MB, Falk E. Primary prevention with statins in the elderly. J Am Coll Cardiol. 2018;71(1):85–94. https://doi.org/10.1016/j.jacc.2017.10.080.
57. Goldstein JL, Brown MS. A century of cholesterol and coronaries from plaques to genes to statins. Cell. 2015;161:161–72. https://doi.org/10.1016/j.cell.2015.01.036.
58. Ference BA, Ginsberg HN, Graham I, et al. Low-density lipoproteins cause atherosclerotic cardiovascular disease. 1. Evidence from genetic, epidemiologic, and clinical studies. A consensus statement from the European Atherosclerosis Society Consensus Panel. Eur Heart J. 2017;38:2459–72. https://doi.org/10.1093/eurheartj/ehx144.
59. Chou R, Cantor A, Dana T, Wagner J, Ahmed A, Fu R, et al. Statin use for the primary prevention of cardiovascular disease in adults: a systematic review for the U.S. Preventive Services Task Force [Internet]. Rockville: Agency for Healthcare Research and Quality (US); 2022. Report No.: 22–05291-EF-1.
60. Sarraju A, Spencer-Bonilla G, Chung S, Gomez S, Li J, Heidenreich P, et al. Statin use in older adults for primary cardiovascular disease prevention across a spectrum of cardiovascular risk. J Gen Intern Med. 2022;37(11):2642–9. https://doi.org/10.1007/s11606-021-07107-7.
61. Khan SS, Matsushita K, Sang Y, Ballew SH, Grams ME, Surapaneni A, et al. Development and validation of the American Heart Association's PREVENT equations. Circulation. 2024;149(6):430–49. https://doi.org/10.1161/CIRCULATIONAHA.123.067626.
62. Han BH, Sutin D, Williamson JD, Davis BR, Piller LB, Pervin H, et al. Effect of statin treatment vs usual care on primary cardiovascular prevention among older adults: the ALLHAT-LLT randomized clinical trial. ALLHAT Collaborative Research Group. JAMA Intern Med. 2017;177(7):955–65. https://doi.org/10.1001/jamainternmed.2017.1442.
63. Kulbertus H, Scheen AJ. The PROSPER Study (PROspective study of pravastatin in the elderly at risk). Rev Med Liege. 2002;57(12):809–13. PMID: 12632840.
64. Shepherd J, Blauw GJ, Murphy MB, Bollen EL, Buckley BM, Cobbe SM. Pravastatin in elderly individuals at risk of vascular disease (PROSPER): a randomised controlled trial., et al PROSPER study group. PROspective Study of Pravastatin in the Elderly at Risk. Lancet. 2002;360(9346):1623–30. https://doi.org/10.1016/s0140-6736(02)11600-x.

65. Stone NJ, Robinson JG, Lichtenstein AH, Nerz CNB, Blum CB, Eckel RH, et al. 2013 ACC/AHA guideline on the treatment of blood cholesterol to reduce atherosclerotic cardiovascular risk in adults: a report of the American College of Cardiology/American Heart Association Task Force on Practice Guidelines. J Am Coll Cardiol. 2014;63:2889–934. https://doi.org/10.1016/j.jacc.2013.11.002.
66. DC G Jr, Lloyd-Jones DM, Bennett G, Coady S, D'Agostino RB Sr, Gibbons R, et al. 2013 ACC/AHA guideline on the assessment of cardiovascular risk: a report of the American College of Cardiology/American Heart Association Task Force on Practice Guidelines. J Am Coll Cardiol. 2014;63:2935–59. https://doi.org/10.1016/j.jacc.2013.11.005.
67. Mortensen MB, Afzal S, Nordestgaard BG, Falk E. Primary prevention with statins: ACC/AHA risk-based approach versus trial-based approaches to guide statin therapy. J Am Coll Cardiol. 2015;66(24):2699–709. https://doi.org/10.1016/j.jacc.2015.09.089.
68. FDA www.accessdata.fda.gov/drugsatfda
69. Albasri A, Hattle M, Koshiaris C, Dunnigan A, Paxton B, Fox SE, et al. STRATIFY investigators association between antihypertensive treatment and adverse events: systematic review and meta-analysis. BMJ. 2021;372:n189. https://doi.org/10.1136/bmj.n189.
70. Kahlaee HR, Latt MD, Schneider CR. Association between chronic or acute use of antihypertensive class of medications and falls in older adults. A systematic review and meta-analysis. Am J Hypertens. 2018;31:467–79. https://doi.org/10.1093/ajh/hpx189.
71. Cai A, Calhoun DA. Antihypertensive medications and falls in the elderly. Am J Hypertens. 2018;31:281–3. https://doi.org/10.1093/ajh/hpx203.
72. Hanna IR, Wenger NK. Secondary prevention of coronary heart disease in elderly patients. Am Fam Physician. 2005;71(12):2289–96. PMID: 15999866.
73. Kasiakogias A, Sharma S. Exercise: the ultimate treatment to all ailments? Clin Cardiol. 2020;43(8):817–26. https://doi.org/10.1002/clc.23369.
74. Atar D, Jukema JW, Molemans B, Taub PR, Goto S, Mach F, et al. New cardiovascular prevention guidelines: how to optimally manage dyslipidaemia and cardiovascular risk in 2021 in patients needing secondary prevention? Atherosclerosis. 2021;319:51–61. https://doi.org/10.1016/j.atherosclerosis.2020.12.013.
75. Grundy SM, Stone NJ, Bailey AL, Beam C, Birtcher KK, Blumenthal RS, et al. AHA/ACC/AACVPR/AAPA/ABC/ACPM/ADA/AGS/APhA/ASPC/NLA/PCNA guideline on the management of blood cholesterol: a report of the American College of Cardiology/American Heart Association task force on clinical practice guidelines. Circulation. 2019;139(25):e1082–143. https://doi.org/10.1161/CIR.0000000000000625.
76. Castilla-Guerra L, Fernandez-Moreno MDC, Leon-Jimenez D, Rico-Corral MA. Statins in ischemic stroke prevention: what have we learned in the post-SPARCL (The Stroke Prevention by Aggressive Reduction in Cholesterol Levels) decade? Curr Treat Options Neurol. 2019;21(5):22. https://doi.org/10.1007/s11940-019-0563-4.
77. LMB R, Vallejo-Vaz AJ, Grijalvo OM. Cerebrovascular disease and statins. Front Cardiovasc Med. 2021;8:778740. https://doi.org/10.3389/fcvm.2021.778740.
78. Hegele RA, Tsimikas S. Lipid-lowering agents. Circ Res. 2019;124(3):386–404. https://doi.org/10.1161/CIRCRESAHA.118.313171.
79. Phan BA, Dayspring TD. Toth PP Ezetimibe therapy: mechanism of action and clinical update. Vasc Health Risk Manag. 2012;8:415–27. https://doi.org/10.2147/VHRM.S33664.
80. Ray KK, Corral P, Morales E, Nicholls SJ. Pharmacological lipid-modification therapies for prevention of ischaemic heart disease: current and future options. Lancet. 2019;394(10199):697–708. https://doi.org/10.1016/S0140-6736(19)31950-6.
81. Roth EM, Davidson MH. PCSK9 inhibitors: mechanism of action, efficacy, and safety. Rev Cardiovasc Med. 2018;19(S1):S31–46. https://doi.org/10.3909/ricm19S1S0002.
82. Marston NA, Giugliano RP, Im KA, Silverman MG, O'Donoghue L, Wiviott SD, et al. Association between triglyceride lowering and reduction of cardiovascular risk across multiple lipid-lowering therapeutic classes: a systematic review and meta-regression analysis of randomized controlled trials. Circulation. 2019;140(16):1308–17. https://doi.org/10.1161/CIRCULATIONAHA.119.041998.

83. O'Donoghue ML, Fazio S, Giugliano RP, Stroes ESG, Kanevsky E, Gouni-Berthold I, et al. Lipoprotein(a), PCSK9 inhibition and cardiovascular risk. Circulation. 2019;139(12):1483–92. https://doi.org/10.1161/CIRCULATIONAHA.118.037184.
84. Nurmohamed NS, Kraaijenhof JM, Stroes ESG. Lp(a): a new pathway to target? Curr Atheroscler Rep. 2022;24(11):831–8. https://doi.org/10.1007/s11883-022-01060-4.
85. Libby P, Pasterkamp G, Crea F, Jang IK. Reassessing the mechanisms of acute coronary syndromes. Circ Res. 2019;124(1):150–60. https://doi.org/10.1161/CIRCRESAHA.118.311098.
86. Chapman MJ. From pathophysiology to targeted therapy for atherothrombosis: a role for the combination of statin and aspirin in secondary prevention. Pharmacol Ther. 2007;113(1):184–96. https://doi.org/10.1016/j.pharmthera.2006.08.005.
87. Cho SW, Franchi F, Angiolillo DJ. Role of oral anticoagulant therapy for secondary prevention in patients with stable atherothrombotic disease manifestations. Ther Adv Hematol. 2019; https://doi.org/10.1177/2040620719861475.
88. Huseynov A, Reinhardt J, Chandra L, Dürschmied D, Langer HF. Novel aspects targeting platelets in atherosclerotic cardiovascular disease-a translational perspective. Int J Mol Sci. 2023;24(7):6280. https://doi.org/10.3390/ijms24076280.
89. Koski R, Kennedy B. Comparative review of oral $P2Y_{12}$ inhibitors. P T. 2018;43(6):352–7. PMC5969212.
90. Visseren FLJ, Mach F, Smulders YM, Carballo D, Koskinas KC, Back M, et al. ESC guidelines on cardiovascular disease prevention in clinical practice. Eur Heart J. 2021;42:3227–37. https://doi.org/10.1093/eurheartj/ehab484.
91. Passacquale G, Sharma P, Perera D, Ferro A. Antiplatelet therapy in cardiovascular disease: current status and future directions. Br J Clin Pharmacol. 2022;88(6):2686–99. https://doi.org/10.1111/bcp.15221.
92. Olie RH, Winckers K, Rocca B, Cate HT. Oral anticoagulants beyond warfarin. Annu Rev Pharmacol Toxicol. 2024;64:551–75. https://doi.org/10.1146/annurev-pharmtox-032823-122811.
93. Hirsh J, Fuster V, Ansell J, Halperin JL. American Heart Association/American College of Cardiology Foundation guide to Warfarin Therapy. Circulation. 2003;107(12):1692–711. https://doi.org/10.1161/01.CIR.0000063575.17904.4E.
94. De Rosa R, Piscione F, Galasso G, De Servi S, Savonitto S. Antiplatelet therapy in very elderly and comorbid patients with acute coronary syndromes. J Geriatr Cardiol. 2019;16(2):103–13. https://doi.org/10.11909/j.issn.1671-5411.2019.02.006.
95. By the 2023 American Geriatrics Society Beers Criteria® Update Expert Panel. American Geriatrics Society 2023 updated AGS Beers Criteria® for potentially inappropriate medication use in older adults. J Am Geriatr Soc. 2023 Jul;71(7):2052–81. https://doi.org/10.1111/jgs.18372
96. Steffel J, Eikelboom JW, Anand SS, Shestakovska O, Yusuf S, Fox KAA. The COMPASS trial: net clinical benefit of low-dose rivaroxaban plus aspirin as compared with aspirin in patients with chronic vascular disease. Circulation. 2020;142(1):40–8. https://doi.org/10.1161/CIRCULATIONAHA.120.046048.
97. Gottsäter A. Antithrombotic treatment in lower extremity peripheral arterial disease. Front Cardiovasc Med. 2021;8:773214. https://doi.org/10.3389/fcvm.2021.773214.
98. Heidenreich PA, Bozkurt B, Aguilar D, Allen LA, Byun JJ, Colvin MM, et al. 2022 AHA/ACC/HFSA guideline for the management of heart failure: a report of the American College of Cardiology/American Heart Association Joint Committee on Clinical Practice Guidelines. Circulation. 2022;145(18):e895–e1032. https://doi.org/10.1161/CIR.0000000000001063.
99. Figueroa MS, Peters JI. Congestive heart failure: diagnosis, pathophysiology, therapy, and implications for respiratory care. Respir Care. 2006;51(4):403–12. PMID: 16563194.
100. Tomasoni D, Vishram-Nielsen JKK, Pagnesi M, Adamo M, Lombardi CM, Gustafsson F, et al. Advanced heart failure: guideline-directed medical therapy, diuretics, inotropes, and palliative care. ESC Heart Fail. 2022;9(3):1507–23. https://doi.org/10.1002/ehf2.13859.
101. Cattadori G, Segurini C, Picozzi A, Padeletti L, Anza C. Exercise and heart failure: an update. ESC Heart Fail. 2018;5(2):222–32. https://doi.org/10.1002/ehf2.12225.

102. Yancy CW, Jessup M, Bozkurt B, Butler J, Casey DE Jr, Drazner MH, et al. 2013 ACCF/AHA guideline for the management of heart failure: executive summary: a report of the American College of Cardiology Foundation/American Heart Association Task Force on practice guidelines. Circulation. 2013;128:1810–52. https://doi.org/10.1161/CIR.0b013e31829e8807.
103. Gotto AM Jr. Statins: powerful drugs for lowering cholesterol; advice for patients. Circulation. 2002;105(13):1514–6. https://doi.org/10.1161/01.cir.0000014245.25136.d2.93.
104. Pinal-Fernandez I, Casal-Dominguez M, Mammen AL. Statins: pros and cons. Med Clin (Barc). 2018;150(10):398–402. https://doi.org/10.1016/j.medcli.2017.11.030.
105. Moßhammer D, Schaeffeler E, Schwab M, Mörike K. Mechanisms and assessment of statin-related muscular adverse effects. Br J Clin Pharmacol. 2014;78(3):454–66. https://doi.org/10.1111/bcp.12360.
106. Ganda OP. Statin-induced diabetes: incidence, mechanisms, and implications. F1000Res. 2016;5.:F1000 Faculty Rev-1499 https://doi.org/10.12688/f1000research.8629.1.
107. Manzur-Barbur MC, Mejia-Sanjuanelo AM, Martinez-Avila MC, Manzur-Jattin F, Garcia-Dominguez JC, Orozco-Deba B. Enalapril-induced angioedema: a forgotten adverse event. Clin Case Reports. 2022;10(6):e05944. https://doi.org/10.1002/ccr3.5944.
108. Siegel RL, Giaquinto AN, Jemal A. Cancer statistics, 2024. CA Cancer J Clin. 2024;74(1):12–49. https://doi.org/10.3322/caac.21820.
109. Nolen SC, Evans MA, Fischer A, Corrada MM, Kawas CH, Bota DA. Cancer-incidence, prevalence and mortality in the oldest-old. A comprehensive review. Mech Ageing Dev. 2017;164:113–26. https://doi.org/10.1016/j.mad.2017.05.002.
110. Weir HK, Sherman R, Yu M, Gershman S, Hofer BM, Wu M, et al. Cancer incidence in older adults in the United States: characteristics, specificity, and completeness of the data. J Registry Manag. 2020;47(3):150–60. PMCID: PMC7879958.
111. Torre LA, Siegel RL, Ward EM, Jemal A. Global cancer incidence and mortality rates and trends–an update. Cancer Epidemiol Biomarkers Prev. 2016;25(1):16–27. https://doi.org/10.1158/1055-9965.EPI-15-0578.
112. Matthews HK, Bertoli C, de Bruin RAM. Cell cycle control in cancer. Nat Rev Mol Cell Biol. 2022;23(1):74–88. https://doi.org/10.1038/s41580-021-00404-3.
113. Hanahan D, Monje M. Cancer hallmarks intersect with neuroscience in the tumor microenvironment. Cancer Cell. 2023;41(3):573–80. https://doi.org/10.1016/j.ccell.2023.02.012.
114. Zhang S, Zheng M, Nie D, Xu L, Tian H, Wang M, Liu W, et al. Efficacy of cetuximab plus PD-1 inhibitor differs by HPV status in head and neck squamous cell carcinoma: a systematic review and meta-analysis. J Immunother Cancer. 2022;10(10):e005158. https://doi.org/10.1136/jitc-2022-005158.
115. Rodier F, Campisi J. Four faces of cellular senescence. J Cell Biol. 2011;192(4):547–56. https://doi.org/10.1083/jcb.201009094.
116. Campisi J, d'Adda di Fagagna F. Cellular senescence: when bad things happen to good cells. Nat Rev Mol Cell Biol. 2007;8(9):729–40. https://doi.org/10.1038/nrm2233.
117. Davalos AR, Coppe JP, Campisi J, Desprez PY. Senescent cells as a source of inflammatory factors for tumor progression. Cancer Metastasis Rev. 2010 Jun;29(2):273–83. https://doi.org/10.1007/s10555-010-9220-9.
118. Kwantwi LB. The dual role of autophagy in the regulation of cancer treatment. Amino Acids. 2024;56(1):7. https://doi.org/10.1007/s00726-023-03364-4.
119. Botti J, Djavaheri-Mergny M, Pilatte Y, Codogno P. Autophagy signaling and the cogwheels of cancer. Autophagy. 2006;2(2):67–73. https://doi.org/10.4161/auto.2.2.2458.
120. Jin J, Zhang H, Weyand CM, Goronzy JJ. Lysosomes in T cell immunity and aging. Front Aging. 2021;2:809539. https://doi.org/10.3389/fragi.2021.809539.
121. Wang Y, Dong C, Han Y, Gu Z, Sun C. Immunosenescence, aging and successful aging. Front Immunol. 2022;2(13):942796. https://doi.org/10.3389/fimmu.2022.942796.
122. Liu Z, Liang Q, Ren Y, Guo C, Ge X, Wang L, et al. Immunosenescence: molecular mechanisms and diseases. Signal Transduct Target Ther. 2023;8(1):200. https://doi.org/10.1038/s41392-023-01451-2.

123. https://www.cdc.gov/chronicdisease/resources/publications/factsheets/cancer.htm#cigarette.
124. Lewandowska AM, Rudzki M, Rudzki S, Lewandowski T, Laskowska B. Environmental risk factors for cancer – review paper. Ann Agric Environ Med. 2019;26(1):1–7. https://doi.org/10.26444/aaem/94299.
125. Yu X, Zhao H, Wang R, Chen Y, Ouyang X, Li W, et al. Cancer epigenetics: from laboratory studies and clinical trials to precision medicine. Cell Death Dis. 2024;10(1):28. https://doi.org/10.1038/s41420-024-01803-z.
126. Guo Q, Zhou Y, Xie T, Yuan Y, Li H, Shi W, et al. Tumor microenvironment of cancer stem cells: perspectives on cancer stem cell targeting. Genes Dis. 2023;11(3):101043. https://doi.org/10.1016/j.gendis.2023.05.024.
127. https://www.cancer.gov/about-cancer/treatment.
128. Given B, Given CW. Older adults and cancer treatment. Cancer. 2008;113(12 Suppl):3505–11. https://doi.org/10.1002/cncr.23939.
129. Hamaker M, Lund C, Molder MT, Soubeyran P, Wildiers Van Huis L, et al. Geriatric assessment in the management of older patients with cancer – a systematic review (update). J Geriatr Oncol. 2022;13(6):761–77. https://doi.org/10.1016/j.jgo.2022.04.008.
130. Korc-Grodzicki B, Holmes HM, Shahrokni A. Geriatric assessment for oncologists. Cancer Biol Med. 2015;12(4):261–74. https://doi.org/10.7497/j.issn.2095-3941.2015.0082.
131. Guralnik JM, Simonsick EM, Ferrucci L, Glynn RJ, Berkman LF, Blazer DG, et al. A short physical performance battery assessing lower extremity function: association with self-reported disability and prediction of mortality and nursing home admission. J Gerontol. 1994;49(2):M85–94. https://doi.org/10.1093/geronj/49.2.m85.
132. Nasreddine ZS, Phillips NA, Bedirian V, Charbonneau S, Whitehead V, Collin I, et al. The montreal cognitive assessment, MoCA: a brief screening tool for mild cognitive impairment. J Am Geriatr Soc. 2005;53(4):695–9. https://doi.org/10.1111/j.1532-5415.2005.53221.x.
133. Malone ER, Oliva M, Sabatini PJB, Stockley TL, Siu LL. Molecular profiling for precision cancer therapies. Genome Med. 2020;12(1):8. https://doi.org/10.1186/s13073-019-0703-1.
134. Chu E, Sartorelli AC. Cancer chemotherapy. In: Katzung BG, editor. Basic and clinical pharmacology. New York; 2007. p. 878–907.
135. Kwok C, Nolan M. Cardiotoxicity of anti-cancer drugs: cellular mechanisms and clinical implications. Front Cardiovasc Med. 2023;10:1150569. https://doi.org/10.3389/fcvm.2023.1150569.
136. Pottier C, Fresnais M, Gilon M, Jerusalem G, Longuespee R, Sounni NE. Tyrosine kinase inhibitors in cancer: breakthrough and challenges of targeted therapy. Cancers (Basel). 2020;12(3):731. https://doi.org/10.3390/cancers12030731.
137. Zahavi D, Weiner L. Monoclonal antibodies in cancer therapy. Antibodies (Basel). 2020;9(3):34. https://doi.org/10.3390/antib9030034.
138. Hargadon KM, Johnson CE, Williams CJ. Immune checkpoint blockade therapy for cancer: an overview of FDA-approved immune checkpoint inhibitors. Int Immunopharmacol. 2018;62:29–39. https://doi.org/10.1016/j.intimp.2018.06.001.
139. Postow MA, Callahan MK, Wolchok JD. Immune Checkpoint Blockade in Cancer Therapy. J Clin Oncol. 2015;33(17):1974–82. https://doi.org/10.1200/JCO.2014.59.4358.
140. Baldo P, Fornasier G, Ciolfi L, Sartor I, Francescon S. Pharmacovigilance in oncology. Int J Clin Pharm. 2018;40(4):832–41. https://doi.org/10.1007/s11096-018-0706-9.
141. Zeien J, Qiu W, Triay M, Dhaibar HA, Cruz-Topete D, Cornett EM, et al. Clinical implications of chemotherapeutic agent organ toxicity on perioperative care. Biomed Pharmacother. 2022;146:112503. https://doi.org/10.1016/j.biopha.2021.112503.
142. Akbarali HI, Muchhala KH, Jessup DK, Cheatham S. Chemotherapy induced gastrointestinal toxicities. Adv Cancer Res. 2022;155:131–66. https://doi.org/10.1016/bs.acr.2022.02.007.
143. Banach M, Juranek JK, Zygulska AL. Chemotherapy-induced neuropathies-a growing problem for patients and health care providers. Brain Behav. 2016;7(1):e00558. https://doi.org/10.1002/brb3.558.
144. Cardinale D, Iacopo F, Cipolla CM. Cardiotoxicity of anthracyclines. Front Cardiovasc Med. 2020;7:26. https://doi.org/10.3389/fcvm.2020.0002.

145. Baldo BA. Adverse reactions to targeted and non-targeted chemotherapeutic drugs with emphasis on hypersensitivity responses and the invasive metastatic switch. Cancer Metastasis Rev. 2013;32(3–4):723–61. https://doi.org/10.1007/s10555-013-9447-3.
146. Sales GTM, Foresto RD. Drug-induced nephrotoxicity. Rev Assoc Med Bras (1992). 2020;66(Suppl 1):s82–90. https://doi.org/10.1590/1806-9282.66.S1.82.
147. Testart-Paillet D, Girard P, You B, Freyer G, Pobel C, Tranchand B. Contribution of modelling chemotherapy-induced hematological toxicity for clinical practice. Crit Rev Oncol Hematol. 2007;63(1):1–11. https://doi.org/10.1016/j.critrevonc.2007.01.005.
148. Lyman GH, Kuderer NM, Aapro M. Improving outcomes of chemotherapy: established and novel options for myeloprotection in the COVID-19. Era Front Oncol. 2021;11:697908. https://doi.org/10.3389/fonc.2021.697908.
149. Kaddoura R, Dabdoob WA, Ahmed K, Yassin MA. A practical guide to managing cardiopulmonary toxicities of tyrosine kinase inhibitors in chronic myeloid leukemia. Front Med (Lausanne). 2023;10:1163137. https://doi.org/10.3389/fmed.2023.1163137.
150. Catalano A, Iacopetta D, Ceramella J, Scumaci D, Giuzio F, Saturnino C, et al. Multidrug resistance (MDR): a widespread phenomenon in pharmacological therapies. Molecules. 2022;27(3):616. https://doi.org/10.3390/molecules27030616.
151. Mansoori B, Mohammadi A, Davudian S, Shirjang S, Baradaran B. The different mechanisms of cancer drug resistance: a brief review. Adv Pharm Bull. 2017;7(3):339–48. https://doi.org/10.15171/apb.2017.041.
152. Alexander JL, Wilson ID, Teare J, Marchesi JR, Nicholson JK, Kinross JM. Gut microbiota modulation of chemotherapy efficacy and toxicity. Nat Rev Gastroenterol Hepatol. 2017;14(6):356–65. https://doi.org/10.1038/nrgastro.2017.20.
153. Brenowitz WD, Hubbard RA, Keene CD, Hawes SE, Longstreth WT Jr, Woltjer RL, et al. Mixed neuropathologies and estimated rates of clinical progression in a large autopsy sample. Alzheimers Dement. 2017;13(6):654–62. https://doi.org/10.1016/j.jalz.2016.09.015.
154. Rajan KB, Weuve J, Barnes LL, McAninch EA, Wilson RS, Evans DA. Population estimate of people with clinical AD and mild cognitive impairment in the United States (2020–2060). Alzheimers Dement. 2021;17(12):1966–75. https://doi.org/10.1002/alz.12362.
155. Tom SE, Hubbard RA, Crane PK, Haneuse S, Bowen J, McCormick WC, et al. Characterization of dementia and Alzheimer's disease in an older population: updated incidence and life expectancy with and without dementia. Am J Public Health. 2015 Feb;105(2):408–13. https://doi.org/10.2105/AJPH.2014.301935.
156. Hebert LE, Weuve J, Scherr PA, Evens DA. Alzheimer disease in the United States (2010–2050) estimated using the 2010 census. Neurology. 2013;80(19):1778–83. https://doi.org/10.1212/WNL.0b013e31828726f5.
157. Gouras GK, Olsson TT, Hansson O. β-Amyloid peptides and amyloid plaques in Alzheimer's disease. Neurotherapeutics. 2015;12(1):3–11. https://doi.org/10.1007/s13311-014-0313-y.
158. Venegas C, Kumar S, Franklin BS, Dierkes T, Brinkschulte R, Tejera D, et al. Microglia-derived ASC specks cross-seed amyloid-beta in Alzheimer's disease. Nature. 2017;552(7685):355–61. https://doi.org/10.1038/nature25158.
159. Koper MJ, Van Schoor E, Ospitalieri S, Vandenberghe R, Vandenbulche M, Arnim CAF, et al. Necrosome complex detected in granulovacuolar degeneration is associated with neuronal loss in Alzheimer's disease. Acta Neuropathol. 2020;139(3):463–84. https://doi.org/10.1007/s00401-019-02103-y.
160. Long JM, Holtzman DM. Alzheimer disease: an update on pathobiology and treatment strategies. Cell. 2019;179(2):312–39. https://doi.org/10.1016/j.cell.2019.09.001.
161. Giannakopoulos P, Herrmann FR, Bussiere T, Bouras C, Kövari E, Perl DP, et al. Tangle and neuron numbers, but not amyloid load, predict cognitive status in Alzheimer's disease. Neurology. 2003;60(9):1495–500. https://doi.org/10.1212/01.wnl.0000063311.58879.01.
162. Nelson PT, Alafuzoff I, Bigio EH, Bouras C, Braak H, Cairns NJ, et al. Correlation of Alzheimer disease neuropathologic changes with cognitive status: a review of the literature. J Neuropathol Exp Neurol. 2012;71(5):362–81. https://doi.org/10.1097/NEN.0b013e31825018f7.

163. DeVos SL, Corjuc BT, Oakley DH, Nobuhara CK, Bannon RN, Chase A, et al. Synaptic Tau seeding precedes Tau pathology in human Alzheimer's disease brain. Front Neurosci. 2018;12:267. https://doi.org/10.3389/fnins.2018.00267.
164. Kunkle BW, Grenier-Boley B, Sims R, Bis JC, Damotte V, Naj AC, et al. Genetic meta-analysis of diagnosed Alzheimer's disease identifies new risk loci and implicates Aβ, tau, immunity and lipid processing. Nat Genet. 2019;51(3):414–30. https://doi.org/10.1038/s41588-019-0358-2.
165. Roses AD. Apolipoprotein E alleles as risk factors in Alzheimer's disease. Annu Rev Med. 1996;47:387–400. https://doi.org/10.1146/annurev.med.47.1.387.
166. Lashley T, Schott JM, Weston P, Murray CE, Wellington H, Keshavan A, et al. Dis Model Mech. 2018;11(5):dmm031781. https://doi.org/10.1242/dmm.031781.
167. Maharjan R, Bustamante LD, Ghattas KN, Ilyas S, Al-Refai R, Khan S. Role of lifestyle in neuroplasticity and neurogenesis in an aging brain. Cureus. 2020;12(9):e10639. https://doi.org/10.7759/cureus.10639.
168. Sikora E, Bielak-Zmijewska A, Dudkowska M, Krzystyniak A, Mosieniak G, Wesierska M, et al. Front Aging Neurosci. 2021;13:646924. https://doi.org/10.3389/fnagi.2021.646924.
169. Bettio LE, Rajendran L, Gil-Mohapel J. The effects of aging in the hippocampus and cognitive decline. Neurosci Biobehav Rev. 2017;79:66–86. https://doi.org/10.1016/j.neubiorev.2017.04.030.
170. Yankova G, Bogomyakova O, Tulupov A. The glymphatic system and meningeal lymphatics of the brain: new understanding of brain clearance. Rev Neurosci. 2021;32(7):693–705. https://doi.org/10.1515/revneuro-2020-0106.
171. Benveniste H, Liu X, Koundal S, Sanggaard S, Lee H, Wardlaw J. The glymphatic system and waste clearance with brain aging: a review. Gerontology. 2019;65(2):106–19. https://doi.org/10.1159/000490349.
172. Ma Q, Ineichen BV, Detmar M, Proulx ST. Outflow of cerebrospinal fluid is predominantly through lymphatic vessels and is reduced in aged mice. Nat Commun. 2017;8(1):1434. https://doi.org/10.1038/s41467-017-01484-6.
173. Ju Y-ES, Ooms SJ, Sutphen C, Macauley SL, Zangrilli MA, Jerome G, et al. Slow wave sleep disruption increases cerebrospinal fluid amyloid-β levels. Brain. 2017;140(8):2104–11. https://doi.org/10.1093/brain/awx148.
174. Fortea J, Zaman SH, Hartley S, Rafii MS, Head E, Carmona-Iragui M. Alzheimer's disease associated with Down syndrome: a genetic form of dementia. Lancet Neurol. 2021;20(11):930–42. https://doi.org/10.1016/S1474-4422(21)00245-3.
175. Wolters FJ, van der Lee SJ, Koudstaal PJ, van Duijn CM, Hofman A, Ikam MK, et al. Parental family history of dementia in relation to subclinical brain disease and dementia risk. Neurology. 2017;88(17):1642–9. https://doi.org/10.1212/WNL.0000000000003871.
176. Loughrey DG, Kelly ME, Kelley GA, Brennan S, Lawlor BA. Association of age-related hearing loss with cognitive function, cognitive impairment, and dementia: a systematic review and meta-analysis. JAMA Otolaryngol Head Neck Surg. 2018;144(2):115–26. https://doi.org/10.1001/jamaoto.2017.2513.
177. Brewster KK, Deal JA, Lin FR. Rutherford BR considering hearing loss as a modifiable risk factor for dementia. Expert Rev Neurother. 2022;22(9):805–13. https://doi.org/10.1080/14737175.2022.2128769.
178. Bartus RT, Dean RL III, Beer B, Lippa AS. The cholinergic hypothesis of geriatric memory dysfunction. Science. 1982;217(4558):408–14. https://doi.org/10.1126/science.7046051.
179. Sharma K. Cholinesterase inhibitors as Alzheimer's therapeutics (Review). Mol Med Rep. 2019;20(2):1479–87. https://doi.org/10.3892/mmr.2019.10374.
180. Jacobson SA, Sabbagh MN. Donepezil: potential neuroprotective and disease-modifying effects. Expert Opin Drug Metab Toxicol. 2008;4:1363–9. https://doi.org/10.1517/17425255.4.10.1363.
181. Rogers SL, Farlow MR, Doody RS, Mohs R, Friedhoff LT. A 24 week double blind placebo controlled trial of donepezil in patients with Alzheimer's disease. Donepezil study group. Neurology. 1998;50:136–45. https://doi.org/10.1212/wnl.50.1.136.

182. Corey-Bloom J, Anand R, Veach J. A randomized trial evaluating the efficacy and safety of ENA 713 (rivastigmine tartrate), a new acetylcholinesterase inhibitor, in patients with mild to moderately severe Alzheimer's disease. Int J Geriatr Psychopharmacol. 1998;1:55–65. https://www.cochranelibrary.com/central/doi/10.1002/central/CN-00211022/full.
183. Mehta M, Adem A, Sabbagh M. New acetylcholinesterase inhibitors for Alzheimer's disease. Int J Alzheimers Dis. 2012:728983. https://doi.org/10.1155/2012/728983.
184. Marucci G, Buccioni M, Ben DD, Lambertucci C, Volpini R, Amenta F. Efficacy of acetylcholinesterase inhibitors in Alzheimer's disease. Neuropharmacology. 2021;190:108352. https://doi.org/10.1016/j.neuropharm.2020.108352.
185. Reisberg B, Doody R, Stöffler A, Schmitt F, Ferris S, Möbius HJ. Memantine in moderate-to-severe Alzheimer's disease. Memantine Study Group. N Engl J Med. 2003;348(14):1333–41. https://doi.org/10.1056/NEJMoa013128.
186. Guo J, Wang Z, Liu R, Huang Y, Zhang N, Zhang R. Memantine, Donepezil, or combination therapy-what is the best therapy for Alzheimer's disease? A network meta-analysis. Brain Behav. 2020;10(11):e01831. https://doi.org/10.1002/brb3.1831.
187. Wang Y, Alzheimers Dement (N Y). An insider's perspective on FDA approval of aducanumab. 2023 Apr–Jun; 9(2): e12382. https://doi.org/10.1002/trc2.12382
188. https://www.nia.nih.gov/news/nia-statement-report-lecanemab.
189. Lee AY. Vascular dementia. Chonnam Med J. 2011;47(2):66–71. https://doi.org/10.4068/cmj.2011.47.2.66.
190. Wong EC, Chui HC. Vascular cognitive impairment and dementia. Continuum (Minneap Minn). 2022;28(3):750–80. https://doi.org/10.1212/CON.0000000000001124.
191. Pantoni L, Poggesi A, Diciotti S, Valenti R, Orsolini S, Rocca ED, et al. Effect of attention training in mild cognitive impairment patients with subcortical vascular changes: the RehAtt study. J Alzheimers Dis. 2017;60(2):615–24. https://doi.org/10.3233/JAD-170428.
192. https://www.who.int/health-topics/diabetes#tab=tab_1.
193. Beckman JA, Paneni F, Cosentino F, Creager MA. Diabetes and vascular disease: pathophysiology, clinical consequences, and medical therapy: part II. Eur Heart J. 2013;34(31):2444–52. https://doi.org/10.1093/eurheartj/eht142.
194. International Diabetes Federation 2021 IDF.org- attachment 29.
195. https://www.cdc.gov/diabetes/data/statistics-report/index.html.
196. Galicia-Garcia U, Benito-Vicente A, Jebari S, Larrea-Sebal A, Siddiqi H, Uribe KB, et al. Pathophysiology of Type 2 diabetes mellitus. Int J Mol Sci. 2020;21(17):6275. https://doi.org/10.3390/ijms21176275.
197. Petersen MC, Vatner DF, Shulman GI. Regulation of hepatic glucose metabolism in health and disease. Nat Rev Endocrinol. 2017;13(10):572–87. https://doi.org/10.1038/nrendo.2017.80.
198. Jiang G, Zhang BB. Glucagon and regulation of glucose metabolism. Am J Physiol Endocrinol Metab. 2003 Apr;284(4):E671–8. https://doi.org/10.1152/ajpendo.00492.2002
199. Carey VJ, Walters EE, Colditz GA, Solomon CG, Willet WC, Rosner BA, et al. Body fat distribution and risk of non-insulin-dependent diabetes mellitus in women: the nurses' health study. Am J Epidemiol. 1997;145(7):614–9. https://doi.org/10.1093/oxfordjournals.aje.a009158.
200. Pavlou V, Cienfuegos S, Lin S, Ezpeleta M, Ready K, Corapi S, et al. Effect of time-restricted eating on weight loss in adults with Type 2 diabetes: a randomized clinical trial. JAMA Netw Open. 2023;6(10):e2339337. https://doi.org/10.1001/jamanetworkopen.2023.39337.
201. Si K, Hu Y, Wang M, Apovian CM, Chavarro JE, Sun Q. Weight loss strategies, weight change, and Type 2 diabetes in US health professionals: a cohort study. PLoS Med. 2022;19(9):e1004094. https://doi.org/10.1371/journal.pmed.1004094.
202. Kahn BB, Flier JS. Obesity and insulin resistance. J Clin Invest. 2000;106(4):473–81. https://doi.org/10.1172/JCI10842.
203. Lopes HF, Correa-Giannella ML, Consolim-Colombo FM, Egan BM. Visceral adiposity syndrome. Diabetol Metab Syndr. 2016;8:40. https://doi.org/10.1186/s13098-016-0156-2.

204. Patterson R, McNamara E, Tainio M, de Sá TH, Smith AD, Sharp SJ, et al. Sedentary behaviour and risk of all-cause, cardiovascular and cancer mortality, and incident type 2 diabetes: a systematic review and dose response meta-analysis. Eur J Epidemiol. 2018;33(9):811–29. https://doi.org/10.1007/s10654-018-0380-1.
205. Thyfault JP, Booth FW. Lack of regular physical exercise or too much inactivity. Curr Opin Clin Nutr Metab Care. 2011;14(4):374–8. https://doi.org/10.1097/MCO.0b013e3283468e69.
206. Venkatasamy VV, Pericherla S, Manthuruthil S, Mishra S, Hanno R. Effect of physical activity on insulin resistance, inflammation and oxidative stress in diabetes mellitus. J Clin Diagn Res. 2013;7(8):1764–6. https://doi.org/10.7860/JCDR/2013/6518.3306.
207. Reynolds LJ, Williams TM, Harden JE, Twiddy HM, Kearney ML. Short-term removal of exercise impairs glycemic control in older adults: a randomized trial. Phys Rep. 2023;11(2):e15591. https://doi.org/10.14814/phy2.15591.
208. Celli A, Barnouin Y, Jiang B, Blevins D, Colleluori G, Mediwala S, et al. Lifestyle intervention strategy to treat diabetes in older adults: a randomized controlled trial. Diabetes Care. 2022;45(9):1943–52. https://doi.org/10.2337/dc22-0338.
209. Kirwan JP, Sacks J, Nieuwoudt S. The essential role of exercise in the management of type 2 diabetes. Cleve Clin J Med. 2017;84(7 Suppl 1):S15–21. https://doi.org/10.3949/ccjm.84.s1.03.
210. Martín-Peláez S, Fito M, Castaner O. Mediterranean diet effects on type 2 diabetes prevention, disease progression, and related mechanisms. A review. Nutrients. 2020;12(8):2236. https://doi.org/10.3390/nu12082236.
211. Esposito K, Chiodini P, Maiorino MI, Bellastella G, Panagiotakos D, Giugliano D. Which diet forprevention of type 2 diabetes? A meta-analysis of prospective studies. Endocrine. 2014;47(1):107–16. https://doi.org/10.1007/s12020-014-0264-4.
212. Chen Z, Liu XA, Kenny PJ. Central and peripheral actions of nicotine that influence blood glucose homeostasis and the development of diabetes. Pharmacol Res. 2023;194:106860. https://doi.org/10.1016/j.phrs.2023.106860.
213. Palmer AK, Tchkonia T, Kirkland JL. Senolytics: potential for alleviating diabetes and its complications. Endocrinology. 2021;162(8):bqab058. https://doi.org/10.1210/endocr/bqab058.
214. Gunasekaran U, Gannon M. Type 2 diabetes and the aging pancreatic beta cell. Aging (Albany NY). 2011;3(6):565–75. https://doi.org/10.18632/aging.100350.
215. Zhu M, Liu X, Liu W, Lu Y, Cheng J, Chen Y. Beta cell aging and age-related diabetes. Aging (Albany NY). 2021;13(5):7691–706. https://doi.org/10.18632/aging.202593.
216. Kim KS, Park KS, Kim MJ, Kim SK, Cho YW, Park SW. Type 2 diabetes is associated with low muscle mass in older adults. Geriatr Gerontol Int. 2014;14(Suppl 1):115–21. https://doi.org/10.1111/ggi.12189.
217. Pearson ER. Type 2 diabetes: a multifaceted disease. Diabetologia. 2019;62(7):1107–12. https://doi.org/10.1007/s00125-019-4909-y.
218. Goyal R, Singhal M, Jialal. I Type 2 diabetes. 2023 Jun 23. In: StatPearls [Internet]. Treasure Island (FL): StatPearls Publishing; 2024 Jan–. PMID: 3002062.
219. Knowler WC, Barrett-Connor E, Fowler SE, Diabetes Prevention Program Research Group, et al. Reduction in the incidence of type 2 diabetes with lifestyle intervention or metformin. N Engl J Med. 2002;346(6):393–403. https://doi.org/10.1056/NEJMoa012512.
220. Diabetes Prevention Program Research Group, Knowler WC, Fowler SE, Hamman RF, et al. 10-year follow-up of diabetes incidence and weight loss in the Diabetes Prevention Program Outcomes Study. Lancet. 2009;374(9702):1677–86. https://doi.org/10.1016/S0140-6736(09)61457-4.

221. Perreault L, Pan Q, Mather KJ, Watson KE, Hamman RF, Kahn SE, Diabetes Prevention Program Research Group. Effect of regression from prediabetes to normal glucose regulation on long-term reduction in diabetes risk: results from the Diabetes Prevention Program Outcomes Study. Lancet. 2012;379(9833):2243–51. https://doi.org/10.1016/S0140-6736(12)60525-X.
222. Tuso P. Prediabetes and lifestyle modification: time to prevent a preventable disease. Perm J. 2014;18(3):88–93. https://doi.org/10.7812/TPP/14-002.
223. Uusitupa M, Khan TA, Viguiliouk E, Kahleova H, Rivellese AA, Hermansen K, et al. Prevention of type 2 diabetes by lifestyle changes: a systematic review and meta-analysis. Nutrients. 2019;11(11):2611. https://doi.org/10.3390/nu11112611.
224. Chaudhury A, Duvoor C, Dendi VSR, Kraleti S, Chada A, Ravilla R, et al. Prediabetes and lifestyle modification: time to prevent a preventablendisease. Front Endocrinol (Lausanne). 2017;8:6. https://doi.org/10.3389/fendo.2017.00006.
225. Padhi S, Nayak AK, Behera A. Type II diabetes mellitus: a review on recent drug based therapeutics. Biomed Pharmacother. 2020;131:110708. https://doi.org/10.1016/j.biopha.2020.110708.
226. Viollet B, Guigas B, Garcia N, Leclerc J, Foretz M, Andreelli F. Cellular and molecular mechanisms of metfromin: an overview. Clin Sci (Lond). 2012;122(6):253–70. https://doi.org/10.1042/CS20110386.
227. Fogelman Y, Kitai E, Blumberg G, Golan-Cohen A, Rapoport M, Carmeli E. Vitamin B12 screening in metformin-treated diabetics in primary care: were elderly patients less likely to be tested? Aging Clin Exp Res. 2017;29(2):135–9. https://doi.org/10.1007/s40520-016-0546-.
228. Wang J-Y, Wang Q-W, Yang X-Y, Yang W, Li D-R, Jin J-Y et al. GLP-1 receptor agonists for the treatment of obesity: Role as a promising approach Front Endocrinol (Lausanne). 2023 Feb 1:14:1085799. https://doi.org/10.3389/fendo.2023.1085799.
229. Proks P, Reimann F, Green N, Gribble F, Ashcroft F. Sulfonylurea stimulation of insulin secretion. Diabetes. 2002;51(Suppl 3):S368–76. https://doi.org/10.2337/diabetes.51.2007.S368.
230. de Wet H, Proks P. Molecular action of sulphonylureas on KATP channels: a real partnership between drugs and nucleotides. Biochem Soc Trans. 2015;43(5):901–7. https://doi.org/10.1042/BST20150096.
231. Wright EM. SGLT2 inhibitors: physiology and pharmacology. Kidney 360. 2021;2(12):2027–37. https://doi.org/10.34067/KID.0002772021.
232. Halimi S, Verges B. Adverse effects and safety of SGLT-2 inhibitors. Diabetes Metab. 2014;40(6 Suppl 1):S28–34. https://doi.org/10.1016/S1262-3636(14)72693-X.
233. Yang S, Liu Y, Zhang S, Wu F, Liu D, Wu Q, et al. Risk of diabetic ketoacidosis of SGLT2 inhibitors in patients with type 2 diabetes: a systematic review and network meta-analysis of randomized controlled trials. Front Pharmacol. 2023;14:1145587. https://doi.org/10.3389/fphar.2023.1145587.
234. Semple RK, Chatterjee VK, O'Rahilly S. PPAR gamma and human metabolic disease. J Clin Invest. 2006;116(3):581–9. https://doi.org/10.1172/JCI28003.
235. Yakaryılmaz FD, Öztürk ZA. Treatment of type 2 diabetes mellitus in the elderly. World J Diabetes. 2017;8(6):278–85. https://doi.org/10.4239/wjd.v8.i6.278.
236. Buzzetti R, FadiniGP NA, Larosa M, Rossi MC, Cucinotta D. Comparative effectiveness of Glargine 300 U/mL vs. Degludec 100 U/mL in patients with type 2 diabetes switching from 1° generation basal insulins. Nutr Metab Cardiovasc Dis. 2022;32(9):2255–63. https://doi.org/10.1016/j.numecd.2022.06.003.
237. Rendell M. Technosphere inhaled insulin (Afrezza). Drugs Today (Barc). 2014;50(12):813–27. https://doi.org/10.1358/dot.2014.50.12.2233894.
238. Meier M, Hummel M. Cardiovascular disease and intensive glucose control in type 2 diabetes mellitus: moving practice toward evidence-based strategies. Vasc Health Risk Manag. 2009;5:859–71. https://doi.org/10.2147/vhrm.s4808.

239. Sesti G, Antonelli Incalzi R, Bonora E, Consoli A, Giaccari A, Maggi S, et al. Management of diabetes in older adults. Nutr Metab Cardiovasc Dis. 2018;28(3):206–18. https://doi.org/10.1016/j.numecd.2017.11.007.
240. Kirkman MS, Briscoe VJ, Clark N, Florez H, Haas LB, Halter JB, et al. Diabetes in older adults. Diabetes Care. 2012;35:2650e64. https://doi.org/10.2337/dc12-1801.
241. Ishikawa T, Koshizaka M, Maezawa Y, Takemoto M, Tokuyama Y, Saito T, et al. Continuous glucose monitoring reveals hypoglycemia risk in elderly patients with type 2 diabetes mellitus. J Diabetes Investig. 2018;9(1):69–74. https://doi.org/10.1111/jdi.12676.
242. Longo M, Bellastella G, Maiorino MI, Meier JJ, Esposito K. Giugliano D diabetes and aging: from treatment goals to pharmacologic therapy. Front Endocrinol (Lausanne). 2019;10:45. https://doi.org/10.3389/fendo.2019.00045.
243. Munshi M, Blair E, Ganda OP, Gabbay, RA, Members of the Joslin Clinical Oversight Committee. CHAPTER 4. Guideline for the care of the older adult with diabetes. Am J Manag Care 2018;24 (7 Spec No.):SP240-SP252. PMID: 29938997.

Medication Use in Major Age-Related Diseases: Chronic Obstructive Pulmonary Disease, Chronic Kidney Disease, and Parkinson's Disease

Abbreviations

ACEI	angiotensin-converting enzyme inhibitor
ACh	acetylcholine
ACR	albumin to creatinine ratio
ADLs	activities of daily living
ARB	angiotensin receptor blocker
ATP	adenosine triphosphate
BEC	blood eosinophil count
BMI	body mass index
BP	blood pressure
CAT	COPD Assessment Test
CD-LD	carbidopa/levodopa
CKD	chronic kidney disease
CNS	central nervous system
COPD	chronic obstructive pulmonary disease
CPS	calcium polystyrene sulfonate
CR	controlled release
CT	computed topography
CV	cardiovascular
DALYs	disability-adjusted life years
DAT	dopamine transporter
DPI	dry powder inhalers
eGFR	estimated glomerular filtration rate
ER	extended release
ESKD	end-stage kidney disease
FVC	forced vital capacity
FEC_1	forced expiratory capacity in one second
g/kg body wt	grams per kilogram body weight

GFR	glomerular filtration rate
GI	gastrointestinal
HIC	high-income countries
ICS	inhaled corticosteroid
IR	immediate release
K+	potassium
LABA	long-acting beta2-adrenergic receptor agonists
LAMA	long-acting muscarinic acetylcholine receptor antagonists
LMIC	low- and middle-income countries
LVRS	lung volume reduction surgery
m2	metered squared
mAChR-antagonists	muscarinic acetylcholine receptor antagonists
MDI	metered-dose inhalers
MDS-UPDRS	motor disorder society—unified Parkinson's disease rating scale
mg/mmol	milligram per millimole
mmol/l	millimoles per liter
mMRC	modified Medical Research Council dyspnea scale
MPTP	1-methyl-4-phenyl-1,2,3,6-tetrahydropyridine
NMDA receptor	N-methyl-D-aspartate receptor
NSAIDs	nonsteroidal anti-inflammatory drugs
nsMRA	nonsteroidal mineralocorticoid receptor antagonist
OTC	over-the-counter
Pa O2	partial pressure of oxygen in arterial blood
PCBs	polychlorinated biphenyls
PIM	potentially inappropriate medication
PSC	patiromer sorbitex calcium
QoL	quality of life
RAAS	renin-angiotensin-aldosterone-system
RBD	idiopathic rapid eye movement (REM) behavior disorder
RCT	randomized clinical trial
ROS	reactive oxygen species
SABA	short-acting beta2-adrenergic receptor agonists
sCr	serum creatinine
sCys	serum cystatin-c
SGLT2I	sodium-glucose cotransporter 2 inhibitor
SGRQ	St Georges Respiratory Questionnaire
SPS	sodium polystyrene sulfonate
SZC	sodium zirconium cyclosilicate
T2DM	type 2 diabetes mellitus
TCE	trichloroethylene
UPDRS	Unified Parkinson's Disease Rating Scale
β_2-AR agonists	beta2-adrenergic receptor agonists
β-ARB	beta-adrenergic receptor blocker

Chronic obstructive pulmonary disease (COPD), chronic kidney disease (CKD), and Parkinson's disease are progressive deteriorative diseases with no cure. These are also age-dependent diseases whose prevalence will continue to augment with an increase in life expectancy. Consequently, they exact a substantial social and economic cost worldwide. Older adults with these chronic illnesses are the heaviest users of health care; the greater their comorbidities, the greater the use. Caregiver strain is also a big concern, as well as the cost of prescription drugs. The pathology of these diseases involves the interaction of environmental toxins and genetics with age changes. Fortunately, both pharmacological and non-pharmacological therapies manage these diseases for many years. Currently prescribed drugs are detailed in Tables 5.1, 5.2, 5.3, and 5.4, although there is a dearth of clinical data supporting use in older adults. Nevertheless, with disease progression, serious attention is required to avoid polypharmacy, drug interactions, and adverse effects. Importantly, COPD and CKD are considered preventable diseases, so awareness and removal of their causal modifiable risk factors are critical.

In addition to drug use in these major diseases, this chapter also presents the pathophysiology, prevalence, risk factors, and important assessment tools for these diseases. Tables 5.1, 5.2, 5.3, and 5.4 provide a summary for the narrative.

Chronic Obstructive Pulmonary Disease

Chronic Obstructive Pulmonary Disease. Introduction The Global Initiatives For Chronic Obstructive Lung Disease [81, 82] have redefined COPD in an effort to better utilize the information on this disease gathered over the past 30 years and to decrease the COPD-associated morbidity and mortality, worldwide. Thus, "COPD is a heterogeneous lung condition characterized by chronic respiratory symptoms (dyspnea, cough, expectoration) due to persistent abnormalities of the airways (bronchitis, bronchiolitis), alveoli (emphysema), and/or pulmonary vessels, confirmed by spirometrically determined airflow limitation and/or objective evidence of structural or physiological pulmonary dysfunction" [83, 84].

In other words, COPD is a lung disease with specific symptoms that vary from individual to individual (heterogeneous), probably due to the complexity of its etiology [82]. COPD is defined by abnormal structural and functional changes in the lungs that reduce respiratory function and the ability to breathe normally. Structural changes occur in the airways, alveoli (tissue of gas exchange), and pulmonary vessels induced by several inflammatory conditions of bronchitis, bronchiolitis, and emphysema. Important symptoms are difficulty in breathing or "shortness of breath" during everyday activities (dyspnea) and persistent cough, with or without discharge of mucous material. Additionally, COPD is characterized by pulmonary function measurements (breathing test) with a spirometer, an instrument that measures the amount of air taken in on a single forced inspiration and expelled within one second on forced expiration. The total of forced inspiration and expiration is termed forced vital capacity (FVC) and the forced expiration in one second is termed forced expiratory capacity (FEC_1). The ratio of FEC_1/FVC determines the degree of pulmonary obstruction. In support of a COPD diagnosis, FEC_1/FVC is ≤0.7, generally determined after administration of a bronchodilator (drug to open the airways). Other tests, such as a computed tomography (CT) of the chest, can identify structural changes such as the presence of emphysema (damaged lung tissue with enlarged air sacs) and abnormal widening of the bronchi and bronchioli (bronchiectasis) [85], essentially a second type of COPD. A CT scan is highly recommended for COPD patients with repeat exacerbations that basically define a state of acute respiratory distress requiring hospitalization and immediate medical attention [83].

COPD is considered a "common, preventable and treatable disease" [85]. It is proposed that with this current practical and broader definition, early stages of COPD may be identified and appropriately treated to prevent progression [83].

Chronic Obstructive Pulmonary Disease. Prevalence The global prevalence of COPD, as assessed in a systematic review and modeling study of 65 countries in adults 30–70 years of age, is 10.3% using the diagnostic standard of FEV_1/FVC of <0.7 [86]. Prevalence is age-dependent with 21.9% of 65–69-year-olds and 32.6% of 70–79-year-olds with COPD in high-income countries (HIC) and slightly higher percentages in these age groups in low- and middle-income countries (LMIC) [86]. The global burden of COPD through 2050, based on modeling and prevalence of established risk factors, is expected to increase worldwide, more dramatically in women in LMIC [87]. In the United States, prevalence in adults >18 years of age is 6% but in those ≥65, prevalence doubles to ~12% [88].

Chronic Obstructive Pulmonary Disease. Risk Factors COPD is considered a complex respiratory disease that is driven by the interaction of environmental, genetic, and pulmonary growth trajectory factors, inducing aging [85]. The major environmental risk factor for COPD is tobacco smoking ([89]; see also Chap. 8). Results from the Framingham Offspring 23-year longitudinal study with measurements in teenagers to older adults showed that smoking significantly accelerated the rate of decline in lung function and also early smoking cessation ameliorated this decline [89]. Tobacco smoking before the age of 15 is highly associated with late-life onset of COPD [90]. Since approximately 20–40% of patients with COPD were never smokers, exposure to other environmental toxins perturbs lung function leading to COPD, although the degree and rate of lung deterioration appear slightly less than with tobacco smoking [91]. Significant environmental risk factors in never smokers that increase the risk of COPD are exposure to passive smoking [92], indoor air pollution due to burning of biomass such as wood or charcoal [92, 93] especially prevalent in women in LMIC [94], and exposure to occupational toxic gases, dust, and fumes [95, 96]. Outdoor air pollution with particulate matter, ozone, nitrogen, and sulfur oxides may not initiate COPD, but it definitely worsens COPD once established [97].

A second component of COPD is genetics with an estimated heritability of 40–60% as reviewed by Silverman (2020) [98]. Thus far, a genetic deficiency of alpha-1 antitrypsin (AAT) is the only mutation (gene SERPINA1) associated with COPD [99]. AAT is a protease (enzyme that destroys proteins) that circulates in the plasma and inhibits another enzyme, elastase found in neutrophil granules [100]. If left unchecked, elastase destroys lung tissue [100]. The progression to emphysema with AAT deficiency, additionally, depends on years of tobacco smoking [99]. Genome-wide association studies have identified a number of genes that appear relevant in animal models of COPD and in the future could provide insight into the pathophysiology of COPD [98].

The third component of COPD relates to the development, maturation, and aging of the pulmonary system, called lung function trajectories [101]. Lung trajectories below normal are associated with reduced lung function and increased risk of COPD [85, 102]. Reduced normal lung function trajectories depend on abnormal developmental factors, chronic exposure to respiratory infections, and accelerated pulmonary aging, all of which elevate the risk for COPD [85]. Normal age changes implicate a decline in beta-2 adrenergic receptor (β2AR) affinity [103] that would favor bronchoconstriction, an increased presence of cell senescence, low-grade inflammaging [104, 105], and immunosenescence [106]. These are changes that promote lung dysfunction.

Chronic Obstructive Pulmonary Disease. Pharmacotherapy Specific age-related pharmacotherapy for the older adult with COPD is primarily extrapolated from randomized clinical trials (RCTs) enrolling younger patients [2]. One reason for this is the elevated prevalence of older COPD patients with comorbidities [107] and generally, these are comorbidities such as diseases of the cardiovascular system that automatically exclude them from RCTs [2]. Thus, in the presence of a paucity of RCT data, caregivers need to apply drug use considerations regarding age-related changes in pharmacokinetics (PK) and pharmacodynamics (PD) (see Chap. 2), effects of comorbidities, e.g., cardiovascular and dementia (see Chap. 4), potential drug–drug interactions (DDIs) (see Chap. 3), and reduced organ function (see Chap. 10). This advice also applies to drug use in CKD and Parkinson's disease, discussed below.

Pharmacotherapy initiation and selection are based on several parameters, including the assessment of lung function obstruction (spirometric measurements) and the presence of symptoms of dyspnea and exacerbations. Lung obstruction is divided into four categories (GOLD 1–4) based on decreasing range of percent FEV_1 predicted post-bronchodilation. It can range from Gold 1, mild at >80% to Gold 4 at <30% predicted. Dyspnea is determined with the modified Medical Research Council dyspnea scale (mMRC). The mMRC is a scale from 0 to 4, which measures breathlessness "breathless with strenuous exercise as 0 and too breathless to leave the house as 4" [108]. The COPD assessment test (CAT) determines quality of life (QoL) with eight questions rated 0–5 and scores of 0–40, with higher numbers indicating worsening condition [109]. Results correlate well with a more extensive questionnaire such as the St. Georges Respiratory Questionnaire (SGRQ) [110]. The number and seriousness (need for hospitalization) of exacerbations are also recorded. Exacerbations are defined as "an event characterized by increased

Table 5.1 Recommendations for treatment of chronic obstructive pulmonary disease[a]

Drug class	Class members	Disease criteria
Bronchodilator	β2-AR agonist— salmeterol, formoterol, olodaterol, vilanterol mAChR- antagonists— tiotropium, ipratropium, umeclidinium	COPD assessment test (CAT[b]) <10; modified Medical Record Council (mMRC[c])0–1 0–1 exacerbations, no hospitalizations
Combined long-acting beta agonist (LABA) plus long-acting muscarinic antagonist (LAMA)	Umeclidinium/vilanterol Indacaterol/ glycopyrronium	CAT ≥10 mMRC ≥2 0–1 exacerbations, no hospitalizations
LABA plus LAMA plus inhaled corticosteroid	Fluticasone furoate/ umeclidinium/vilanterol	≥2 exacerbations with ≥1 leading to hospitalization

β2-AR agonist—beta2-adrenergic receptor agonist: mAChR-antagonist—muscarinic acetylcholine receptor antagonist
[a]Summary from Ref. [1]
[b]CAT-Patient response to questions on quality of life and burden of symptoms (score 0–10 = mild impact); higher scores, higher impact
[c]mMRC—measures dyspnea with score of 0–4 (increasing severity)

dyspnea and/or cough and sputum that worsens in <14 days which may be accompanied by tachypnea (abnormally rapid breathing) and/or tachycardia (rapid heart rate) and is often associated with increased local and systemic inflammation caused by infection, pollution, or other insult to the airways" [84].

Just as the definition of COPD is evolving for the better, so are the recommendations for COPD therapy [1]. As summarized in Table 5.1, *three classes of drugs* are useful in the treatment of COPD. They are:

1. $β_2$-adrenergic receptor agonists ($β_2$-AR agonists) that are classed as ultra-long-acting $β_2$-AR agonists (ultra-LABA, 24 h), e.g., indacaterol, long-acting (LABA, 12 h), e.g., salmeterol, formoterol, olodaterol, vilanterol, and short-acting $β_2$-AR agonists (SABA, 4–6 h), e.g., salbutamol, terbutaline [111].
2. Long-acting muscarinic acetylcholine receptor antagonists (mAChR-antagonists) (LAMA), e.g., tiotropium, ipratropium, umeclidinium.
3. Inhaled corticosteroid (ICS), e.g., fluticasone furoate, mometasone, beclomethasone, budesonide, flunisolide. The advantages and disadvantages of COPD pharmacotherapy are presented in Table 5.2 [2].

$β_2$-AR Agonists $β_2$-AR agonists produce bronchodilation by stimulating the $β_2$-ARs of the airway smooth muscle cells causing them to relax and open the airways [111]. Although LABA and ultra-LABA are drugs of choice, SABA are used as needed and in emergencies [82]. LAMA blocks the ability of neurotransmitter, acetylcholine (ACh) to stimulate muscarinic receptors in the lungs. MChR stimulation

Table 5.2 Pharmacotherapy for chronic obstructive pulmonary disease in the older adult. (Reprinted with permission from Matera et al. [2])

Drug class	Advantages	Disadvantages
β2-AR agonist	Indacaterol acutely reduced lung hyperinflation with improvements in right cardiac chamber compliance indices and contractility in 40 patients, aged 50–80 [3] Indacaterol is effective in improving FEV_1 across age groups (<65, ≥65, and ≥75 years), pooled analysis of 11 clinical trials [4]	Newly prescribed LABA associated with higher incidence of cardiovascular events among older adults [5, 6] Formoterol and salmeterol are more effective in improving FEV_1 in patients aged <65 years [4]
mChR-antagonists	Older adults (aged >60 years) respond better than younger patients to ipratropium [7] Bronchodilator response to β-agonist following methacholine-induced bronchoconstriction does not change with age [8]	Increased risk of acute urinary retention when treating older patients with evidence of benign prostatic hyperplasia, both short and long-acting mChR antagonists [9]
Dual bronchodilators	Effectiveness of UMEC/VI across all age groups (<65, ≥65, and ≥75 years, post hoc of seven clinical trials [10] Indacaterol/glycopyrronium in patients aged ≥80 years (n = 30), acceptable cardiac profile without an increase in short term pro-arrhythmic risk in very old [11]	Difference in FEV_1 changes with UMEC/VI vs LAMA less pronounced in subjects aged ≥75 years [10] Bronchodilator effect most evident in subjects aged 40 to <65 years and trend to smaller effects in subjects aged ≥75 years [12]
ICS, LABA/ICS, ICS/LABA/LAMA	**ICS/LABA/LAMA (FF/UMEC/VI) vs ICS/LABA and LABA/LAMA greater improvement in lung function and health [13]** **ICS/LABA/LAMA (FF/UMEC/VI) vs ICS/LABA and LABA/LAMA greater reduction in rate of exacerbations regardless of age but best response in 65–74 and ≥75 years subgroups [13]** Long-term use of ICS not associated with osteoporosis or fractures [14] ICS use associated with reduced hospitalization for those <75 years of age [15]	Corticosteroid doses that appear safe in younger people may place older patients at risk of infection [16] Patients aged >75 years and frail subjects at a greater risk of hospitalization when taking ICSs [15] Increased risk of fractures with ICS/LABA and ICS/LABA/LAMA for ≥65 years of age, ≥12 months use; in particular, ↑fracture risk with budesonide (320 µg bid, MDI inhalation device) [17]
PDE4 inhibitors	**Small benefit on lung function; use only as add-on in subset resistant to above therapies [18]**	Adverse effect of GI disturbances, weight loss, psychotic events, insomnia, depressed mood, ave age 64 [18]
Macrolides	Azithromycin is most effective in patients (>65 years), with a significant interaction between age and treatment effect on the risk of exacerbation [19] Network meta-analysis—prophylactic use of macrolides (64–75 years of age) reduces time to next exacerbations with best safety profile compared to tetracyclines and quinolones [118]	One year azithromycin use associated with measurable hearing loss [20] Response to macrolides (3–12 month) decreases with age (> 65 years) [21]

β2-AR agonist beta 2 adrenergic receptor agonist, *FEV* forced expiratory volume in 1 second, *mChR antagonists* muscarinic cholinergic receptor antagonists, *UMEC/VI* umeclidinium/vilanterol, *LAMA* Long-acting muscarinic acetylcholine receptor antagonists, *ICS* inhaled corticosteroid, *LABA* Long-acting beta adrenergic receptor agonists, *FF* fluticasone furoate, *MDI* metered dose inhaler, *PDE4 inhibitors* phosphodiesterase 4 inhibitors leads not only to airway bronchoconstriction but also to mucus production, vascular dilation, and inflammation [112]. ACh is released from the parasympathetic nerves innervating the lungs and cells such as epithelial [113] and endothelial cells [112]. Blockage of ACh-dependent effects improves lung function in COPD [112]. ICS act by suppressing certain inflammatory pathways and are successful in COPD patients with ≥300 blood eosinophil count (BEC) [114]. Eosinophils (white cells) are used as a biomarker that predicts the success of ICS in treating COPD [115].

LABA and LAMA LABA and LAMA are used as a monotherapy in COPD where mMRC is 0–1 and CAT is <10 (see Table 5.1). It is recommended that COPD patients with these characteristics be treated with long-acting bronchodilators. Patients with a greater degree of breathlessness and one moderate exacerbation per year should be treated with dual LABA and LAMA, shown to be effective at all ages (see Table 5.2). Patients with ≥2 exacerbations per year or ≥1 leading to hospitalization, dual LABA and LAMA plus inhaled corticosteroid is recommended [81, 84]. In the older adult, a post hoc analysis of the IMPACT trial showed that triple therapy of ICS/LABA/LAMA was superior to dual therapy (either ICS/LABA or LABA/LAMA [13] and a meta-analysis of four randomized controlled trials concluded that triple therapy produced overall better outcomes than dual therapy for COPD patients [116].

Other drugs such as phosphodiesterase 4 (PDE4) inhibitors (roflumilast, oral) and macrolides (azithromycin, erythromycin, clarithromycin, roxithromycin) are also used with the above to treat COPD (see Table 5.2). Roflumilast acts to elevate the concentration of cyclic AMP by blocking its breakdown. Elevated cyclic AMP levels exert anti-inflammatory effects by inhibiting the expression of important mediators of inflammation [116]. In a review of 47 RCTs using roflumilast in COPD, only a small beneficial effect was observed but with numerous adverse effects [18]. Macrolides are antimicrobial drugs that inhibit bacterial protein synthesis but also exert anti-inflammatory activities [118]. Macrolides outperform other antibiotics (tetracycline, quinolones) in prophylactically reducing the time to exacerbations, improving QoL, and exhibiting the best safety profile [119].

Chronic Obstructive Pulmonary Disease. Adverse Drug Reactions Although the safety profile of LABA and LAMA as monotherapy, dual therapy, or combined with ICS is acceptable and comparable to placebo in numerous RCTs [3, 10], COPD patients with newly prescribed LABA or LAMA have a higher risk of hospitalizations or emergency room visits due to cardiac events according to a retrospective case-nested study [5]. Expected adverse effects of β2-AR agonists include elevation in resting heart rate, tremors, possible arrhythmias, hypokalemia (low level of potassium in blood) (especially with concurrent use of thiazide diuretics), and an increase in oxygen consumption at rest although the latter two adverse effects lessen with time [82].

Drugs with anticholinergic effects, e.g., LAMA, theoretically are a concern for the older adult due to their many effects, e.g., dry mouth, urinary retention, blurred vision, and cardiac effects, including palpitations, tachycardia, and arrhythmia [120] and are additive to many other drugs with anticholinergic effects (see Chap. 3). However, since the mAChR antagonists are poorly absorbed and mainly stay within the lungs, the main adverse effect is a dry mouth [82]. However, an epidemiological study compared COPD patients on tiotropium HandiHaler to those on LABA and found a small increased risk of angina, myocardial infarction, and stroke with the use of LAMA [121]. Also, population-based data of acute urinary retention (surgery, hospital, emergency visits) showed an elevated risk of acute urinary retention in older men using either SAMA or LAMA and an even greater risk in men with benign hyperplasia [9]. Causality in this study was not established [82].

Use of corticosteroids poses a hazard for the older adult due to the elevated risk of infection, e.g., pneumonia [122, 123], greater risk of hospitalizations, especially if older than 75 years and frail [15], increased risk of fracture [96], adverse gastrointestinal (GI) and central nervous system (CNS) effects [119], and possible glaucoma and cataracts [124]. Also, long-term use of ICS increases the bacterial load, especially in COPD patients with low eosinophil count [125]. Regarding COPD patients using macrolides long term, it is recommended that they be monitored for antibiotic resistance, hearing loss, and QTc prolongation (abnormal electrical activity in the heart) [126, 127].

The presence of comorbidities in COPD patients is high. Approximately 79% of COPD patients have one co-morbidity, and 48% have three or more co-morbidities [107], creating an elevated risk of polypharmacy and drug–drug interactions. GOLD2024's recommendation is to treat comorbidities as if COPD is not present. Comorbidities related to the cardiovascular system (heart failure, ischemic heart disease, arrhythmias) are common [107] (see Chap. 4). It is estimated that almost 30% of older adults with COPD (>75 years) also suffer from heart failure [128]. Other comorbid conditions include lung cancer, osteoporosis, depression, diabetes, gastroesophageal disease [82], and frailty (see Chap. 7).

Selective β1 adrenergic receptor antagonists (e.g., metoprolol, bisoprolol, or nebivolol) are drugs of choice to reduce morbidity and mortality in heart failure and are not contraindicated in COPD [129] but should not be used to reduce exacerbations [130]. LABA and LAMA bronchodilators are considered safe in patients with cardiovascular comorbidities [131]. Use of antibacterial drugs (β-lactam, macrolide, tetracycline, quinolone, sulfonamide, and others, e.g., trimethoprim) to treat exacerbations of COPD patients may interact with a large number of drugs used to treat comorbidities of cardiovascular disease, diabetes, CNS disorders, and others [132]. For example, macrolides (CYP3A4 inhibitors) block the metabolism of antihypertensive calcium channel blockers (CYP3A4 substrate), leading to a serious fall in blood pressure. Other interactions such as spironolactone or angiotensin-converting enzyme inhibitor (ACEI) and trimethoprim/sulfamethoxazole, direct oral anticoagulant (DOAC), and macrolides are discussed in Chap. 3.

Chronic Obstructive Pulmonary Disease. Inhalers There is an abundance of aerosol drug delivery devices available for the treatment of COPD [133]. These range from nebulizers, metered-dose inhalers (MDIs), breath-activated MDIs, and dry powder inhalers (DPIs) [82]. There are "basic principles for appropriate inhalation device choice" [1]. Appropriate inhalation device choice and education and training on its use are essential because "errors in device use are common and are mainly related to inspiratory flow (such as peak inspiratory flow rate), inhalation duration, coordination, dose preparation, exhalation maneuver prior to inhalation, and a breath hold following inhalation" [1]. Use of inhalers requires *three* conditions: normal cognition, strength, and dexterity, some of which may be compromised with age. A forceful inspiration is required for DPIs, and MDIs require coordination between device triggering and inhalation and ability to maintain a slow deep inhalation [1]. A nebulizer is a possible choice if DPIs or MDIs cannot be properly used [1].

The following are the steps taught to patients on the use of the inhaler: remove the cover; shake the canister; inhale and exhale completely; place the inhaler between your teeth and seal your lips around it; inhale and depress the canister simultaneously; hold your breath for 5–10 s; exhale slowly. Pharmacotherapy is not achieved if the inhaler is used incorrectly, so choice, training, education, and continual reassessment are required for optimal COPD pharmacotherapy [1].

Chronic Obstructive Pulmonary Disease. Non-pharmacotherapy There are several non-pharmacological therapies for the prevention and treatment of COPD. First and foremost is tobacco (and cannabis) smoking cessation, as smoking is the major risk factor for COPD, and its cessation reduces COPD mortality [1]. Avoidance of environmental and occupational respiratory toxins is advisable. Second, engagement in pulmonary rehabilitation with an appropriately monitored physical activity program, such as one designed by the American Thoracic Society and the European Respiratory Society [134]. Third, relevant vaccinations are recommended to include influenza, pneumococcal, SARS-Cov-2 (COVID-19), respiratory syncytial virus, herpes zoster (shingles), and Tdap for pertussis (whooping cough), tetanus, diphtheria if not vaccinated as youth [82]. Other measures such as long-term oxygen use, ventilatory support, and lung volume reduction surgery are appropriate for select subgroups [82]. In the presence of partial pressure of arterial oxygen at Pa O_2 ≤55 mmHg or Pa O_2 55–60 mmHg with other conditions, e.g., pulmonary hypertension, edema, and hematocrit >55%, long-term oxygen use increases survival. Ventilatory support is beneficial for patients with very severe stable COPD. Those with upper lobe emphysema and low exercise capacity benefit from lung volume reduction surgery (LVRS) [135]. Structural changes of LVRS reduce hyperinflation, improve elastic recoil, increase expiratory flow, improve lung function, and QoL [82].

Chronic Kidney Disease

Chronic Kidney Disease. Introduction CKD is described as a complex, multifaceted disease that ideally requires guidance from a multidisciplinary medical team [38, 136]. CKD is generally diagnosed at late stages of pathology, during which significant negative interactions with diabetes and cardiovascular disease are evident, leading to reduced QoL and early mortality [136]. Diagnosis of CKD in initial stages of development would significantly slow disease progression, reduce its promotional effects on other morbidities, and reduce mortality [136]. Although there is no cure, CKD is treatable and preventable [137].

Chronic Kidney Disease. Prevalence Globally, CKD was the 12th leading cause of death as of 2017 [137]. The prevalence of CKD worldwide ranges from 8.5–9.8% [137] to 11–13% [138]. The discrepancy relates to "methodological approach and data inclusion criteria" [137]. In the analysis by Hill et al. (2016) [138], 79% of those with CKD were late stage, suggesting that the inclusion of underdiagnosed early stage CKD would further increase prevalence. According to the Global Burden of Diseases, Injuries, and Risk Factors Study 2017, global CKD prevalence has remained constant from 1990 to 2017 in association with an increase in the use of dialysis and renal transplantation [137].

A US prevalence of 15% was derived from the National Health and Nutrition Examination Survey and the CKD Epidemiology Collaboration in adults >18 years of age from 2015 to 2018 [136]. This data excluded late-stage kidney failure and used the 2019 population census. CKD is age dependent with the highest prevalence (38%) in those $\geq$65 years of age [139]. Differences in prevalence by gender (males 14%; females 12%) and ethnicities (adults: non-Hispanic blacks 16%; Hispanics 14%; non-Hispanic whites 13%; non-Hispanic Asians 13%) are modest [139].

Chronic Kidney Disease. Pathophysiology "CKD is defined as abnormalities of kidney structure or function, present for a minimum of 3 months, with implications for health" [140]. KDIGO, 2024 guidelines determine CKD if (1) estimated glomerular filtration rate (eGFR) is <60 ml/min per 1.73 m^2 or (2) there is a presence of kidney biomarkers to include "albuminuria (ACR $\geq$30 mg/g [$\geq$3 mg/mmol]), urine sediment abnormalities, persistent hematuria (RBCs in urine), electrolytes, and other abnormalities due to tubular disorders, abnormalities detected by histology, structural abnormalities detected by imaging, history of kidney transplantation." [140] GFR is broken down into categories (G1,G2,G3a,G3b,G4,G5, formerly stages) depending on the filtration rate with G1 at $\geq$90 ml/min per 1.73 m^2 as normal or high and G5 at <15 as kidney failure [140]. Albuminuria, the presence of albumin, a plasma protein in the urine indicative of filtration leakage, is measured as a ratio to creatinine (albumin to creatinine ratio, ACR) and is divided into three categories A1–A3 where A1 is <3 mg/mmol as normal to mildly increased and A3 at >30 mg/mmol as severely increased.

The pathophysiology of CKD is complex because it is heavily intertwined with pathological changes of cardiovascular disease [141] and type 2 diabetes mellitus (T2DM) [142]. The "final common pathway" is renal fibrosis in which abnormal matrix proteins over time replace normal tissue of the glomeruli and tubules [143, 144]. Fibrosis is a normal kidney repair response following acute injury. However, with chronic injury of epithelial cells or endothelial cells, factors are secreted that allow for the development of a new cell type called a myofibroblast. Myofibroblasts secrete unwanted matrix proteins, pro-inflammatory factors and inhibit normal tissue repair, activities responsible for the destruction of the kidney [143].

Chronic Kidney Disease. Risk Factors There are basically *two* major risk factors for CKD. They are *hypertension* [145, 146] and *hyperglycemia* leading to T2DM [147, 148]. The complex pathophysiology of each is interactive and eventually leads to inflammatory and fibrotic destruction of the glomeruli and tubules [149]. Hypertension and hyperglycemia are modifiable but when uncontrolled, they participate in a vicious downward depression of renal function [148]. In essence, they are both a cause and a consequence of CKD [143]. Forty percent of adult diabetics have CKD, and diabetic kidney disease is the major cause of end-stage kidney failure [147]. As noted before (see Chap. 4), hypertension is a major cardiovascular risk factor that raises the probability of coronary heart disease, peripheral arterial disease, stroke, arrhythmias, and heart failure. The addition of CKD worsens these outcomes and increases cardiovascular mortality [141, 151]. Other risk factors for CKD include obesity [152], tobacco smoking [153], and dyslipidemia (high LDL-cholesterol and triglycerides) [154].

Alert: Modifiable risk factors for chronic kidney disease are hypertension and hyperglycemia.

Chronic Kidney Disease. Aging Effects on Diagnosis Drugs whose effects are terminated by renal elimination produce adverse drug reactions (ADRs) in individuals with reduced kidney function and hence require a reduction in dose or selection of an alternative drug with a different route of elimination (see Chaps. 2 and 3). Since ample data show that kidney structure and function decline with age independent of disease [155, 156], measurement of kidney function (as with eGFR) is a prerequisite prior to drug use [140]. However, age-associated kidney decline (eGFR of 0.75 ml/min/1.73m^2 per year after the age of 50) occurs in some but not all older adults as revealed by the results of the Baltimore Longitudinal Study in which kidney function, measured over many years remained constant in 30% of the older adults [157].

However, when present, normal age-associated decline in kidney function complicates the diagnosis of CKD [156, 158, 159]. The question is whether the age-dependent renal impairment should dictate a diagnosis of early stage CKD [156, 159, 160]. Results of several population studies demonstrate that the absolute and relative mortality rates in older adults with a modest reduction in eGFR are weaker in older adults compared to younger individuals with similar eGFR [160]. Similarly, in an 8-year cohort study using the established cutoff points [140], adults 65 years and older with eGFR of 45–59 mL/min/1.73 m^2 with normal/mild albuminuria diagnosed with CKD exhibited risks of kidney failure and death comparable to those without CKD (eGFR at 60 mL/min/1.73 m^2) [159]. These data support a call for age-adapted definition of CKD that would prevent over diagnosis and unnecessary treatment in the older population [159, 161].

An additional concern relevant to aging of the kidney is the use of serum creatinine (sCr) to calculate eGFR. The KDIGO (2024) [140] recommends sCr measurements as "appropriate for diagnosis, staging, and monitoring the progression of CKD". However, creatinine clearance declines with age [155]. Thus, in association with sCr measurement and for more in-depth analysis, use of GFR estimating equations that incorporate age and sex is required as a valued adjustment [140]. Additionally, another issue is the presence of age- and frailty-associated sarcopenia, an acute loss of muscle mass that reduces the availability of creatinine (source of creatinine) and jeopardizes the accuracy of eGFR [152]. In place of creatinine, serum cystatin-c (sCys), an endogenous protein marker of filtration, is considered an appropriate alternate and even more accurate than creatinine [163]. However, the sCys assay is not perfect and is associated with issues of standardization, interference from steroids, systemic inflammation, and thyroid dysfunction [164]. Nevertheless, use of both sCr and sCys is considered better than use of either one alone [163]. However, they are inappropriate for morbidities such as malnutrition, cancer, heart failure, cirrhosis, where more invasive assessment of clearance with endogenous or radioactive compounds is prescribed [140].

Chronic Kidney Disease. Pharmacotherapy Use of inhibitors of the renin-angiotensin-aldosterone-system (RAAS) is highly recommended as pharmacotherapy for CKD in stages G1–4 without diabetes and stages G1–4 with albuminuria at A2–A3 with diabetes [140]. Combinations of angiotensin-converting enzyme inhibitor (ACEI), angiotensin receptor blocker (ARB), or direct renin inhibitors with or without diabetes in CKD are contraindicated. As shown in Table 5.3, a maximal tolerated dose of an RAAS inhibitor provides renoprotection (decreasing albuminuria, slowing progression) [22, 23, 27], reduces cardiovascular (CV) events [24] and all-cause mortality [24, 25, 28]. The frequent monitoring of blood pressure (BP), sCr, and serum potassium is recommended. The hyperkalemia associated with RAAS inhibitors is best treated with potassium exchange compounds [42] or diet rather than dose reduction. Dose reduction or discontinuation is needed with the development of hypotension, uncontrolled hyperkalemia (even when treated) or with uremia (elevation of nitrogen-containing toxins in blood) (eGFR<15 ml/min per 1.73 m^2) [140].

Table 5.3 Pharmacotherapy for chronic kidney disease in the older adult

Risk factor	Drug class	Advantages	Disadvantages
Hypertension and CV complications, diabetes	ACEI ARB	Losartan (ARB) + other antihypertensives, ↓ composite endpoints of proteinuria, improved kidney function in DCKD: no effect on mortality, RENAAL, ave. age 60) [22]	
		Irbesartan provides renoprotection independent of BP control (IDNT ave. age 59 years) [23]	↑ incidence of hyperkalemia [23]
		Intense ↓ BP <120 mm Hg systolic ↓ CVEs and all-cause mortality (subgroup analysis SPRINT, 43% >75 years) [24]	↑ risk of hypokalemia, hyperkalemia and ARF with intense therapy [24]
		Maximal dose tolerable of ACEI decrease mortality in DCKD, ↓ risk of ESKD and albuminuria improvements; meta-analysis of RCTs [25]	↑ risk of hyperkalemia with ARB [25]
		Discontinuation of RAASI during episode of hyperkalemia in CKD- ↑ risk of CV events and death [26]	
		eGFR ↓ least with ramipril (ACEI), ↑ in urinary albumin excretion was less with telmisartan (ARB) 1 year [27]	No advantage of ARB in ACE-intolerant CKD with vascular complications [27]
		RAASI associated with lower risk of ESKD and death independent of age (CKD-REIN cohort study [28]	Combination of ACEI and ARB not as good as each alone in pts >55 years with CV or diabetic CKD [28]
Potential for blood clot formation	Anticoagulants	Lower risk of VTE and major bleeding with DOAC (apixaban) compared to warfarin in systematic review [29]	AF and anticoagulation with CKD must be determined on individual basis [29]
Diabetes (hyperglycemia)	SGLT2 inhibitors	Canagliflozin lowers primary outcomes (ESKD, 2x sCr, death), ~30% in CKD with diabetes +RAASI; reduction in CV events (2.6 years CREDENCE trial) [30]	SGLT2 inhibitors—risk of urinary tract infections, diabetic ketoacidosis [33]
		Dapagliflozin greater efficacy in CKD (<30 ml/min/1.73 m2) with or without diabetes—effective in broader group of pts (2 years, ave. age 62 DAPA-CKD trial) [31]	Meta analysis of RCTs of SGLT2I in CKD, ↑ risk of diabetic ketoacidosis, genital infection, and volume depletion [34]
		Empagliflozin ↓ cardiorenal outcomes in CKD with and without diabetes including pts with urinary albumin: creatinine ratio <30 mg/g and eGFR to as low as 15–20 mL/min/1.73 m² (Empa-Kidney) [32]	

Cardiorenal protection	sMRA (spironolactone, eplerenone) nsMRA (finerenone)	Use limited to eGFR >45 ml/min/1.73 m² in pts resistant to antihypertensive treatment [35]	↑ hyperkalemia and not to be used with nsMRAs
		Slowed progression with ↓ kidney failure, reduced ↓ eGFR and ↓ death due to renal causes (FIDELIO-DKD 2.6 years, ave. age 65 years) [36]	Possible hyperkalemia; numerous DDIs with CYP3A4 inhibitors/inducers and drugs producing hyperkalemia (RAASI, NSAIDs, heparin, ketoconazole, amiloride, triamterene, trimethoprim, lithium) (review of RCTs) [38]
		Improves cardiac outcomes in pts with DCKD, albuminuria and taking ACEI or ARB (ave age 64 years, 3.6 years trial FIGARO-DKD) [37]	
Hyperkalemia	Potassium exchange compounds		
	Sodium polystyrene sulfonate (SPS)	Small study, 1 week, SPS lowers mild hyperkalemia > placebo [39]	SPS review—electrolyte changes (hypokalemia, hypomagnesemia and hypokalemia) and GI disturbances; may ↑ sodium level and cause fluid retention; contraindicated in heart failure, severe hypertension and marked edema [44]
	Calcium polystyrene suffocate (CPS)	Small study 3 days showed CPS and SPS comparable in lowering mild hyperkalemia in CKD [40]	
	Patiromer.	DCKD with mild-moderate hyperkalemia, patiromer ↓ K⁺ 4–52 weeks (phase 2) [36]	Hypomagnesemia: mild-moderate constipation, diarrhea, nausea [42]
		Patiromer allows CKD + resistant hypertension to remain on spironolactone with ↓ hyperkalemia (phase 2, AMBER, phase 2) [41]	
		Patiromer ↓ hyperkalemia in CKD + RAAS (OPAL-HK, phase 3, ave age 65 years) [42]	
	Sodium-zirconium-cyclosilicate (SZC)	Normalizes and maintains K⁺ with SZC in pts with eGFR<60 ml/min per 1.73 m², and RAASI (12 mos ave age 64 years, phase 3) [43].	Hyperkalemia and edema (KDIGO, 2024), mild GI disorders—nausea, constipation, vomiting, diarrhea [43]

ACEI Angiotensin-converting enzyme inhibitor, *ARB* angiotensin receptor blocker, *DCKD* diabetic chronic kidney disease, *ave* average, *CVEs* cardiovascular events, *ARF* acute renal failure, *ESKD* end-stage renal disease, *RAAS* renal angiotensin aldosterone system inhibitors, *VTE* venous thromboembolism, *DOAC* direct oral anticoagulants, *AF* atrial fibrillation, *sCr* serum creatinine, *pts* patients, *eGFR* estimated glomerular filtration rate, *sMRA* steroidal mineralocorticoid receptor antagonist, *nsMRA* nonsteroidal mineralocorticoid receptor antagonist, *SPRINT* Systolic blood pressure intervention trial, *RENAAL* Reduction of endpoints in non-insulin-dependent diabetes mellitus with the angiotensin II antagonist losartan study, *IDNT* Irbesartan diabetic nephropathy trial, *EMPA-KIDNEY* The study of heart and kidney protection with Empagliflozin, *CREDENCE* Canagliflozin and renal events in diabetes with established nephropathy clinical evaluation, *DAPA-CKD* A study to evaluate the effect of Dapagliflozin on renal outcomes and cardiovascular mortality in patients with chronic kidney disease, ↑ increase, ↓ decrease

Another important first-line therapy for CKD is the sodium-glucose cotransporter 2 inhibitors (SGLT2Is) (canagliflozin, dapagliflozin, empagliflozin), originally developed to increase urinary excretion of glucose in T2DM but in cardiovascular trials, this class of drugs showed a favorable slowing of kidney decline and a convincing safety profile [165]. As shown in Table 5.3, clinical trials with SGLT2I therapy over 2 years or more are renoprotective by lowering the composite endpoints leading to end-stage kidney disease (ESKD), by decreasing expected doubling of sCr, and by reducing mortality [30–32]. SGLT2I benefits a wide range of patients with CKD with or without diabetes and low eGFR as evident with results from the EMPA-kidney trial [32]. KDIGO (2024) [140] recommends the use of SGLT2I for CKD regardless of the level of albuminuria. Because of the risk of ketoacidosis with SGLT2I [33], KDIGO additionally recommends "withholding SGLT2I during times of prolonged fasting, surgery or critical medical illness."

The nonsteroidal mineralocorticoid receptor antagonist (nsMRA), finerenone, is a reasonable addition to RAAS inhibitor and SGLT2 inhibitor therapy and is specifically for individuals "with T2DM, eGFR >25 ml/min/1.73m^2, normal potassium concentration and albuminuria (>30 mg/g [>3 mg/mmol])" [140]. Clinical trial results support addition of finerenone to slow progression of kidney disease and improve CV outcomes [36, 37]. Of concern is the risk of hyperkalemia that must be monitored frequently after finerenone initiation. The use of steroidal MRAs, e.g., spironolactone or eplerenone, that are beneficial in heart failure, refractory hypertension, and hyperaldosteronism, may be harmful in CKD [140].

Chronic Kidney Disease. Managing Hyperkalemia As kidney function declines, the potential risk of hyperkalemia (>5.0 mmol/l of potassium) increases although not in direct accord with depressed eGFR [140]. Furthermore, many drugs beneficial to CKD (see Table 5.3) also elevate potassium, potentially adding to hyperkalemia. Additionally, drugs used to treat comorbidities, e.g., β-ARB, potassium-sparing diuretics, heparin, digitalis glycoside, NSAIDs, sMRA, also produce hyperkalemia [140]. Hyperkalemia is an important issue because potassium in association with sodium and calcium maintains the essential energy gradient across cell membranes and among other things, regulates the excitability of cells [166]. Thus, elevated potassium perturbs normal excitability and fosters arrhythmias, muscle cramps and weakness, metabolic acidosis and can be fatal [167]. Managing hyperkalemia involves three levels of approach: a) consider the need of non-RAAS inhibitors (given above), review dietary intake of potassium-rich foods (especially meat-based and processed foods), consider changes, and seek help from a knowledgeable dietician; b) medication considerations include appropriate use of diuretics to increase potassium excretion, optimize sodium bicarbonate levels to suppress metabolic acidosis, and use potassium exchange drugs according to label instructions; c) least desired due to increase in adverse CV events is to reduce dose or discontinue RAAS inhibitors or nsMRA, which may possibly be re-prescribed later [140]. It is also important that considerable care be taken in the measurement of hyperkalemia, as many factors may inadvertently elevate potassium levels, such as a tourniquet that is too tight, an increase in plasma osmolarity (number of particles in plasma) due to dehydration or hyperglycemia, uncontrolled diabetes, constipation with severe CKD, biological diurnal variation, slightly higher serum values compared to plasma values, and an elevation in postprandial hyperkalemia with kidney decline [140].

There are four oral potassium-binding drugs used to lower hyperkalemia in CKD. Each one is slightly different in its mechanism of action, onset, and duration. The first in use were sodium polystyrene sulfonate (SPS) and calcium polystyrene sulfonate (CPS), resins that bind potassium, calcium, and magnesium in exchange for sodium. Newer potassium exchange agents are patiromer sorbitex calcium (PSC), a polymer that binds potassium, magnesium, and phosphate in exchange for sodium and calcium, and sodium zirconium cyclosilicate (SZC), a crystalline compound that binds potassium [167]. The gut is the site of action and they are excreted in the feces [167]. Not surprisingly, these drugs cause gastrointestinal (GI) upsets (Table 5.3). A systematic review and network meta-analysis concluded that use of these potassium binders depends on the clinical situation but that SZC can produce short- and long-term decrease in potassium, as needed, with minimal GI adversity compared to other potassium-binding drugs [168]. However, it remains unproven whether potassium binders effectively blunt postprandial hyperkalemia and thus obviate the need for a low-potassium diet [169].

Chronic Kidney Disease. Non-pharmacological Management KDIGO, 2024 [140] recommends that individuals with CKD engage in (1) physical activity of moderate intensity (150 min/week) comparable to individual CV tolerance, (2) eat a healthy diet favoring plant-based foods, avoiding processed foods with protein intake of 0.8 g/kg body weight and maintain a healthy weight (BMI preferable target <25 kg/m^2), and (3) quit smoking or using tobacco products. Referrals to qualified providers in these areas should be readily given. For the older adult with sarcopenia or frailty, higher protein intakes (1.0–1.2 g/kg body weight) are suggested to avert muscle loss and prevent malnutrition [170] but should be followed based on the rate of CKD progression.

Parkinson's Disease

Parkinson's Disease. Introduction Parkinson's disease is a progressive neurodegenerative disease that together with abnormal motor and non-motor symptoms creates years-long disability and eventual death [171, 172].

Parkinson's Disease. Prevalence Globally, Parkinson's disease prevalence, disability, and deaths have doubled from 1990 to 2015, attributed largely to the increase in life expectancy and harmful impact of industry-generated toxins, although newer methodologies in tracking diseases and a decrease in smoking (considered "protective") may have contributed to this increase [173]. The prevalence of Parkinson's disease increases with age up to a peak at 85–89 years and is slightly higher in males than females (1.6% males; 1.2% females) [173]. It is the second most common neurological disorder in older adults after Alzheimer's Disease. Disability-adjusted life years (DALYs), a value generated from the addition of the number of years with a disability and number of years lost to premature mortality, also increased globally [173].

As of 2016, 6 million individuals worldwide and over 700,000 in the United States had Parkinson's disease [173]. Parkinson's disease prevalence in the United States is expected to increase to 1.2 million by 2030 [174].

Parkinson's Disease. Pathophysiology A scientific consensus on the etiology of Parkinson's disease has not be established. However, major features of its pathology are known. Disease pathology entails the gradual structural and functional loss of dopaminergic neurons located in a specific region of the brain termed the substantia nigra pars compacta (part of the midbrain above the brain stem). Dopaminergic neurons project to other brain areas such as the striatum, a critical part of the basal ganglia (collection of diverse neurons) and the (pre)frontal cortex. Dopaminergic neurons modulate nerve traffic through the striatum by the release of the neurotransmitter dopamine, which stimulates dopamine receptors (D1–3) [175]. Since the basal ganglia coordinates motor output and motor learning operations, deficiencies in dopaminergic function produce the undesired motor dysfunction characteristic of Parkinson's disease.

Another pathological finding (on autopsy) is the presence of Lewy bodies and Lewy neurites, which are abnormal collections of misfolded proteins in cells or their projections, such as axons [176]. One protein in particular, α-synuclein, is prominent in Lewy pathology and supports the description of Parkinson's disease as a synucleinopathy [177]. The contribution of Lewy pathology to Parkinson's disease is not fully known, although the presence of misfolded proteins is considered a hallmark of aging [178], suggesting one path whereby aging elevates the risk for Parkinson's disease.

Parkinson's Disease. Motor Abnormalities Parkinson's disease produces several classic motor abnormalities and lesser-known non-motor abnormalities (see Fig. 5.1) [172]. The main diagnostic features of Parkinson's disease according to the Movement Disorder Society Parkinson's disease Criteria are bradykinesia, in addition to rest tremor or rigidity [179]. Bradykinesia is slowness of movement revealed as difficulty in initiating a movement, e.g., rising from a chair; reduced automatic movements, e.g., blinking or arm movement when walking; slowness in physical actions; and/or decrease in facial expression [180]. Rest tremor is defined as shaking at 4–6 Hz (cycle per second) frequency, and rigidity is impedance to passive joint movement independent of velocity of movement [181]. With the progression of Parkinson's disease, other motor disturbances of postural instability and difficulty in walking appear along with dysphasia (swallowing difficulty) and dysarthria (speaking difficulty) [177].

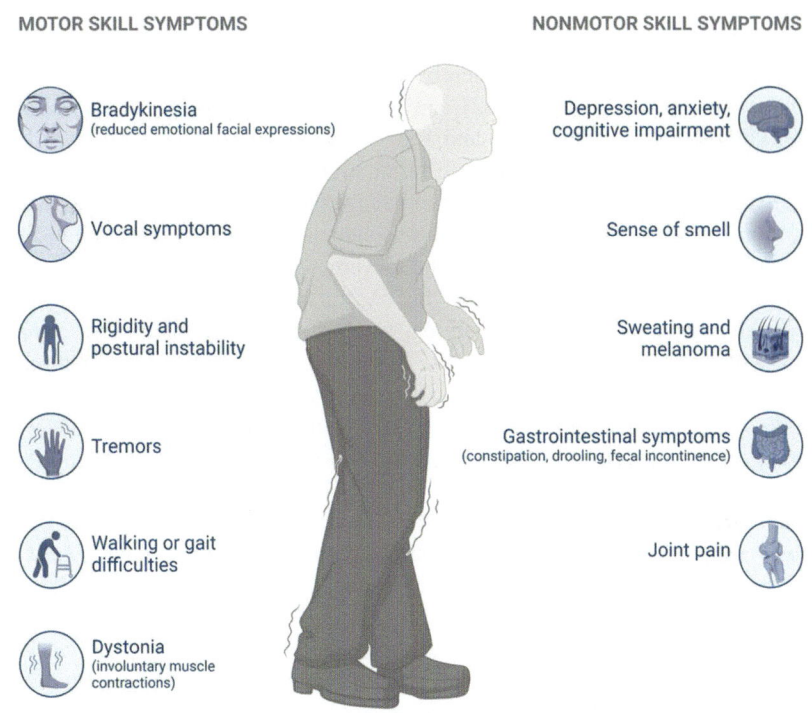

Fig. 5.1 Symptoms of Parkinson's disease. (Reproduced with permission from Prajjwal et al. [172])

Parkinson's Disease. Non-motor Symptoms Associated with Parkinson's disease are several non-motor symptoms that occur years prior to a diagnosis and that significantly impact QoL [171]. These early occurring symptoms, termed prodromal symptoms, include hyposmia (loss of sense of smell) [182], constipation [183], idiopathic rapid eye movement (REM) behavior disorder (RBD) ("sleep walking loosely") [184, 185] and cognitive impairment in executive function and some aspects of memory [185]. Other prodromal changes involve hallucinations, sensory and neuritic pain [187], and a range of autonomic nervous system dysfunctions such as excessive salivation, urinary incontinence, orthostatic hypotension [171]. The etiology of prodromal symptoms is not clear. Some (cognitive and autonomic dysfunction, pain, RBD) appear to be at least partially dopamine-dependent since medications optimizing dopamine and its effects ameliorate these symptoms to some degree. Others (hyposmia, depression, orthostatic hypotension) are possibly driven by deficiencies in other neurotransmitters such as serotonin, acetylcholine, or norepinephrine [171]. It is postulated that prodromal symptoms result from the growing presence of abnormal α-synuclein deposits (Lewy pathology) that appear initially in the dorsal motor nucleus of the vagus nerve and spread eventually to the brain [176, 188, 189] and engage negatively and positively with innate and adaptive immunity [190].

Parkinson's Disease. Diagnosis/Assessment To obtain an accurate diagnosis of Parkinson's disease, clinimetric scales are used to assess balance, gait, and arm/hand use [191]. The two most frequently used scales are the Hoehn and Yahr stages of progression of the disease [192] and the Unified Parkinson's Disease Rating Scale (UPDRS) [47]. The Hoehn and Yahr scale describes disease progress from Stages 1 to 5. The Parkinson's disease foundation describes these changes as follows: Stages 1–2 begin with mild symptoms in walking, posture, and facial expression, tremor, and movement disorder on one side of the body, progressing to Stage 2 with bilateral involvement in tremor and movement disorders, presence of rigidity, and difficulty with activities of daily living (ADLs that include essential daily tasks e.g. eating, washing, dressing, grooming, using the toilet); Stage 3 worsening of motor symptoms, falls are common due to instability in balance, still able to live independently; Stage 4 progresses to worsening symptoms, walking and standing requires a cane or other support and assistance with ADLs; Stage 5 is characterized by muscle stiffness, requiring wheelchair and full-time assistance.

Another important rating scale used in RCTs is the UPDRS (see details in Online UPDRS). There are four parts of (1) mental activity, behavior, and mood, (2) ADLs, (3) motor examination, and (4) complications of therapy (in past week) each with a series of questions requiring a 0–4-level response. An updated revision, the MDS-UPDRS, sorts inquiries into four main categories of "I: Non-motor Experiences of Daily Living; II: Motor Experiences of Daily Living; III: Motor Examination; IV: Motor Complications [193]. These revisions were developed to provide clinicians with a reliable procedure to diagnose Parkinson's disease by its motor dysfunction but also to assess the non-motor symptoms and to exclude misdiagnosis with "red flags," e.g., lack of motor dysfunction progression over 5 years [179]. Also emphasized is the core feature of Parkinson's disease, which is bradykinesia and one other motor abnormality of rigidity or rest tremor [179].

Parkinson's Disease. Risk Factors. Aging Age is the major risk factor for Parkinson's disease, although environmental toxins and genetics also contribute but to lesser extents [194, 195]. Data from animal studies, human cell cultures, and human autopsy findings support the working hypothesis that Parkinson's disease results from uncontrolled oxidative stress that creates a milieu culminating in death and disappearance of dopaminergic neurons [195]. Oxidative dysfunction permits many other changes, chief of which is the unwanted oxidation and phosphorylation of α-synuclein, a protein involved in the importation of iron into the nerve and equally necessary for this synthesis, release, and reuptake of dopamine [196]. The accumulation of damaged α-synuclein into Lewy bodies and Lewy neurites is considered a hallmark of disease [197]. Neuronal cell death and disappearance (apoptosis) is a consequence of this environment filled with elevated cell stressors such as reactive oxygen species (ROS) [195]. Thus far, however, administration of antioxidants, e.g., α-tocopherol or coenzyme Q and others from 3 weeks to 3 years in early Parkinson's disease has failed to suppress disease symptoms [195]. This is attributed to the inability of these compounds to enter the brain in sufficient amounts and/or to the varied source of ROS in the brain [195]. Future research hopes to sort this out.

Parkinson's Disease. Genetic Contribution Mutated genes have been identified that are non-modifiable causal factors for Parkinson's disease [172]. They contribute about 25% to the risk of the disease [198]. There are two general categories of gene mutations: (1) monogenic or rare variants in single genes directly causing Parkinson's disease, e.g., PARK7 and PRKN, variants that cause mitochondrial dysfunction, and (2) polygenic or common variants in many genes that contribute modestly to disease risk, e.g., SNCA producing slight abnormalities of α-synuclein and other neuronal functions [199]. There is continuing and extensive research into the genetics of Parkinson's disease because an understanding of genetic causes will more accurately define Parkinson's disease pathology, allow more targeted therapies, and overall support better disease management [199].

Parkinson's Disease. Environmental Contribution The discovery that the neurotoxin, 1-methyl-4-phenyl-1,2,3,6-tetrahydropyridine (MPTP) selectively damages dopaminergic neurons of the substantia nigra raised the possibility that there exist environmental risk factors for Parkinson's disease [200]. Currently, there is considerable interest in specifically identifying these environmental toxins since they represent modifiable risk factors that could significantly reduce the global burden of Parkinson's disease [201]. In large case-controlled studies, findings show exposure to pesticides increases the risk for Parkinson's disease [202, 203]. However, although the number of pesticides is large, including herbicides, insecticides, fungicides, and rodenticides, the two most studied pesticides are paraquat, an agricultural herbicide, and rotenone, an all-purpose insecticide to which exposure significantly elevates the risk for Parkinson's disease [202, 204]. There is suggestive support for other potential Parkinson's disease-inducing environmental toxins that include the polychlorinated biphenyls (PCBs), solvents, e.g., trichloroethylene (TCE), toluene, acetone, and metals, e.g., copper, iron, lead [205]. The challenge in assessing toxin risk for Parkinson's disease is the heterogeneity of human genetics with the potential to metabolize toxins to different extents, especially evident with genetic mutations [206].

> *Alert*: Risk factors for Parkinson's disease are age and genetics; modifiable risk factors are environmental toxins.

Parkinson's Disease. Pharmacotherapy The development of Parkinson's disease pharmacotherapy rests heavily on the results of RCTs (see the finding of select trials in Table 5.4). It is necessary to note that these trials included adults ≥30 years of age with Parkinson's disease, achieving an average age for most trials at 63 years of age. Thus, with a few exceptions, drug use in the older adult rests on extrapolation.

Table 5.4 Pharmacotherapy of Parkinson's disease in the older adult

Drug class	Advantages	Disadvantages
Dopamine replacement	Efficacy of CD-LD over LD; significant improvement in Parkinson's disease motor function at 6 mos up to 2 years [45]	With time (years), ↓ ON time and ↑ OFF time; involuntary motor activity [45]
CD-LD IR	CD-LD CR efficacy comparable to CD-LD IR in 75 year olds with Parkinson's disease [46]	Insomnia [46]
CD-LD CR	CD-LD IR in a dose response improves symptoms (UPDRS); 9 mos ELLDOPA study; ave. age 65 years [47]	High dose (600 mg) produces dyskinesia, nausea, infection, hypertonia, and headache [47]
CD-LD ER	CD-LD ER reduces "OFF" time compared to IR by more than 1 hr ADVANCE-PD; ave. age of 63 years [48]	Insomnia, nausea, falls [48]
	Post hoc analysis of ADVANCE-PD - ER ↑ "ON" time compared to IR [49]	Dizziness, nausea, hypertension to mild degree in all groups [50]
	ER compared to IR and CR - longer duration of effect based on MDS-UPDRS part III scores compared with IR CD-LD [50] ave. age 66	Mild-moderate nausea during conversion from CD-LD IR or CLE; discontinued due to dyskinesia, anxiety, dizziness [51]
	Conversion from CD-LD IR or CLE to CD-LD ER decreases "OFF" time; ↑ "ON" time with no ↑ dyskinesia ave. age 64 years [51]	Nausea, vomiting, falls, upper respiratory tract infection on conversion; incidence reduced during treatment [218]
	IR ↓ % "OFF" time; Advanced Parkinson's disease trial compared to CD-LD + CLE, 64 years [218]	

Nonergoline dopamine receptor agonists		
Ropinirole	6 mos efficacy (improved UPDRS compared to placebo early Parkinson's disease, ave. age 62.8 years [53] Ropinirole compared to CD-LD in early disease over 5 years, ↓ risk of dyskinesia (20% vs 40%) ave. age 63 years [54] Comparison of 24 h release (1x) vs immediate release (3x) early Parkinson's disease monotherapy, 12 weeks titration; 8 weeks maintenance—comparable efficacy (EASE-PD), [52] 24 h release as adjunct to LD, advanced disease ↓ "OFF" time, ↑ "ON" time without dyskinesia, ↑ADLs, QoL, (EASE-PD Adjunct), [55] Long-term safety study; 73-month study, early and advanced disease with 24 hrs. ropinirole with other medications [56]	Hypotension, GI effects [53] Hallucinations higher in ropinirole treatment group [54] Dyskinesia, nausea, dizziness, somnolence, hallucinations, and orthostatic hypotension [55] 87% with at least 1 AE, e.g., back pain (14%), hallucinations (13%), somnolence (11%), and peripheral edema (11%) [56]
Rotigotine (transdermal patch)	Comparison of oral ropinirole and transdermal rotigotine shows comparable efficacy with ↓ "OFF" time, ave. age 65–67 years [57] Early Parkinson's disease, Pram BID (total daily dose of 1–1.5 mg) vs TID (0.5 mg) with comparable efficacy [58] ER comparable efficacy (UPDRS pt. II pt. III) to IR in early disease monotherapy for 33 weeks [59] ER in advanced disease improves UPDRS and "OFF" time compared to placebo, 33 weeks [60] 15 mos with treatment at start or delayed 6–9 mos; no difference in efficacy or neuroimaging of striatal dopamine transporter binding; PROUD study, age range 39–79 years [61]	Application site reaction in 58% pts. [57] Somnolence, fatigue, nausea, constipation, and peripheral edema not dose dependent [58]
Pramipexole		
Apomorphine	3–66 mos, SC or infusion of APO ↓ "OFF" time, no effect on dyskinesia, age range 42–80 years [62] Transdermal APO adjunct to LD improved UPDRSIII score, ↓ "OFF" time [63] Large multicenter 12 week 16 hrs. daily infusion in poorly controlled disease—significantly ↓ "OFF" time [64]	Nausea, hallucinations, and orthostatic hypotension [61] Reaction site; psychiatric issues [62]

(continued)

Table 5.4 (continued)

Drug class	Advantages	Disadvantages
COMTI Entacapone Opicapone Tolcapone	14 pts.; entacapone adjunct to CD-LD CR or IR ↑ duration of efficacy [65] Once daily 50 mg capsule for 3 or 6 mos improves global perception of motor fluctuations by clinicians and pts; QoL also improved (OPTIPARK open label study) ave. age 68 years. [66] Analysis of two RCT phase 3 with 1 year opicapone ↓ "OFF" time and ↑ "ON" time without dyskinesia, ave. age 63–65 years [67] 3 mos tolcapone adjunct ↓ "OFF" time, ↑ "ON" time, ↓ LD dose [68]	75% of pts with TEAEs; most frequent dyskinesia, dry mouth, dizziness, diarrhea [66] No effect on dyskinesia: expected dopaminergic effects; diarrhea [68]
MAO-B inhibitors Rasagiline Selegiline	Early disease, oral rasagiline vs placebo improvement in MDS-UPDRS Part II + III at 26 wks, ave. age 67 years [69] Slight improvement in motor functions and ↓ "OFF" time with selegiline adjuvant in pts poorly responsive to LD, at 8 weeks [70] Monotherapy early disease, 12 weeks ↓ UPDRS I,II, III total score, ave. age 64 years [71]	Nasopharyngitis, eczema [69] Better response in 50–59 years with early stage disease compared to older pts [70] No safety issues but short study [71]
MAO-Bi + CCI Safinamide	2 years benefit mid-late disease as adjunct to LD for ↑ "ON" time (absent dyskinesia), ↓ "OFF" time, ↑ ADL, ↑ QoL, and ↓ symptoms of depression ave. age 60 years [72]	↓ dyskinesia in patients with moderate dyskinesia at baseline [72]

NMDA receptor antagonist Amantadine IR Amantadine ER capsules	27 day crossover study, amantadine daily in advanced disease, shows suppression of dyskinesia (RDRS) in >60% patients, ave. age 63 [73] 300 mg/day significantly ↓ LID in 30 days, ave. age 63 [74] ER adjunct to LD ↓ dyskinesia (UPDRS) and ↓ "OFF" time by 1 hr./day (pooled results of 2 Phase III trials) [75]	Efficacy lost after 8 months [74] Hallucination, dizziness, dry mouth, peripheral edema, constipation, falls, and orthostatic hypotension [75]
Adenosine 2A receptor antagonist Istradefylline	Istradefylline added to standard therapy significantly ↓ "OFF" time, ↑ "ON" time over 12 wks, ave. age 66 [76]	Mild-moderate dyskinesia not dose related [76]
Serotonin 5HT-2A inverse agonist Pimavanserin	28 day treatment of pimavanserin in LD or DA-induced psychosis -improves psychosis (some not all aspects) without change in motor function, sedation or hypotension; ave. age 71 years [77]	Sedation, confusion [78]
Serotonin 5HT-2A receptor antagonist Clozapine	6-mos–2-year study; clozapine improves Parkinson's disease psychosis at 1 year without worsening disease [78] Low dose (25 mg/day) clozapine significantly improves disease psychosis without worsening motor function, no anticholinergic effects, ave. age 72 years [79] 28 day study low dose clozapine improves psychosis without effects on memory or disease; ave. age 71 years [80]	2 cases neutropenia but no agranulocytosis Somnolence [80]

CD-LD carbidopa/levodopa, *IR* immediate release, *CR* controlled release, *ER* extended release, *Mos* months, ↑ increase, ↓ decrease, *UPDRS* Unified Parkinson's disease rating scale, *ave* average, *ELLDOPA* Earlier versus later levodopa therapy in Parkinson disease, *CLE* carbidopa, levodopa, entacapone, *RDRS* Rush dyskinesia rating scale, *ADLs* activities of daily living, *QoL* quality of life, *EASE-PD* efficacy and safety evaluation in PD, *AE* adverse event, *APO* apomorphine, *COMTI* catechol-o-methyltransferase inhibitor, *TEAEs* treatment emergent adverse events, *CCI* calcium channel inhibitor, *LID* levodopa-induced dyskinesia, *Pram* pramipexole, *RCT* randomized clinical trial, *DA* dopamine, *hrs* hours, *SC* subcutaneous

Carbidopa/Levodopa The central component of Parkinson's disease therapy is replacement treatment with the combination of carbidopa/levodopa (CD-LD) that slows disease progression [47, 207, 208]. Levodopa (L-dopa) is the chemical precursor of dopamine, whose deficiency produces the motor dysfunction of Parkinson's disease. However, oral L-dopa is rapidly converted to dopamine in the periphery by the enzyme dopa-decarboxylase [190] preventing sufficient amounts of L-dopa from reaching the brain. The addition of carbidopa, an inhibitor of dopa-decarboxylase, blocks peripheral conversion and enables appropriate levels of L-dopa to reach the brain and hence elevate dopamine sufficiently in the substantia nigra pars compacta to correct motor dysfunction.

Nonergoline Dopamine Agonists A second successful monotherapy is the use of nonergoline dopamine agonists, ropinirole, pramipexole, apomorphine, and rotigotine that are selective for dopamine receptors [209]. The nonergoline dopamine agonists differ chemically from the early ergoline dopamine agonists (e.g., bromocriptine) associated with cardiovascular adverse effects [210] but still pose safety concerns with sudden sleep attacks and impulse control disorder [209].

Both of these therapies successfully correct motor dysfunction from many years [181]. As the disease progresses, motor fluctuations occur, characterized by more time "OFF" in which motor symptoms reoccur and less time "ON" with sufficient normalization of symptoms and additionally, in some patients, the onset of levodopa-induced dyskinesia (LID), involuntary spastic-type jerky movements [181]. Motor fluctuations and LID occur in about 40% of patients within 4–6 years post-diagnosis [211]. The origin of motor fluctuations is not completely understood but attributed to "younger age at onset, worse disease severity, and higher levodopa dose" [181]. LID is attributed to oscillating levels of dopamine with reduced dopaminergic neurons to accommodate levodopa uptake [181].

As evidenced in Table 5.4, there is considerable effort to develop therapies that minimize motor fluctuations and LID. For example, the CD-LD ER, extended release, assures dopamine levels throughout the day and significantly increases "ON" time without the presence of dyskinesia [49–51]. Ropinirole and pramipexole are effective monotherapies for symptoms of Parkinson's disease [181]. As shown in Table 5.4, adjunct therapy with rotigotine (transdermal patch) and subcutaneous injection or intravenous infusions of apomorphine are additionally useful to decrease "OFF" time. Furthermore, ropinirole in a 5-year treatment study of early Parkinson's disease (Stages 1–3) cut the risk of dyskinesia in half compared to CD-LD [54]. The NMDA receptor antagonist, amantadine ER, is a benefit as a monotherapy as well as an adjunct to CD-LD therapy [181] and as an adjunct ER capsule, it reduces dyskinesia and "OFF" time [75]. With the exception of rasagiline, the other monoamine oxidase inhibitors, the COMT inhibitors, and istradefylline, an adenosine 2A receptor antagonist, are considered adjunct therapies to treat motor fluctuations. On the other hand, rasagiline is an acceptable monotherapy in early Parkinson's disease [181]. Two other drugs, affecting the serotonin receptor, pimavanserin and clozapine improve Parkinson's disease psychosis without worsening motor symptoms (Table 5.4).

Parkinson's Disease. Adverse Effects The most common adverse effects with Parkinson's disease drugs, either as monotherapy or adjunct therapy, are nausea, hypotension, and hallucinations, all of which potentially add to the non-motor symptoms of disease. Safety is a big concern, so clients are taught to change positions slowly. Other instructions are to take their medicine with food in the early morning, limit protein until the evening, and report any irregular or fast heartbeat.

Polypharmacy is common in Parkinson's disease due to the necessity to (1) correct motor dysfunction, (2) reduce motor fluctuations, (3) reduce LID, and (4) ameliorate non-muscle symptoms. Vigilance is needed to go slow with the lowest dose possible. Potentially inappropriate medication (PIM) is also common in the older adults with Parkinson's disease. Based on data from beneficiaries of Medicare part A,B,D, excluding OTC products and in-hospital prescriptions, approximately 36% of Parkinson's disease patients ≥65 years of age received at least 1 PIM in 2014 [212]. PIMs also nearly double hospital stays for patients [213]. Use of drugs with strong anticholinergic activity (see Chap. 3 for a list of drugs with anticholinergic effects) should be avoided in Parkinson's disease due to the risk of confusion, dry mouth, constipation that would exacerbate Parkinson's disease symptoms. Specifically, according to the Beers Criteria® Update (2023) [33], this would encompass the first-generation antihistamines, e.g., diphenhydramine; ineffective antiparkinson drugs, e.g., benztropine and trihexyphenidyl; antispasmodic, e.g., scopolamine; skeletal muscle relaxants, e.g., cyclobenzaprine and methocarbamol; antidepressants, e.g., tricyclic antidepressants (amitriptyline) and some antipsychotics, e.g., risperidone and quetiapine with the exception of clozapine and pimavanserin (Table 5.4). Additionally, there are a number of antiemetic/antipsychotic drugs that are dopamine antagonists and hence are to be avoided in Parkinson's disease. Examples include amisulpride, droperidol, and chlorpromazine.

Parkinson's Disease. Non-pharmacotherapy Several lifestyle choices are proposed as helpful non-pharmacotherapy for Parkinson's disease and also as early prevention. In general, these include wise dietary choices such as the Mediterranean diet [214], physical activity of all types, and avoidance of head trauma [202, 215, 216]. Specifically, rehabilitation physical exercises have received considerable attention. In a meta-analysis of over 150 relatively small RCTs of Parkinson's disease patients exercising compared to passive controls, physical exercise provided essential benefits compared to controls [217]. As determined by UPDRS and other assessments, motor symptoms and QoL improved with several types of exercise, e.g., dance, aqua-based, gait/balance/functional exercises, multi-domain training, and endurance exercises, although the differences between them were small, suggesting physical exercise is key, but the exact one is not [217].

Guidance
1. Until there is a cure, pharmacotherapy for chronic obstructive pulmonary disease (COPD), chronic kidney disease (CKD), and Parkinson's disease has the potential to manage disease symptoms for many years. Mainstay, first-line drugs are:
   (a) COPD—β2-adrenergic receptor agonists (short, long, and ultra-long acting), muscarinic acetylcholine receptor antagonists (long-acting) and inhaled corticosteroids; used as mono, dual, or triple therapy depending on disease progression; macrolides are the antibiotics of choice but to be used with caution. Co-morbidities are treated separately as if COPD was absent.
   (b) CKD—Angiotensin-converting enzyme inhibitors, angiotensin receptor inhibitors, sodium glucose cotransporter 2 inhibitors and nonsteroidal mineralocorticoid receptor antagonist; hyperkalemia is best treated with potassium exchange compounds or diet.
   (c) Parkinson's Disease—Carbidopa/levodopa (immediate, controlled, and extended release); nonergoline dopamine receptor agonists; motor fluctuation and levodopa-induced dyskinesia require adjunct drug use with NMDA receptor antagonist, monoamine oxidase inhibitors, and others.
2. General concerns and potential adverse effects.
   (a) COPD—First-time use of long-acting β2-adrenergic receptor agonists in COPD associated with adverse cardiovascular events; long-acting muscarinic acetylcholine receptor antagonists produce dry mouth and some evidence of other anticholinergic effects, e.g., acute urinary retention; long-term use of corticosteroids poses risks of infections requiring hospitalizations, fractures, adverse gastrointestinal and central nervous system effects.

   Age changes in cognition, strength, and dexterity affect the selection and use of inhalers for COPD and must be considered to achieve efficacy in the treatment of COPD

   (b) CKD—Reduced kidney function has implications for all drugs eliminated by this route - requires lower dose or different drug choice.

   Age-associated decline in estimated glomerular filtration rate should be considered to avoid over diagnosis of CKD in the older adult; in the presence of age or frailty-induced sarcopenia, consider cystatin-c as an alternative to creatinine or direct measurement of glomerular filtration

   Risk of hyperkalemia is high with CKD drugs and additive to the drugs used to treat cardiovascular disease; consider alternate ways to lower potassium (diet, diuretics, remove nonessential drugs); ketoacidosis may occur with sodium-glucose cotransporter 2 inhibitors

   (c) Parkinson's disease—Nausea, hypotension, and hallucinations expected with Parkinson's disease drugs - select drugs that lack anticholinergic

(continued)

effects and dopamine receptor antagonism. Supply safety instructions to avoid falls, when best to take medication, and report side effects.

Treatment of comorbidities in these diseases is challenging. Vigilance is required to avoid polypharmacy and potential inappropriate medications

3. Non-pharmacological therapies.
   (a) COPD—Smoking cessation and avoidance of indoor biomass burning, industrial fumes/dust, outdoor pollution; participation in pulmonary rehabilitation program, vaccinations against lung pathogens.
   (b) CKD—Control hypertension, hyperglycemia and dyslipidemia, weight reduction and smoking cessation, participate in physical exercise as cardiovascular system allows.
   (c) Parkinson's disease—Avoid exposure to pesticides especially paraquat and rotenone; participate in physical exercise of choice, select a healthy diet and avoid head trauma.

References

1. Terry PD, Dhand R. The 2023 GOLD report: updated guidelines for inhaled pharmacological therapy in patients with stable COPD. Pulm Ther. 2023;9(3):345–57. https://doi.org/10.1007/s41030-023-00233-z.
2. Matera MG, Hanania NA, Maniscalco M, Cazzola M. Pharmacotherapies in older adults with COPD: challenges and opportunities. Drugs Aging. 2023;40(7):605–19. https://doi.org/10.1007/s40266-023-01038-0.
3. Santus P, Radovanovic D, Di Marco S, Valenti V, Raccanelli R, Blasi F, et al. Effect of indacaterol on lung deflation improves cardiac performance in hyperinflated COPD patients: an interventional, randomized, double-blind clinical trial. Int J Chron Obstruct Pulmon Dis. 2015;10:1917–23. https://doi.org/10.2147/COPD.S91684. eCollection 2015
4. Girodet PO, Jasnot JY, Le Gros V, Decuypere L, Cao W, Devouassoux G. Efficacy and safety of indacaterol in patients with chronic obstructive pulmonary disease aged over 65 years: a pooled analysis. Respir Med. 2017;128:92–101. https://doi.org/10.1016/j.rmed.2017.05.010.
5. Gershon A, Croxford R, Calzavara A, To T, Stanbrook MB, Upshur R, et al. Cardiovascular safety of inhaled long-acting bronchodilators in individuals with chronic obstructive pulmonary disease. JAMA Intern Med. 2013;173(13):1175–85. https://doi.org/10.1001/jamainternmed.2013.1016.
6. Au DH, Curtis JR, Every NR, McDonell MB, Fihn SD. Association between inhaled beta-agonists and the risk of unstable angina and myocardial infarction. Chest. 2002;121(3):846–51.
7. van Schayck CP, Folgering H, Harbers H, Maas KL, van Weel C. Effects of allergy and age on responses to salbutamol and ipratropium bromide in moderate asthma and chronic bronchitis. Thorax. 1991;46(5):355–9. https://doi.org/10.1136/thx.46.5.355.
8. Parker AL. Aging does not affect beta-agonist responsiveness after methacholine-induced bronchoconstriction. J Am Geriatr Soc. 2004;52(3):388–92. https://doi.org/10.1111/j.1532-5415.2004.52110.x.
9. Stephenson A, Seitz D, Bell CM, Gruneir A, Gershon AS, Austin PC, et al. Inhaled anticholinergic drug therapy and the risk of acute urinary retention in chronic obstructive pulmonary disease: a population-based study. Arch Intern Med. 2011;171(10):914–20. https://doi.org/10.1001/archinternmed.2011.170.

10. Ray R, Tombs L, Naya I, Compton C, Lipson DA, Boucot I. Efficacy and safety of the dual bronchodilator combination umeclidinium/vilanterol in COPD by age and airflow limitation severity: a pooled post hoc analysis of seven clinical trials. Pulm Pharmacol Ther. 2019;57:101802. https://doi.org/10.1016/j.pupt.2019.101802.
11. Spannella F, Giulietti F, Cesari V, Francioso A, Cocci G, Landi L, et al. Combination therapy of inhaled Indacaterol/Glycopyrronium for chronic obstructive pulmonary disease in the very elderly: is it safe? An electrocardiographic evaluation. Respiration. 2018;95(Suppl 1):22–9. https://doi.org/10.1159/000487182.
12. Ferguson GT, Karpel JP, Clerisme-Beaty E, Gronke L, Vos F, Buhl R. Efficacy and safety of tiotropium + olodaterol maintenance treatment in patients with COPD in the TONADO R and OTEMTO R studies: a subgroup analysis by age. Int J Chron Obstruct Pulmon Dis. 2016;11:2701–10. https://doi.org/10.2147/COPD.S108758.
13. Hanania NA, Caveney S, Soule T, Tombs L, Lettis S, Crim C, et al. Effect of age on efficacy and safety of fluticasone furoate/vilanterol (FF/VI), umeclidinium (UMEC), and UMEC + FF/VI in patients with chronic obstructive pulmonary disease: analyses of five randomized clinical trials. Int J Chron Obstruct Pulmon Dis. 2021;24(16):1925–38. https://doi.org/10.2147/COPD.S302864.
14. Caramori G, Ruggeri P, Arpinelli F, Salvi L, Girbino G. Long-term use of inhaled glucocorticoids in patients with stable chronic obstructive pulmonary disease and risk of bone fractures: a narrative review of the literature. Int J Chron Obstruct Pulmon Dis. 2019;14:1085–97. https://doi.org/10.2147/COPD.S190215.
15. Kendzerska T, Aaron SD, To T, Licskai C, Stanbrook M, Vozoris NT, et al. Effectiveness and safety of inhaled corticosteroids in older individuals with chronic obstructive pulmonary disease and/or asthma: a population study. Ann Am Thorac Soc. 2019;16(10):1252–62. https://doi.org/10.1513/AnnalsATS.201902-126OC.
16. Bowie MW, Slattum PW. Pharmacodynamics in the older adult. A review. Am J Geriatr Pharmacother. 2007;5(3):263–303. https://doi.org/10.1016/j.amjopharm.2007.10.001.
17. Peng S, Tan C, Du L, Niu Y, Liu X, Wang R. Effect of fracture risk in inhaled corticosteroids in patients with chronic obstructive pulmonary disease: a systematic review and meta-analysis. BMC Pulm Med. 2023;23(1):304. https://doi.org/10.1186/s12890-023-02602-5.
18. Janjua S, Fortescue R, Poole P. Phosphodiesterase-4 inhibitors for chronic obstructive pulmonary disease. Cochrane Database Syst Rev. 2020;5(5):CD002309. https://doi.org/10.1002/14651858.CD002309.pub6.
19. Han MK, Tayob N, Murray S, et al. Predictors of chronic obstructive pulmonary disease exacerbation reduction in response to daily azithromycin therapy. Am J Respir Crit Care Med. 2014;189(12):1503–8. https://doi.org/10.1164/rccm.201402-0207OC.
20. Albert RK, Connett J, Bailey WC, Casaburi R, Cooper JA Jr, Criner GJ, et al. COPD clinical research network. Azithromycin for prevention of exacerbations of COPD. N Engl J Med. 2011;365(8):689–98. https://doi.org/10.1056/NEJMoa1104623.
21. Cao Y, Xuan S, Wu Y, Yao X. Effects of long-term macrolide therapy at low doses in stable COPD. Int J Chron Obstruct Pulmon Dis. 2019;14:1289–98. https://doi.org/10.2147/COPD.S205075.
22. Brenner BM, Cooper ME, de Zeeuw D, Keane WF, Mitch WE, Parving HH, et al. Effects of losartan on renal and cardiovascular outcomes in patients with type 2 diabetes and nephropathy. N Engl J Med. 2001;345(12):861–9. https://doi.org/10.1056/nejmoa011161.
23. Lewis EJ, Hunsicker LG, Clarke WR, Berl T, Pohl MA, Lewis JB, et al. Renoprotective effect of the angiotensin-receptor antagonist irbesartan in patients with nephropathy due to type 2 diabetes. N Engl J Med. 2001;345(12):851–60. https://doi.org/10.1056/nejmoa011303.
24. Cheung AK, Rahman M, Reboussin DM, Craven TE, Greene T, Kimmel PL, et al. Effects of intensive BP control in CKD. J Am Soc Nephrol. 2017;28(9):2812–23. https://doi.org/10.1681/ASN.2017020148.

25. Strippoli GFM, Bonifati C, Craig M, Navaneethan SD, Craig JC. Angiotensin converting enzyme inhibitors and angiotensin II receptor antagonists for preventing the progression of diabetic kidney disease. Cochrane Database Syst Rev. 2006;2006(4):CD006257. https://doi.org/10.1002/14651858.CD006257.
26. Leon SJ, Whitlock R, Rigatto C, Komenda P, Bohm C, Sucha E, et al. Hyperkalemia-related discontinuation of Renin-Angiotensin-Aldosterone system inhibitors and clinical outcomes in CKD: a population-based cohort study. Am J Kidney Dis. 2022;80(2):164–73.e1. https://doi.org/10.1053/j.ajkd.2022.01.002.
27. Mann JFE, Schmieder RE, McQueen M, Dyal L, Schumacher H, Pogue J, et al. Renal outcomes with telmisartan, ramipril, or both, in people at high vascular risk (the ONTARGET study): a multicentre, randomised, double-blind, controlled trial. Lancet. 2008;372(9638):547–53. https://doi.org/10.1016/S0140-6736(08)61236-2.
28. Villain C, Metzger M, Liabeuf S, Hamroun A, Laville S, Mansencal N, et al. Effectiveness and tolerance of renin-angiotensin system inhibitors with aging in chronic kidney disease. J Am Med Dir Assoc. 2022;23(6):998–1004.e7. https://doi.org/10.1016/j.jamda.2021.10.019.
29. Parker K, Hartemink J, Saha A, Mitra R, Lewis P, Power A, et al. A systematic review of the efficacy and safety of anticoagulants in advanced chronic kidney disease. J Nephrol. 2022;35(8):2015–33. https://doi.org/10.1007/s40620-022-01413-x.
30. Perkovic V, Jardine MJ, Neal B, Bompoint S, Heerspink HJL, Charytan DM, et al. Canagliflozin and renal outcomes in type 2 diabetes and nephropathy. N Engl J Med. 2019;380(24):2295–306. https://doi.org/10.1056/NEJMoa1811744.
31. Heerspink HJL, Stefánsson BV, Correa-Rotter R, Chertow GM, Greene T, Hou FF, et al. Dapagliflozin in patients with chronic kidney disease. N Engl J Med. 2020;383(15):1436–46. https://doi.org/10.1056/NEJMoa2024816.
32. Fernández-Fernandez B, Sarafidis P, Soler MJ, Ortiz A. EMPA-KIDNEY: expanding the range of kidney protection by SGLT2 inhibitors. Clin Kidney J. 2023;16(8):1187–98. https://doi.org/10.1093/ckj/sfad082.
33. By the 2023 American Geriatrics Society Beers Criteria® Update Expert Panel. American Geriatrics Society 2023 updated AGS Beers Criteria® for potentially inappropriate medication use in older adults. J Am Geriatr Soc. 2023;71(7):2052–81. https://doi.org/10.1111/jgs.18372.
34. Qiu M, Ding LL, Zhang M, Lin JH, Gu JS, Zhou X, et al. SGLT2 inhibitors for prevention of cardiorenal events in people with type 2 diabetes without cardiorenal disease: a meta-analysis of large randomized trials and cohort studies. Pharmacol Res. 2020;161:105175. https://doi.org/10.1016/j.phrs.2020.105175.
35. de Boer IH, Khunti K, Sadusky T, et al. Diabetes management in chronic kidney disease: a consensus report by the American Diabetes Association (ADA) and kidney disease: improving global outcomes (KDIGO). Kidney Int. 2022;102(5):974–89. https://doi.org/10.1016/j.kint.2022.08.012.
36. Bakris GL, Agarwal R, Anker SD, Pitt B, Ruilope LM, Rossing P, et al. Effect of finerenone on chronic kidney disease outcomes in type 2 diabetes. N Engl J Med. 2020;383(23):2219–29. https://doi.org/10.1056/NEJMoa2025845.
37. Pitt B, Filippatos G, Agarwal R, Anker SD, Bakris GL, Rossing P, et al. Cardiovascular events with finerenone in kidney disease and type 2 diabetes. N Engl J Med. 2021;385(24):2252–63. https://doi.org/10.1056/NEJMoa2110956.
38. Ashjian E, Clarke M, Pogue K. Pharmacotherapy considerations with finerenone in the treatment of chronic kidney disease associated with type 2 diabetes. Am J Health Syst Pharm. 2023;80(23):1708–21. https://doi.org/10.1093/ajhp/zxad192.
39. Lepage L, Dufour AC, Doiron J, Handfield K, Desforges K, Bell R, et al. Randomized clinical trial of sodium polystyrene sulfonate for the treatment of mild hyperkalemia in CKD. Clin J Am Soc Nephrol. 2015;10(12):2136–42. https://doi.org/10.2215/CJN.03640415.
40. Nasir K, Ahmad A. Treatment of hyperkalemia in patients with chronic kidney disease: a comparison of calcium polystyrene sulphonate and sodium polystyrene sulphonate. J Ayub Med Coll Abbottabad. 2014;26(4):455–8.

41. Agarwal R, Rossignol P, Budden J, Mayo MR, Arthur S, Williams B, et al. Patiromer and Spironolactone in resistant hypertension and advanced CKD: analysis of the randomized AMBER trial. Kidney 360. 2021;2(3):425–34. https://doi.org/10.34067/KID.0006782020.
42. Weir MR, Bakris GL, Bushinsky DA, Mayo MR, Garza D, Stasiv Y, et al. OPAL-HK investigators. Patiromer in patients with kidney disease and hyperkalemia receiving RAAS inhibitors. N Engl J Med. 2015;372(3):211–21. https://doi.org/10.1056/NEJMoa1410853.
43. Spinowitz BS, Fishbane S, Pergola PE, Roger SD, Lerma EV, Butler J, et al. Sodium zirconium cyclosilicate among individuals with hyperkalemia: a 12-month phase 3 study. Clin J Am Soc Nephrol. 2019;14(6):798–809. https://doi.org/10.2215/CJN.12651018. Epub 2019 May 20
44. Rahman S, Marathi R. Sodium polystyrene sulfonate 2024. https://www.ncbi.nlm.nih.gov/books/NBK559206/#__NBK559206_dtls__.
45. Lieberman A, Goodgold A, Jonas S, Leibowitz M. Comparison of dopa decarboxylase inhibitor (carbidopa) combined with levodopa and levodopa alone in Parkinson's disease. Neurology. 1975;25(10):911–6. https://doi.org/10.1212/wnl.25.10.911.
46. Manyam BV, Hare TA, Robbs R, Cubberley VB. Evaluation of equivalent efficacy of sinemet and sinemet CR in patients with Parkinson's disease applying levodopa dosage conversion formula. Clin Neuropharmacol. 1999;22(1):33–9. https://doi.org/10.1097/00002826-199901000-00007.
47. Fahn S, Oakes D, Shoulson I, Kieburtz K, Rudolph A, Lang A, et al. Levodopa and the progression of Parkinson's disease. N Engl J Med. 2004;351(24):2498–508. https://doi.org/10.1056/NEJMoa033447.
48. Hauser RA, Hsu A, Kell S, Espay AJ, Sethi K, Stacy M, et al. Extended-release carbidopa-levodopa (IPX066) compared with immediate-release carbidopa-levodopa in patients with Parkinson's disease and motor fluctuations: a phase 3 randomised, double-blind trial. Lancet Neurol. 2013;12(4):346–56. https://doi.org/10.1016/S1474-4422(13)70025-5.
49. Hauser RA, Zeitlin L, Fisher S, D'Souza R. Duration of benefit per dose: Carbidopa-Levodopa immediate release vs. extended release capsules (Rytary). Parkinsonism Relat Disord. 2021;82:133–7. https://doi.org/10.1016/j.parkreldis.2020.12.002.
50. Modi NB, Mittur A, Rubens R, Khanna S, Gupta S. Single-dose pharmacokinetics and pharmacodynamics of IPX203 in patients with advanced parkinson disease: a comparison with immediate-release Carbidopa-Levodopa and with extended-release Carbidopa-Levodopa capsules. Clin Neuropharmacol. 2019;42(1):4–8. https://doi.org/10.1097/WNF.0000000000000314.
51. Nausieda PA, Hsu A, Elmer L, Gil RA, Spiegel J, Singer C, et al. Conversion to IPX066 from standard levodopa formulations in advanced Parkinson's disease: experience in clinical trials. J Parkinsons Dis. 2015;5(4):837–45. https://doi.org/10.3233/JPD-150622.
52. Stocchi F, Hersh BP, Scott BL, Nausieda PA, Giorgi L, Ease PD, Monotherapy Study Investigators. Ropinirole 24-hour prolonged release and ropinirole immediate release in early Parkinson's disease: a randomized, double-blind, non-inferiority crossover study. Curr Med Res Opin. 2008;24(10):2883–95. https://doi.org/10.1185/03007990802387130.
53. Adler CH, Sethi KD, Hauser RA, Davis TL, Hammerstad JP, Bertoni J, et al. Ropinirole for the treatment of early Parkinson's disease. Neurology. 1997;49(2):393–9. https://doi.org/10.1212/wnl.49.2.393.
54. Rascol O, Brooks DJ, Korczyn AD, DeDeyn PP, Clarke CE, Lang AE. A five-year study of the incidence of dyskinesia in patients with early Parkinson's disease who were treated with ropinirole or levodopa. N Engl J Med. 2000;342(20):1484–91. https://doi.org/10.1056/NEJM200005183422004.
55. Lieberman A, Olanow CW, Sethi K, Swanson P, Waters CH, Fahn S, Ropinirole Study Group, et al. A multicenter trial of ropinirole as adjunct treatment for Parkinson's disease. Neurology. 1998;51(4):1057–62. https://doi.org/10.1212/wnl.51.4.1057.
56. Makumi CW, Asgharian A, Ellis J, Shaikh S, Jimenez T, VanMeter S. Long-term, open-label, safety study of once-daily ropinirole extended/prolonged release in early and advanced

Parkinson's disease. Int J Neurosci. 2016;126(1):30–8. https://doi.org/10.3109/00207454.2014.991924.
57. Mizuno Y, Nomoto M, Hasegawa K, Hattori N, Kondo T, Murata M, et al. Rotigotine vs ropinirole in advanced stage Parkinson's disease: a double-blind study. Parkinsonism Relat Disord. 2014;20(12):1388–93. https://doi.org/10.1016/j.parkreldis.2014.10.005.
58. Kieburtz K, The Parkinson Study Group PRAMIBID Investigators. Twice-daily, low-dose pramipexole in early Parkinson's disease: a randomized, placebo-controlled trial. Mov Disord. 2011;26(1):37–44. https://doi.org/10.1002/mds.23396.
59. Poewe W, Rascol O, Barone P, Hauser RA, Mizuno Y, Haaksma M, et al. Extended-release pramipexole in early Parkinson disease: a 33-week randomized controlled trial. Neurology. 2011;77(8):759–66. https://doi.org/10.1212/WNL.0b013e31822affb0.
60. Schapira AH, Barone P, Hauser RA, Mizuno Y, Rascol O, Busse M, et al. Extended-release pramipexole in advanced Parkinson disease: a randomized controlled trial. Neurology. 2011;77(8):767–74. https://doi.org/10.1212/WNL.0b013e31822affdb.
61. Schapira AHV, McDermott MP, Barone P, Comella CL, Albrecht S, Hsu HH, et al. Pramipexole in patients with early Parkinson's disease (PROUD): a randomised delayed-start trial. Lancet Neurol. 2013;12(8):747–55. https://doi.org/10.1016/S1474-4422(13)70117-0.
62. Pietz K, Hagell P, Odin P. Subcutaneous apomorphine in late stage Parkinson's disease: a long term follow up. J Neurol Neurosurg Psychiatry. 1998;65(5):709–16. https://doi.org/10.1136/jnnp.65.5.709.
63. Priano L, Albani G, Brioschi A, Calderoni S, Lopiano L, Rizzone M, et al. Transdermal apomorphine permeation from microemulsions: a new treatment in Parkinson's disease. Mov Disord. 2004;19(8):937–42. https://doi.org/10.1002/mds.20054.
64. Katzenschlager R, Poewe W, Rascol O, Trenkwalder C, Deuschl G, Chaudhuri KR, et al. Apomorphine subcutaneous infusion in patients with Parkinson's disease with persistent motor fluctuations (TOLEDO): a multicentre, doubleblind, randomised, placebo-controlled trial. Lancet Neurol. 2018;17(9):749–59. https://doi.org/10.1016/S1474-4422(18)30239-4.
65. Piccini P, Brooks DJ, Korpela K, Pavese N, Karlsson M, Gordin A. The catechol-O-methyltransferase (COMT) inhibitor entacapone enhances the pharmacokinetic and clinical response to Sinemet CR in Parkinson's disease. J Neurol Neurosurg Psychiatry. 2000;68(5):589–94. https://doi.org/10.1136/jnnp.68.5.589.
66. Reichmann H, Lees A, Rocha JF, Magalhães D, Soares-da-Silva P, OPTIPARK investigators. Effectiveness and safety of opicapone in Parkinson's disease patients with motor fluctuations: the OPTIPARK open-label study. Transl Neurodegener. 2020;9(1):9. https://doi.org/10.1186/s40035-020-00187-1.
67. Ferreira JJ, Lees A, Rocha JF, Poewe W, Rascol O, Soares-da-Silva P. Long-term efficacy of opicapone in fluctuating Parkinson's disease patients: a pooled analysis of data from two phase 3 clinical trials and their open-label extensions. Eur J Neurol. 2019;26(7):953–60. https://doi.org/10.1111/ene.13914.
68. Baas H, Beiske AG, Ghika J, Jackson M, Oertel WH, Poewe W, et al. Catechol-O-methyltransferase inhibition with tolcapone reduces the "wearing off" phenomenon and levodopa requirements in fluctuating parkinsonian patients. J Neurol Neurosurg Psychiatry. 1997;63(4):421–8. https://doi.org/10.1136/jnnp.63.4.421.
69. Hattori N, Takeda A, Takeda S, Nishimura A, Kitagawa T, Mochizuki H, et al. Rasagiline monotherapy in early Parkinson's disease: a phase 3, randomized study in Japan. Parkinsonism Relat Disord. 2019;60:146–52. https://doi.org/10.1016/j.parkreldis.2018.08.024.
70. Takahashi M, Yuasa R, Imai T, Tachibana H, Yorifuji S, Nakamura Y, et al. Selegiline (L-deprenyl) and L-dopa treatment of Parkinson's disease: a double-blind trial. Intern Med. 1994;33(9):517–24. https://doi.org/10.2169/internalmedicine.33.517.
71. Mizuno Y, Hattori N, Kondo T, Nomoto M, Origasa H, Takahashi R. A randomized doubleblind placebo-controlled phase III trial of Selegiline monotherapy for early Parkinson disease. Clin Neuropharmacol. 2017;40(5):201–7. https://doi.org/10.1097/WNF.0000000000000239.

72. Borgohain R, Szasz J, Stanzione P, Meshram C, Bhatt MH, Chirilineau D, et al. Two-year, randomized, controlled study of safinamide as add-on to levodopa in mid to late Parkinson's. Mov Disord. 2014;29(10):1273–80. https://doi.org/10.1002/mds.25961.
73. Sawada H, Oeda T, Kuno S, Nomoto M, Yamamoto K, Yamamoto M, et al. Amantadine for dyskinesias in Parkinson's disease: a randomized controlled trial. PLoS One. 2010;5(12):e15298. https://doi.org/10.1371/journal.pone.0015298.
74. Thomas A, Iacono D, Luciano AL, Armellino K, Di Iorio A, Onofrj M. Duration of amantadine benefit on dyskinesia of severe Parkinson's disease. J Neurol Neurosurg Psychiatry. 2004;75(1):141–3.
75. Elmer LW, Juncos JL, Singer C, Truong DD, Criswell SR, Parashos S, et al. Pooled analyses of phase III studies of ADS-5102 (Amantadine) extended-release capsules for Dyskinesia in Parkinson's disease. CNS Drugs. 2018;32(4):387–98. https://doi.org/10.1007/s40263-018-0498-4.
76. Mizuno Y, Kondo T, Japanese Istradefylline Study Group. Adenosine A2A receptor antagonist istradefylline reduces daily OFF time in Parkinson's disease. Mov Disord. 2013;28(8):1138–41. https://doi.org/10.1002/mds.25418.
77. Meltzer HY, Mills R, Revell S, Williams H, Johnson A, Bahr D, et al. Pimavanserin, a serotonin(2A) receptor inverse agonist, for the treatment of parkinson's disease psychosis. Neuropsychopharmacology. 2010;35(4):881–92. https://doi.org/10.1038/npp.2009.176.
78. Factor SA, Brown D, Molho ES, Podskalny GD. Clozapine: a 2-year open trial in Parkinson's disease patients with psychosis. Neurology. 1994;44(3 Pt 1):544–6. https://doi.org/10.1212/wnl.44.3_part_1.544.
79. Parkinson Study Group. Low-dose clozapine for the treatment of drug-induced psychosis in Parkinson's disease. N Engl J Med. 1999;340(10):757–63. https://doi.org/10.1056/NEJM199903113401003.
80. Pollak P, Tison F, Rascol O, Destée A, Péré JJ, Senard JM, et al. Clozapine in drug induced psychosis in Parkinson's disease: a randomised, placebo controlled study with open follow up. J Neurol Neurosurg Psychiatry. 2004;75(5):689–95. https://doi.org/10.1136/jnnp.2003.029868.
81. Global Initiative for Chronic Obstructive Lung Disease (GOLD). Global strategy for the diagnosis, management, and prevention of chronic obstructive pulmonary disease: 2023 report. Available from: https://goldcopd.org/wp-content/uploads/2022/11/GOLD-2023-ver-1.0-14Nov2022_WMV.pdf.
82. Global Strategy for Prevention, Diagnosis and Management of Copd: 2024 Report https://goldcopd.org/2024-gold-report/
83. Celli B, Fabbri L, Criner G, Martinez FJ, Mannino D, Vogelmeiers C, et al. Definition and nomenclature of chronic obstructive pulmonary disease time for its revision. Am J Respir Crit Care Med. 2022;206(11):1317–25. https://doi.org/10.1164/rccm.202204-0671PP.
84. Global Initiative for Chronic Obstructive Lung Disease 2023 Report: GOLD Executive Summary.
85. Agustí A, Celli BR, Criner GJ, Halpin D, Anzueto A, Barnes P, et al. Global Initiative for Chronic Obstructive Lung Disease 2023 Report: GOLD Executive Summary Eur Respir J. 2023;61(4):2300239. https://doi.org/10.1183/13993003.00239-2023.
86. Adeloye D, Song P, Zhu Y, Campbell H, Sheikh A, Rudan I. NIHR RESPIRE global respiratory health unit. Global, regional, and national prevalence of, and risk factors for, chronic obstructive pulmonary disease (COPD) in 2019: a systematic review and modelling analysis. Lancet Respir Med. 2022;10(5):447–58. https://doi.org/10.1016/S2213-2600(21)00511-7.
87. Boers E, Barrett M, Su JG, Benjafield AV, Sinha S, Kaye L, et al. Global Burden of Chronic Obstructive Pulmonary Disease Through 2050 JAMA Netw Open. 2023;6(12):e2346598. https://doi.org/10.1001/jamanetworkopen.2023.46598.
88. Liu D, Meister M, Zhang S, Vong CI, Wang S, Fang R, et al. Impact of the spirometric definition on comorbidities in chronic obstructive pulmonary disease. Respir Res. 2020;21(1):242. https://doi.org/10.1186/s12931-020-01507-9.

89. Kohansal R, Martinez-Camblor P, Agusti A, Buist AS, Mannino DM, Soriano JB. The natural history of chronic airflow obstruction revisited: an analysis of the Framingham offspring cohort. Am J Respir Crit Care Med. 2009;180(1):3–10. https://doi.org/10.1164/rccm.200901-0047OC.
90. Sargent JD, Halenar M, Steinberg AW, Ozga J, Tang Z, Stanton CA, et al. Childhood cigarette smoking and risk of COPD in older U.S. adults. Am J Respir Crit Care Med. 2023;208(4):428–34. https://doi.org/10.1164/rccm.202303-0476OC.
91. Yang IA, Jenkins CR, Salvi SS. Chronic obstructive pulmonary disease in never-smokers: risk factors, pathogenesis, and implications for prevention and treatment. Lancet Respir Med. 2022;10(5):497–511. https://doi.org/10.1016/S2213-2600(21)00506-3.
92. Pando-Sandoval A, Ruano-Ravina A, Candal-Pedreira C, Rodriguez-Garcia C, Represas-Represas C, Golpe R, et al. Risk factors for chronic obstructive pulmonary disease in never-smokers: a systematic review. Clin Respir J. 2022;16(4):261–75. https://doi.org/10.1111/crj.13479.
93. Orozco-Levi M, Garcia-Aymerich J, Villar J, Ramırez-Sarmiento A, Anto JM, Gea J. Wood smoke exposure and risk of chronic obstructive pulmonary disease. Eur Respir J. 2006;27:542–6. https://doi.org/10.1183/09031936.06.00052705.
94. Kamal R, Srivastava AK, Kesavachandran CN, Bihari V, Singh A. Chronic obstructive pulmonary disease (COPD) in women due to indoor biomass burning: a meta analysis. Int J Environ Health Res. 2022 Jun;32(6):1403–17. https://doi.org/10.1080/09603123.2021.1887460.
95. Becklake MR. Occupational exposures: evidence for a causal association with chronic obstructive pulmonary disease. Am Rev Respir Dis. 1989;140(3 Pt 2):S85–91. https://doi.org/10.1164/ajrccm/140.3_Pt_2.S85.
96. Peng C, Yan Y, Li Z, Jiang Y, Cai Y. Chronic obstructive pulmonary disease caused by inhalation of dust: a meta-analysis Medicine (Baltimore) 2020;99(34):e21908. https://doi.org/10.1097/MD.0000000000021908.
97. Berend N. Contribution of air pollution to COPD and small airway dysfunction. Respirology. 2016;21(2):237–44. https://doi.org/10.1111/resp.12644.
98. Silverman EK. Genetics of COPD. Annu Rev Physiol. 2020;82:413–31. https://doi.org/10.1146/annurev-physiol-021317-121224.
99. Mostafavi B, Diaz S, Piitulainen E, Stoel BC, Wollmer P, Tanash HA. Lung function and CT lung densitometry in 37- to 39-year-old individuals with alpha-1-antitrypsin deficiency. Int J Chron Obstruct Pulmon Dis. 2018;13:3689–98. https://doi.org/10.2147/COPD.S167497.
100. Meseeha M, Sankari A, Attia M. Alpha-1 antitrypsin deficiency. In: StatPearls [Internet]. Treasure Island: StatPearls Publishing; 2024. Jan. 2024 Aug 17.
101. Agusti A, Faner R. Lung function trajectories in health and disease. Lancet Respir Med. 2019;7(4):358–64. https://doi.org/10.1016/S2213-2600(18)30529-0.
102. Stern DA, Morgan WJ, Wright AL, Guerra S, Martinez FD. Poor airway function in early infancy and lung function by age 22 years: a nonselective longitudinal cohort study. Lancet. 2007;370(9589):758–64. https://doi.org/10.1016/S0140-6736(07)61379-8.
103. Scarpace PJ, Tumer N, Mader SL. Beta-adrenergic function in aging. Basic mechanisms and clinical implications. Drugs Aging. 1991;1(2):116–29. https://doi.org/10.2165/00002512-199101020-00004.
104. Budinger GRS, Kohanski RA, Gan W, Kobor S, Amaral LA, Armanios M, et al. The intersection of aging biology and the pathobiology of lung diseases: a joint NHLBI/NIA workshop. J Gerontol A Biol Sci Med Sci. 2017;72(11):1492–500. https://doi.org/10.1093/gerona/glx090.
105. Yanagi S, Tsubouchi H, Miura A, Matsuo A, Matsumoto N, Nakazato M. The impacts of cellular senescence in elderly pneumonia and in age-related lung diseases that increase the risk of respiratory infections. Int J Mol Sci. 2017;18(3):503. https://doi.org/10.3390/ijms18030503.
106. Li Y, Wang C, Peng M. Aging immune system and its correlation with liability to severe lung complications. Front Public Health. 2021;9:735151. https://doi.org/10.3389/fpubh.2021.735151.

107. Negewo NA, Gibson PG, McDonald VM. COPD and its comorbidities: Impact, measurement and mechanisms. Respirology. 2015;20(8):1160–71. https://doi.org/10.1111/resp.12642.
108. Perez T, Burgel PR, Paillasseur JL, Caillaud D, Deslée G, Chanez P et al. Modified Medical Research Council scale vs Baseline Dyspnea Index to evaluate dyspnea in chronic obstructive pulmonary disease. Int J Chron Obstruct Pulmon Dis. 2015;10:1663–72. https://doi.org/10.2147/COPD.S82408
109. Jones PW, Harding G, Berry P, Wiklund I, Chen W-H, Leidy NK. Development and first validation of the COPD Assessment. Test Eur Respir J. 2009;34(3):648–54. https://doi.org/10.1183/09031936.00102509.
110. Jones PW, Quirk FH, Baveystock CM, Littlejohns P. A self-complete measure of health status for chronic airflow limitation. The St. George's respiratory questionnaire. Am Rev Respir Dis. 1992;145(6):1321–7. https://doi.org/10.1164/ajrccm/145.6.1321.
111. Billington CK, Penn RB, Hall IP. $β_2$-agonists. Handb Exp Pharmacol. 2017;237:23–40. https://doi.org/10.1007/164_2016_64.
112. Buels KS, Fryer AD. Muscarinic receptor antagonists: effects on pulmonary function. Handb Exp Pharmacol. 2012;208:317–41. https://doi.org/10.1007/978-3-642-23274-9_14.
113. Proskocil BJ, Sekhon HS, Jia Y, Savchenko V, Blakely RD, Lindstrom J, et al. Acetylcholine is an autocrine or paracrine hormone synthesized and secreted by airway bronchial epithelial cells. Endocrinology. 2004;145(5):2498–506. https://doi.org/10.1210/en.2003-1728.
114. Lea S, Higham A, Beech A, Singh D. How inhaled corticosteroids target inflammation in COPD. Eur Respir Rev. 2023;32(170):230084. https://doi.org/10.1183/16000617.0084-2023.
115. Siddiqui SH, Pavord ID, Barnes NC, Guasconi A, Lettis S, Pascoe S, et al. Blood eosinophils: a biomarker of COPD exacerbation reduction with inhaled corticosteroids. Int J Chron Obstruct Pulmon Dis. 2018;13:3669–76. https://doi.org/10.2147/COPD.S179425.
116. Calzetta L, Ritondo BL, de Marco P, Cazzola M, Rogliani P. Evaluating triple ICS/LABA/LAMA therapies for COPD patients: a network meta-analysis of ETHOS, KRONOS, IMPACT, and TRILOGY studies. Expert Rev Respir Med. 2021;15(1):143–52. https://doi.org/10.1080/17476348.2020.1816830.
117. Crocetti L, Floresta G, Cilibrizzi A, Giovannoni MP. An overview of PDE4 inhibitors in clinical trials: 2010 to early 2022. Molecules. 2022;27(15):4964. https://doi.org/10.3390/molecules27154964.
118. Kanoh S, Rubin BK. Mechanisms of action and clinical application of macrolides as immunomodulatory medications. Clin Microbiol Rev. 2010;23(3):590–615. https://doi.org/10.1128/CMR.00078-09.
119. Janjua S, Mathioudakis AG, Fortescue R, Walker RA, Sharif S, Threapleton CJ, et al. Prophylactic antibiotics for adults with chronic obstructive pulmonary disease: a network meta-analysis. Cochrane Database Syst Rev. 2021;1(1):CD013198. https://doi.org/10.1002/14651858.CD013198.pub2.
120. Mintzer J, Burns A. Anticholinergic side-effects of drugs in elderly people. Soc Med. 2000;93(9):457–62. https://doi.org/10.1177/014107680009300903.
121. Jara M, Wentworth C 3rd, Lanes SA. New user cohort study comparing the safety of long-acting inhaled bronchodilators in COPD. BMJ Open. 2012;2(3):e000841. https://doi.org/10.1136/bmjopen-2012-000841.
122. Yang IA, Clarke MS, Sim EHA, Fong KM. Inhaled corticosteroids for stable chronic obstructive pulmonary disease. Cochrane Database Syst Rev. 2012, 2012;(7):CD002991. https://doi.org/10.1002/14651858.CD002991.pub3.
123. Hespanhol V, Bárbara C. Pneumonia mortality, comorbidities matter? Pulmonology. 2020;26(3):123–9. https://doi.org/10.1016/j.pulmoe.2019.10.003.
124. Wang JJ, Rochtchina E, Tan AG, Cumming RG, Leeder SR, Mitchell P. Use of inhaled and oral corticosteroids and the long-term risk of cataract. Ophthalmology. 2009;116(4):652–7. https://doi.org/10.1016/j.ophtha.2008.12.001.
125. Contoli M, Pauletti A, Rossi MR, Spanevell A, Casolari P, Marcellini A, et al. Long-term effects of inhaled corticosteroids on sputum bacterial and viral loads in COPD. Eur Respir J. 2017;50(4):1700451. https://doi.org/10.1183/13993003.00451-2017.

References

126. Albertson TE, Louie S, Chan AL. J Am Geriatr Soc. 2010;58(3):570–9. https://doi.org/10.1111/j.1532-5415.2010.02741.x.
127. Herath SC, Normansell R, Maisey S, Poole P. Prophylactic antibiotic therapy for chronic obstructive pulmonary disease (COPD). Cochrane Database Syst Rev. 2018;10(10):CD009764. https://doi.org/10.1002/14651858.CD009764.pub3.
128. Olschewski H, Canepa M, Kovacs G. Pulmonary and cardiac drugs: clinically relevant interactions. Herz. 2019;44(6):517–21. https://doi.org/10.1007/s00059-019-4834-3.
129. Ponikowski P, Voors AA, Anker SD, Bueno H, Cleland JGF, Coats AJS, et al. 2016 ESC guidelines for the diagnosis and treatment of acute and chronic heart failure: the task force for the diagnosis and treatment of acute and chronic heart failure of the European Society of Cardiology (ESC) developed with the special contribution of the heart failure association (HFA) of the ESC. Eur Heart J. 2016;37(27):2129–200. https://doi.org/10.1093/eurheartj/ehw128.
130. Dransfield MT, Garner JL, Bhatt SP, Slebos D-J, Klooster K, Sciurba FC, et al. LIBERATE study group. Effect of Zephyr endobronchial valves on dyspnea, activity levels and quality of life at one year: results from a randomized clinical trial. Ann Am Thorac Soc. 2020;17(7):829–38. https://doi.org/10.1513/AnnalsATS.201909-666OC.
131. Andreas S. Effects of LAMA/LABA alone and in combination on cardiac safety. Int J Chron Obstruct Pulmon Dis. 2020;(15):1931–3. https://doi.org/10.2147/COPD.S246356.
132. Wang Y, Bahar MA, Jansen AME, Kocks JWH, Alffenaar JC, Hak E, et al. Improving antibacterial prescribing safety in the management of COPD exacerbations: systematic review of observational and clinical studies on potential drug interactions associated with frequently prescribed antibacterials among COPD patients. J Antimicrob Chemother. 2019;74(10):2848–64. https://doi.org/10.1093/jac/dkz221.
133. Pleasants RA, Hess DR. Aerosol delivery devices for obstructive lung diseases. Respir Care. 2018;63(6):708–33. https://doi.org/10.4187/respcare.06290.
134. Vogiatzis I, Rochester CL, Spruit MA, Troosters T, Clini EM. American Thoracic Society/European Respiratory Society task force on policy in pulmonary rehabilitation. Increasing implementation and delivery of pulmonary rehabilitation: key messages from the new ATS/ERS policy statement. Eur Respir J. 2016;47(5):1336–41. https://doi.org/10.1183/13993003.02151-2015.
135. Fishman A, Martinez F, Naunheim K, Piantadosi S, Wise R, Ries A, et al. National Emphysema Treatment Trial Research Group. N Engl J Med. 2003;348(21):2059–73. https://doi.org/10.1056/NEJMoa030287.
136. Evans M, Lewis RD, Morgan AR, Whyte MB, Hanif W, Bain SC, et al. A narrative review of chronic kidney disease in clinical practice: current challenges and future perspectives. Adv Ther. 2022;39(1):33–43. https://doi.org/10.1007/s12325-021-01927-z.
137. GBD Chronic Kidney Disease Collaboration. Global, regional, and national burden of chronic kidney disease, 1990–2017: a systematic analysis for the Global Burden of Disease Study 2017. Lancet. 2020;395(10225):709–33. https://doi.org/10.1016/S0140-6736(20)30045-3.
138. Hill NR, Fatoba ST, Oke JL, Hirst JA, O'Callaghan CA, Lasserson DS, et al. Global prevalence of chronic kidney disease–a systematic review and meta-analysis. PLoS One. 2016;11(7):e0158765. https://doi.org/10.1371/journal.pone.0158765.
139. Centers for Disease Control and Prevention. Chronic Kidney Disease in the United States, 2021. Atlanta: US Department of Health and Human Services, Centers for Disease Control and Prevention; 2021.
140. KDIGO. Clinical practice guideline for the evaluation and management of chronic kidney disease. Kidney Disease: Improving Global Outcomes (KDIGO) CKD Work Group. Kidney Int. 2024;105(4S):S117–314. https://doi.org/10.1016/j.kint.2023.10.018.
141. Jankowski J, Floege J, Fliser D, Böhm M, Marx N. Cardiovascular disease in chronic kidney disease: pathophysiological insights and therapeutic options. Circulation 2021;143(11):1157–72. https://doi.org/10.1161/CIRCULATIONAHA.120.050686.

142. Jha V, Garcia-Garcia G, Iseki K, Li Z, Naicker S, Plattner B, et al. Chronic kidney disease: global dimension and perspectives. Lancet. 2013;382(9888):260–72. https://doi.org/10.1016/S0140-6736(13)60687-X.
143. Humphreys BD. Mechanisms of renal fibrosis. Annu Rev Physiol. 2018;80:309–26. https://doi.org/10.1146/annurev-physiol-022516-034227.
144. Braga PC, Alves MG, Rodrigues AS. Oliveira PF mitochondrial pathophysiology on chronic kidney disease. Int J Mol Sci. 2022;23(3):1776. https://doi.org/10.3390/ijms23031776.
145. De Bhailis ÁM, Kalra PA. Hypertension and the kidneys. Br J Hosp Med (Lond). 2022;83(5):1–11. https://doi.org/10.12968/hmed.2021.0440.
146. Burnier M, Damianaki A. Hypertension as cardiovascular risk factor in chronic kidney disease. Circ Res. 2023;132(8):1050–63. https://doi.org/10.1161/CIRCRESAHA.122.321762.
147. Vallianou NG, Mitesh S, Gkogkou A, Geladari E. Chronic kidney disease and cardiovascular disease: is there any relationship? Curr Cardiol Rev. 2019;15(1):55–63. https://doi.org/10.2174/1573403X14666180711124825.
148. Lytvyn Y, Bjornstad P, van Raalte DH, Heerspink HL, Cherney DZI. The new biology of diabetic kidney disease—mechanisms and therapeutic implications. Endocr Rev. 2020;41(2):202–31. https://doi.org/10.1210/endrev/bnz010.
149. Chaudhuri A, Ghanim H, Arora P. Improving the residual risk of renal and cardiovascular outcomes in diab. Diabetes Obes Metab. 2022;24(3):365–76. https://doi.org/10.1111/dom.14601.
150. US Centers for Disease Control and Prevention. National diabetes statistics report, 2020. https://www.cdc.gov/diabetes/pdfs/data/statistics/national-diabetes-statistics-report.pdf.
151. Gansevoort RT, Correa-Rotter R, Hemmelgarn BR, Jafar TH, Heerspink HJL, Mann JF, et al. Chronic kidney disease and cardiovascular risk: epidemiology, mechanisms, and prevention. Lancet. 2013;382(9889):339–52. https://doi.org/10.1016/S0140-6736(13)60595-4.
152. Jiang Z, Wang Y, Zhao X, Cui H, Han M, Ren X, et al. Obesity and chronic kidney disease. Am J Physiol Endocrinol Metab. 2023;324(1):E24–41. https://doi.org/10.1152/ajpendo.00179.2022.
153. Hall ME, Wang W, Okhomina V, Agarwal M, Hall JE, Dreisbach AW, et al. Cigarette smoking and chronic kidney disease in African Americans in the Jackson Heart Study. J Am Heart Assoc. 2016;5(6):e003280. https://doi.org/10.1161/JAHA.116.003280.
154. Choudhury D, Tuncel M, Levi M. Disorders of lipid metabolism and chronic kidney disease in the elderly. Semin Nephrol. 2009;29(6):610–20. https://doi.org/10.1016/j.semnephrol.2009.07.006.
155. Epstein M. Aging and the kidney. J Am Soc Nephrol. 1996;7(8):1106–22. https://doi.org/10.1681/ASN.V781106.
156. Glassock RJ, Rule AD. Aging and the kidneys: anatomy, physiology and consequences for defining chronic kidney disease. Nephron. 2016;134(1):25–9. https://doi.org/10.1159/000445450.
157. Lindeman RD, Shock NW. Longitudinal studies on the rate of decline in renal function with age. J Am Geriatr Soc. 1985;33(4):278–85. https://doi.org/10.1111/j.1532-5415.1985.tb07117.x.
158. Nitta K, Okada K, Yanai M, Takahashi S. Aging and chronic kidney disease. Kidney Blood Press Res. 2013;38(1):109–20. https://doi.org/10.1159/000355760.
159. Liu P, Quinn RR, Lam NN, Elliott MJ, Xu Y, James MT, et al. Accounting for age in the definition of chronic kidney disease. JAMA Intern Med. 2021;181(10):1359–66. https://doi.org/10.1001/jamainternmed.2021.4813.
160. O'Hare AM, Choi AI, Bertenthal D, Bacchetti P, Garg AX, Kaufman JS, et al. Age affects outcomes in chronic kidney disease. J Am Soc Nephrol. 2007;18(10):2758–65. https://doi.org/10.1681/ASN.2007040422.
161. Delanaye P, Jager KJ, Bökenkamp A, Christensson A, Dubourg L, Odvar B, et al. CKD: a call for an age-adapted definition. J Am Soc Nephrol. 2019;30(10):1785–805. https://doi.org/10.1681/ASN.2019030238.

References

162. Cruz-Jentoft AJ, Bahat G, Bauer J, Boirie Y, Bruyère O, Cederholm T, et al. Sarcopenia: revised European consensus on definition and diagnosis. Age Ageing. 2019;48(1):16–31. https://doi.org/10.1093/ageing/afy169.
163. Levey AS, Inker LA, Coresh J. GFR estimation: from physiology to public health. Am J Kidney Dis. 2014;63(5):820–34. https://doi.org/10.1053/j.ajkd.2013.12.006.
164. Chen DC, Potok OA, Rifkin D, Estrella MM. Advantages, limitations, and clinical considerations in using cystatin C to estimate GFR. Kidney 360. 2022;3(10):1807–14. https://doi.org/10.34067/KID.0003202022.
165. Thomas MC, Neuen BL, Twigg SM, Cooper ME, Badve SV. SGLT2 inhibitors for patients with type 2 diabetes and CKD: a narrative review. Endocr Connect. 2023;12(8):e230005. https://doi.org/10.1530/EC-23-0005.
166. Wright SH. Generation of resting membrane potential. Adv Physiol Educ. 2004;28(1–4):139–42. https://doi.org/10.1152/advan.00029.2004.
167. Palmer BF, Carrero JJ, Clegg DJ, Colbert GB, Emmett M, Fishbane S, et al. Clinical management of hyperkalemia. Mayo Clin Proc. 2021;96(3):744–62. https://doi.org/10.1016/j.mayocp.2020.06.014.
168. Dong L, Xu W, Deng Y, Tan J, Qin W. Efficacy and safety of potassium binders in the treatment of patients with chronic kidney disease and hyperkalemia. Eur J Pharmacol. 2022;(931):175174. https://doi.org/10.1016/j.ejphar.2022.175174.
169. St-Jules DE, Clegg DJ, Palmer BF, Carrero JJ. Can novel potassium binders liberate people with chronic kidney disease from the low-potassium diet? A cautionary tale. Clin J Am Soc Nephrol. 2022;17(3):467–72. https://doi.org/10.2215/CJN.09660721.
170. Volkert D, Beck AM, Cederholm T, Cruz-Jentoft A, Hooper L, Kiesswetter E, et al. ESPEN practical guideline: clinical nutrition and hydration in geriatrics. Clin Nutr. 2022;41(4):958–89. https://doi.org/10.1016/j.clnu.2022.01.024.
171. Schapira AHV, Chaudhuri KR, Jenner P. Non-motor features of Parkinson disease. Nat Rev Neurosci. 2017;18(7):435–50. https://doi.org/10.1038/nrn.2017.62.
172. Prajjwal P, Flores Sanga HS, Acharya K, Tango T, John J, Rodriguez RSC, et al. Parkinson's disease updates: addressing the pathophysiology, risk factors, genetics, diagnosis, along with the medical and surgical treatment. Ann Med Surg (Lond). 2023;85(10):4887–902. https://doi.org/10.1097/MS9.0000000000001142.
173. GBD 2016 Parkinson's Disease Collaborators*. Global, regional, and national burden of Parkinson's disease, 1990–2016: a systematic analysis for the Global Burden of Disease Study 2016. Lancet Neurol. 2018;17(11):939–53. https://doi.org/10.1016/S1474-4422(18)30295-3.
174. https://www.parkinson.org/understanding-parkinsons/statistics.
175. Groenewegen HJ. The basal ganglia and motor control. Neural Plast. 2003;10(1–2):107–20. https://doi.org/10.1155/NP.2003.107.
176. Goedert M, Spillantini MG, Tredici KD, Baraak H. 100 years of Lewy pathology. Nat Rev Neurol. 2013;9(1):13–24. https://doi.org/10.1038/nrneurol.2012.242.
177. Tolosa E, Garrido A, Scholz SW, Poewe W. Challenges in the diagnosis of Parkinson's disease. Lancet Neurol. 2021;20(5):385–97. https://doi.org/10.1016/S1474-4422(21)00030-2.
178. López-Otín C, Blasco MA, Partridge L, Serrano M, Kroemer G. Hallmarks of aging: an expanding universe. Cell. 2023;186(2):243–78. https://doi.org/10.1016/j.cell.2022.11.001.
179. Postuma RB, Berg D, Stern M, Poewe W, Olanow CW, Oertel W, et al. MDS clinical diagnostic criteria for Parkinson's disease. Mov Disord. 2015;30(12):1591–601. https://doi.org/10.1002/mds.26424.
180. Parkinson's Foundation. https://www.parkinson.org/understanding-parkinsons/movement-symptoms/bradykinesia#:~:text=Bradykinesia%20means%20slowness%20of%20movement,Parkinson's%20diagnosis%20to%20be%20considered.
181. Aradi SD, Hauser RA. Medical management and prevention of motor complications in Parkinson's Disease. Neurotherapeutics. 2020;17(4):1339–65. https://doi.org/10.1007/s13311-020-00889-4.

182. Bohnen NI, Studenski SA, Constantine GM, Moore RY. Diagnostic performance of clinical motor and non-motor tests of Parkinson disease: a matched case-control study. Eur J Neuro. 2008;15(7):685–91. https://doi.org/10.1111/j.1468-1331.2008.02148.x.
183. Chen Z, Li G, Liu J. Autonomic dysfunction in Parkinson's disease: implications for pathophysiology, diagnosis, and treatment. Neurobiol Dis. 2020;134:104700. https://doi.org/10.1016/j.nbd.2019.104700.
184. Reijnders JSAM, Ehrt U, Weber WEJ, Aarsland D, Leentjens AFG. A systematic review of prevalence studies of depression in Parkinson's disease: the prevalence of depression in PD. Mov Disord. 2008;23(2):183–9. https://doi.org/10.1002/mds.21803.
185. Iranzo A, Santamaria J, Tolosa E. Idiopathic rapid eye movement sleep behaviour disorder: diagnosis, management, and the need for neuroprotective interventions. Lancet Neurol. 2016;15(4):405–19. https://doi.org/10.1016/S1474-4422(16)00057-0.
186. Chahine LM, Weintraub D, Hawkins KA, Siderowf A, Eberly S, Oakes D, et al. Cognition in individuals at risk for Parkinson's: Parkinson associated risk syndrome (PARS) study findings. Mov Disord. 2016 Jan;31(1):86–94. https://doi.org/10.1002/mds.26373.
187. Wasner G, Deuschl G. Pains in Parkinson disease–many syndromes under one umbrella. Nat Rev Neurol. 2012;8(5):284–94. https://doi.org/10.1038/nrneurol.2012.54.
188. Braak H, Tredici KD, Rüb U, de Vos RAI, Steur ENHJ, Braak E. Staging of brain pathology related to sporadic Parkinson's disease. Neurobiol Aging. 2003;24(2):197–211. https://doi.org/10.1016/S0197-4580(02)00065-9.
189. Braak H, Ghebremedhin E, Rüb U, Bratzke H, Tredici KD. Stages in the development of Parkinson's disease-related pathology. Cell Tissue Res. 2004;318(1):121–34. https://doi.org/10.1007/s00441-004-0956-9.
190. Zhu B, Yin D, Zhao H, Zhang L. The immunology of Parkinson's disease. Semin Immunopathol. 2022;44(5):659–72. https://doi.org/10.1007/s00281-022-00947-3.
191. Opara J, Małecki A, Małecka E, Socha T. Motor assessment in Parkinson's disease. Ann Agric Environ Med. 2017;24(3):411–5. https://doi.org/10.5604/12321966.1232774.
192. Hoehn MM, Yahr MD. Parkinsonism: onset, progression and mortality. Neurology. 1967;17(5):427–42. https://doi.org/10.1212/wnl.17.5.427.
193. Goetz CG, Tilley BC, Shaftman SR, Stebbins GT, Fahn S, Martinez-Martin P, et al. Movement disorder society-sponsored revision of the unified Parkinson's disease rating scale (MDS-UPDRS): scale presentation and clinimetric testing results. Mov Disord. 2008;23(15):2129–70. https://doi.org/10.1002/mds.22340.
194. Pang SY, Ho PW, Liu HF, Leung CT, Li L, Chang EES, et al. The interplay of aging, genetics and environmental factors in the pathogenesis of Parkinson's disease. Transl Neurodegener. 2019;8:23. https://doi.org/10.1186/s40035-019-0165-9.
195. Trist BG, Hare DJ, Double KL. Oxidative stress in the aging substantia nigra and the etiology of Parkinson's disease. Aging Cell. 2019;18(6):e13031. https://doi.org/10.1111/acel.13031.
196. Duce JA, Wong BX, Durham H, Devedjian JC, Smith DP, Devos D. Post translational changes to alpha-synuclein control iron and dopamine trafficking; a concept for neuron vulnerability in Parkinson's disease. Mol Neurodegener. 2017;12(1):45. https://doi.org/10.1186/s13024-017-0186-8.
197. Fayyad M, Salim S, Majbour N, Erskine D, Stoops E, Mollenhauer B, OMA E-A, et al. Parkinson's disease biomarkers based on alpha-synuclein. J Neurochem. 2019;150(5):626–36. https://doi.org/10.1111/jnc.14809.
198. Goldman SM, Marek K, Ottman R, Meng C, Comyns K, Chan P, et al. Concordance for Parkinson's disease in twins: a 20-year update. Ann Neurol. 2019;85(4):600–5. https://doi.org/10.1002/ana.25441.
199. Day JO, Mullin S. The genetics of Parkinson's disease and implications for clinical practice. Genes (Basel). 2021;12(7):1006. https://doi.org/10.3390/genes12071006.
200. Langston JW, Langston EB, Irwin I. MPTP-induced parkinsonism in human and non-human primates–clinical and experimental aspects. Acta Neurol Scand Suppl. 1984;100:49–54. PMID: 6333134

201. De Miranda BR, Goldman SM, Miller GW, Greenamyre JT, Dorsey ER. Preventing Parkinson's disease: an environmental agenda. J Parkinsons Dis. 2022;12(1):45–68. https://doi.org/10.3233/JPD-212922.
202. Dick FD, De Palma G, Ahmadi A, Scott NW, Prescott GJ, Bennett J, et al. Environmental risk factors for Parkinson's disease and parkinsonism: the Geoparkinson study. Occup Environ Med. 2007;64(10):666–72. https://doi.org/10.1136/oem.2006.027003.
203. Pezzoli G, Cereda E. Exposure to pesticides or solvents and risk of Parkinson disease. Neurology. 2013;80(22):2035–41. https://doi.org/10.1212/WNL.0b013e318294b3c8.
204. Tanner CM, Goldman SM, Ross GW, Grate SJ. The disease intersection of susceptibility and exposure: chemical exposures and neurodegenerative disease risk. Alzheimers Dement. 2014;10(3 Suppl):S213–25. https://doi.org/10.1016/j.jalz.2014.04.014.
205. Steenland K, Hein MJ, Cassinelli RT 2nd, Prince MM, Nilsen NB, Whelan EA, et al. Polychlorinated biphenyls and neurodegenerative disease mortality in an occupational cohort. Epidemiology. 2006;17(1):8–13. https://doi.org/10.1097/01.ede.0000190707.51536.2b.
206. Fitzmaurice AG, Rhodes SL, Lulla A, Murphy NP, Lam HA, O'Donnell KC, et al. Aldehyde dehydrogenase inhibition as a pathogenic mechanism in Parkinson disease. Proc Natl Acad Sci USA. 2013;110(2):636–41. https://doi.org/10.1073/pnas.1220399110.
207. Olanow CW, Stern MB, Sethi K. The scientific and clinical basis for the treatment of Parkinson disease. Neurology. 2009;72(21 Suppl 4):S1–136. https://doi.org/10.1212/WNL.0b013e3181a1d44c.
208. Fox SH, Katzenschlager R, Lim SY, Ravina B, Seppi K, Coelho M, et al. The movement disorder society evidence-based medicine review update: treatments for the motor symptoms of Parkinson's disease. Mov Disord. 2011;26(Suppl 3):S2–41. https://doi.org/10.1002/mds.23829.
209. Alonso Cánovas A, Luquin Piudo R, García Ruiz-Espiga P, Burguera JA, Campos Arillo V, Castro A, et al. Dopaminergic agonists in Parkinson's disease. Neurologia. 2014;29(4):230–41. https://doi.org/10.1016/j.nrl.2011.04.012.
210. Quinn N, Illas A, Lhermitte F, Agid Y. Bromocriptine in Parkinson's disease: a study of cardiovascular effects. J Neurol Neurosurg Psychiatry. 1981 May;44(5):426–9. https://doi.org/10.1136/jnnp.44.5.426.
211. Ahlskog JE, Muenter MD. Frequency of levodopa-related dyskinesias and motor fluctuations as estimated from the cumulative literature. Mov Disord. 2001;16(3):448–58. https://doi.org/10.1002/mds.1090.
212. Abraham DS, Pham Nguyen TP, Hennessy S, Weintraub D, Gray SL, Xie D, et al. Frequency of and risk factors for potentially inappropriate medication use in Parkinson's disease. Age Ageing. 2020;49(5):786–92. https://doi.org/10.1093/ageing/afaa033.
213. Cox N, Louie JM, Sederholm BH. Inappropriate medication use in hospitalized patients diagnosed with Parkinson's disease. Pharmacy (Basel). 2018;6(3):100. https://doi.org/10.3390/pharmacy6030100.
214. Bisaglia M. Mediterranean diet and Parkinson's disease. Int J Mol Sci. 2022;24(1):42. https://doi.org/10.3390/ijms24010042.
215. Flach A, Jaegers L, Krieger M, Bixler E, Kelly P, Weiss EP, et al. Endurance exercise improves function in individuals with Parkinson's disease: a meta-analysis. Neurosci Lett. 2017;(659):115–9. https://doi.org/10.1016/j.neulet.2017.08.076.
216. Marras C, Canning CG, Goldman SM. Environment, lifestyle, and Parkinson's disease: implications for prevention in the next decade. Mov Disord. 2019;34(6):801–11. https://doi.org/10.1002/mds.27720.
217. Ernst M, Folkerts AK, Gollan R, Lieker E, Caro-Valenzuela J, Adams A, et al. Physical exercise for people with Parkinson's disease: a systematic review and network meta-analysis. Cochrane Database Syst Rev. 2023;1(1):CD013856. https://doi.org/10.1002/14651858.CD013856.pub2.
218. Stocchi F, Hsu A, Khanna S, Ellenbogen A, Mahler A, Liang G, et al. Comparison of IPX066 with carbidopa-levodopa plus entacapone in advanced PD patients. Parkinsonism Relat Disord. 2014;20(12):1335–40. https://doi.org/10.1016/j.parkreldis.2014.08.004.

Medication Use in Infectious Diseases

Abbreviations

A. baumannii	*Acinetobacter baumannii-calcoaceticus complex*
ACE2	Angiotensin converting enzyme 2
ACEI	Angiotensin converting enzyme inhibitor
ADR	Adverse drug reaction
AFB	Acid-fast bacilli
AKI	Acute kidney injury
AMR	Antimicrobial resistance
AMS	Antimicrobial stewardship
ARDS	Acute respiratory distress syndrome
ASB	Asymptomatic bacteriuria
ATS	American Thoracic Society
BPaL	Pretomanid + bedaquiline + linezolid
C. difficile	*Clostridioides difficile*
CAP	Community acquired immunity
CPT	Convalescent plasma therapy
CYP P450	Cytochrome P450
DNA	Deoxyribonucleic acid
eGFR	Estimated glomerular filtration rate
EMB	Ethambutol
EPI	Epinephrine
FDC	Fixed dose combination
HP	Hospital-acquired pneumonia
ICU	Intensive care unit
IDSA	Infectious Diseases Society of America
IFN	Interferon
IGRA	Interferon-γ release assay
IL	Interleukin

© The Author(s), under exclusive license to Springer Nature Switzerland AG 2025
G. E. Bilder, P. Brown-O'Hara, *Drug Use in the Older Adult*, https://doi.org/10.1007/978-3-031-84831-5_6

INH	Isoniazid
LTBI	Latent TB infection
LTCF	Long term care facilities
MDR	Multidrug resistance
MDRO	Multidrug resistant organisms
MERS	Middle east respiratory syndrome
MRSA	Methicillin-resistant *Staphylococcus aureus*
Mtb- *M. tuberculosis*	*Mycobacterium tuberculosis*
NE	Norepinephrine
OTC	Over-the-counter
P. aeruginosa	*Pseudomonas aeruginosa*
PD	Pharmacodynamics
P-gp	P-glycoprotein
PK	Pharmacokinetics
Ply	Pneumolysin
PSI	Pneumonia Severity Index
PZA	Pyrazinamide
RDV	Remdesivir
RIF	Rifampin
RNA	Ribonucleic acid
RSV	Respiratory syncytial virus
S protein	Spike protein
S. pneumoniae	*Streptococcus pneumoniae*
SARS	Serious acute respiratory syndrome
Spp	Many species
TB	Tuberculosis
TST	Tuberculosis skin test
UTI	Urinary tract infection
VAP	Ventilatory-acquired pneumonia
VP	Vasopressin

Introduction Infectious diseases are caused by pathogens that are classified as bacteria, viruses, fungi and parasites. Bacteria are microorganisms, single cells, various shapes with a small percentage harmful to humans. Many bacteria reside in the gastrointestinal tract, the gut microbiota, and provide structural, metabolic and protective effects of significance [1]. In contrast, for example, pathogenic bacteria cause pneumonia (*Streptococcus pneumoniae)*, urinary tract infections *(Escherichia coli, Klebsiella pneumoniae*), diarrhea (*Clostridioides difficile*), tuberculosis (*Mycobacterium tuberculosis*) and ulcers and possible cancer (*Helicobacter pylori*).

Viruses are subcellular entities driven by encapsulated segments of DNA or RNA [2]. Viruses cause diseases relevant to the older adult such as influenza (Influenza A-C viruses), COVID-19 (SARS-CoV-2 virus), hepatitis (Hepatitis A, B, C virus), and chicken pox and latent emergence, shingles (varicella-zoster virus) [2].

Fungi (yeast and molds) are both unicellular and multicellular organisms that are especially helpful supporters of plant growth. Among the plentiful and various fungi, only a few are pathogenic, largely in immunocompromised individuals or those with steroid-suppressed immunity. Serious fungal infections are candidiasis (*C. albicans, C. auris, C glabrata* and others), and aspergillosis (*A. fumigatus, A. flavus, A. terreus* and others) [3]. *C. auris* candidiasis is considered a global threat due to drug-resistance and high transmissibility (skin-to-skin), especially in nursing homes [4].

Parasites are complex organisms that maintain their survival by extracting nutrients from other organisms (their so-called host). Parasites are transmitted to humans through insect bites, improperly prepared food or contaminated food or water. Examples of food-transmitted parasites are roundworms (*Trichinella spp, Anisaki spp*), tapeworms (*Diphyllobothrium* spp., *Taenia* spp.) and protozoans, (*Cryptosporidium* spp., *Giardia intestinalis, Toxoplasma gondii* and *Cyclospora cayetanensis*). Diseases caused by parasites commonly found in contaminated water are Guinea worm disease (*Dracunculus medinensis*), schistosomiasis (trematode worms), amebiasis (*Entamoeba histolytica*) and cryptosporidiosis (*Cryptosporidium spp*) and giardiasis (*Giardia intestinalis*). Many of these are transmitted in undercooked seafood and meats and contaminated raw vegetables and plants [5].

Societal advancements in sanitation, clean water, sulfa drugs, antibiotics and vaccines in the early twentieth century exerted the greatest impact on life expectancy, producing a remarkable doubling of life expectancy from 40 years to close to 80 years of age [6]. These improvements allowed more individuals, mainly children, to survive deadly infectious diseases and achieve adulthood. As older adults, infectious disease again becomes challenging, exacting a high mortality toll [7]. This high cost results from complexity of issues. Of major importance is immunosenescence in which age changes in immunity put the older adult at greater susceptibility to pathogens and reduce their responsiveness to vaccines [8]. Secondly, infections in the older adult are frequently diagnosed late because symptoms are absent or atypical [9, 10]. Thirdly, aging markedly influences the pharmacokinetics (PK) and pharmacodynamics (PD) of all drugs (see Chap. 2), including antimicrobials, which can lead to incorrect or inappropriate dosing that fails to kill invading microbes or produces serious adverse drug reactions (ADRs) [11]. Furthermore, antimicrobial drugs are seldom assessed in randomized clinical trials (RCT) comprised of older adults (see Tables 6.1 and 6.4), limiting reliable drug use in this age category. Fourthly, another issue is that the older adult with co-morbidities will be exposed to environments, e.g., critical care hospital departments or long-term care facilities (LTCF) more frequently than younger individuals without co-morbidities and thus encounter a higher risk of exposure to pathogens that are antimicrobial drug-resistant and hence difficult to treat [12]. Results of a recent review concluded that one of the many benefits of home-based primary care was a reduction in hospitalizations, reducing unnecessary exposure to infectious pathogens [13].

This chapter discusses drug use in major infective diseases (COVID-19; pneumonia, influenza, urinary tract infections, tuberculosis, sepsis) significant for the older adult. Tables 6.1, 6.2, 6.3, and 6.4 provide a summary of the narrative.

Infectious Diseases

Infectious Diseases. Prevalence Prior to the start of the pandemic in December 2019, lower respiratory infections ranked sixth as a cause of mortality worldwide, followed by tuberculosis (TB), diarrheal diseases, and HIV (9th) [14]. These conclusions were drawn from estimates of the Disability Adjusted Life Years (DALYs) metric that assesses the lost years of healthy life [14]. At that same time, within the USA, the CDC reported that influenza and pneumonia placed ninth in mortality among the older adult [15]. However, the assessment of mortality causes in the older adult thereafter positioned COVID-19 in third place, influenza and pneumonia in 11th place and septicemia in 13th [7]. These prominent infectious diseases and urinary tract infections (UTI) and tuberculosis (TB) will be discussed in this chapter.

Infectious Diseases. Risk Factors. Age Changes Despite the wealth of antimicrobial drugs, infectious diseases from which the younger individual readily recovers prove more serious and life-threatening in the older adult. As expressed in the Introduction, there are several reasons for this. One critical reason is the aging of the immune system termed immunosenescence that normally protects the individual from invading pathogens through its composite system of anatomical and physiological barriers, innate immunity and adaptive immunity [16]. Barriers such as skin, cilia of the lungs, acid of the stomach, and innate immunity encompassing circulating white cells and assisting protein cascades and resident macrophages provide the first line of defense against invading pathogens. With age, barrier function declines and innate cell function becomes suboptimal [16]. Adaptive immunity, although of considerable complexity and sophistication, exhibits reduced robustness, in large part, driven by loss of diversity among the two cell types, the antibody-producing B-cells and the cytokine-producing T-cells [8, 17]. Reduced B- and T-cell diversity alters adaptive immunity in many ways but primarily impedes the quick and forceful response to "new" pathogens not previously experienced. The older individual is protected from pathogens formerly encountered in youth due to the creation of cells with long-term "memory" but is poorly protected from "new" pathogens [17]. This accounts for the older adults' poor response, in general, to vaccinations [18] and to the enhanced susceptibility and serious outcomes of the older adult to, for example, the SARS-CoV-2 virus and also to many other pathogens [19, 20].

Increased susceptibility to respiratory infections relies heavily on age changes specific to the pulmonary system. Pulmonary reserve declines with age because just about every cell type in the trachea, bronchi, bronchioles and alveolar sacs exhibits reduced function [21]. This minimizes protective mechanisms, for example, provided by ciliated epithelial cells and mucous-producing cells in clearing pathogenic debris and prevents effective cross-talk with innate resident immune cells such as macrophages essential for a robust immune response [21]. A reduction in thoracic compliance (chest wall stiffness) impedes the cough reflex [22] and shifts gas exchange to the upper chest, promoting a favorable anaerobic environment for pathogens in the lower lung [23].

The older adult may experience serious consequences from infectious diseases if pharmacotherapy is either inappropriate or initiated at an incorrect dose that produces an adverse reaction or is insufficient, thus possibly favoring pathogen resistance [24]. For drugs eliminated by the kidneys, age-dependent reduction in kidney function needs accurate assessment (see Chap. 3 and discussion below) that is often inaccurate with simple serum creatinine measurement. Infections also suppress the function of hepatic cytochrome P450 (CYP P450), drug-metabolizing enzymes, and, although age-independent, nevertheless remain an important issue [25].

Infectious Diseases. Risk Factor. Altered Symptoms Another important factor that leads to an elevated risk of infectious diseases in the older individual is the transformation of the clearly defined disease symptoms expressed in young individuals to atypical or absent symptoms in the older individual [9, 10]. In the older adult, symptoms are non-specific and characterized by "confusion, frequent falls, difficulty ambulating, reduced food intake, dysphagia, incontinence, weight loss and failure to thrive" [10]. For example, 30% of older adults with pneumonia, a common infectious disease in this age group, exhibit impaired febrile response [26] and absent leucocytosis (increase in white cell count) [9], both common in the young person. These uncharacteristic symptoms may be complicated by dementia and polypharmacy with the overall effect of delaying a diagnosis, preventing essential pharmacological care and failing to achieve a good outcome [10].

Infectious Diseases. Comorbidities As with dementia, other co-morbidities that include cardiovascular disease, diabetes mellitus, cancers, chronic kidney disease and chronic obstructive pulmonary disease, increase the individual's vulnerability to infectious diseases [10]. Additionally, some of these conditions require medical devices, e.g., pacemakers, infusion lines, heart valves, and prosthetic implants that are prime sites for infections. Moreover, malnutrition and peripheral vascular disease, conditions that slow wound healing, increase susceptibility to infections [10].

COVID-19

COVID-19. Prevalence The most prominent viral infection in recent history is that produced by the beta-corona virus, SARS-CoV-2, causing the serious acute respiratory syndrome, COVID-19. Originating in Wuhan, China, its enhanced transmissibility and pathogenicity killed over seven million individuals worldwide from April 2020–January 2024 [27]. As exemplified by statistics from the CDC, of the over one million Americans who died from COVID-19 (2020–2024), more than half were 75 years and older, ~22% were 65–74 years and ~18% were 50–64 years of [28]. Clearly, older adults were the most vulnerable to the pathogenicity of the SARS-CoV-2 virus.

COVID-19. Pathophysiology The COVID-19 pandemic was preceded by two earlier coronavirus outbreaks, SARS-CoV (serious acute respiratory syndrome, (2002–2003) and Middle East respiratory syndrome (MERS-CoV) (2012–2013) of higher lethality but lesser transmissibility [29]. All three coronaviruses are considered zoonotic, that is, of animal origin, mutating sufficiently to infect humans. However, that theory has not been confirmed for SARS-CoV-2. Emerging data show that, in fact, SARS-CoV-2 accidentally escaped from a research laboratory in Wuhan, China, developed experimentally with man-made viral mutations [30].

The SARS-CoV-2 virus infects alveolar epithelial cells [31], gaining entry through a cell membrane enzyme ACE2 (angiotensin-converting enzyme 2, modulator of vasoconstriction of angiotensin 1 and II). With an incubation period of 3–7 days, the viral entry, viral replication, and continued infection with viral release induce an extensive inflammatory response [32, 33] and continued lung damage. Inflammatory reactions irritate nerve endings, initiating the cough reflex [34] and increasing vascular permeability, leading to edema and dyspnea (shortness of breath), all classic symptoms of COVID-19 infection [35]. The presence of ACE2 in other tissues (heart, blood vessels, kidneys) allows the virus to invade and damage these tissues [33]. In the older adult with age-related lung structure and functional changes and immunosenescence, serious outcomes include "acute respiratory distress syndrome, septic shock, metabolic acidosis, and coagulation dysfunction, which may ultimately lead to multiple organ failure and even death" [33].

COVID-19. Pharmacotherapy There exist *three main treatment protocols* for COVID-19. They are vaccines (see Table 6.4), antiviral drugs (see Table 6.1) and convalescent plasma therapy (CPT) (a type of passive immunization) [36]. The first two have achieved moderate success while CPT, to date, has been less well studied [36]. Of interest are the antiviral drugs remdesivir (RDV), paxlovid, and molnupiravir (see Table 6.1). RDV(intravenous) and molnupiravir (oral) are prodrugs that are metabolized to nucleoside analogs disrupting viral RNA synthesis; paxlovid is comprised of nirmatrelvir and ritonavir, the former is a viral protease inhibitor preventing viral replication and the latter is required to inhibit the rapid hepatic CYP P450 metabolism of nirmatrelvir [37].

Antiviral Drugs These antiviral drugs have been evaluated in numerous randomized clinical trials (RCTs), some of which are presented in Table 6.1. It is apparent that although the older adult is the prime target of SARS-CoV-2, these therapy trials barely included this population. Generally, antiviral drugs are given within 3–5 days of the onset of COVID-19 symptoms and for a short period of 3–5 days to reduce hospitalization and death in at-risk patients.

Specifically, RDV produced positive results in several studies [38–40] but had no efficacy in others [41–43]. Further, Patnaik et al. (2023) [44] reviewed 5 RCTs with RDV and showed that RDV had no benefit on mortality but did decrease the need for mechanical ventilation and extracorporal oxygenation. RDV is approved for use without dose adjustment even with reduced kidney function (estimated glomerular filtration rate, eGFR<30 ml/min) and in the presence of dialysis [37]. Since RDV is given IV, it may cause infusion site rash and hypersensitivity [37].

Table 6.1 Infectious diseases, pharmacotherapy, efficacy and adverse reactions

Infectious disease (pathogen)	Recommended pharmacotherapy	Efficacy/Adverse Reactions
COVID-19 (SARS-CoV-2 coronavirus, variants)	Remdesivir (RDV) IV	RCTs with >1000 pts —Shortens time to recovery in hospitalized pts with Covid-19, ave. age 59 yrs [38]. Modest effect, 55–77 yrs, reduced need for mechanical ventilation [183]. RCT ~500 pts, no effect at 5 or 10 days of therapy, 45–66 yrs [41]. RCT open label <1000 pts, no effect, 54–73 yrs [42]. ~8000 pts worldwide, no effect on mortality [43] 3 days treatment in non-hospitalized pts ↓ (87%) risk of hospitalization or death; ave. age 50 yrs [39]. Common adverse effects are nausea, vomiting, and transaminase elevations [11]
	Paxlovid (nirmatrelvir plus ritonavir) oral	RCT >2000 pts, 89% ↓ risk of hospitalization or death of unvaccinated COVID pts with risk of progression compared to placebo by day 28, 18–86 yrs [46]. Similar trial design, 45% ↓ risk of hospitalization or death in high-risk vaccinated 49–56 yrs [45]. ↓hospitalization and death in 65 and older COVID-19 pts treated with paxlovid evaluated during omicron surge; subgroup analysis [47]. Pt reports on AE include disease recurrence at 16.23%, dysgeusia at 6.05%, and diarrhea at 3.04%, ave. age 58 yrs [191].
	Molnupiravir	RCT >1000 at-risk unvaccinated pts 32% > 50 yrs - ↓ incidence of hospitalization or death; no safety issues; quicker resolution of symptoms (shortness of breath, cough, loss of taste/smell, fatigue) compared to placebo [52, 53]. >20,000 inpts, comparison of paxlovid with molnupiravir, 75 yrs ave. age – both ↓ all-cause mortality, but not ICU admission or ventilatory need [51]. Small RCT trial of 200 unvaccinated pts, ~5% >65 yrs shows enhanced clearance of the virus [54]. Common adverse effects are headaches, diarrhea, and nausea [11].
Pneumonia (bacteria, viruses)	B-lactams (amoxicillin, amoxicillin/clavulanate)	Amoxicillin shown superior to penicillin in 10 day dosing CAP but enrollment <50 pts, ave. age 49 yrs [192]. 3-day therapy with beta-lactam efficacious as 8-day therapy [193]. Hepatotoxicity (cholestasis and jaundice) is a common adverse effect for amoxicillin-clavulanic acid and flucloxacillin [11]. Neurotoxicity (seizures to hyperactivity) higher in older adults [11].

(continued)

Table 6.1 (continued)

Infectious disease (pathogen)	Recommended pharmacotherapy	Efficacy/Adverse Reactions
	Tetracyclines (doxycycline)	Small RCT with doxycycline compared to levofloxacin-similar efficacy in CAP requiring hospitalization; reduced stay with doxycycline [194]. Known adverse effects of tetracyclines are photosensitivity, cutaneous infections, esophagitis, and hepatotoxicity but data lacking in older adults [11].
	Macrolides (azithromycin clarithromycin)	Three-day course of azithromycin has efficacy comparable to amoxicillin/clavulanate for 7 days in outpt CAP. GI symptoms with both treatments [195]. Efficacy is 88.5–93.5% (cure rate) in 2 large multinational RCTs of mild-moderate CAP outpts (24–30% > 65 yrs) [196]. Avoid in older adults with hearing loss as macrolides associated with ototoxicity; concern for arrhythmias is controversial [11].
	Fluoroquinolones (levofloxacin)	Efficacy of 96.3% (52/54) for CAP with MDRSP and 95.1% (347/365) for non-MDRSP, pathogen eradication equally high in both groups [197]. Efficacy is 86.6% (cure rate) in small RCT of moderate to severe CAP; 46% with adverse GI events 17% ≥ 65 yrs [198]. ≥ 65 yrs, associated with the highest risk of *C. difficile* 90 days after antibiotic use [199]. Fluoroquinolones associated with tendinopathy (Achilles tendon rupture and tendinitis) [200] and CNS effects (>80 yrs) [201].
	Others for MRSA, P. aeruginosa. (vancomycin, cephalosporins, carbapenem)	Cephalosporins and carbapenems associated with neurotoxicities (delirium, psychosis) in older adults [202].
Influenza (Influenza virus Type A, Type B)	Antiviral neuraminidase inhibitors: (oseltamivir phosphate (oral); zanamivir (inhaled); peramivir (IV); endonuclease inhibitor: baloxavir marboxil (not for complicated illness or hospitalizations).	Comparable efficacy (shortening time to recovery and ↓ viral titers) with peramivir and oseltamivir in high-risk influenza pts ave. age 70–72 [86]. Large RCT baloxavir marboxil vs placebo vs oseltamivir; greater effectiveness with baloxavir and less adverse side effects, 20% ≥65–74 yrs, 7% ≥75 yrs [87]. Side effects-nausea and vomiting (oseltamivir), bronchospasm (zanamivir); diarrhea (peramivir).

Tuberculosis (TB)	Isoniazid (INH), rifampin (RIF), pyrazinamide (PZA) and ethambutol (EMB) Drug resistant pulmonary TB—Pretomanid, bedaquiline and linezolid (BPaL)	Thirteen RCTs show comparable efficacy of first-line therapy as fixed dose or single dose in newly diagnosed pulmonary TB. Most studies with a cutoff age of 50 yrs [102]. BPaL efficacious in small trials (<100 pts) with MDR or XMDR, no control [107]. First-line therapy compared with rifapentine replacing RIF shows rifapentine produces a greater number of microbiological negative sputum cultures, age range of 18–76 yrs [203]. Linezolid associated with thrombocytopenia with long duration and low platelet count [143]. ADRs for first-line treatment vary 8–85% from mild GI upsets to serious hepatotoxicity, ototoxicity and neurotoxicity [204].
Urinary tract infections (UTI)	Cystitis—nitrofurantoin or fosfomycin; pyelonephritis-ciprofloxacin or levofloxacin; High risk of MDR—oral β-lactams and fluoroquinolones for cystitis; ceftriaxone or ertapenem and trimethoprim-sulfamethoxazole, Augmentin or a third-generation cephalosporin	Five-day nitrofurantoin compared to 1 dose fosfomycin was more efficacious in resolving uncomplicated UTI (age 21–64 yrs) [205]. Low-intensity intervention in LTCF ↑ appropriate antibiotic prescribing for uncomplicated UTI [206]. In presence of low antibiotic resistance, fosfomycin, nitrofurantoin, TMP-SMX, and fluoroquinolones show equal efficacy in acute uncomplicated cystitis, ages 18–65; rapid urine test reduces antibiotic use by 10% [207]. Three-day amoxicillin/clavulanic acid better than 1-day treatment only in women with recurrent UTI 18–87 yrs [208]. Comparable efficacy with 3-day cefixime and ofloxacin on cure rate and reduction of bacteriuria [209] Cefepime/enmetazobactam superior (79.1% cure rate) to piperacillin/tazobactam (58.9% cure rate) in complicated UTI or acute pyelonephritis due to gram-negative pathogens; 40% >65 yrs [210]. TMP-SMX associated with neurotoxicity, GI upsets, hypersensitivity, and dermatologic reactions [11]. Nitrofurantoin associated with the highest risk of *C. difficile* [199] and neurotoxicity (headache, dizziness) in older adults [11].

(continued)

Table 6.1 (continued)

Infectious disease (pathogen)	Recommended pharmacotherapy	Efficacy/Adverse Reactions
Sepsis; septic shock	Common choices: Piperacillin/tazobactam; amoxicillin/clavulanate; Ceftriaxone	Choice depends on the infection site: pulmonary, urinary, CNS, abdominal, skin, gyn, undefined [136]. Additional therapy—balanced crystalloids, vasopressors NE, VP, oxygen, other: heparin, insulin Addition of albumin to crystalloid resuscitation is safe but has no advantage over crystalloid use, 70 yrs median age [142]. Use of biomarker, PCT guidance reduces adverse events associated with infection, 28-day mortality, and cost of hospitalization, ave. age 79 yrs [211]. Use of crystalloid reduced 30-day in-hospital mortality compared to saline, ave. age 60 yrs [212]. Mortality outcome not changed with EGDT vs usual care in early septic shock, ave. age 64–66 yrs [213]

EGDT early goal-directed therapy, *RCT* randomized clinical trial, *ave* average; *yrs* years; *pts* patients; *AE* adverse events; *inpts* inpatients; *outpts* outpatients, *ICU* intensive care unit, *CAP* community acquired pneumonia, *MDR* multidrug resistance, *MDRSP* multidrug resistant *Streptococcus pneumoniae*, *LTCF* long term care facilities, *Augmentin* amoxicillin/clavulanate, *TMP-SMX* trimethoprim-sulfamethoxazole, *gyn* gynecological, *PCT* procalcitonin, *NE* norepinephrine, *VP* vasopressin, *UTI* urinary tract infection, *XMDR* extensively multidrug resistance

Paxlovid therapy appears more promising, with trial results demonstrating decreased risk of hospitalization or death in the order of 45% [45] to 89% [46]. In a subgroup analysis of the EPIC-HR trial [46], it was reported that patients 65 years and older exposed to the omicron surge (SARS-CoV-2 variant) benefited from paxlovid with decreased hospitalizations and deaths [47]. A large retrospective cohort study of an Israeli database reported that paxlovid given to at-risk patients, 65 years on average, was highly effective in reducing the risk of severe COVID-19 or death [48]. A serious issue with paxlovid is CYP3A4 inhibition by ritonavir. While essential to assure adequate drug levels of nirmatrelvir, ritonavir can elevate the concentration of many other drugs that require this enzyme for metabolism (see Chap. 3) and hence produce serious toxicity [49]. Therefore, before treatment with paxlovid, all drug usage, including over-the-counter (OTC) drugs, biologicals, and herbal substances, needs assessment and adjustment [37]. One unusual nonserious side effect is dysgeusia, a metallic taste [50].

Wan et al. [51] reported that in a large study comparing paxlovid and molnupiravir in the older adult, both reduced all-cause mortality but not intensive care unit (ICU) admissions or ventilatory need. Other studies with younger at-risk patients treated with molnupiravir show a decreased incidence of hospitalization or death [52], quicker resolution of symptoms [53] and enhanced viral clearance [54].

Pneumonias

Pneumonias. Incidence Pneumonia is a leading cause of death in the older adult [55]. Pneumonia is generally classified as to where it is acquired [9] since this aids with empirical decisions on diagnosis and treatment when needed [56]. The most common designation is community-acquired pneumonia (CAP) [57], accounting for a large percentage of hospitalizations [58]. CAPs may include those with and without risk of pneumonia to multidrug-resistant organisms (MDRO). Additionally, residents of LTCF are at risk of CAP with or without MDRO [57]. Other classifications are hospital-acquired pneumonia (HP) and ventilatory-acquired pneumonia (VAP) [59]. Knowing the classification gives a reasonable indication of the pathogenic cause [56].

The incidence of CAP rises with age and is highest in those over 80 years of age [60]. The primary causative pathogen of CAP is *Streptococcus pneumoniae* (*S. pneumoniae*) [61]. Other pathogens in order of causation incidence are *Haemophilus influenzae*, *Staphylococcus aureus* and Gram-negative bacilli, with viruses contributing to 10–30% of cases [61]. Common CAP viruses are influenza, rhinovirus and respiratory syncytial virus (RSV) [55].

Alert: Pneumonias are the leading cause of death in older adults.

Pneumonias. Pathophysiology *S. pneumoniae* and *Staphylococcus aureus* are gram-positive bacteria that become destructive when entering the lower respiratory airways. Here the bacteria thwart host immunity by suppressing alveolar macrophage function [62]. Lung damage and subsequent dissemination of bacteria to other organs is mediated in large part by pneumolysin (Ply), a pore-forming cytolysin and toxin produced by the bacteria [63]. Ply interaction with alveolar macrophages and dendritic cells negates normal innate immunity and suppresses the needed proinflammatory actions that usually contain and kill pathogens [64]. Ply also depresses the maturation of dendritic cells and communication with adaptive immunity, preventing activation of essential T-cells (CD4+) [62]. Many other Ply-mediated effects occur, including epithelial and endothelial cell death, increased permeability, platelet activation and microvascular occlusions [62].

Pneumonias. Atypical Symptoms As noted above, a diagnosis of infectious disease in the older adult is often difficult due to atypical symptoms and the presence of co-morbidities producing pneumonia-like symptoms [9]. The classic clinical presentation of chest pain on breathing, fever, cough or leucocytosis may be absent and replaced by falls, reduced appetite, or change in functional and mental status [65].

Pneumonias. Assessment Tools The American Thoracic Society (ATS) and Infectious Diseases Society of America (IDSA) provide a comprehensive summation and recommendation on the diagnosis and therapy of CAP [66]. Similar guidelines are provided by the British Thoracic Society, the European Respiratory Society/European Society of Clinical Microbiology and Infectious Diseases [67] and the National Institute for Health and Care Excellence [68].

There are several validated assessment tools to diagnose the severity of pneumonia and assist with treatment options [65]. They are the Pneumonia Severity Index (PSI), the CURB65 and the CRB65. All three are comparable in predicting mortality at 30 days, but the PSI has a slight advantage in the identification of low-risk patients while the other two exhibit strength in the identification of high-risk patients [69]. PSI assessment evaluates 20 variables [69]. CURB65 uses 5 variables (one point for each variable) that are confusion, urea, respiratory rate, blood pressure and age ≥ 65 years [70] and CRB65 omits the urea value and is appropriate for outpatient assessment [65]. Using CURB65 or CRB65, a score of 0 or 1 suggests low-risk and outpatient therapy while a higher score of 3 or more suggests hospitalization [65]. The ATS and IDSA prefer the use of PSI because clinical trial results show efficacy and safety of identifying and treating low-risk patients on an outpatient basis with PSI [66]. However, treatment plans should also include, in addition to clinical judgment and education, the financial and social concerns of the patient [66].

Pneumonias. Pharmacotherapy Therapy guidelines recommend empirical treatment for common pathogens, "*Streptococcus pneumoniae, Haemophilus influenzae, Mycoplasma pneumoniae, Staphylococcus aureus, Legionella species, Chlamydia pneumoniae, and Moraxella catarrhalis*" [66]. Gram staining of sputum and cultures is only recommended for severe CAP. There is further discussion of this below regarding antimicrobial stewardship (AMS).

Pneumonias. Amoxicillin and Others Amoxicillin (β-lactam) is the drug of choice for outpatient treatment of CAP without co-morbidities and absent risk for methicillin-resistant *Staphylococcus aureus* (MRSA) or *Pseudomonas aeruginosa* [71]. The choice of doxycycline (tetracycline), azithromycin, or clarithromycin (both macrolides, if pneumococcal resistance <25%) is possible. Outpatients with co-morbidities require amoxicillin/clavulanate (clavulanate fortifies amoxicillin by blocking pathogens producing β-lactamases) or a cephalosporin (β-lactam subgroup) along with doxycycline or a macrolide or given alone fluoroquinolones, e.g., levofloxacin [68, 71]. For inpatients with nonsevere CAP (PSI criteria), β-lactams (e.g., amoxicillin, cefotaxime, ceftriaxone) plus a macrolide (azithromycin or clarithromycin) or a respiratory fluoroquinolone (levofloxacin) are recommended. Severe CAP therapy consists of a β-lactam plus a macrolide or β-lactam plus a fluoroquinolone [71]. The presence of resistant pathogens, MRSA and *P. aeruginosa* should be confirmed with laboratory tests and treated with vancomycin (glycopeptide) or linezolid (oxazolidinone) (against MRSA) and piperacillin-tazobactam (penicillins), cefepime, ceftazidime (cephalosporins), imipenem (carbapenem) (against *P. aeruginosa*). Prior history of these pathogens requires treatment until tests indicate no current presence [71].

Xacduro The FDA recently (2023) approved xacduro for the treatment of hospital-acquired bacterial pneumonia, HABP) and ventilator-acquired bacterial pneumonia (VABP) due to carbapenem-resistant *Acinetobacter baumannii (A. baumannii)* [72]. Xacduro, comprised of sulbactam similar in structure to penicillin and durlobactam, a drug that prevents bacterial enzymes from destroying sulbactam, is cytotoxic for *A. baumannii-calcoaceticus* complex, a prominent causative agent of HABP and VABP. In the clinical trial leading to this FDA approval, slightly more than 50% of participants were ≥65 years and xacduro reduced mortality compared to colistin therapy [73].

Clinical trials with antibiotics have been criticized for lack of studies definitively determining antibiotic superiority, mortality outcomes, or treatment failures [71] (see Table 6.1). The conclusions reached in a meta-analysis of 11 RCTs (1991–2012) comparing one antibiotic with another for the treatment of CAP were that the efficacy of antibiotics (e.g., levofloxacin, azithromycin, amoxicillin, clarithromycin, ceftriaxone) are comparable and with a few exceptions, the adverse effects are also similar [74]. Additionally, few studies in this analysis and in other studies included the older adult [65]. Mortality from CAP depends largely on age, co-morbidities and exposure to resistant pathogens, all significant for the older adult [75]. Therefore, lacking precise therapeutic data, the clinician, to maximize efficacy and minimize adverse effects, also needs to consider the age-associated changes in PK (see Chap. 2 and section below), the impact of co-morbidities (see Chaps. 4 and 5), frailty (see Chap. 7) and polypharmacy (see Chap. 3) [67].

Influenza

Introduction. Influenza Influenza, commonly termed the flu, is a respiratory infection of the nose, throat and lungs caused by RNA influenza type A and type B virus [76]. Influenza is highly transmissible and in the older adult and those with comorbidities, can be deadly. Influenza causes an estimated 290,000 to 650,000 respiratory deaths each year worldwide [77]. In the USA, 21,000 deaths and 31 million with symptoms of the illness were estimated for 2022–2023 [78].

Influenza. Atypical Symptoms The symptoms of influenza (fever in most but not all), cough, sore throat, muscle aches, headaches, and fatigue share similarities with COVID-19 symptoms. The different causative viruses can be distinguished with PCR analysis. As with COVID-19 and pneumonia, the older adult may experience modified symptoms that result in a late diagnosis, ineffective therapy and complications [79, 80]. Those complications include pneumonia, inflammation of the heart, brain and muscles, multi-organ failure and sepsis [78]. Annual influenza vaccination is the best way to prevent influenza (see Table 6.4), but for the older adult, immunization provides less than optimal protection and many older adults refuse vaccinations [81].

Influenza. Pharmacotherapy The FDA has approved four antiviral drugs for influenza therapy. These drugs block two pathogenic mechanisms of the influenza virus. Influenza viruses are classified according to their surface glycoproteins, hemagglutinin (HA) and neuraminidase (NA) [82]. The virus uses HA and NA proteins to enter the epithelial cells of the respiratory tract, passing through the mucous layer and attaching to *N*-acetylneuraminic (sialic) acid of the epithelial cells. Inside the cell, the virus usurps metabolic pathways to make viral RNA similar to host RNA [82].

Antiviral Drugs Three of the approved antiviral drugs, oseltamivir, zanamivir and peramivir are neuraminidase inhibitors (inhibiting sialic acid) needed for virus entry and exit from the host cell [83]. The fourth antiviral drug, baloxavir marboxil, is a prodrug and an endonuclease inhibitor, preventing viral transcription (copying of more viral RNA) [84]. In a systematic and network meta-analysis of 26 RCTs comparing these antiviral drugs with each other and a placebo, Liu et al. (2021) [85] concluded that while they all shortened the time to alleviation of influenza symptoms, zanamivir exhibited the greatest effect and the risk for influenza-related complications was the lowest with baloxavir. Some of these trials focused on children, so the overall average age was approximately 33 years. RCTs included in Table 6.1 enrolled the older adult and reported the efficacy of peramivir and oseltamivir in high-risk patients [86] and baloxavir to be more effective than oseltamivir with fewer side effects [87].

Tuberculosis

Tuberculosis. Introduction Tuberculosis (TB) is a highly contagious lung disease that may involve thoracic lymph nodes as well as other organs [88]. It is caused by the bacterium *Mycobacterium tuberculosis (M. tuberculosis)* (M.tb) and related species and spreads in tiny airborne droplets via a cough, speaking or singing from an infected individual [88]. It is a heterogeneous disease with quiescent subclinical features in some to mild-severe disease presentation and death in others [89]. Traditionally, TB is categorized as either latent TB infection (LTBI) or active TB. This is because the pathogenesis of TB is complicated and depends on the extensive host immune response and the M.tb production of virulent factors [90]. On exposure to droplets with M.tb, the alveolar macrophages may (a) kill the pathogen (clearance) and (b) engulf it, with immune cells forming a granuloma that prevents replication (LTBI) or allows colonization, replication, and dissemination depending on the capabilities of the host (active TB) [90]. In active TB the individual is sick with persistent cough, chest pains, expelling bloody sputum, fever, chills, fatigue, weight loss and night sweats [88].

Tuberculosis. Incidence The global incidence of active TB in 2021 was estimated to be 10.6 million individuals, a 4.5% increase from 2020 [91]. The highest number of cases were in South-East Asia (45%) and Africa (23%). TB mortality reached 1.6 million in 2021 worldwide. Mortality rates had been falling since 2005 but reversed following the pandemic [91]. In the USA, TB cases numbered 8331 in 2022, an approximate 5.5% increase in incidence from the year before [92]. The CDC also reported that an estimated 13 million individuals in the United States are living with LTBI [92].

Tuberculosis. Diagnosis Guidelines have been established for the effective diagnosis and treatment of TB [93]. The strategy is two-fold in that eradicating the M.tb in the infected individual not only leads to a cure for the patient but also benefits society by eliminating the spread. Diagnostics include assessing those at high risk of exposure as well as those who are ill. Clinical evaluation, laboratory tests, radiographic analysis, and patient input are essential for a diagnosis. It is also recommended that TB be treated ahead of culture results if clinical expertise strongly suspects TB [93]. Two screening tests, interferon-γ release assay (IGRA) or tuberculosis skin test (TST) are recommended for diagnosis of LTBI in those at risk of TB [94]. The preference is for the use of IGRA unless " IGRA is not available, too costly, or too burdensome" [93]. Both tests measure a cell-mediated immunity response. The FDA-approved IGRA tests (QuantiFERON®-TB Gold Plus (QFT-Plus) and T-SPOT®.TB test (T-Spot) require a phlebotomy to determine the isolated T-cell response to specific M.tb antigens; the TST measures the delay hypersensitivity (inflammatory) response to skin injection of bacilli antigen (purified protein derivative of M.tb) [95]. There is scant evidence as to which screening test is superior [96]. However, the older adult is less responsive to the TST, making test results unreliable in detecting LTBI [97, 98]. Also needed for a diagnosis are results from an acid-fast bacilli (AFB) smear microscopy in sputum (3 specimens, 5–10 ml), considered a "fast, safe, inexpensive, sensitive and specific diagnostic test" and, in other words, an invaluable tool [99].

Tuberculosis. Pharmacotherapy Drug therapy for active TB and LTBI consists of 4 medications given for 2 months followed by continuation of 2 of the 4 drugs for an additional 4 months. First-line medications are isoniazid (INH), rifampin (RIF), pyrazinamide (PZA) and ethambutol (EMB) for 2 months, after which INH and RIF are continued for 4 additional months [93]. Pyridoxine (vitamin B_6) is given to counter potential neuropathy by these drugs [100, 101]. First-line therapy for pulmonary TB is highly effective whether given in fixed-dose combination (FDC) or as single doses according to a meta-analysis of 13 trials (1989–2015) in newly diagnosed pulmonary TB in high-risk populations [102]. It is interesting to note that the older adult was excluded from most of these trials, with two possible exceptions, including patients up to 70 years.

Adverse Drug Reactions According to the CDC, the most serious adverse effect of first-line TB therapy is hepatitis, which requires frequent tests of hepatic enzymes. This is especially important for the older adults in which data show hepatotoxicity with TB therapy both active and latent increases with age [103]. The seriousness of adverse effects of TB drug therapy raises the issue of whether the older adult should be treated for LTBI since only 10% of LTBI convert to overt TB [104] and hepatotoxicity may be worse than TB [103]. An alternative argument favors treatment to reduce TB spread and treatment of those with known frequent exposure to active TB and those with an increased risk of overt TB [103].

Drug-Resistant Tuberculosis Treatment of drug-resistant TB is difficult. Extensive drug resistance is defined as "tuberculosis caused by *M. tuberculosis* strains with resistance to rifampin and isoniazid, any fluoroquinolone, and at least one additional group A drug (levofloxacin, moxifloxacin, bedaquiline, and linezolid) [105]. Using this updated definition, a systematic review (2005–2023) assessed 94 studies (mostly observational but some RCTs) from 26 countries of >10,000 patients with extensive drug-resistant TB. Successful outcomes encompassing treatment completion or cure reached 44.2%, which needs improvement [106]. In 2019, the FDA approved the use of pretomanid combined with bedaquiline and linezolid (BPaL) (26–39 weeks) for drug-resistant pulmonary TB in adults [107]. Additional studies (systematic analysis of 8 RCTs including Conradie et al. [107]) found pretomanid in combination with moxifloxacin and pyrazinamide was highly effective in the treatment of patients with rifampin-resistant tuberculosis [108]. Of importance is that the average age of study participants was 30–35 years. Several adverse effects e.g. peripheral neuropathy, optic neuritis, myelosuppression, hepatotoxicity, pancreatitis, QT prolongation, and lactic acidosis were observed with these new drug combinations [107].

Urinary Tract Infections

Urinary Tract Infections. Introduction The presence of bacteria in the urinary tract is termed either a symptomatic urinary tract infection (UTI) [109] or an asymptomatic urinary tract infection, also termed asymptomatic bacteriuria (ASB) [110]. In both cases, laboratory analysis with a dipstick, microscope, and cultures of urine confirms uropathogen presence [111]. Uropathogens enter the urethra to colonize the bladder, creating UTI termed cystitis; subsequent spread of pathogens through the ureters to the kidneys initiates UTI termed pyelonephritis [112]. The entrance of these pathogens into the bloodstream creates bacteremia, leading to sepsis and septic shock (see below). Although UTI is treatable, it can become deadly [109].

Urinary Tract Infections. Incidence and Risk Factors The incidence of UTI increases with age and is much more common among premenopausal women than men [113]. However, in a population-based study of 598 community-dwelling women ≥65 years of age (average age of 72 years), 16% of older women were diagnosed with UTI on their first primary care visit [114]. By age 85, the incidence increases to approximately 30% [115]. UTI is uncommon in men aged 60 or younger [116] but increases with age such that the incidence of UTI is similar in both men and women ≥80 years [117]. UTI caused by instrumentation (generally catheter insertion) is labeled healthcare-associated UTI and is ranked fifth as the most common healthcare-associated infection [118]. Approximately 30–40% of healthcare-associated infections in LTCF are UTIs [119, 120]. In addition to age and urinary tract procedures, additional risk factors for UTI are a history of UTI, diabetes and conditions that create voiding irregularities inhibiting self-hygiene, e.g., dementia, Parkinson's disease and stroke [109].

Urinary Tract Infections. Pathogens The most common pathogens are uropathogenic strains of *Escherichia coli (E. coli)* found in 70–95% of outpatients with UTI [121]. *Staphylococcus saprophyticus* is the causative agent in a smaller number (5–15%) of outpatients with UTIs. Other pathogens, *Klebsiella pneumoniae*, *Proteus spp*, *Enterococcus faecalis* and *Streptococcus agalactiae* (Group B Streptococci) may also be causative pathogens [121].

Urinary Tract Infections. Diagnosis The diagnosis of UTI in the older adult is a challenge [109]. This is because the classic symptoms of UTI in young adults (cystitis: painful/ burning urination; frequent urination, bloody urine, pressure groin/ lower abdomen; pyelonephritis: fever, chills, lower back pain, nausea/vomiting) [122] may or may not be present but frequently are replaced with atypical or general symptoms (lower abdominal pain, back pain, and constipation) [123]. Additionally, distinguishing between UTI and ASB (asymptomatic bacteriuria) in which pathogens are present in the urine in a defined amount but symptoms are absent, represents a difficult problem [109]. Both ASB and UTI increase dramatically with age [124], but antibiotic treatment is not recommended for ASB [110].

Urinary Tract Infections. Pharmacotherapy In uncomplicated UTIs, the data suggest that a delay in antibiotic treatment yields benefits. Results of a prospective cohort study showed that a delay (maximum of 7 days) in antibiotic initiation led to a decrease in antibiotic use, and of those who opted to delay treatment, 71% reported clinical improvement or cure [125]. When antibiotics are used, guidelines suggest nitrofurantoin or fosfomycin for low-risk cystitis (low multi-drug resistance) and ciprofloxacin or levofloxacin for low-risk pyelonephritis (see Table 6.1). High risk multidrug resistant cystitis due to extended hospital stay or recent antibiotic use may be treated with oral beta-lactams and fluoroquinolones; high-risk pyelonephritis therapy consists of ceftriaxone or ertapenem and trimethoprim-sulfamethoxazole, amoxicillin/clavulanate or a third-generation cephalosporin [112].

Sepsis, Septic Shock

Sepsis, Septic Shock. Introduction Sepsis is a "life-threatening organ dysfunction caused by a dysregulated host response to infection" [126]. It is a syndrome that essentially mediates the "final common pathway for all infectious diseases" [127]. Septic shock is the deteriorative component of sepsis, producing overwhelming circulatory depression with a high risk of death [126].

Sepsis. Incidence Using vital death records from the Global Burden of Diseases, Injuries, and Risk Factors Study (GBD) 2017 [127], Rudd et al. (2020) [128] estimated the incidence of sepsis from 1990 to 2017. Global incidence decreased from 60 million to 48·nine million cases, declining approximately 37%. 11 million individuals died in 2017 from sepsis worldwide, with the most common cause being lower respiratory infection [128]. However, in the USA, septic shock has increased (1997–2017) as have the associated hospitalization costs [129]. It is the older adult who experiences the highest incidence and mortality rate for sepsis and septic shock. Seventy-five percent of all sepsis deaths occur in those ≥65 years of age, with an eight-fold greater number of deaths in those ≥85 years of age [130, 131].

Sepsis. Risk Factors Several reasons are offered for the high incidence of sepsis mortality in the older adult, including "suboptimal quality of care, an inadequate health infrastructure, poor infection prevention measures in place, late diagnosis, and inappropriate clinical management" [127]. Other factors include antimicrobial resistance and high-risk populations such as those in ICUs. Adding to this are the presence of comorbidities [132], immunosenescence [129], atypical presentation of symptoms leading to late diagnosis and treatment [133, 134], higher exposure to pathogens with more frequent surgical procedures and possibly higher rates of exposure to gram-negative pathogens [129].

Sepsis is preventable [135] but it must be promptly diagnosed and treated. However, this can be formidable. A recent update on the management of sepsis and septic shock in the emergency department describes in detail the requisite therapy and issues [136]. The essential first step is the immediate initiation of empiric antimicrobial therapy [136]. A delay in therapy onset is associated with an increase in septic shock mortality [134]. Common pathogens are *Staphylococcus aureus* and *S. pneumoniae* (gram-positive pathogens*), Escherichia coli, Klebsiella* and *Pseudomonas spp* (gram-negative pathogens) and *Candida spp* (fungus) [136].

Sepsis. Diagnosis Diagnosing sepsis and septic shock in the older adult is exceptionally challenging [137]. Symptoms are nonspecific, ranging from a change in mental state and appetite, lethargy, weakness, dizziness, falls, and incontinence [137]. Consequently, it is impossible to get an accurate health history [138]. Other symptoms, such as temperature change, are unreliable since core temperature and thermoregulation decline with age [139] and only become useful if there exists baseline data [137]. Overall, the older adult most likely will not experience a fever for the reasons just mentioned but also because of immunosenescence and malnutrition effects. Biomarkers such as procalcitonin [140] associated with systemic bacteremia are of value but more reliable if there also is a baseline value [137].

Sepsis. Pharmacotherapy The choice of antibiotics depends on many factors. These factors are the site of the infection, e.g., lungs, skin, urinary tract, etc.; the identified pathogen, if not possible, local epidemiology is useful; whether the patient has a high risk for resistant pathogens, e.g., MRSA, *P. aeruginosa* if exposed to these pathogens within the last year or used multiple antibiotics within the last 4 weeks or is immunosuppressed or on chemotherapy. It is essential to achieve the minimal inhibitory concentration (MIC), generally with a loading dose but followed by adjustments based on kidney/liver assessments. For septic shock, a multidrug antimicrobial approach is beneficial [136]. See Table 6.1 for commonly used antimicrobials.

The second aspect of therapy is a readjustment of fluids to achieve normal blood pressure. Vasoplegia (profound vasodilation) due to a damaged and porous endothelial layer (specifically the glycocalyx) is considered the mechanism for septic shock [141]. The use of crystalloids rather than colloids or albumin with continuous hemodynamic monitoring is recommended [142]. The third component of therapy is the use of vasoactive drugs, such as norepinephrine (NE), to achieve a mean arterial pressure of 60–65 mmHg. NE may be tempered with the use of vasopressin (VP) to avoid excessive NE effects, and epinephrine (EPI) is of value if NE and VP fail to achieve the required mean arterial pressure [136]. Three other therapies are useful:

oxygen via a respiratory mask to achieve SpO_2 94–98% (oxygen saturation) or less if there is a risk of hypercapnic respiratory failure (increase in arterial CO_2); heparin to prevent thrombotic events; insulin to stabilize glucose levels; sodium bicarbonate for severe metabolic/lactic acidosis [136].

Safety of Antimicrobials

Safety of Antimicrobial Drugs. Issues There is an awareness among clinicians that the use of antimicrobials among patients of all ages must proceed cautiously and with relevant medical information. Specifically, "antimicrobial stewardship (AMS) interventions to help clinicians improve the appropriateness and safety of antimicrobial prescriptions" have been developed [11]. These are discussed in detail below. In treating infectious diseases in the older adult, the number of important variables is legion. Variables such as age-related changes in PK/PD, comorbidities, atypical presentation of symptoms, and the need to extrapolate treatment doses/efficacy/adverse effects from RCTs of young adults due to the paucity of data with the older adults, all complicate drug use in the older adult with infectious diseases and create an increased risk of antimicrobial drug resistance, adverse effects and mortality [11].

Antimicrobial Drugs. Pharmacokinetics. Absorption Consideration of age-related changes in PK is an essential first step to the prudent use of antimicrobials in the older adult [143]. Age-related changes in absorption, distribution, metabolism and excretion are described in detail in Chap. 2. In relation to antimicrobial drug use, it is important to reemphasize key points. Chronic use of proton pump inhibitors (e.g., omeprazole) or calcium carbonate increases stomach pH and retards absorption (bioavailability) of several classes of antimicrobials (alkaline) to include β-lactams, macrolides azoles, and atazanavir [144] whereas other drugs, e.g., raltegravir become more soluble and are 3–4 times more bioavailability [145]. An additional complication is the blockade of intestinal P-glycoprotein (P-gp) transporters by proton pump inhibitors that increase the bioavailability of antiviral drugs such as saquinavir with ritonavir [146] and conversely, antimicrobials can inhibit P-gp transporters from increasing the concentration of nonmicrobial drugs.

Antimicrobial Drugs. Distribution Because of the age-associated change in body composition, the increase in fat volume assures lipophilic drugs (macrolides, fluoroquinolones, rifampin, and tetracyclines) enjoy a larger volume of distribution and hence longer half-life and residence in the body. This change leads to lower drug concentrations and a lack of efficacy [147]. Water volume tends to decrease with age such that concentration of hydrophilic (water soluble) drugs (β-lactams, glycopeptides, aminoglycosides, and antifungal azoles) achieve higher concentrations in the older adult compared to the younger adult [11]. Generally, interactions of drugs at the site of protein binding lack clinical relevance unless the drugs are highly protein bound (>90%), have a narrow therapeutic window, have a high hepatic extraction ratio and if the drug is given IV [148]. An exception is antimicrobial drug use in the critically ill may lead to displacement of essential protein-bound drugs by an antimicrobial drug and initiate adverse effects (see Table 6.3 phenytoin and sulfonylureas displaced by trimethoprim-sulfamethoxazole) [11].

Antimicrobial Drugs. Metabolism and Excretion Metabolism and excretion are two PK aspects of major concern for antimicrobial drug use in the older adult [11, 149]. Except with liver disease [150], hepatic CYP P450 enzymes change very little with age. However, liver size and blood flow may decline significantly with age, resulting in a reduction in drugs undergoing first-pass and high-capacity extraction, hence increasing their bioavailability [151–153]. This applies to fluoroquinolones, macrolides, antifungal azoles and antiretrovirals [154]. CYP P450 enzymes are critically important since antimicrobial drugs, like all drugs, may be substrates, inducers and/or inhibitors of hepatic enzymes and compete with one another and other drugs (see Chaps. 2 and 3). An age-related decline in CYP2C19 and CYP3A4 has been reported in patients with sarcopenia, exposing them to a whole complex of drug interaction and adverse effects [149].

A large number of antimicrobial drugs are eliminated by the kidneys (beta-lactams, aminoglycosides, glycopeptides, fluoroquinolones (except moxifloxacin), lipoglycopeptides, lipopeptides (daptomycin), and trimethoprim/sulfamethoxazole [154]. Although an age-associated decline in kidney function does not occur in all older adults, kidney function should be assessed prior to antimicrobial use [143]. A decline in kidney function increases the bioavailability of these drugs, producing a higher-than-needed drug level and requires dosage or interval changes depending on whether the pathogen killing is concentration dependent (increase dosing interval) or time-dependent (decrease the dose but keep interval) [11, 155]. Concentration-dependent drugs are aminoglycosides, metronidazole, fluoroquinolones, daptomycin, and tetracyclines; and time-dependent drugs are β-lactams, clindamycin, and vancomycin [11]. Values of eGFR derived from serum creatinine are frequently used to assess kidney function but suffer from bias and overestimation of GFR (see Chap. 3). Additional assessment with cystatin C is helpful [156] although for those in acute-care hospitals, LTCF or with chronic kidney disease, measurement of urine creatinine clearance is necessary to avoid incorrect dosing [143, 157]. Additionally, disregard for reduced kidney function is permissive for nephrotoxicity, a serious adverse effect of many microbial drugs [149] (see Table 6.2). The greatest rate of acute kidney injury (AKI) occurs with the use of penicillins (piperacillin, tazobactam, cloxacillin, flucloxacillin) and vancomycin [158, 159].

Antimicrobial Drugs. Adverse Drug Reactions As emphasized by Soraci et al. (2023) [11], all classes of antimicrobials have the potential to cause adverse drug reactions (ADRs), with the most frequent ADRs being nephrotoxicity, ototoxicity, and neurotoxicity (see Table 6.2). Other serious ADRs reported with treatment of

Table 6.2 Adverse drug reactions to antimicrobial drugs in the older adult (reproduced with permission from Socrai et al. [11])

Antimicrobial drugs	Common adverse reactions	Adverse reactions at increased risk in older adults
Antbiotics		
Aminoglycosides [160, 224–226]	Nephrotoxicity, ototoxicity	Nephrotoxicity, ototoxicity
Tetracyclines [227, 228]	Photosensitivity, cutaneous infections, esophagitis, hepatotoxicity, pancreatitis	
Sulfonamides and trimethoprim [225, 226]	Nephrotoxicity, gastrointestinal intolerance, hypersensitive reactions, dermatologic reactions	Nephrotoxicity, neurotoxicity
Polymyxins [143, 229]	Nephrotoxicity and neurotoxicity	Nephrotoxicity
Oxazolidinones [143, 202]	Thrombocytopenia, neurotoxicity	
Macrolides [157, 201, 227]	Gastrointestinal intolerance, hepatotoxicity, cardiotoxicity, ototoxicity	Ototoxicity, neurotoxicity
Glycopeptide [201, 225]	Nephrotoxicity, ototoxicity, red man syndrome	Nephrotoxicity
Lipopeptides [230]	Nausea, muscle toxicity, eosinophilic pneumonia	
β-Lactams [225, 226, 231–239]	Hypersensitive reactions, gastrointestinal intolerance	Nephrotoxicity, neurotoxicity *Clostridioides difficile* infection (broad-spectrum penicillins and combinations, third/fourth-generation cephalosporins, carbapenems)
Fluoroquinolones [200, 240, 241]	Tendinopathy, *Clostridioides difficile* infection, cardiotoxicity	Tendinopathy, neurotoxicity, *Clostridioides difficile* infection
Nitroimidazoles [202]	Neurotoxicity, cardiotoxicity	
Nitrofurans [143, 202]	Neurotoxicity	Neurotoxicity
Lincosamides [201, 234]	*Clostridioides difficile* infection	*Clostridioides difficile* infection
Antimyobacterial		
Flucytosine [242]	Inhibition of the bone marrow, hepatotoxicity	

(continued)

Table 6.2 (continued)

Antimicrobial drugs	Common adverse reactions	Adverse reactions at increased risk in older adults
Isoniazid [201, 235, 242]	Hepatotoxicity	Hepatotoxicity, neurotoxicity
Rifampin [201, 225, 235]	Red-orange discoloration of urine, tears, and sweat	Nephrotoxicity, hepatotoxicity (association with isoniazid)
Antivirals		
Nucleosides/nucleotides excluded reverse transcriptase inhibitors [244–249]	Nephrotoxicity, gastrointestinal intolerance	Neurotoxicity
Derivatives of phosphonic acid [225, 250]	Nephrotoxicity	Nephrotoxicity
Neuraminidase inhibitors [251, 252]	Gastrointestinal intolerance	
Interferon-α [253, 254]	Influenza-like symptoms, nausea, headache, depression, alopecia	
Nucleoside/nucleotide reverse transcriptase inhibitors [255, 256]	Mitochondrial toxicity	Nephrotoxicity, bone toxicity
Non-nucleoside reverse transcriptase inhibitors [257, 258]	Dermatologic reactions, hepatotoxicity	
Protease inhibitors [259, 260]	Hyperlipidemia, lipodystrophy, hyperglycemia, insulin resistance	
Antifungals		
Echinocandins [261, 262]	Nausea, hepatotoxicity, skin rash, phleitis	
Triazoles [242, 261, 262]	Gastrointestinal intolerance, skin rash, hepatotoxicity	Hepatotoxicity, neurotoxicity
Amphotericin B [261, 263, 264]	Infusion-related reactions, hepatotoxicity, hematological effects, nephrotoxicity	

C. difficile infection are hepatoxicity and hypersensitivity reactions specific to different drug subclasses. Nephrotoxicity, ototoxicity, and neurotoxicity take a particularly greater toll on the older adult by adding to existing age changes in the kidneys, ears and brain that not only diminish QoL but require additional healthcare and longer hospital stays [154]. Sadly, for the older adult, high-quality data on the use of antimicrobial drugs in the older population is generally lacking [11, 154]. This limits the ability of healthcare providers in their capacity to assure safe and efficacious therapy for infectious diseases in the older adult [154]. There exists one systematic and meta-analysis that determined the risk of organ (kidney, liver and tissue) damage with antimicrobial use in the older adult, 65 years and older [160]. Among 29 studies included for systematic review and 25 of those for meta-analysis (predominately retrospective cohort studies), the absolute risk of nephrotoxicity was 15.1%, 19.1% and 0.3% for aminoglycosides, glycopeptides, and macrolides, respectively [160]. AKI was also reported for cephalosporins, penicillins, quinolones, trimethoprim and nitrofurantoin; hepatoxicity was reported for antimycobacterial drugs and tendon rupture with quinolones [160]. Although controversial, long-term treatment (more than 7 days) of aminoglycosides or glycopeptides appeared not to be a factor in the incidence of AKI among these studies [160]. It is evident that the risk for AKI may be higher in specific populations such as those hospitalized or critically ill [161, 162].

> *Alert*: The most frequent ADRs for antimicrobials are nephrotoxicity, ototoxicity and neurotoxicity.

Antimicrobial Drugs. Drug-Drug Interactions (DDIs) Soraci et al. (2023) [11] has summarized important drug interactions of antimicrobials with a range of medications used to treat common diseases (see Table 6.3). Most of the data is obtained from each drug package insert. However, several of these interactions are reinforced with Beers Criteria® Analysis which cautions the combined use of trimethoprim-sulfamethoxizole and phenytoin [163] due to CYP2C9 enzyme competition that produces phenytoin toxicity [164]. Also, the concurrent use of trimethoprim-sulfamethoxizole and angiotensin-converting enzyme inhibitors (ACEIs) increases the risk of hyperkalemia [163]. Another serious DDI of concern for the older adult is the simultaneous use of ciprofloxacin and theophylline in which the former blocks the metabolism (CYP1A2) of the latter, producing theophylline toxicity. Ciprofloxacin, macrolides and trimethoprim-sulfamethoxizole also interact with warfarin to increase the risk of bleeding [163]. Although conducted in adults 25 years of age, a small RCT showed that voriconazole, an antifungal agent used in conjunction with warfarin, increases the risk of bleeding [165]. Several antimicrobials (clarithromycin, erythromycin, tetracyclines) increase the bioavailability of digoxin and hence produce toxicity [166] and do so by inhibition of P-gp transporters [167]. Awareness that linezolid may increase the concentration of serotonin relates significantly to those individuals taking a selective serotonin reuptake inhibitor because the result may be the induction of a rare but fatal serotonin syndrome [168]. There is an extended list of drugs with nephrotoxicity potential to include many of the antimicrobials as well as loop diuretics, cisplatin, cyclosporine and tacrolimus so that using two concurrently assures AKI [169].

ANTIMICROBIAL STEWARDSHIP Antimicrobial stewardship (AMS) originated more than 20 years ago as the Consensus Principles developed by expert clinicians from several nations concerned with the development of antimicrobial resistance (AMR) due to inappropriate antimicrobial drug use [24]. "The objectives

Table 6.3 Antimicrobial drug interactions (Reproduced with permission from Socrai et al. [11])

Antimicrobial drug	Interacting drugs → adverse side effects
Aminoglycosides [265]	Amphotericin B, cyclosporin, cisplatin, loop diuretics, tacrolimus, vancomycin → ↑ nephrotoxicity
Amoxicillin, ampicillin [266, 267]	Allopurinol → rash
Fluoroquinolones [268–271]	Medications containing aluminum, iron, magnesium, or zinc; antacids; sucralfate → ↓ absorption of fluoroquinolones
Ciprofloxacin	Antiarrhythmics → ventricular arrhythmias Calcium-containing supplements ↓ absorption of ciprofloxacin Theophylline → ↑ theophylline concentration Warfarin → ↑ bleeding risk
Linezolid [272]	Serotoninergic drugs (MAOIs, TCAs, SSRIs) → serotonin syndrome
Azithromycin [273]	Drugs containing aluminum or magnesium → ↓ azithromycin absorption
Clarithromycin and erythromycin [274–276]	Calcium channel blockers, HMG-Co-A reductase inhibitors, cyclosporine, digoxin, theophylline, and warfarin; DOACs → ↑ concentration of interacting drugs; ↑ concentration of the antibiotic (calcium channel blockers).
Metronidazole [132, 277]	Warfarin → ↑ bleeding risk Alcohol → disulfiram-like reaction
Rifampin [133, 278]	Antacids → ↓ rifampin concentration Antiarrhythmics, benzodiazepines, calcium channel blockers, corticosteroids, digoxin, enalapril, estrogens and/or progestins, methadone, phenytoin, tamoxifen, theophylline, valproate, voriconazole, warfarin, DOACs → ↓ concentration of the interacting drugs
Tetracyclines [279–283]	Drugs containing aluminum, calcium, iron or magnesium; bismuth subsalicylate → ↓ tetracycline absorption Digoxin → ↑ digoxin toxicity
Triazole antifungals [242, 261, 262]	Carbamazepine, phenobarbital, phenytoin and rifampin → ↓ concentration of antifungals Antiarrhythmics, benzodiazepines, calcium channel blockers, corticosteroids, digoxin, HMG-CoA reductase inhibitors, sulfonylureas, warfarin, DOACs → ↑ concentration of interacting drugs
Itraconazole, ketoconazole	Antacids, H2-receptor antagonists, PPIs → ↓ antifungal absorption
Voriconazole	Phenytoin, PPIs → ↑ concentration of interacting drugs
Trimethoprim-sulfamethoxazole [284]	Phenytoin → ↑ phenytoin concentration Sulfonylureas → hypoglycemia Warfarin → ↑ bleeding risk ACE inhibitors, potassium-sparing diuretics → hyperkalemia

ACE angiotensin-converting enzyme, *DOACs* direct oral anticoagulants, *HMG-CoA* 3-hydroxy-3-methylglutaryl coenzyme A, *MAOIs* monoamine oxidase inhibitors, *PPIs* proton pump inhibitor, *SSRIs* selective serotonin reuptake inhibitors, *TCAs* tricyclic antidepressants, *H2 receptor antagonist* histamine type 2 blocker; ↑ increase; ↓ decrease, → cause of the Consensus Group were to optimize antibiotic therapy in order to reduce morbidity, therapeutic failure and consequent added cost and prevent resistance emergence" [24]. Today the view remains that inappropriate drug use results in poor outcomes and antimicrobial drug resistance [170]. Consider the data presented in Table 6.2 and the development of resistant pathogens including (a) the extended-spectrum β-lactamase enterobacteriales (ESBL-E) (resistance to penicillins, cephalosporins, and aztreonam), (b) AmpC β-lactamase enterobacteriales (AmpC-E) (resistant to ceftriaxone, cefotaxime, and ceftazidime), (c) carbapenem-resistant enterobacteriales (CRE) (resistant to carbapenem, meropenem or imipenem), (d) MDR-P. aeruginosa difficult to treat and resistant to multiple classes of antibiotics, and (e) carbapenem-resistant *Acinetobacter baumannii* (CRAB) (resistant to carbapenem and most other antibiotics) [171–173].

The challenge is how to change prescribing behavior to achieve the goals of the Consensus Principles. The original principles set forth by Ball et al. [174], as they relate to antibiotic use, are as follows: (1) treat only bacterial infections with antibiotics, (2) optimize diagnosis and severity assessment, (3) maximize bacterial eradication, (4) recognize (and act on) local resistance prevalence, (5) utilize pharmacodynamics to assist in the choice of effective agents and dosing and (6) integrate local resistance, efficacy and cost-effectiveness. To assist with the Consensus Principles, the WHO developed a classification database of antibiotics to evaluate and monitor use [175]. Antibiotics are classified into three groups by WHO: (1) "Access" category includes drugs with low resistance potentially effective against common pathogens. Some examples are amoxicillin/clavulanic-acid, first-generation cephalosporins, select penicillins, nitrofurantoin, (2) "Watch" category includes drugs with higher resistance potential and limited use such as azithromycin, second and third generation cephalosporins, ciprofloxacin, clarithromycin, erythromycin, and (3) "Reserve" category include drugs for use with suspected or confirmed multidrug resistance (MDR) pathogens such as aztreonam, fifth generation cephalosporins, daptomycin, linezolid, and colistin.

In reference to the older adult, Soraci et al. (2023) [11] proposed the following in support of AMS: (1) Avoidance of inappropriate empirical antimicrobial prescribing. Pathogen identification by laboratory cultures and assays is essential prior to prescribing in stable or asymptomatic patients. The empirical approach is appropriate for unstable patients who may require immediate therapy. (2) Adherence to proven guidelines of the appropriate duration of therapy. Data show that the use of 7 days or less for bacterial infections, 5 days or less for uncomplicated UTI and respiratory infections and 15 days or less for fungal skin conditions are sufficient for efficacious outcomes. Continuing clinical assessment during treatment is important. (3) Special management teams for antibiotic use in end-stage illness or advanced dementia. (4) "watch and wait" approach and no routine urine culture for asymptomatic bacteriuria. (5) Upper respiratory tract infections or acute bronchitis requires differential diagnosis for bacterial or viral infection prior to treatment. (6) Avoidance of quinolones as first-line empirical therapy of UTI in consideration of adverse effects and induction of gram-negative resistance. (7) Gastroenteritis requires pathogen determination prior to therapy with empirical antimicrobial treatment in severe cases or those with no clinical improvement. (8) Chronic ulcers or skin lesions should be treated for underlying causes and only in verified cases of cellulitis, deep soft tissue, or bone infection [11]. These recommendations are supported by ample data with the older adult.

Vaccines

Vaccines. Introduction Vaccinations are a successful means of prevention of infectious diseases. The CDC has established a comprehensive immunization program with specific schedules and booster shots from birth to 15 months and 18 months to 18 years that include immunizations for diphtheria, tetanus and acellular pertussis, respiratory syncytial virus (RSV), poliovirus, hepatitis A and B virus, rotavirus, Hemophilus influenza type B, measles, mumps, rubella, varicella, pneumococcal pneumonia and human papilomavirus [176]. Vaccines given annually are for the prevention of influenza and COVID-19 and additionally, for the older adult, the CDC recommends vaccination against latent varicella virus (chicken pox with late expression as shingles), and depending on earlier vaccinations, pneumococcal pneumonia, and RSV vaccination (see Table 6.4).

Vaccines. Age Effects Immunological response to newly encountered pathogens in the older adult is generally less than optimal while immunological activation against pathogenic antigens confronted in younger years remains strong [177]. Immunosenescence encompasses deficits in both innate and adaptive immunity with poorly functioning antigen-processing cells (macrophages and dendritic cells), a limited number of naive B and T cells, and functional decline in current subsets of antibody-producing B and cytokine-producing T cells. The result of these changes leads to a weakened response to new antigens (as in vaccines) and a shorter duration of protection [8, 17]. Thus, it is recognized that efficacy of immunizations in the older adult is lower than in younger individuals [17] and is a serious problem in older adults with comorbidities, enhancing the risk of poor outcomes in the face of deadly pathogens [178]. Nevertheless, immunization overall provides numerous health benefits, not only in disease prevention in the young but also in long-term disability prevention and reduction of health care costs [179]. For the older adult, vaccine efficacy has improved with the use of increased dosage and modified antigenic composition of vaccines [180, 181].

Table 6.4 Vaccines for the older adult

Disease	Efficacy	Issues/recommendations
COVID-19—mRNA vaccines against SARS-CoV-2 viral variants 1. COMIRNATY (Pfizer-BioNTech) 2. SPIKEVAX (Moderna) Protein subunit vaccine for COVID-19 3. Novavax COVID-29 Vaccine, Adjuvant	COMIRNATY: 94.5% prevention of symptomatic COVID-19; efficacious against severe COVID-19 (grouped as 15 yrs and older) [214] SPIKEVAX (main dose, 2 boosters)—82.4% ≥65 < 74; 100% ≥75 yrs [215] Novavax—90.4% protection of symptomatic COVID-19; 100% protective of mod-severe COVID-19; ~12% ≥ 65 yrs in assessment [183].	Recommended for 65 and older as of February 2021—mRNA, and protein subunit vaccines; targets Omicron variant lineage XBB; serious ADRs are rare but may be myocarditis or pericarditis [216]
Pneumonia (*Streptococcus pneumoniae* bacteria) 1. Pneumococcal conjugate vaccines (PCV15 and PCV20) 2. Pneumococcal polysaccharide vaccine (PPSV23)	PCV 20 or PVC15 in series with PPSV23 comparable efficacy to standard PCV13 but effective against additional serotypes and more cost-effective [180] PPSV23 effectiveness of 45% against PPSV23-type IPD (9 studies) and 18% against PPSV23-type PP (5 studies) (meta-analysis of most studies with 65 and older pts) [186].	CDC recommendations: PV15 or PV20, followed by PPSV23 for 65 yrs and older; if vaccinated earlier with PV13, may replace with PV20 if also vaccinated with PPSV23. Mild reactions of pain/redness at injection site; fever, muscle aches [217]
Influenza 2024–2025 season Egg-based or Cell/recombinant-based targeted: H1N1, H3N2, and B/Victoria lineage	Efficacy over 10 yr [218] or 12 yr pd [181] of high dose tri or quadrivalent vaccine in those 65 and older superior to standard dose. Meta-analysis shows efficacy in older adults~ 30–50% [219]	High-dose inactivated influenza vaccine (trivalent or quadrivalent) more efficacious in older adults in preventing influenza-like illness and associated hospitalization [181] CDC recommends annual immunization with either egg-based or cell/recombinant vaccines [220]

(continued)

Table 6.4 (continued)

Disease	Efficacy	Issues/recommendations
Respiratory syncytial virus 3 RSV vaccines (GSK, Pfizer, Moderna) approved by FDA	81.38% efficacy from systemic/meta-analysis of 5 RCTs to prevent lower respiratory disease; age > 60 yrs; 61% efficacy with 1 yr follow up [187]	CDC recommends RSV vaccine for those 75 and older or 60–74 yrs with comorbidities [221]
Herpes zoster (shingles) Shingrix (recombinant herpes zoster vaccine)	97.2% efficacy in preventing the emergence of the latent varicella-zoster virus, RCT results in those >50 yrs [222]. 68–89% efficacious in >80 yrs [185]	CDC recommends Shingrix for those 50 yrs and older, since 99% have been exposed to chicken pox [223]
Tuberculosis Bacillus Calmette-Guerin (BCG)	Variable with reduced disease progression [188]	Use of alternate routes of administration hold promise to improve efficacy [189]. Booster vaccine shows 49.7% efficacy in active TB prevention (3 yrs) in pts with latent TB, oldest pt was 44 yrs [190]

ADR adverse drug reaction, *IPD* invasive pneumococcal disease, *PP* pneumococcal pneumonia, *CDC* Center for Disease Control, *pts* patients, *RCT* randomized clinical trial, *yrs* years

Vaccines. Recommendations by the Center for Disease Control CDC vaccine recommendations for the older adult are presented in Table 6.4. Presently, COVID-19 vaccines are the most efficacious (82.4–94.5%) vaccines with the capability of targeting the most prevalent SARS-CoV-2 viral variants [182, 183]. However, the duration of efficacy is only about 6 months and new variants continue to arise, necessitating updated vaccines [184]. Herpes zoster (Shingrix) vaccine is highly efficacious but drops to 68–89% in those older than 80 years [185]. Pneumococcal vaccines PV15 and PV20 (conjugated forms) are more efficacious than the earlier PPVS23 [186]. Also the use of high-dose influenza vaccine in the older adult improved efficacy [181]. Currently, RSV vaccines, recommended for those 75 years and older and those younger with comorbidities, are 81% effective. However, this efficacy is transient and drops to 61% after the first year [187]. There is considerable interest in developing a highly effective vaccine against TB [89]. The only available vaccine, Bacillus Calmette-Guerin (BCG), reduces disease progression but does not prevent the disease [188]. Modification of the route of administration has proven successful in animal models of TB [189] and administration of a novel booster (M72/AS01$_E$) proved 46.7% efficacious in preventing TB for 3 years in those with LTBI [190].

Guidance
Although infectious diseases are generally considered preventable and treatable (Tables 6.1 and 6.4), for the older adult, age changes in organ function, primarily in the immune, pulmonary and renal systems, and the presence of comorbidities create an increased vulnerability to pathogens and a higher risk for a poor outcome.

I. To improve outcomes, awareness of the following issues is advised:
   A. In the older adult, classical symptoms of infectious diseases are replaced by atypical symptoms. This delays diagnosis and treatment. For example:
      1. Pneumonia symptoms of fever, cough, and chest pain are replaced by falls, reduced appetite or change in functional and mental status.
      2. UTI symptoms of painful/ burning urination, frequent urination, bloody urine, pressure groin/lower abdomen in cystitis and fever, chills, lower back pain, nausea/vomiting in pyelonephritis are replaced with general symptoms of lower abdominal pain, back pain, and constipation.
      3. Sepsis and septic shock symptoms in the older adult are anomalous and range from a change in mental state, lethargy, weakness, dizziness, falls, and incontinence.
      4. Influenza and COVID-19 symptoms of fever, cough, sore throat, muscle aches, headaches may present with shortness of breath or no consistent pattern.
   B. There exists an abundance of antimicrobial drugs but appropriate use requires an understanding of age-related changes in the pharmacokinetics of the older adult and pharmacodynamics of pathogens:
      1. Absorption of some antimicrobial drugs (β-lactams, macrolides azoles, and atazanavir) may decrease in the presence of chronic use of proton pump inhibitors while absorption of raltegravir is increased.
      2. The age-associated increase in body fat and decrease in body water affects antimicrobial drug concentrations such that macrolides, fluoroquinolones, rifampin, and tetracyclines (fat-loving drugs) reside in the body longer but at lower concentrations than expected and hence may not be efficacious. β-lactams, glycopeptides, aminoglycosides, and antifungal azoles (water-loving drugs) reach higher than expected concentrations and may induce toxicity.
      3. Age-related reduction in liver function may diminish the metabolism of the fluoroquinolones, macrolides, antifungal azoles and antiretrovirals, producing higher than expected concentrations.

(continued)

4. Accurate assessment of kidney function is essential for appropriate antimicrobial drug use and avoidance of adverse reactions. Serum creatinine measurement tends to overestimate kidney function and urine creatinine clearance measurement is preferred. Many drugs are excreted by the kidneys to include beta-lactams, aminoglycosides, glycopeptides, fluoroquinolones (except moxifloxacin), lipoglycopeptides, lipopeptides (daptomycin), and trimethoprim/sulfamethoxazole.
5. Pathogens require either a certain minimal concentration for killing or a certain minimal duration of killing. Hence, antimicrobial drugs, e.g., aminoglycosides, metronidazole, fluoroquinolones, daptomycin, and tetracyclines are concentration-dependent and antimicrobial drugs, e.g., β-lactams, clindamycin, and vancomycin are time-dependent. Reduced kidney function requires increasing dosing intervals for the former and decreasing dose but no change of interval for the latter drugs.

C. Strict adherence to the above is necessary to minimize adverse reactions to antimicrobials in the older adult. Most antimicrobials have the potential to cause nephrotoxicity, ototoxicity, and neurotoxicity (Table 6.2).
D. The presence of comorbidities in the older adult requires wise selection of antimicrobial therapy as medications used to treat morbidities may be affected (generally through competitive hepatic metabolism) by concurrent use, yielding reduced efficacy or adverse reactions (Table 6.3).

II. Vaccinations are the best way to prevent infectious diseases for individuals of all ages. The CDC recommends, in addition to those received at a younger age, immunization to prevent COVID-19, influenza, bacterial pneumonia, respiratory syncytial virus and herpes zoster (Table 6.4).

III. Antimicrobial drug resistance is a serious worldwide problem. To address this problem, Antimicrobial Stewardship proposes the following practices:

A. Avoidance of inappropriate empirical antimicrobial prescribing unless absolutely necessary for seriously ill unstable patients.
B. Adherence to proven guidelines of appropriate duration of therapy.
C. Special management teams for antibiotic use in end-stage illness or advanced dementia.
D. "Watch and wait" approach and no routine urine culture for asymptomatic bacteriuria.
E. Upper respiratory tract infections or acute bronchitis requires differential diagnosis for bacterial or viral infection prior to treatment.
F. Avoidance of quinolones as first-line empirical therapy of UTI.

References

1. Adak A, Khan MR. An insight into gut microbiota and its functionalities. Cell Mol Life Sci. 2019;76(3):473–93. https://doi.org/10.1007/s00018-018-2943-4.
2. Pellett PE, Mitra S, Holland TC. Basics of virology. Handb Clin Neurol. 2014;123:45–66. https://doi.org/10.1016/B978-0-444-53488-0.00002-X.
3. Martins-Santana L, Rezende CP, Rossi A, Martinez-Rossi NM, Almeida F. Addressing microbial resistance worldwide: challenges over controlling life-threatening fungal infections. Pathogens. 2023;12(2):293. https://doi.org/10.3390/pathogens12020293.
4. Chowdhary A, Jain K, Chauhan N. *Candida auris* genetics and emergence. Ann Rev Microbiol. 2023;77:583–602. https://doi.org/10.1146/annurev-micro-032521-015858.
5. https://www.cdc.gov/parasites/causes
6. Kinsella KG. Changes in life expectancy 1900–1990. Am J Clin Nutr. 1992;55(6 Suppl):1196S–202S. https://doi.org/10.1093/ajcn/55.6.1196S.
7. CDC, vital statistics. http://wonder.cdc.gov/ucd-icd10-expanded.html
8. Bilder GE. Human biological aging from macromolecules to organ systems. Hoboken, NJ: Wiley Blackwell; 2016. p. 303–18.
9. Cunha BA. Pneumonia in the elderly. Clin Microbiol Infect. 2001;7(11):581–8. https://doi.org/10.1046/j.1198-743x.2001.00328.x.
10. Liang SY. Sepsis and other infectious disease emergencies in the elderly. Emerg Med Clin North Am. 2016;34(3):501–22. https://doi.org/10.1016/j.emc.2016.04.005.
11. Soraci L, Cherubini A, Paoletti L, Filippelli G, Luciani F, Laganà P, et al. Safety and tolerability of antimicrobial agents in the older patient. Drugs Aging. 2023;40(6):499–526. https://doi.org/10.1007/s40266-023-01019-3.
12. Dumyati G, Stone ND, Nace DA, Crnich CJ, Jump RL. Challenges and strategies for prevention of multidrug-resistant organism transmission in nursing homes. Curr Infect Dis Rep. 2017;19(4):18. https://doi.org/10.1007/s11908-017-0576-7.
13. Sabetfakhri NN. Homebound older adult, caregiver, and provider perspectives on the benefits of home-based primary care: a narrative review. J Patient Cent Res Rev. 2023;10(4):239–46. https://doi.org/10.17294/2330-0698.2048.
14. https://www.who.int/news-room/fact-sheets/detail/the-top-10-causes-of-death
15. https://www.cdc.gov/nchs/data/hus/2020-2021/LCODAge.pdf
16. Turvey SE, Broide DH. Innate immunity. J Allergy Clin Immunol. 2010;125(2 Suppl 2):S24–32. https://doi.org/10.1016/j.jaci.2009.07.016.
17. Allen JC, Toapanta FR, Chen W, Tennant SM. Understanding immunosenescence and its impact on vaccination of older adults. Vaccine. 2020;38(52):8264–72. https://doi.org/10.1016/j.vaccine.2020.11.002.
18. Crooke SN, Ovsyannikova IG, Poland GA, Kennedy RB. Immunosenescence and human vaccine immune responses. Immun Ageing. 2019;16:25. https://doi.org/10.1186/s12979-019-0164-9.
19. Williamson EJ, Walker AJ, Bhaskaran K, Bacon S, Bates C, Morton CE, et al. Factors associated with COVID-19-related death using OpenSAFELY. Nature. 2020;584(7821):430–6. https://doi.org/10.1038/s41586-020-2521-4.
20. Chen Y, Klein SL, Garibaldi BT, Li H, Wu C, Osevala NM, et al. Aging in COVID-19: vulnerability, immunity and intervention. Ageing Res Rev. 2021;65:101205. https://doi.org/10.1016/j.arr.2020.101205.
21. Schneider JL, Rowe JH, Garcia-de-Alba C, Kim CF, Sharpe AH, Haigis MC. The aging lung: physiology, disease, and immunity. Cell. 2021;184(8):1990–2019. https://doi.org/10.1016/j.cell.2021.03.005.
22. Mouton CP, Bazaldua OV, Pierce B, Espino DV. Common infections in older adults. Am Fam Physician. 2001;63(2):257–68.
23. Cho SJ, Stout-Delgado HW. Aging and lung disease. Annu Rev Physiol. 2020;82:433–59. https://doi.org/10.1146/annurev-physiol-021119-034610.

24. Canton R, Akova M, Langfeld K, Torumkuney D. Relevance of the consensus principles for appropriate antibiotic prescribing in 2022. J Antimicrob Chemother. 2022;77(Suppl_1):i2–9. https://doi.org/10.1093/jac/dkac211.
25. de Jong LM, Jiskoot W, Swen JJ, Manson ML. Distinct effects of inflammation on cytochrome P450 regulation and drug metabolism: lessons from experimental models and a potential role for pharmacogenetics. Genes (Basel). 2020;11(12):1509. https://doi.org/10.3390/genes11121509.
26. Norman DC. Fever in the elderly. Clin Infect Dis. 2000;31(1):148–51. https://doi.org/10.1086/313896.
27. https://www.worldometers.info/coronavirus
28. https://covid.cdc.gov/covid-data-tracker/#demographics
29. Al-Osail AM, Al-Wazzah MJ. The history and epidemiology of Middle East respiratory syndrome corona virus. Multidiscip Respir Med. 2017;12:20. https://doi.org/10.1186/s40248-017-0101-8.
30. https://oversight.house.gov/release/covid-origins-hearing-wrap-up-facts-science-evidence-point-to-a-wuhan-lab-leak%EF%BF%BC/
31. Yi Y, Lagniton PNP, Ye S, Li E, Xu R-H. What has been learned and to be learned about the novel coronavirus disease. Int J Biol Sci. 2020;16(10):1753–66. https://doi.org/10.7150/ijbs.45134.
32. Liu J, Zheng X, Tong Q, Li W, Wang B, Sutter K, et al. Overlapping and discrete aspects of the pathology and pathogenesis of the emerging human pathogenic coronaviruses SARS-CoV, MERS-CoV, and 2019-nCoV. J Med Virol. 2020;92(5):491–4. https://doi.org/10.1002/jmv.25709.
33. Rahman S, Montero MTV, Rowe K, Kirton R, Kunik F Jr. Epidemiology, pathogenesis, clinical presentations, diagnosis and treatment of COVID-19: a review of current evidence. Expert Rev Clin Pharmacol. 2021;14(5):601–21. https://doi.org/10.1080/17512433.2021.1902303.
34. Hu G, Christman JW. Editorial: alveolar macrophages in lung inflammation and resolution. Front Immunol. 2019;10:2275. https://doi.org/10.3389/fimmu.2019.02275.
35. Fahey E, Doyle SL. IL-1 family cytokine regulation of vascular permeability and angiogenesis. Front Immunol. 2019;10:1426. https://doi.org/10.3389/fimmu.2019.01426.
36. Chavda VP, Bezbaruah R, Dolia S, Shah N, Verma S, Savale S, et al. Convalescent plasma (hyperimmune immunoglobulin) for COVID-19 management: an update. Process Biochem. 2023;127:66–81. https://doi.org/10.1016/j.procbio.2023.01.018.
37. COVID-19 Treatment Guidelines Panel. Coronavirus Disease 2019 (COVID-19) Treatment Guidelines. National Institutes of Health. Available at https://www.covid19treatmentguidelines.nih.gov/. RCT - randomized clinical trials.
38. Beigel JH, Tomashek KM, Dodd LE, Mehta AK, Zingman BS, Kalil AC, et al. Remdesivir for the treatment of Covid-19 - final report. N Engl J Med. 2020;383(19):1813–26. https://doi.org/10.1056/NEJMoa2007764.
39. Gottlieb RL, Vaca CE, Paredes R, Mera J, Wevv BJ, Perez G, et al. Early remdesivir to prevent progression to severe covid-19 in outpatients. N Engl J Med. 2021;386(4):305–15. https://doi.org/10.1056/NEJMoa2116846.
40. Ali K, Azher T, Baqi M, Binnie A, Borgia S, Carrier FM, et al. Remdesivir for the treatment of patients in hospital with COVID-19 in Canada: a randomized controlled trial. CMAJ. 2022;194(7):E242–51. https://doi.org/10.1503/cmaj.211698.
41. Spinner CD, Gottlieb RL, Criner GJ, Lopez JRA, Cattelan AM, Viladmiu AS, et al. Effect of remdesivir vs standard care on clinical status at 11 days in patients with moderate COVID-19. JAMA. 2020;324(11):1–10. https://doi.org/10.1001/jama.2020.16349.
42. Ader F, Bouscambert-Duchamp M, Hites M, Peiffer-Smadja N, Poissy J, Belhadi D, et al. Remdesivir plus standard of care versus standard of care alone for the treatment of patients admitted to hospital with COVID-19 (DisCoVeRy): a phase 3, randomised, controlled, open-label trial. Lancet Infect Dis. 2022;22(2):209–21. https://doi.org/10.1016/S1473-3099(21)00485-0.

43. WHO Solidarity Trial Consortium. Remdesivir and three other drugs for hospitalised patients with COVID-19: final results of the WHO solidarity randomised trial and updated meta-analyses. Lancet. 2022;399(10339):1941–53. https://doi.org/10.1016/S0140-6736(22)00519-0.
44. Patnaik R, Chandramouli T, Mishra SB. A systematic review and meta-analysis of randomized controlled trials with trial sequence analysis of remdesivir for COVID-19 treatment. Int J Crit Illn Inj Sci. 2023;13(4):184–91. https://doi.org/10.4103/ijciis.ijciis_23_2.
45. Ganatra S, Dani SS, Ahmad J, Kumar A, Shah J, Abraham GM, et al. Oral nirmatrelvir and ritonavir in non-hospitalized vaccinated patients with COVID-19. Clin Infect Dis. 2023;76(4):563–72. https://doi.org/10.1093/cid/ciac673.
46. Hammond J, Leister-Tebbe H, Gardner A, Abreu P, Bao W, Wisemandle W, et al. Oral nirmatrelvir for high-risk, nonhospitalized adults with COVID-19. N Engl J Med. 2022;386(15):1397–408. https://doi.org/10.1056/NEJMoa2118542.
47. Arbel R, Wolff Sagy Y, Hoshen M, Battat E, Lavie G, Sergienko R, et al. Nirmatrelvir use and severe Covid-19 outcomes during the omicron surge. N Engl J Med. 2022;387(9):790–8. https://doi.org/10.1056/NEJMoa2204919.
48. Najjar-Debbiny R, Gronich N, Weber G, Khoury J, Amar M, Stein N, et al. Effectiveness of Paxlovid in reducing severe COVID-19 and mortality in high risk patients. Clin Infect Dis. 2023;76(3):e342–9. https://doi.org/10.1093/cid/ciac443.
49. Loos NHC, Beijnen JH, Schinkel AH. The mechanism-based inactivation of CYP3A4 by ritonavir: what mechanism? Int J Mol Sci. 2022;23(17):9866. https://doi.org/10.3390/ijms23179866.
50. Brooks JK, Song JH, Sultan AS. Paxlovid-associated dysgeusia. Oral Dis. 2023;29(7):2980–1. https://doi.org/10.1111/odi.14312.
51. Wan EYF, Yan VKC, Mok AHY, Wang B, Xu W, Cheng FWT, et al. Effectiveness of Molnupiravir and Nirmatrelvir-Ritonavir in hospitalized patients With COVID-19: a target trial emulation study. Ann Intern Med. 2023;176(4):505–14. https://doi.org/10.7326/M22-3057.
52. Jayk Bernal A, Gomes da Silva MM, Musungaie DB, Kovalchuk E, Gonzalez A, Delos Reyes V, et al. Molnupiravir for oral treatment of Covid-19 in nonhospitalized patients. N Engl J Med. 2022;386(6):509–20. https://doi.org/10.1056/NEJMoa2116044.
53. Guan Y, Puenpatom A, Johnson MG, Zhang Y, Zhao Y, Surber J, et al. Impact of Molnupiravir treatment on patient-reported COVID-19 symptoms in the phase 3 MOVe-OUT trial: a randomized, placebo-controlled trial. Clin Infect Dis. 2023;77(11):1521–30. https://doi.org/10.1093/cid/ciad409.
54. Fischer WA 2nd, Eron JJ Jr, Holman W, Cohen MS, Fang L, Szewczyk LJ, et al. A phase 2a clinical trial of molnupiravir in patients with COVID-19 shows accelerated SARS-CoV-2 RNA clearance and elimination of infectious virus. Sci Transl Med. 2022;14(628):eabl7430. https://doi.org/10.1126/scitranslmed.abl7430.
55. Ferreira-Coimbra J, Sarda C, Rello J. Burden of community-acquired pneumonia and unmet clinical needs. Adv Ther. 2020;37(4):1302–18. https://doi.org/10.1007/s12325-020-01248-7.
56. Lanks CW, Musani AI, Hsia DW. Community-acquired pneumonia and hospital-acquired pneumonia. Med Clin North Am. 2019;103(3):487–501. https://doi.org/10.1016/j.mcna.2018.12.008.
57. Henig O, Kaye KS. Bacterial pneumonia in older adults. Infect Dis Clin N Am. 2017;31(4):689–713. https://doi.org/10.1016/j.idc.2017.07.015.
58. DeFrances CJ, Lucas CA, Buie VC. 2006 National hospital discharge survey. Natl Health Stat Rep. 2008;5:1–20.
59. Modi AR, Kovacs CS. Hospital-acquired and ventilator-associated pneumonia: diagnosis, management, and prevention. Cleve Clin J Med. 2020;87(10):633–9. https://doi.org/10.3949/ccjm.87a.19117.
60. Broulette J, Yu H, Pyenson B, Iwasaki K, Sato R. The incidence rate and economic burden of community-acquired pneumonia in a working-age population. Am Health Drug Benefits. 2013;6(8):494–503.

61. Shoar S, Musher DM. Etiology of community-acquired pneumonia in adults: a systematic review. Pneumonia (Nathan). 2020;12:11. https://doi.org/10.1186/s41479-020-00074-3.
62. Anderson R, Feldman C. The global burden of community-acquired pneumonia in adults, encompassing invasive pneumococcal disease and the prevalence of its associated cardiovascular events, with a focus on and macrolide antibiotics in pathogenesis and therapy. Int J Mol Sci. 2023;24(13):11038. https://doi.org/10.3390/ijms241311038.
63. Anderson R, Nel JG, Feldman C. Multifaceted role of pneumolysin in the pathogenesis of myocardial injury in community-acquired pneumonia. Int J Mol Sci. 2018;19(4):1147. https://doi.org/10.3390/ijms19041147.
64. Subramanian K, Neill DR, Malak HA, Spelmink L, Khandaker S, Dalla Libera Marchiori G, et al. Pneumolysin binds to the mannose receptor C type 1 (MRC-1) leading to anti-inflammatory responses and enhanced pneumococcal survival. Nat Microbiol. 2019;4(1):62–70. https://doi.org/10.1038/s41564-018-0280-x.
65. Grief SN, Loza JK. Guidelines for the evaluation and treatment of pneumonia. Prim Care. 2018;45(3):485–503. https://doi.org/10.1016/j.pop.2018.04.001.
66. Metlay JP, Waterer GW, Long AC, Anzueto A, Brozek J, Crothers K, et al. Diagnosis and treatment of adults with community-acquired pneumonia an official clinical practice guideline of the American Thoracic Society and Infectious Diseases Society of America. Am J Respir Crit Care Med. 2019;200(7):e45–67. https://doi.org/10.1164/rccm.201908-1581ST.
67. Cilloniz C, Rodriguez-Hurtado D, Torres A. Characteristics and management of community-acquired pneumonia in the era of global aging. Med Sci (Basel). 2018;6(2):35. https://doi.org/10.3390/medsci6020035.
68. NICE. National Institute for Health and Care Excellence; 2019. https://www.nice.org.uk/guidance/ng138
69. Chalmers J, Singanayagam A, Akram A. Severity assessment tools for predicting mortality in hospitalised patients with community-acquired pneumonia. Systematic review and meta-analysis. Thorax. 2010;65(10):878–83. https://doi.org/10.1136/thx.2009.133280.
70. Lim WS, van der Eerden MM, Laing R, Boersma WG, Karalus N, Town GI, et al. Defining community acquired pneumonia severity on presentation to hospital: an international derivation and validation study. Thorax. 2003;58(5):377–82. https://doi.org/10.1136/thorax.58.5.377.
71. ATS/IDSA; 2019. https://www.idsociety.org/practice-guideline/community-acquired-pneumonia-cap-in-adults/
72. https://www.fda.gov/news-events/press-announcements/fda-approves-new-treatment-pneumonia-caused-certain-difficult-treat-bacteria
73. https://clinicaltrials.gov/study/NCT03894046
74. Pakhal S, Mulpuru S, Verheii TJM, Kochen MM, Rohde GU, Bjerre LM, et al. Antibiotics for community-acquired pneumonia in adult outpatients. Cochrane Database Syst Rev. 2014;2014(10):CD002109. https://doi.org/10.1002/14651858.CD002109.pub4.
75. Cillóniz C, Polverino E, Ewig S, Aliberti S, Gabarrús A, Menéndez R, et al. Impact of age and comorbidity on cause and outcome in community-acquired pneumonia. Chest. 2013;144(3):999–1007. https://doi.org/10.1378/chest.13-0062.
76. CDC. https://www.cdc.gov/flu/about/index.html
77. WHO. https://www.who.int/news-room/fact-sheets/detail/influenza-(seasonal)
78. https://www.cdc.gov/flu/about/burden-prevented/2022-2023.htm#:~:text=Preliminary%20estimates%20of%20the%20burden,21%2C000%20flu%20deaths%20(9)
79. Choi SH, Chung JW, Kim T, Park KH, Lee MS, Kwak YG. Late diagnosis of influenza in adult patients during a seasonal outbreak. Korean J Intern Med. 2018;33(2):391–6. https://doi.org/10.3904/kjim.2016.226.
80. Ambrosch A, Luber D, Klawonn F, Kabesch M. Focusing on severe infections with the respiratory syncytial virus (RSV) in adults: risk factors, symptomatology and clinical course compared to influenza A/B and the original SARS-CoV-2 strain. J Clin Virol. 2023;161:105399. https://doi.org/10.1016/j.jcv.2023.105399.

81. Wilhelm M. Influenza in older patients: a call to action and recent updates for vaccinations. Am J Manag Care. 2018;24(2 Suppl):S15–24.
82. Kumari R, Sharma SD, Kumar A, Ende Z, Mishina M, Wang Y, et al. Antiviral approaches against influenza virus. Clin Microbiol Rev. 2023;36(1):e0004022. https://doi.org/10.1128/cmr.00040-22.
83. Yang J, Liu S, Du L, Jiang S. A new role of neuraminidase (NA) in the influenza virus life cycle: implication for developing NA inhibitors with novel mechanism of action. Rev Med Virol. 2016;26(4):242–50. https://doi.org/10.1002/rmv.1879.
84. Todd B, Tchesnokov EP, Gotte M. The active form of the influenza cap-snatching endonuclease inhibitor baloxavir marboxil is a tight binding inhibitor. J Biol Chem. 2021;296:100486. https://doi.org/10.1016/j.jbc.2021.100486.
85. Liu JW, Lin SH, Wang LC, Chiu HY, Lee JA. Comparison of antiviral agents for seasonal influenza outcomes in healthy adults and children: a systematic review and network meta-analysis. JAMA Netw Open. 2021;4(8):e2119151. https://doi.org/10.1001/jamanetworkopen.2021.19151.
86. Nakamura S, Miyazaki T, Izumikawa K, Kakeya H, Saisho Y, Yanagihara K, et al. Efficacy and safety of intravenous peramivir compared with oseltamivir in high-risk patients infected with influenza a and b viruses: a multicenter randomized controlled study. Open Forum Infect Dis. 2017;4(3):ofx129. https://doi.org/10.1093/ofid/ofx129.
87. Ison MG, Portsmouth S, Yoshida Y, Shishido T, Mitchener M, Tsuchiya K, et al. Early treatment with baloxavir marboxil in high-risk adolescent and adult outpatients with uncomplicated influenza (CAPSTONE-2): a randomised, placebo-controlled, phase 3 trial. Lancet Infect Dis. 2020;20(10):1204–14. https://doi.org/10.1016/S1473-3099(20)30004-9.
88. https://www.cdc.gov/tb/hcp/clinical-overview/index.html
89. Flynn JL, Chan J. Immune cell interactions in tuberculosis. Cell. 2022;185(25):4682–702. https://doi.org/10.1016/j.cell.2022.10.025.
90. Abbasnia S, Hashem Asnaashari AM, Sharebiani H, Soleimanpour S, Mosavat A, Rezaee SA. Mycobacterium tuberculosis and host interactions in the manifestation of tuberculosis. J Clin Tuberc Other Mycobact Dis. 2024;36:100458. https://doi.org/10.1016/j.jctube.2024.100458.
91. World Health Organization. Global tuberculosis report 2023. Geneva: 2023. ISBN: 9789240083851.
92. https://www.cdc.gov/tb/statistics/reports/2022/national_data.htm
93. Lewinsohn DM, Leonard MK, LoBue PA, Cohn DL, Daley CL, Desmond DE, et al. Official American Thoracic Society/Infectious Diseases Society of America/Centers for Disease Control and Prevention Clinical Practice Guidelines: Diagnosis of Tuberculosis in Adults and Children. Clin Infect Dis. 2017;64(2):e1–e33. https://doi.org/10.1093/cid/ciw694.
94. US Preventive Services Task Force, Mangione CM, Barry MJ, Nicholson WK, Cabana M, Chelmow D, Coker TR, et al. Screening for latent tuberculosis infection in dults: US Preventive Services Task Force recommendation statement. JAMA. 2023;329(17):1487–94. https://doi.org/10.1001/jama.2023.4899.
95. No authors listed. Targeted tuberculin testing and treatment of latent tuberculosis infection. Am J Respir Crit Care Med. 2000;161(4 Pt 2):S221–47. https://doi.org/10.1164/ajrccm.161.supplement_3.ats600.
96. Auguste P, Tsertsvadze A, Pink J, Court R, McCarthy N, Sutcliffe P. Comparing interferon-gamma release assays with tuberculin skin test for identifying latent tuberculosis infection that progresses to active tuberculosis: systematic review and meta-analysis. BMC Infect Dis. 2017;17(1):200. https://doi.org/10.1186/s12879-017-2301-4.
97. Agius E, Lacy KE, Mukmanovic-Stejic M, Jagger AL, Papageorgiou A-P, Hall S, et al. Decreased TNF-alpha synthesis by macrophages restricts cutaneous immunosurveillance by memory CD4+ T cells during aging. J Exp Med. 2009;206(9):1929–40. https://doi.org/10.1084/jem.20090896.

References

98. Zhou G, Luo Q, Luo S, He J, Chen N, Zhang Y, et al. Positive rates of interferon-gamma release assay and tuberculin skin test in detection of latent tuberculosis infection: a systematic review and meta-analysis of 200,000 head-to-head comparative tests. Clin Immunol. 2022;245:109132. https://doi.org/10.1016/j.clim.2022.109132.
99. Bayot ML, Mirza T, Sharma S. Acid fast bacteria. Treasure Island (FL): StatPearls Publishing; 2024.
100. Snider DE Jr. Pyridoxine supplementation during isoniazid therapy. Tubercle. 1980;61(4):191–6. https://doi.org/10.1016/0041-3879(80)90038-0.
101. Visser ME, Texeira-Swiegelaar C, Maartens G. The short-term effects of antituberculosis therapy on plasma pyridoxine levels in patients with pulmonary tuberculosis. Int J Tuberc Lung Dis. 2004;8(2):260–2.
102. Gallardo CR, Rigau Comas D, Valderrama Rodríguez A, Roqué i Figuls M, Parker LA, Caylà J, et al. Fixed-dose combinations of drugs versus single-drug formulations for treating pulmonary tuberculosis. Cochrane Database Syst Rev. 2016;2016(5):CD009913. https://doi.org/10.1002/14651858.CD009913.pub2.
103. Hosford JD, von Fricken ME, Lauzardo M, Chang M, Dai Y, Lyon JA, et al. Hepatotoxicity from antituberculous therapy in the elderly: a systematic review. Tuberculosis (Edinb). 2015;95(2):112–22. https://doi.org/10.1016/j.tube.2014.10.006.
104. https://www.cdc.gov/tb/media/pdfs/Latent-TB-Infection-A-Guide-for-Primary-Health-Care-Providers.pdf
105. WHO meeting report; 2020. https://www.who.int/publications/i/item/9789240018662
106. Pedersen OS, Holmgaard FB, Mikkelsen MKD, Lange C, Sotgiu G, Lillebaek T, et al. Global treatment outcomes of extensively drug-resistant tuberculosis in adults: a systematic review and meta-analysis. J Infect. 2023;87(3):177–89. https://doi.org/10.1016/j.jinf.2023.06.014.
107. Conradie F, Diacon AH, Ngubane N, Howell P, Everitt D, Crook AM, et al. Treatment of highly drug-resistant pulmonary tuberculosis. N Engl J Med. 2020;382(10):893–902. https://doi.org/10.1056/NEJMoa1901814.
108. Gils T, Lynen L, de Jong BC, Van Deun A, Decroo T. Pretomanid for tuberculosis: a systematic review. Clin Microbiol Infect. 2022;28(1):31–42. https://doi.org/10.1016/j.cmi.2021.08.007.
109. Rowe TA, Juthani-Mehta M. Diagnosis and management of urinary tract infection in older adults. Infect Dis Clin N Am. 2014;28(1):75–89. https://doi.org/10.1016/j.idc.2013.10.004.
110. Colgan R, Jaffe GA, Nicolle LE. Asymptomatic bacteriuria. Am Fam Physician. 2020;102(2):99–104.
111. Chu CM, Lowder JL. Diagnosis and treatment of urinary tract infections across age groups. Am J Obstet Gynecol. 2018;219(1):40–51. https://doi.org/10.1016/j.ajog.2017.12.231.
112. Klein RD, Hultgren SJ. Urinary tract infections: microbial pathogenesis, host-pathogen interactions and new treatment strategies. Nat Rev Microbiol. 2020;18(4):211–26. https://doi.org/10.1038/s41579-020-0324-0.
113. Deltourbe L, Mariano LL, Hreha TN, Hunstad DA, Ingersoll MA. The impact of biological sex on diseases of the urinary tract. Mucosal Immunol. 2022;15(5):857–66. https://doi.org/10.1038/s41385-022-00549-0.
114. Marques LP, Flores JT, de Barros O Jr, Rodrigues GB, de Medeiros MC, Moreira RMP. Epidemiological and clinical aspects of urinary tract infection in community-dwelling elderly women. Braz J Infect Dis. 2012;16(5):436–41. https://doi.org/10.1016/j.bjid.2012.06.025.
115. Eriksson I, Gustafson Y, Fagerstrom L, Olofsson B. Prevalence and factors associated with urinary tract infections (UTIs) in very old women. Arch Gerontol Geriatr. 2010;50(2):132–5. https://doi.org/10.1016/j.archger.2009.02.013.
116. https://www.ncbi.nlm.nih.gov/books/NBK572335/
117. Schaeffer AJ, Nicolle LE. Urinary tract infections in older men. N Engl J Med. 2016;374(6):562–71. https://doi.org/10.1056/NEJMcp1503950.
118. https://www.cdc.gov/nhsn/pdfs/pscmanual/7pscauticurrent.pdf

119. Tsan L, Langberg R, Davis C, Phillips Y, Pierce J, Hojlo C, et al. Nursing home-associated infections in Department of Veterans Affairs community living centers. Am J Infect Control. 2010;38(6):461–6. https://doi.org/10.1016/j.ajic.2009.12.009.
120. Cotter M, Donlon S, Roche F, Byrne H, Fitzpatrick F. Healthcare-associated infection in Irish long-term care facilities: results from the First National Prevalence Study. J Hosp Infect. 2012;80(3):212–6. https://doi.org/10.1016/j.jhin.2011.12.010.
121. Bettcher CM, Campbell E, Pretty LA, Rew KT, Zelnik JC, Lane GI, et al. Urinary Tract Infection [Internet]. Ann Arbor (MI): Michigan Medicine University of Michigan; 2021. Bookshelf ID: NBK572335
122. https://www.cdc.gov/uti/about/index.html
123. Arinzon Z, Shabat S, Peisakh A, Berner Y. Clinical presentation of urinary tract infection (UTI) differs with aging in women. Arch Gerontol Geriatr. 2012;55(1):145–7. https://doi.org/10.1016/j.archger.2011.07.012.
124. Nicolle LE. Asymptomatic bacteriuria in the elderly. Infect Dis Clin N Am. 1997;11(3):647–62. https://doi.org/10.1016/s0891-5520(05)70378-0.
125. Knottnerus BJ, Geerlings SE, Moll Van Charante EP, ter Riet G. Women with symptoms of uncomplicated urinary tract infection are often willing to delay antibiotic treatment: a prospective cohort study. BMC Fam Pract. 2013;14:71. https://doi.org/10.1186/1471-2296-14-71.
126. Singer M, Deutschman CS, Seymour CW, Shankar-Hari M, Annane D, Bauer M, et al. The third international consensus definitions for sepsis and septic shock (Sepsis-3). JAMA. 2016;315(8):801–10. https://doi.org/10.1001/jama.2016.0287.
127. WHO. Global report on the epidemiology and burden of sepsis: current evidence, identifying gaps and future directions. Geneva, Switzerland: World Health Organization; 2020.
128. Rudd KE, Johnson SC, Agesa KM, Shackelford KA, Tsoi D, Kievlan DR, et al. Global, regional, and national sepsis incidence and mortality, 1990–2017: analysis for the global burden of disease study. Lancet. 2020;395(10219):200–11. https://doi.org/10.1016/S0140-6736(19)32989-7.
129. Kingren MS, Starr ME, Saito H. Divergent sepsis pathophysiology in older adults. Antioxid Redox Signal. 2021;35(16):1358–75. https://doi.org/10.1089/ars.2021.005.
130. NCHS Data Brief. https://www.cdc.gov/nchs/products/databriefs/db422.htm.
131. National vital statistics system, United States, 2021. MMWR Morb Mortal Wkly Rep. 2023;72:1043. https://doi.org/10.15585/mwr7238a5
132. Esper AM, Moss M, Lewis CA, Nisbet R, Mannino DM, Martin GS. The role of infection and comorbidity; factors that influence disparities in sepsis. Crit Care Med. 2006;34(10):2576–82. https://doi.org/10.1097/01.CCM.0000239114.50519.0E.
133. Kumar A, Roberts D, Wood KE, Light B, Parrillo JE, Sharma S, et al. Duration of hypotension before initiation of effective antimicrobial therapy is the critical determinant of survival in human septic shock. Crit Care Med. 2006;34(6):1589–96. https://doi.org/10.1097/01.CCM.0000217961.75225.E9.
134. Ferrer R, Martin-Loeches I, Phillips G, Osborn TM, Townsend S, Dellinger RP, et al. Empiric antibiotic treatment reduces mortality in severe sepsis and septic shock from the first hour: results from a guideline-based performance improvement program. Crit Care Med. 2014;42(8):1749–55. https://doi.org/10.1097/CCM.0000000000000330.
135. WHO. https://www.who.int/news-room/fact-sheets/detail/sepsis#:~:text=lack%20of%20urination.-,Prevention,home%20and%20in%20healthcare%20settings
136. Guarino M, Perna B, Cesaro AE, Maritati M, Spampinato MD, Contini C, et al. Update on sepsis and septic shock in adult patients: management in the emergency department. J Clin Med. 2023;12(9):3188. https://doi.org/10.3390/jcm12093188.
137. Clifford KM, Dy-Boarman EA, Haase KK, Maxvill K, Pass SE, Alvarez CA. Challenges with diagnosing and managing sepsis in older adults. Expert Rev Anti-Infect Ther. 2016;14(2):231–41. https://doi.org/10.1586/14787210.2016.1135052.
138. van Duin D. Diagnostic challenges and opportunities in older adults with infectious disease. Clin Infect Dis. 2012;54(7):973–8. https://doi.org/10.1093/cid/cir927.

139. Downton JH, Andrews K, Puxty JA. 'Silent' pyrexia in the elderly. Age Ageing. 1987;16(1):41–4. https://doi.org/10.1093/ageing/16.1.41.
140. Assicot M, Gendrel D, Carsin H, Raymond J, Guilbaud J, Bohuon C. High serum procalcitonin concentrations in patients with sepsis and infection. Lancet. 1993;341(8844):515–8. https://doi.org/10.1016/0140-6736(93)90277-n.
141. Belousoviene E, Kiudulaite I, Pilvinis V, Pranskunas A. Links between endothelial glycocalyx changes and microcirculatory parameters in septic patients. Life. 2021;11(8):790. https://doi.org/10.3390/life11080790.
142. Caironi P, Tognoni G, Masson S, Fumagalli R, Pesenti A, Romero M, et al. Albumin replacement in patients with severe sepsis or septic shock. N Engl J Med. 2014;370:1412–21. https://doi.org/10.1056/NEJMoa1305727.
143. Falcone M, Paul M, Tiseo G, Yahav D, Prendki V, Friberg LE, et al. Considerations for the optimal management of antibiotic therapy in elderly patients. J Glob Antimicrob Resist. 2020;22:325–33. https://doi.org/10.1016/j.jgar.2020.02.022.
144. Mazzei T. The difficulties of polytherapy: examples from antimicrobial chemotherapy. Intern Emerg Med. 2011;6 Suppl 1:103–9. https://doi.org/10.1007/s11739-011-0680-x.
145. Iwamoto M, Wenning LA, Nguyen BY, Teppler H, Moreau AR, Rhodes RR, et al. Effects of omeprazole on plasma levels of raltegravir. Clin Infect Dis. 2009;48(4):489–92. https://doi.org/10.1086/596503.
146. Winston A, Back D, Fletcher C, Robinson L, Unsworth J, Tolowinska I, et al. Effect of omeprazole on the pharmacokinetics of saquinavir-500 mg formulation with ritonavir in healthy male and female volunteers. AIDS. 2006;20(10):1401–6. https://doi.org/10.1097/01.aids.0000233573.41597.8a.
147. Ulldemolins M, Rello J. The relevance of drug volume of distribution in antibiotic dosing. Curr Pharm Biotechnol. 2011;12(12):1996–2001. https://doi.org/10.2174/138920111798808365.
148. Rolan PE. Plasma protein binding displacement interactions—why are they still regarded as clinically important? Br J Clin Pharmacol. 1994;37(2):125–8. https://doi.org/10.1111/j.1365-2125.1994.tb04251.x.
149. Butranova OL, Ushkalova EA, Zyryanv SK, Chunkurov MS, Baybulatova EA. Pharmacokinetics of antibacterial agents in the elderly: the body of evidence. Biomedicines. 2023;11(6):1633. https://doi.org/10.3390/biomedicines11061633.
150. Drozdzik M, Lapczuk-Romanska J, Wenzel C, Skalski L, Szeląg-Pieniek S, Post M, et al. Protein abundance of drug metabolizing enzymes in human hepatitis C livers. Int J Mol Sci. 2023;24(5):4543. https://doi.org/10.3390/ijms24054543.
151. Zeeh J, Platt D. The aging liver: structural and functional changes and their consequences for drug treatment in old age. Gerontology. 2002;48(3):121–7. https://doi.org/10.1159/000052829.
152. Wynne H. Drug metabolism and ageing. J Br Menopause Soc. 2005;11(2):51–6. https://doi.org/10.1258/136218005775544589.
153. Davies EA, O'Mahony MS. Adverse drug reactions in special populations—the elderly. Br J Clin Pharmacol. 2015;80(4):796–807. https://doi.org/10.1111/bcp.12596.
154. Giarratano A, Green SE, Nicolau DP. Review of antimicrobial use and considerations in the elderly population. Clin Interv Aging. 2018, Apr 17;13:657–67. https://doi.org/10.2147/CIA.S133640.
155. Noreddin AM, Haynes V. Use of pharmacodynamic principles to optimise dosage regimens for antibacterial agents in the elderly. Drugs Aging. 2007;24(4):275–92. https://doi.org/10.2165/00002512-200724040-00002.
156. Shlipak MG, Mattes MD, Peralta CA. Update on cystatin C: incorporation into clinical practice. Am J Kidney Dis. 2013;62(3):595–603. https://doi.org/10.1053/j.ajkd.2013.03.027.
157. Pea F. Antimicrobial treatment of bacterial infections in frail elderly patients: the difficult balance between efficacy, safety and tolerability. Curr Opin Pharmacol. 2015;24:18–22. https://doi.org/10.1016/j.coph.2015.06.006.

158. Robertson AD, Li C, Hammond DA, Dickey TA. Incidence of acute kidney injury among patients receiving the combination of vancomycin with piperacillin-Tazobactam or Meropenem. Pharmacotherapy. 2018;38:1184–93.
159. Crochette R, Ravaiau C, Perez L, Coindre JP, Piccoli GB, Blanchi S. Incidence and risk factors for acute kidney injury during the treatment of methicillin-sensitive staphylococcus aureus infections with Cloxacillin based antibiotic regimens: a French retrospective study. J Clin Med. 2021;10(12):2603. https://doi.org/10.3390/jcm10122603.
160. Chinzowu T, Roy S, Nishtala PS. Risk of antimicrobial-associated organ injury among the older adults: a systematic review and meta-analysis. BMC Geriatr. 2021;21(1):617. https://doi.org/10.1186/s12877-021-02512-3.
161. Selby NM, Shaw S, Woodier N, Fluck RJ, Kolhe NV. Gentamicin-associated acute kidney injury. QJM. 2009;102(12):873–80. https://doi.org/10.1093/qjmed/hcp143.
162. Oliveira JF, Silva CA, Barbieri CD, Oliveira GM, Zanetta DM, Burdmann EA. Prevalence and risk factors for aminoglycoside nephrotoxicity in intensive care units. Antimicrob Agents Chemother. 2009;53(7):2887–91. https://doi.org/10.1128/AAC.01430-08.
163. By the 2023 American Geriatrics Society Beers Criteria® Update Expert Panel. American Geriatrics Society 2023 updated AGS Beers Criteria® for potentially inappropriate medication use in older adults. J Am Geriatr Soc. 2023;71(7):2052–81. https://doi.org/10.1111/jgs.18372.
164. Antoniou T, Gomes T, Mamdani MM, Juurlink DN. Trimethoprim/sulfamethoxazole-induced phenytoin toxicity in the elderly: a population-based study. Br J Clin Pharmacol. 2011;71(4):544–9. https://doi.org/10.1111/j.1365-2125.2010.03866.x.
165. Purkins L, Wood N, Kleinermans D, Nichols D. Voriconazole potentiates warfarin-induced prothrombin time prolongation. Br J Clin Pharmacol. 2003;56(Suppl 1):24–9. https://doi.org/10.1046/j.1365-2125.2003.01995.x.
166. Rodin SM, Johnson BF. Pharmacokinetic interactions with digoxin. Clin Pharmacokinet. 1988;15(4):227–44. https://doi.org/10.2165/00003088-198815040-00003.
167. Rengelshausen J, Göggelmann C, Burhenne J, Riedel KD, Ludwig J, Weiss J, et al. Contribution of increased oral bioavailability and reduced nonglomerular renal clearance of digoxin to the digoxin-clarithromycin interaction. Br J Clin Pharmacol. 2003;56(1):32–8. https://doi.org/10.1046/j.1365-2125.2003.01824.x.
168. Elli C, Novella A, Pasina L. Serotonin syndrome: a pharmacovigilance comparative study of drugs affecting serotonin levels. Eur J Clin Pharmacol. 2024;80(2):231–7. https://doi.org/10.1007/s00228-023-03596-z.
169. Dobrek L. A synopsis of current theories on drug-induced nephrotoxicity. Life (Basel). 2023;13(2):325. https://doi.org/10.3390/life13020325.
170. Hung Y-P, Chen P-L, Ho C-Y, Hsieh C-C, Lee C-H, Lee C-C, Ko W-C. Prognostic effects of inappropriate empirical antimicrobial therapy in adults with community-onset bacteremia: age matters. Front Med (Lausanne). 2022;9:861032. https://doi.org/10.3389/fmed.2022.861032.
171. Jacobson KL, Cohen SH, Inciardi JF, King JH, Lippert WE, Iglesias T, et al. The relationship between antecedent antibiotic use and resistance to extended-spectrum cephalosporins in group I beta-lactamase-producing organisms. Clin Infect Dis. 1995;21(5):1107–13. https://doi.org/10.1093/clinids/21.5.1107.
172. Castanheira M, Kimbrough JH, DeVries S, Mendes RE, Sader HS. Trends of beta-lactamase occurrence among Escherichia coli and Klebsiella pneumoniae in United States hospitals during a 5-year period and activity of antimicrobial agents against isolates stratified by beta-lactamase type. Open Forum Infect Dis. 2023;10(2):ofad038. https://doi.org/10.1093/ofid/ofad038.
173. IDSA. https://www.idsociety.org/practice-guideline/amr-guidance
174. Ball P, Baquero F, Cars O, File T, Garau, Klugman K, et al. Antibiotic therapy of community respiratory tract infections: strategies for optimal outcomes and minimized resistance emergence. J Antimicrob Chemother. 2002;49(1):31–40. https://doi.org/10.1093/jac/49.1.31.
175. https://www.who.int/publications/i/item/2021-aware-classification
176. https://www.cdc.gov/vaccines/schedules/hcp/imz/child-adolescent.html

References

177. Swanson KA, Schmitt HJ, Jansen KU, Anderson AS. Adult vaccination. Hum Vaccin Immunother. 2015;11(1):150–5. https://doi.org/10.4161/hv.35858.
178. Del Riccio M, Boccalini S, Cosma C, Vaccaro G, Bonito B, Zanella B, et al. Effectiveness of pneumococcal vaccination on hospitalization and death in the adult and older adult diabetic population: a systematic review. Expert Rev Vaccines. 2023;22(1):1179–84. https://doi.org/10.1080/14760584.2023.2286374.
179. Remy V, Zollner Y, Heckmann U. Vaccination: the cornerstone of an efficient healthcare system. J Mark Access Health Policy. 2015;3:27041. https://doi.org/10.3402/jmahp.v3.27041.
180. Kobayashi M, Farrar JL, Gierke R, Britton A, Childs L, Leidner AJ, et al. Use of 15-valent pneumococcal conjugate vaccine and 20-valent pneumococcal conjugate vaccine among U.S. adults: updated recommendations of the Advisory Committee on Immunization Practices—United States, 2022. MMWR Morb Mortal Wkly Rep. 2022;71(4):109–17. https://doi.org/10.15585/mmwr.mm7104a1.
181. Lee JKH, Lam GKL, Yin JK, Loiacono MM, Samson SI. High-dose influenza vaccine in older adults by age and seasonal characteristics: systematic review and meta-analysis update. Vaccine X. 2023;14:100327. https://doi.org/10.1016/j.jvacx.2023.100327.
182. https://www.cdc.gov/vaccines/schedules/hcp/imz/adult.html
183. Dunkle LM, Kotloff KL, Gay CL, Anez G, Adelglass JM, Barrat AQ, et al. Efficacy and safety of NVX-CoV2373 in adults in the United States and Mexico. N Engl J Med. 2022;386(6):531–43. https://doi.org/10.1056/NEJMoa2116185.
184. Fiolet T, Kherabi Y, MacDonald CJ, Ghosn J, Peiffer-Smadja N. Comparing COVID-19 vaccines for their characteristics, efficacy and effectiveness against SARS-CoV-2 and variants of concern: a narrative review. Clin Microbiol Infect. 2022;28(2):202–21. https://doi.org/10.1016/j.cmi.2021.10.005.
185. Marra Y, Lalji F. Prevention of herpes zoster: a focus on the effectiveness and safety of herpes zoster vaccines. Viruses. 2022;14(12):2667. https://doi.org/10.3390/v14122667.
186. Farrar JL, Childs L, Ouattara M, Akhter F, Britton A, Pilishvili T, et al. Systematic review and meta-analysis of the efficacy and effectiveness of pneumococcal vaccines in adults. Pathogens. 2023;12(5):732. https://doi.org/10.3390/pathogens12050732.
187. Riccò M, Cascio A, Corrado S, Bottazzoli M, Marchesi F, Gili R, et al. Efficacy of respiratory syncytial virus vaccination to prevent lower respiratory tract illness in older adults: a systematic review and meta-analysis of randomized controlled trials. Vaccines (Basel). 2024;12(5):500. https://doi.org/10.3390/vaccines12050500.
188. Khader SA, Divangahi M, Hanekom W, Hill PC, Maeurer M, Makar KW, et al. Targeting innate immunity for tuberculosis vaccination. J Clin Invest. 2019;129:3482–91. https://doi.org/10.1172/JCI128877.
189. Qu M, Zhou X. Li H BCG vaccination strategies against tuberculosis: updates and perspectives. Hum Vaccin Immunother. 2021;17(12):5284–95. https://doi.org/10.1080/21645515.2021.2007711.
190. Tait DR, Hatherill M, Van Der Meeren O, Ginsberg AM, Van Brakel E, Salaun B, et al. Final analysis of a trial of M72/AS01E vaccine to prevent tuberculosis. N Engl JMed. 2019;381(25):2429–39. https://doi.org/10.1056/NEJMoa1909953.
191. Lv B, Gao X, Zeng G, Guo H, Li F. Safety profile of Paxlovid in the treatment of COVID-19. Curr Pharm Des. 2024;30(9):666–75. https://doi.org/10.2174/0113816128280987240214103432.
192. Llor C, Perez A, Carandel E, Garci-Sangenis A, Rezola J. Efficacy of high doses of penicillin versus amoxicillin in the treatment of uncomplicated community acquired pneumonia in adults. A non-inferiority controlled clinical trial. Aten Primaria. 2019;51(1):32–9. https://doi.org/10.1016/j.aprim.2017.08.003.
193. Dinh A, Ropers J, Duran C, Davido B, Deconinck L, Matt M, et al. Discontinuing beta-lactam treatment after 3 days for patients with community-acquired pneumonia in non-critical care wards (PTC): a double-blind, randomised, placebo-controlled, non-inferiority trial. Pneumonia Short Treatment (PTC) Study Group. Lancet. 2021;397(10280):1195–203.

194. Mokabberi R, Haftbaradaran A, Ravakhah KJ. Doxycycline vs. levofloxacin in the treatment of community-acquired pneumonia. Clin Pharm Ther. 2010;35(2):195–200. https://doi.org/10.1111/j.1365-2710.2009.01073.x.
195. Paris R, Confalonieri M, Dal Negro R, Ligia GP, Mos L, Todisco T, et al. Efficacy and safety of azithromycin 1 g once daily for 3 days in the treatment of community-acquired pneumonia: an open-label randomised comparison with amoxicillin-clavulanate 875/125 mg twice daily for 7 days. J Chemother. 2008;20(1):77–86. https://doi.org/10.1179/joc.2008.20.1.77.
196. English ML, Fredericks CE, Milanesio NA, Rohowsky N, Xu Z-Q, Jenta TRJ, et al. Cethromycin versus clarithromycin for community-acquired pneumonia: comparative efficacy and safety outcomes from two double-blinded, randomized, parallel-group, multicenter, multinational noninferiority studies. Antimicrob Agents Chemother. 2012;56(4):2037–47. https://doi.org/10.1128/AAC.05596-11.
197. Peterson J, Yektashenas B, Fisher AC. Levofloxacin for the treatment of pneumonia caused by Streptococcus pneumoniae including multidrug-resistant strains: pooled analysis. Curr Med Res Opin. 2009;25(3):559–68. https://doi.org/10.1185/03007990802694741.
198. Oldach D, Clark K, Schranz J, Das A, Craft JC, Scott D, et al. Randomized, double-blind, multicentre phase 2 study comparing the efficacy and safety of oral solithromycin (CEM-101) to those of oral levofloxacin in the treatment of patients with community-acquired bacterial pneumonia. Antimicrob Agents Chemother. 2013;57(6):2526–34. https://doi.org/10.1128/AAC.00197-13.
199. Zhang J, Chen L, Gomez-Simmonds A, Yin MT, Freedberg DE. Antibiotic-specific risk for community-acquired *Clostridioides difficile* infection in the United States from 2008 to 2020. Antimicrob Agents Chemother. 2022;66(12):e01129–2. https://doi.org/10.1128/aac.01129-22.
200. Stahlmann R, Lode H. Safety considerations of fluoroquinolones in the elderly: an update. Drugs Aging. 2010;27:193–209. https://doi.org/10.2165/11531490-000000000-00000.
201. Faulkner CM, Cox HL, Williamson JC. Unique aspects of antimicrobial use in older adults. Clin Infect Dis. 2005;40:997–1004. https://doi.org/10.1086/428125.
202. Mattappalil A, Mergenhagen KA. Neurotoxicity with antimicrobials in the elderly: a review. Clin Ther. 2014;36:1489–511.e4. https://doi.org/10.1016/j.clinthera.2014.09.020.
203. Dorman SE, Savic RM, Goldberg S, Stout JE, Schluger N, Muzanyi G, et al. Daily rifapentine for treatment of pulmonary tuberculosis. A randomized, dose-ranging trial. Am J Respir Crit Care Med. 2015;191(3):333–43. https://doi.org/10.1164/rccm.201410-1843OC.
204. Prasad R, Singh A, Gupta N. Adverse drug reactions in tuberculosis and management. Indian J Tuberc. 2019;66(4):520–32. https://doi.org/10.1016/j.ijtb.2019.11.005.
205. Huttner A, Kowalczyk A, Turjeman A, Babich T, Brossier C, Eliakim-Raz N. Effect of 5-day nitrofurantoin vs single-dose Fosfomycin on clinical resolution of uncomplicated lower urinary tract infection in women: a randomized clinical trial. JAMA. 2018;319(17):1781–9. https://doi.org/10.1001/jama.2018.3627.
206. Hanlon JT, Perera S, Schweon S, Drinka P, Crnich C, Nace DA. Improvements in antibiotic appropriateness for cystitis in older nursing home residents: a quality improvement study with randomized assignment. J Am Med Dir Assoc. 2021;22(1):173–7. https://doi.org/10.1016/j.jamda.2020.07.040.
207. Etienne M, Lefebvre E, Frebourg N, Hamel H, Pestel-Caron M, Caron F, et al. Antibiotic treatment of acute uncomplicated cystitis based on rapid urine test and local epidemiology: lessons from a primary care series. BMC Infect Dis. 2014;14:137. https://doi.org/10.1186/1471-2334-14-137.
208. Raz R, Rottensterich E, Boger S, Potasman I. Comparison of single-dose administration and three-day course of amoxicillin with those of clavulanic acid for treatment of uncomplicated urinary tract infection in women. Antimicrob Agents Chemother. 1991;35(8):1688–90. https://doi.org/10.1128/AAC.35.8.1688.

209. Raz R, Rottensterich E, Leshem Y, Tabenkin H. Double-blind study comparing 3-day regimens of cefixime and ofloxacin in treatment of uncomplicated urinary tract infections in women. Antimicrob Agents Chemother. 1994;38(5):1176–7. https://doi.org/10.1128/AAC.38.5.1176.
210. Kaye KS, Belley A, Barth P, Lahlou O, Knechtle P, Motta P. Effect of cefepime/enmetazobactam vs piperacillin/tazobactam on clinical cure and microbiological eradication in patients with complicated urinary tract infection or acute pyelonephritis: a randomized clinical trial. JAMA. 2022;328(13):1304–14. https://doi.org/10.1001/jama.2022.17034.
211. Kyriazopoulou E, Liaskou-Antoniou L, Adamis G, Panagaki A, Melachroinopoulos N, Drakou E, et al. Procalcitonin to reduce long-term infection-associated adverse events in sepsis. A randomized trial. Am J Respir Crit Care Med. 2021;203(2):202–10. https://doi.org/10.1164/rccm.202004-1201OC.
212. Brown RM, Wang L, Coston TD, Krishnan NI, Casey JD, Wanderer J, et al. Balanced crystalloids versus saline in sepsis. A secondary analysis of the SMART clinical trial. Am J Respir Care Med. 2019;200(12):1487–95. https://doi.org/10.1164/rccm.201903-0557OC.
213. Mouncey PR, Osborn TM, Power GS, Harrison DA, Sadique MZ, Grieve RD. Trial of early, goal-directed resuscitation for septic shock. N Engl J Med. 2015;372(14):1301–11. https://doi.org/10.1056/NEJMoa1500896.
214. https://www.fda.gov/media/151707/download?attachment
215. https://www.fda.gov/vaccines-blood-biologics/spikevax
216. CDC. https://www.cdc.gov/coronavirus/2019-ncov/vaccines/different-vaccines/overview-COVID-19-vaccines.html
217. https://www.cdc.gov/vaccines/vpd/pneumo/index.html
218. Lee JKH, Lam GKL, Shin T, Samson SI, Greenberg DP, Chit A. Efficacy and effectiveness of high-dose influenza vaccine in older adults by circulating strain and antigenic match: an updated systematic review and meta-analysis. Vaccine. 2021;39 Suppl 1:A24–35. https://doi.org/10.1016/j.vaccine.2020.09.004.
219. Osterholm MT, Kelley NS, Sommer A, Belongia EA. Efficacy and effectiveness of influenza vaccines: a systematic review and meta-analysis. Lancet Infect Dis. 2012;12(1):36–44. https://doi.org/10.1016/S1473-3099(11)70295-X.
220. https://www.cdc.gov/flu/season/faq-flu-season-2024-2025.htm
221. https://www.cdc.gov/vaccines/vpd/rsv/hcp/older-adults.(html#:~:text=The%20RSV%20vaccine%20is%20not,risk%20of%20severe%20RSV%20disease
222. Shah RA, Limmer AL, Nwannunu CE, Patel RR, Mui UN, Tyring SK. Shingrix for herpes zoster: a review. Skin Therapy Lett. 2019;24(4):5–7. PMID: 31339679
223. https://www.cdc.gov/vaccines/vpd/shingles/hcp/shingrix/recommendations.html
224. Mörike K, Schwab M, Klotz U. Use of aminoglycosides in elderly patients. Pharmacokinetic and clinical considerations. Drugs Aging. 1997;10:259–77. https://doi.org/10.2165/00002512-199710040-00003.
225. Mizokami F, Mizuno T. Acute kidney injury induced by antimicrobial agents in the elderly: awareness and mitigation strategies. Drugs Aging. 2015;32:1–12. https://doi.org/10.1007/s40266-014-0232-y.
226. Khan S, Loi V, Rosner MH. Drug-induced kidney injury in the elderly. Drugs Aging. 2017;34:729–41. https://doi.org/10.1007/s40266-017-0484-4.
227. Al-Hasan MN, Al-Jaghbeer MJ. Use of antibiotics in chronic obstructive pulmonary disease: what is their current role in older patients? Drugs Aging. 2020;37:627–33. https://doi.org/10.1007/s40266-020-00786-7.
228. Maisch NM, Kochupurackal JG, Sin J. Azithromycin and the risk of cardiovascular complications. J Pharm Pract. 2014;27:496–500. https://doi.org/10.1177/0897190013516503.
229. Bangert MK, Hasbun R. Neurological and psychiatric adverse effects of antimicrobials. CNS Drugs. 2019;33:727–53. https://doi.org/10.1007/s40263-019-00649-9.
230. Patel S, Saw S. Daptomycin. Treasure Island: StatPearls Publishing; 2022.
231. Shenoy ES, Macy E, Rowe T, Blumenthal KG. Evaluation and management of penicillin allergy: a review. JAMA.2019;321:188–99. https://doi.org/10.1001/jama.2018.19283.

232. Vardakas KZ, Kalimeris GD, Triarides NA, Falagas ME. An update on adverse drug reactions related to β-lactam antibiotics.Expert Opin Drug Saf. 2018;17:499–508. https://doi.org/10.1080/14740338.2018.1462334.
233. Lagacé-Wiens P, Rubinstein E. Adverse reactions to β-lactam antimicrobials. Expert Opin Drug Saf. 2012;11:381–99. https://doi.org/10.1517/14740338.2012.643866.
234. McDonald LC, Gerding DN, Johnson S, Bakken JS, Carroll KC, Coffin SE, et al. Clinical Practice Guidelines for Clostridium difficile Infection in Adults and Children: 2017 Update by the Infectious Diseases Society of America (IDSA) and Society for Healthcare Epidemiologyof America (SHEA). Clin Infect Dis. 2018;66:987–94. https://doi.org/10.1093/cid/ciy149.
235. Lucena MI, Sanabria J, García-Cortes M, Stephens C, Andrade RJ. Drug-induced liver injury in older people. Lancet Gastroenterol Hepatol. 2020;5:862–74. https://doi.org/10.1016/s2468-1253(20)30006-6.
236. Wang N, Nguyen PK, Pham CU, Smith EA, Kim B, Goetz MB,Graber CJ. Sodium Content of intravenous antibiotic preparations. Open forum Infect Dis. 2019;6:ofz508. https://doi.org/10.1093/ofid/ofz508.
237. Deshayes S, Coquerel A, Verdon R. Neurological adverse effects attributable to β-lactam antibiotics: a literature review. Drug Saf. 2017;40:1171–98. https://doi.org/10.1007/s40264-017-0578-2.
238. Zareifopoulos N, Panayiotakopoulos G. Neuropsychiatric effects of antimicrobial agents. Clin Drug Investig. 2017;37:423–37. https://doi.org/10.1007/s40261-017-0498-z.
239. Payne LE, Gagnon DJ, Riker RR, Seder DB, Glisic EK, Morris JG. Cefepime-induced neurotoxicity: a systematic review. Crit Care. 2017;21:276. https://doi.org/10.1186/s13054-017-1856-1.
240. Alves C, Mendes D, Marques FB. Fluoroquinolones and the risk of tendon injury: a systematic review and meta-analysis.Eur J Clin Pharmacol. 2019;75:1431–43. https://doi.org/10.1007/s00228-019-02713-1.
241. Tanne JH. FDA adds "black box" warning label to fluoroquinolone antibiotics. Br Med J. 2008;337(7662):816. https://doi.org/10.1136/bmj.a816.
242. Dekkers BGJ, Veringa A, Marriott DJE, Boonstra JM, van der Elst KCM, Doukas FF, McLachlan AJ, Alffenaar J-WC. Invasive candidiasis in the elderly: considerations for drug therapy. Drugs Aging. 2018;35:781–9. https://doi.org/10.1007/s40266-018-0576-9.
243. Stine JG, Sateesh P, Lewis JH. Drug-induced liver injury in the elderly. Curr Gastroenterol Rep. 2013;15:299. https://doi.org/10.1007/s11894-012-0299-8.
244. Drew WL, Buhles W, Erlich KS. Herpesvirus infections (cytomegalovirus, herpes simplex virus, varicella-zoster virus). How to use ganciclovir (DHPG) and acyclovir. Infect Dis Clin N Am.1988;2:495–509.
245. US FDA. Zovirax (Aciclovyr) [package insert]. https://www.accessdata.fda.gov/drugsatfda_docs/label/2005/018828s030,020089s019,019909s020lbl.pdf. Accessed 1 Sep 2022.
246. Brandariz-Nunez D, Correas-Sanahuja M, Maya-Gallego S, Martín Herranz I. Neurotoxicity associated with acyclovir and valacyclovir: a systematic review of cases. J Clin Pharm Ther. 2021;46:918–26. https://doi.org/10.1111/jcpt.13464.
247. US FDA. Ganciclovir (Ganciclovir) [package insert]. https://www.accessdata.fda.gov/drugsatfda_docs/label/2017/209347lbl.pdf. Accessed 1 Sep 2022.
248. US FDA. Remdesivir (Veklury) [package insert]. https://www.accessdata.fda.gov/drugsatfda_docs/label/2020/214787Orig1s000lbl.pdf. Accessed 1 Sep 2022.
249. European Medicines Agency. Molnupiravir (Lagevrio) [package insert]. https://www.ema.europa.eu/en/documents/referral/lagevrioalso-known-molnupiravir-mk-4482-covid-19-article-53-procedure-conditions-use-conditions_en.pdf
250. US FDA. Foscarnet (Foscavir) [package insert]. https://www.accessdata.fda.gov/drugsatfda_docs/label/2012/020068s018lbl.pdf. Accessed 1 Sep 2022.
251. US FDA. Oseltamivir (Tamiflu) [package insert]. https://www.accessdata.fda.gov/drugsatfda_docs/label/2011/021087s057lbl.pdf. Accessed 1 Sep 2022.

252. Electronic Medicines Compendium. Zanamivir (Ralenza) [package insert]. https://www.medicines.org.uk/emc/product/3809/smpc. Accessed 1 Sep 2022.
253. Sleijfer S, Bannink M, Van Gool AR, Kruit WH, Stoter G. Side effects of interferon-alpha therapy. Pharm World Sci. 2005;27:423–31. https://doi.org/10.1007/s11096-005-1319-7.
254. Li L, Wang X, Wang R, Hu Y, Jiang S, Lu X. Antiviral Agent therapy optimization in special populations of COVID-19 patients. Drug Des Devel Ther. 2020;14:3001–13. https://doi.org/10.2147/dddt.S259058.
255. Jourjy J, Dahl K, Huesgen E. Antiretroviral treatment efficacy and safety in older HIV-infected adults. Pharmacotherapy. 2015;35:1140–51. https://doi.org/10.1002/phar.1670.
256. Kayaaslan B, Guner R. Adverse effects of oral antiviral therapy in chronic hepatitis B. World J Hepatol. 2017;9:227–41. https://doi.org/10.4254/wjh.v9.i5.227.
257. Benedicto AM, Fuster-Martínez I, Tosca J, Esplugues JV, Blas-García A, Apostolova N. NNRTI and liver damage: evidence of their association and the mechanisms involved. Cells. 2021. https://doi.org/10.3390/cells10071687.
258. US FDA. Epavirenz (Sustiva) [package insert]. https://www.accessdata.fda.gov/drugsatfda_docs/label/2011/020972s038lbl.pdf. Accessed 1 Sep 2022.
259. Tsiodras S, Perelas A, Wanke C, Mantzoros CS. The HIV-1/HAART associated metabolic syndrome—novel adipokines, molecular associations and therapeutic implications. J Infect. 2010;61:101–13. https://doi.org/10.1016/j.jinf.2010.06.002.
260. US FDA. Ritonavir (Norvir) [package insert]. https://www.accessdata.fda.gov/drugsatfda_docs/label/2017/209512lbl.pdf. Accessed 1 Sep 2022.
261. Kyriakidis I, Tragiannidis A, Munchen S, Groll AH. Clinical hepatotoxicity associated with antifungal agents. Expert Opin Drug Saf. 2017;16:149–65. https://doi.org/10.1080/14740338.2017.1270264.
262. Mourad A, Perfect JR. Tolerability profile of the current antifungal armoury. J Antimicrob Chemother. 2018;73:i26–32. https://doi.org/10.1093/jac/dkx446.
263. Kauffman CA. Fungal infections in older adults. Clin Infect Dis. 2001;33:550–5. https://doi.org/10.1086/322685.
264. Soares JR, Nunes MC, Leite AF, Falqueto EB, Lacerda BE, Ferrari TC. Reversible dilated cardiomyopathy associated with amphotericin B therapy. J Clin Pharm Ther. 2015;40:333–5. https://doi.org/10.1111/jcpt.12237.
265. Oliveira JFP, Silva CA, Barbieri CD, Oliveira GM, Zanetta DMT, Burdmann EA. Prevalence and risk factors for aminoglycoside nephrotoxicity in intensive care units. Antimicrob Agents Chemother. 2009;53:2887–91. https://doi.org/10.1128/AAC.01430-08.
266. US FDA. Amoxicillin (Amoxil) [package insert]. https://www.accessdata.fda.gov/drugsatfda_docs/label/2008/050542s24,050754s11,050760s10,050761s10lbl.pdf. Accessed 15 Feb 2023.
267. US FDA. Ampicillin/sulbactam (Unasyn) [package insert]. https://www.accesssdata.fda.gov/drugsatfda_docs/label/2008/050608s029lbl.pdf. Accessed 15 Feb 2023.
268. US FDA. Ciprofloxacin (Cipro IV) [package insert]. https://www.accessdata.fda.gov/drugsatfda_docs/label/2013/019857s062lbl.pdf. Accessed 15 Feb 2023.
269. US FDA. Ciprofloxacin (Cipro) [package insert]. https://www.accessdata.fda.gov/drugsatfda_docs/label/2016/019537s086lbl.pdf. Accessed 15 Feb 2023.
270. US FDA. Levofloxacin (Levaquin) [package insert]. https://www.accessdata.fda.gov/drugsatfda_docs/label/2008/021721s020_020635s57_020634s52_lbl.pdf. Accessed 15 Feb 2023.
271. US FDA. Moxifloxacin (Avelox) [package insert]. https://www.accessdata.fda.gov/drugsatfda_docs/label/2016/021085s063lbl.pdf. Accessed 15 Feb 2023.
272. US FDA. Linezolid (Zyvox) [package insert]. https://www.accessdata.fda.gov/drugsatfda_docs/label/2014/021130s032,021131s026,021132s031lbl.pdf. Accessed 15 Feb 2023.
273. US FDA. Azithromycin (Zitromax) [package insert]. https://www.accessdata.fda.gov/drugsatfda_docs/label/2013/050710s039,050711s036,050784s023lbl.pdf. Accessed 15 Feb 2023.
274. US FDA. Clarithromycin (Biaxin) [package insert]. https://www.accessdata.fda.gov/drugsatfda_docs/label/2009/050662s042,050698s024,050775s013lbl.pdf. Accessed 15 Feb 2023.

275. US FDA. Erythromycin (Ery-Ped)[package insert]. https://www.accessdata.fda.gov/drugsatfda_docs/label/2018/050207s074,050611s036lbl.pdf. Accessed 20 Feb 2023.
276. US FDA. Erythromycin (Erithrocin) [package insert]. https://www.nebraskamed.com/sites/default/files/documents/forproviders/asp/tnmc-anti-infective-renal-dosing-guidelines.pdf. Accessed 15 Feb 2023.
277. US FDA. Metronidazole (Metronidazole) [package insert]. https://www.accessdata.fda.gov/drugsatfda_docs/label/2018/018890s052lbl.pdf. Accessed 15 Feb 2023.
278. US FDA. Rifampin (Rifadin) [package insert]. https://www.accessdata.fda.gov/drugsatfda_docs/label/2010/050420s073,050627s012lbl.pdf. Accessed 15 Feb 2023.
279. US FDA. Tetracycline (Tetracycline) [package insert]. https://www.nebraskamed.com/sites/default/files/documents/for-providers/asp/tnmc-anti-infective-renal-dosing-guidelines.pdf. Accessed 15 Feb 2023.
280. US FDA. Doxycycline (Doryx) [package insert]. https://www.accessdata.fda.gov/drugsatfda_docs/label/2008/050795s005lbl.pdf. Accessed 15 Feb 2023.
281. US FDA. Doxycyline (Vibramycin) [package insert]. https://www.accessdata.fda.gov/drugsatfda_docs/label/2013/050442s016lbl.pdf. Accessed 15 Feb 2023.
282. US FDA.Minocycline (Minocin) [package insert]. https://www.accessdata.fda.gov/drugsatfda_docs/label/2010/050649023lbl.pdf. Accessed 15 Feb 2023.
283. US FDA. Tigecycline (Tigacyl) [package insert]. https://www.accessdata.fda.gov/drugsatfda_docs/label/2010/021821s021lbl.pdf. Accessed 15 Feb 2023.
284. US FDA. Sulfamethoxazole and trimethoprim (Bactrim) [package insert]. https://www.accessdata.fda.gov/drugsatfda_docs/label/2013/017377s068s073lbl.pdf. Accessed 15 Feb 2023.

Geriatric Syndromes: Definition, Assessment, and Effective Therapy

Abbreviations

ACE	Angiotensin converting enzyme
ADLs	Activities of Daily Living
BMI	Body mass index
CAM	Confusion assessment method
CGA	Comprehensive geriatric assessment
CV	Cardiovascular
EWGSOP	European Working Group on Sarcopenia in Older People
FI	Frailty Index
GI	Gastrointestinal
GS	Geriatric syndrome
IADLs	Instrumental Activities of Daily Living
ICDSC	Intensive Care Delirium Screening Checklist
ICU	Intensive care unit
MAGS	Medications against geriatric syndromes
MCI	Mild cognitive impairment
MMSE	Mini mental state exam
MoCA	Montreal Cognitive Assessment
PD	Pharmacodynamics
PIMs	Potentially inappropriate medications
PK	Pharmacokinetics
QoL	Quality of life
RCTs	Randomized clinical trials
SNF	Skilled nursing facility
SNRI	Serotonin/norepinephrine reuptake inhibitor
SSRI	Selective serotonin reuptake inhibitor
UI	Urinary incontinence

Introduction Geriatric syndromes are defined as "clinical conditions in older persons that do not fit into disease categories but are highly prevalent in old age, multifactorial, associated with multiple co-morbidities and poor outcomes and are only treatable when a multidimensional approach is used" [1]. Poor outcomes are chronic disability, longer hospital stays, strain on family members and drain on personal and health care financial resources, all adding to a significant reduction in quality of life (QoL) [2]. The geriatric syndrome (GS) differs dramatically from traditional medical syndromes. Specifically, multiple signs and symptoms result from a single pathological cause in the case of the traditional medical syndrome compared to the *reverse* in which multiple pathological changes converge to produce the GS [3].

The identification and treatment of GSs are immensely important as the growth of the older population continues to expand (see Chap. 1) [4]. *Identification in the early "pre" or vulnerable stage enables prevention* [5–7], but sadly, despite the high prevalence of GSs in the older population [8], a screen for GSs, with the exception of falls, is not routinely practiced in the general older population [9]. Early intervention would lessen the use of valuable resources in the community, hospitals and nursing facilities as well as save lives [5]. The identification of GSs during hospital admissions and/or discharge will impact subsequent decision-making and care that prevents worsening but this also is infrequently done [10].

GSs initially encompassed pressure ulcers (currently termed pressure injuries), incontinence, falls, functional decline, delirium and frailty [11]. Others have identified sarcopenia and unintentional weight loss [8], dysphagia (difficulty swallowing), hearing and visual impairments [12], late-life depression [13] and malnutrition [14] as important GSs.

This chapter will discuss the prevalence, risk factors, assessment tools and interventions (mostly nonpharmacological with pharmacological cautionary advice) of the following GSs: frailty, sarcopenia, falls, cognitive impairment, delirium, urinary incontinence, pressure injuries, malnutrition, eating/feeding problems, unintentional weight loss, sleep disorders, and depression.

FRAILTY Frailty is the "cornerstone of geriatric medicine" [11, 15]. Figure 7.1 illustrates the central position of frailty and its relation to other GSs. Frailty has many definitions. A consensus definition from six international societies, including the USA, specifies frailty as "a medical syndrome with multiple causes and contributors that is characterized by diminished strength, endurance, and reduced physiologic function that increases an individual's vulnerability for developing increased dependency and/or death" [5]. *Frailty is distinct from disability* [16]. Frailty, if not treated, spirals downward to infirmity, helplessness and death [17].

Frailty Prevalence Although limited, global estimates (62 countries) of the prevalence of frailty for those over 50 years of age range from 12% identified by the physical frailty assessments and 24% with the assessment of frailty index (accumulation of deficits) [18]. Results of screening over eleven thousand older adults in the

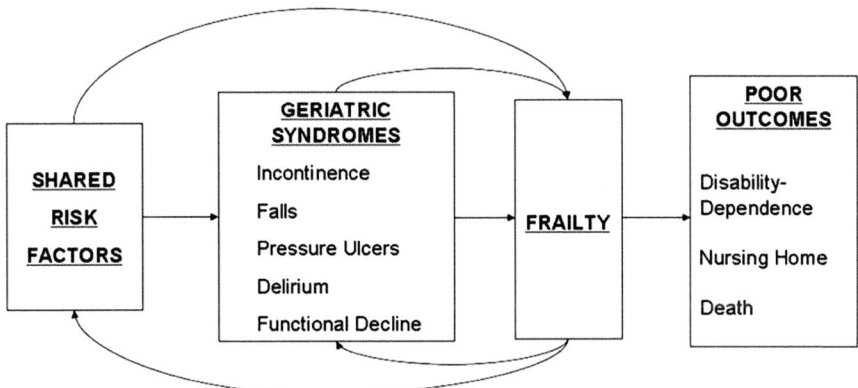

Fig. 7.1 A unifying conceptual model demonstrates that shared risk factors may lead to geriatric syndromes, which may, in turn, lead to frailty, with feedback mechanisms enhancing the presence of shared risk factors and geriatric syndromes. Such self-sustaining pathways may result in poor outcomes involving disability-dependence, nursing home placement, and ultimately death, thus holding important implications for elucidating pathophysiologic mechanisms and designing effective intervention strategies. (Reprinted with permission from Inouye et al. [11])

US with the Rapid Geriatric Assessment (discussed with other assessment tools below) in all settings (community to nursing homes) found the prevalence of frailty to be 30.4% and prefrailty at 41% [8]. Prevalence of frailty in acute care facilities varies between 33.5 and 68.5 [19], with the prevalence of frailty the highest (72.3%) in nursing homes compared to community-dwelling (21.5%) [8].

Frailty Incidence Regarding incidence or new cases over a specified duration, a systemic and meta-analysis of global estimates (28 countries) reported that the incidence of frailty in community-dwellers 60 years and older was 13.6% [20]. Incidence variables included sex (greater in women), country income (high-income countries have the lowest incidence) and diagnostic criteria (Fried phenotype with the lowest incidence) [20]. Of those identified as prefrailty at the start of the study, 18.9% progressed to frailty over the median 3 years [20].

Frailty Risk Factors An extensive review identified a wealth of risk factors for frailty [21]. These were "older age, lower BMI (body mass index), female sex, living alone, low levels of exercise, polypharmacy, smoking status, drinking status, low vitamin D levels, and malnutrition" [21]. Others reported an association of frailty with diabetes, dyslipidemia, cognitive decline, and hypertension [22].

Frailty Assessment Tools Given the high rate of frailty prevalence and incidence and the multiplicity of risk factors, it is essential to screen for frailty. Frailty may be assessed in one of several ways. Two original and well-documented assessments are: (1) the Frailty Index (FI), which considers the accumulation of deficits [23, 24], and (2) the Frailty Phenotype, which considers interlinked reductions in physical weakness, slowness, exhaustion, low activity, and weight loss [25]. The Rapid Geriatric Assessment, mentioned above, is essentially a set of questionnaires that evaluate 4 domains of frailty: state of muscle loss (sarcopenia), nutritional and cognitive status and key questions on the condition of frail [26]. Several other validated frailty screening tools are the Clinical Frailty Scale [5], FRAIL Scale [27], Gait Speed [27], Gérontopôle Frailty Screening Tool [28], PRISMA Questionnaire [29], Time-up-and-Go Test [29] and the Study of Osteoporotic Fractures Frailty Scale [30]. These are discussed in detail in Carlson et al. (2015) [4] and Walston et al. (2018) [15].

Frailty Index (FI) The FI is a comprehensive quantitative evaluation of "deficits in health" [31]. The FI assesses at least 30 variables that relate to the state of health, that increase with age without early plateau, that involve many organ-systems, and that may be repeatedly evaluated in the same individual [23]. Deficits include "signs, symptoms, disabilities and diseases" [31] and would include "restricted activity, disability in Activities of Daily Living (ADLs) (e.g., daily care) and Instrumental ADLs (e.g., handling finances), impairments in general cognition and physical performance (e.g., impaired grip strength, impaired walking), co-morbidity, self-rated health, and depression/mood [23].

Nonpharmacological Intervention. Physical Activity Frailty has the potential for both prevention and reversal [32]. Nonpharmacological interventions for frailty to prevent/minimize functional decline entail physical exercises, optimized nutrition, multicomponent interventions and customized geriatric care [15]. Analysis of high-quality randomized clinical trials (RCTs) on frailty interventions concludes that physical exercise (aerobics, resistance, mixed, mind-body) was the most efficacious, with resistance exercise superior to the others [33]. Resistance exercise improves muscle strength and performance, thereby reducing major components of frailty [34]. It is an inexpensive intervention for which there are numerous validated guidelines that focus on major muscles that require exercise 3 times weekly with increasing demand to achieve a progressively better outcome [35, 36].

Nonpharmacological Intervention. Nutrition Nutrition and frailty are intertwined and complicated as both under nutrition (inadequate ingestion of foods to supply necessary energy and nutrients) and over nutrition (leading to obesity), although distinct conditions, contribute to an increased risk of frailty [37]. Deficiencies in micronutrients, macronutrients, and antioxidants are important, despite the fact that findings in some areas are inconsistent [38]. The strongest data show that tissue deficiency of vitamin B_{12} and reduced serum levels of carotenoids (yellow, orange, and red pigmented compounds in fruits/vegetables), α-tocopherol (one of several forms of vitamin E), 25-hydroxyvitamin D, and vitamin B_6 are associated with a higher risk of frailty [38]. Although more studies are required, a higher intake of protein- and antioxidant-laden foods lowers frailty risk [38].

Clearly, the better the caliber of the diet, the lower the risk of frailty [37]. Fortunately, nutrition is an amendable factor. Despite the need for long-term RCTs that demonstrate causality, results of observational studies suggest interventions such as the Mediterranean dietary pattern, which entails the intake of high amounts of fruits, vegetables, nuts, legumes, seeds, lesser amounts of meats, dairy products, and use of olive oil, lowers the risk of frailty [39–42]. Longitudinal and cross-sectional trial data show a lower risk of frailty with daily higher intakes of protein [43]. Protein intake levels associated with frailty ranged from <43–63 g/day or < 1 g/kg body weight per day [43]. However, protein supplements are recommended only as an adjunct to exercise training, yielding better results in muscle mass and strength in the frail individual compared to exercise alone [44]. While these studies are important, Ni Lochlainn et al. (2018) [37] concluded that "the potential of diet to prevent or treat frailty is therefore not yet clear."

Multicomponent Intervention The combination of multicomponent interventions and customized geriatric care is best exemplified by the interventional RCT, Sarcopenia and Physical Railty IN older people: multicomponenT Treatment strategies (SPRINT-T) project [45] that developed and implemented " long-term structured physical activity and a personalized nutritional intervention, supported by information and communication technology" [46]. The results of this large (760 participants in experimental and control groups with frailty, age 70 years or older) showed that three years of a personalized exercise program of moderate intensity [47] plus actimeter assessments (measures physical activity) and nutritional counseling to achieve established energy and protein requirements [48] in physical frailty and sarcopenia (next section), individuals improved their mobility and women lost less muscle mass and strength compared to controls [49]. This applied to those with an initial score of 3–7 on the short physical performance battery (range 0–12; the higher the number, the better the performance) [50] but not to those with higher scores [49].

SARCOPENIA Sarcopenia is a major component of frailty [51]. A timely definition of sarcopenia that takes in the most recent understanding of sarcopenia states that "sarcopenia is a progressive and generalized skeletal muscle disorder that is associated with increased likelihood of adverse outcomes including falls, fractures, physical disability and mortality" [52]. This is the latest consensus definition from the European Working Group on Sarcopenia in Older People (EWGSOP). Although its emphasis is placed on loss of muscle strength, recommended assessments of sarcopenia also include loss of muscle mass and quality [52].

Sarcopenia is considered a GS because of the multiplicity of factors that interact in poorly understood ways with the aging of skeletal muscles [52]. Progressive changes in skeletal muscles with age, primarily loss of muscle fibers (type and size)

[53], are influenced by lack of physical activity, deficient nutrition and reduced presence of hormones, with muscle loss greatest in women after menopause [54]. However, many other factors come together to accelerate muscle aging such as long-term bed-rest or sedentary lifestyle, morbidities, and medications.

Sarcopenia. Prevalence The prevalence of sarcopenia varies with the setting and the definition of sarcopenia [55]. Globally, the prevalence of sarcopenia is estimated at 0.2–86.5% [55], but others report ranges of 18% in diabetic patients to 66% in patients with inoperable esophageal cancer [56]. Prevalence of 1–29% in community-dwelling older adults, 14–33% in long-term care facilities and 10% in acute hospital care has been recorded [57].

The EWGSOP2 (second conference) developed "an algorithm with specifics on case-finding, making a diagnosis and quantifying severity in practice" [52]. Briefly, this entails a questionnaire or clinical assessment for case-finding, tests for muscle strength (grip strength, chair stand), muscle quality/mass assessment (e.g., dual-energy X-ray absorptiometry (DEXA), MRI) and performance (timed-up-and-go (TUG), timed chair rise, 3 meter walk, return and sit down); 400 meter timed walk.

Sarcopenia. Nonpharmacological Interventions The most effective intervention in older adults to improve muscle strength and performance is a resistance exercise program [57–59]. Additionally, prevention of sarcopenia begins in early life (with physical activities) to maximize muscle mass and strength, followed by maintenance of strength in middle age (continued physical activities) and minimization of loss of strength in older age (persistence in a quality exercise program) according to a proposed life course model [60].

FALLS Falls are intertwined with frailty [61]. Falls are a GS resulting in numerous consequences: fractures, head injuries, hospitalizations, reduced mobility/independence, post-fall anxiety syndrome, untimely long-term care, increased risk of death and elevated healthcare costs [62].

Falls. Incidence According to the National Safety Council, falls commonly occur at a rate of 1 in 4 among community-dwellers 65 and older in the US [63]. Furthermore, hospitalizations due to falls have increased by 43% over the past 10 years and fall-related deaths have increased by 60% [63]. Since the rate of falling increases with age, half of all individuals over 80 years of age have at least one fall per year and fall injuries account for the main injury-related death in this age group [62].

Falls. Risk Factors Although falls are common, they are often unacknowledged as patients are frequently reluctant to share a fall incident and hence fall risk goes untreated. Many of the risk factors for falls, e.g., poor balance, gait, vision, orthostatic hypotension, sarcopenia, footwear, environmental hazards, and osteoarthritis are modifiable while others, e.g., cognitive decline and muscle weakness from medical conditions, remain a challenge [62]. In the home, the most significant factors contributing to falls are clutter, pets, throw rugs, cords/wires, insufficient lighting, items placed too high or too low, shoes without good support and slippery/wet floors [64].

Falls. Nonpharmacological Interventions Poor balance and gait and orthostatic hypotension are likely caused by mediations such as sedatives, antipsychotics, and some antihypertensives (see Table 7.1), which should be cautiously de-prescribed and slowly withdrawn. Sarcopenia, osteoarthritis, and poor balance and gait can be mitigated by a program of resistance and balance exercises [65]. Poor vision, generally cataracts, may be corrected as can unsuitable footwear. Environmental (home) hazards, e.g., throw rugs and clutter, may be removed and increased lighting added. Other risk factors that include muscle weakness due to stroke or Parkinsonism and cognitive decline require additional aids [62].

To assess what intervention(s) really work to decrease the risk of falling, a systemic and network meta-analysis of 192 studies on single and multiple interventions to prevent falls in community-dwelling adults 65 years and older found that exercise was the single most important intervention to reduce the risk of falls and fall-related fractures [66]. Additionally, added to exercise and basic fall risk assessment, multiple interventions noted above also significantly reduce the number of fallers and the rate of falling [66]. However, another large analysis found that multicomponent interventions (e.g., supervised exercise and home safety assessment) in community-dwelling older adults only reduced the rate of falling and not fall-related outcomes [67]. In the hospital setting, a systemic and meta-analysis of studies including two large RCTs [68, 69] focused on fall reduction in hospitals, concluded that education and training (patient and staff) were the most effective interventions to reduce fall rates. Although multicomponent interventions trended to have positive effects, chair/bed alarms, wearable sensors and scored risk assessments were of no value [70]. An assessment of 71 studies of interventions in acute care facilities to reduce the number of falls found nothing of value since the data were low or very low quality, allowing for uncertainty regarding any of the above interventions [71].

COGNITIVE IMPAIRMENT Cognitive decline is not an expected outcome of normal aging. In the absence of disease, some cognitive spheres remain constant (semantic memory, autobiographical memory, automatic memory processes, most aspects of language and emotional processing). Other spheres of cognition exhibit variable degrees of lesser capacity (information processing speed, reward-based behavior, executive function, and certain memory processes, e.g., encoding and retrieval, source finding) [72]. Brain aging can be minimized with life-style modifications of physical exercise, diet and cognitive engagement [73].

Mild cognitive impairment (MCI) is the transition from healthy aging to dementia (see Chap. 4 for discussion of dementia). The global prevalence of MCI is approximately 15% [74] but this can vary between 6.7% and 25.2%, depending on the definition of MCI [75].

Cognitive Impairment. Risk Factors Risk factors of cognitive decline are age, genetics, socioeconomic, and environmental factors, including nutrition and physical activity [76]. Results of birth cohort studies (individuals born at the same time) support this and expand risk factors to include childhood cognition, education, occupation and genetics plus epigenetics (environmental influence on genes) that influence late-life cognitive decline [77].

Cognitive Impairment Assessment There are several tests to evaluate the presence of cognitive impairment [4]. The 3 most frequently used tests are (1) the mini-mental state exam (MMSE, a 30-item test, abnormal cognition is a score ≤ 24), (2) Montreal Cognitive Assessment (MoCA, 30 item test [78]), and (3) Mini-cog (clock drawing, 3 item recall, impairment if one of two is abnormal [79]).

Cognitive Impairment. Interventions Multi-domain interventions that include "dietary counseling, exercise, cognitive training, social activities, and monitoring and management of vascular and metabolic risk factors" improved cognitive test scores, executive function, processing speed, complex memory tasks and reduced risk of cognitive decline in a large 2-year RCT [80]. A second large RCT, lasting 3 years and additionally adding the supplement, omega-3 fatty acid, also showed benefits of a multi-domain intervention on slowing cognitive decline and some small improvements with the supplement [81]. Literature reviews also support aerobic exercise, mental activity, social engagement and control of cardiovascular (CV) risk factors as successful interventions for the prevention of cognitive decline [82].

DELIRIUM "Delirium is a severe neuropsychiatric syndrome that is characterized by acute onset of deficits in attention and other aspects of cognition" [83]. The level of arousal varies from almost stupor to extreme alertness. Disturbed emotions and psychosis with hallucinations may also be present, and these features may fluctuate in time and intensity [83]. It is basically the inability of a susceptible brain to respond adequately to sudden stressors [83]. It incurs "increased hospital expenses, medical complications, and mortality" [84].

Delirium. Initiating Factors and Prevalence Delirium cannot be explained by known cognitive deficits. It is initiated by anyone of several conditions, often more than one [85]. These factors entail serious acute illness (e.g., sepsis, hypoglycemia, stroke), surgery, trauma (e.g., head injury, fracture), drug use/withdrawal (notably benzodiazepines, dihydropyridines, antihistamines, opioids) [86] and psychiatric illnesses. Delirium may last 3 months to a year or more [87]; some patients never recovery [88]. The prevalence of delirium in hospitalized patients varies with the surgical procedures but is generally around 23% [89]. In nursing homes, prevalence may be as high as 36.8% [90] but is very low in the community at 2% [83].

Delirium. Risk Factors Risk factors for delirium are (1) older age, (2) cognitive impairment, (3) frailty, (4) co-morbidities, (5) psychiatric illness, (6) depression, (7) alcohol use, (8) poor nutritional status, (9) visual/hearing loss, and (10) extensive cerebral atrophy [83]. To these acute precipitating factors of delirium, add the above-noted conditions [85]. Worse outcomes are dependent on older age, frailty, duration and severity of the delirium and hypoactive subtype delirium [83]. The pathophysiological mechanisms are poorly understood, although several working hypotheses, cerebral metabolic deficits, systemic inflammation, and reduced neuronal connectivity, are currently under investigation [83].

Delirium. Assessment Delirium is frequently assessed according to the Diagnostic and Statistical Manual of Mental Disorders (DSM) version 5 as a major disruption in attention and awareness (including near coma condition) coupled with one other cognitive deficit of recent development and inexplicable by any established medical conditions [91]. However, with the suspicion of change in attention, environmental awareness, and/or cognition, there exists an abundance of tools, rapid to intensive, to identify delirium [92, 93]. The choice depends on the location. For example, the 4As test, useful in hospitals and considered sensitive and specific, assesses alertness, cognition, attention and evidence of acute changes [94]. In critical care situations, e.g., intensive care units (ICU) or nursing homes, the best (valid and reliable) tools are the Confusion Assessment Method (CAM)-based tools (CAM-ICU) and Intensive Care Delirium Screening Checklist [95]. The former determines delirium by assessment with specific questions on four conditions—acute onset/fluctuating course, inattention, disorganized thinking and altered level of consciousness (alert to coma). If the first two conditions are present plus one other, a diagnosis of delirium is given [95]. The ICDSC measures 8 domains (level of consciousness, inattention, disorientation, hallucinations or delusions, psychomotor activity, inappropriate speech or mood, sleep disturbance and fluctuation of symptoms with a yes equal to 1 and a score of ≥ 4 signifying delirium [96]. Despite these effective assessment tools, delirium is underdiagnosed, possibly due to a lack of educational training for students and graduates on this topic, underappreciated as to the seriousness of the condition and a lack of clarity as to the discipline responsible for assessment and intervention [83].

Delirium. Nonpharmacological Interventions Two consensus guidelines propose effective nonpharmacological interventions for delirium at-risk hospital inpatients [97, 98]. The focus is on "physiotherapy, reorientation, cognitive stimulation, early mobilization, non-pharmacological promotion of sleep, correction of sensory impairments, identification and treatment of underlying causes or postoperative complications, pain management, avoidance of constipation, hydration, nutrition and oxygen delivery" [83].

Delirium. Pharmacological Interventions Pharmacological interventions in delirium are mainly ones of minimal drug use or avoidance. It is recommended that for patients over 60 years of age, deep anesthesia be avoided with careful monitoring [97]. Benzodiazepines and antipsychotic should be avoided [86]. Other drugs to avoid include tricyclic antidepressants, anticholinergic medications, antihistamines and tramadol [99], which overlaps with potentially inappropriate medications (PIMs) of the Beers Criteria® [100]. Pain medications should be used cautiously. Fentanyl and morphine are not significantly linked to delirium but should be used at the lowest dose to avoid side effects [86]. For sedation and agitation reduction in delirium, the current meta-analysis assessment of 8 trial results found dexmedetomidine, an alpha-2 agonist, to be efficacious but with side effects of bradycardia (slowed heart rate) and hypotension [101]. Guidelines suggest that pharmacological intervention be reserved for situations of "intractable stress" or where the safety of patients and others is endangered [97].

URINARY INCONTINENCE Urinary incontinence (UI) is a GS that results from a composite of factors. As with other GSs of delirium, falls, and frailty, UI shares the four risk factors of age, baseline cognitive impairment, baseline functional impairment and impaired mobility [11]. Additionally, age-related changes in the lower urinary tract, complicated by disease and medication, impose a barrier to continence. UI is a GS that negatively impacts the QoL to the greatest extent [102]. However, due to patient embarrassment, many do not get help and sadly are forced into isolation [4]. Untreated UI creates stress on both the patient and caregivers and often results in unnecessary additional health care expenditures for UI products [103].

Urinary Incontinence. Prevalence UI prevalence is high. Nearly 40% of older women worldwide suffer from UI [104]. UI also affects approximately 10–35% of older men, especially related to the pathology of the prostate gland [105]. Prevalence is excessively high (80%) in older adults in long-term care facilities [106].

Urinary Incontinence. Risk Factors Multiple risk factors for UI are comorbidities such as neurological diseases, cardiovascular diseases, diabetes, and obesity [106], the presence of multi-morbidities and frailty [107], and delirium, insomnia, falls, and mobility problems [106]. Certain drugs (e.g., diuretics, muscle relaxants, sedatives, narcotics, antihistamines, and alpha-adrenergic antagonists [108] and inflammation/infection increase the risk of UI [109].

Urinary Incontinence. Classification There are basically *two main types of chronic UI*: stress UI in which there is an involuntary loss of urine during physical exertion or exercise attributed to reduced skeletal muscle sphincter tone and urge UI in which there is an involuntary loss of urine associated with a sudden sense of urgency (sensory or motor dysfunction due to hyper or hypo activity of the detrusor muscle) [110]. Additional types include mixed UI with attributes of both stress and urgency, overflow due to overextended bladder and functional UI with disability prohibiting access to the toilet [4]. Many drugs cause UI including alpha-adrenergic agonists/antagonists, angiotensin-converting enzyme inhibitors, calcium channel blockers, anticholinesterase inhibitors, diuretics, lithium, opioid analgesics, psychotropic drugs, sedatives, hypnotics, selective serotonin reuptake inhibitor, gabapentin, glitazones and nonsteroidal antiinflammatory drugs [111].

Urinary Incontinence. Assessment Use of the validated Three Incontinence Questions [112] and others [4] help identify UI. This may be followed by a comprehensive physical exam (focus on the CV, renal and urinary systems, prostate, neurological function, and gynecological exam), review of current medications (including OTC drugs/herbal supplements), fluid intake/micturition diary, and laboratory tests, e.g., electrolytes, urinalysis, and urine culture [4] to fully understand UI and to individualize therapy. Assessment of the type of UI is critically important.

Urinary Incontinence. Nonpharmacological Therapy Nonpharmacological therapy for UI contains multiple personalized components highly successful if supplied by a multidisciplinary team [113]. Effective therapies are fluid optimization, weight loss, and pelvic floor muscle training [111]. Additionally, there are several proven surgical interventions that may be of value, such as synthetic mid-urethral sling placement or electrical/chemical neuromodulation [111].

Urinary Incontinence. Pharmacological Therapy Medical therapy may be of value as a second line of therapy for UI [111]. However, *available choices are limited for the older adult*. For women, vaginal estrogen, but not systemic estrogen, provides increased blood flow and lessens atrophy that subsequently alleviates UI [114]. For men, the phosphodiesterase inhibitor (PDE5), tadalafil, exhibits efficacy exceeding that of standard anticholinergic agents in treating symptoms of UI and additionally improves QoL and sexual function [115]. Although anticholinergic agents (fesoterodine fumarate, oxybutynin chloride, tolterodine tartrate, trospium chloride, darifenacin, solifenacin succinate) are first choice drugs to treat urgency incontinence because they correct in part the insufficiencies of the detrusor muscle, they are to be avoided in the older adult due to the myriad of side effects, additive to age changes [100]. In place of anticholinergic agents, a beta$_3$-adrenergic agonist (mirabegron) may be used, and although it has fewer side effects, its efficacy is modest and it has the potential to exacerbate hypertension [111].

PRESSURE INJURIES "Pressure injuries are localized damage to the skin and underlying soft tissue, usually occurring over a bony prominence or related to medical devices. They result from prolonged or severe pressure with contributions from shear and friction force" [116]. The older adult is especially sensitive to pressure injuries due to aging of the skin with reduced thickness of the dermis/epidermis and diminution of immune protection [117]. The effect of a pressure injury is devastating as it reduces QoL, increases health care costs and elevates the risk of death [116]. Formerly termed pressure ulcers, pressure injury depends on risk factors of malnutrition, hypo-perfusion of poor circulation and underlying morbidity that prevents mobility [118]. Essentially, a pressure injury occurs above a certain pressure value. Pressure chokes off blood flow, oxygen, and nutrients to the underlying cells and creates clots, cell death, and inflammation [116].

Pressure Injuries. Prevalence The prevalence of pressure injuries has been estimated at 5–15% for hospitalized patients and higher (2.3% to 28%) for those in long-term care facilities [119]. More recently, global pressure injuries in intensive care units were estimated at 16.2%, with increasing severity of the pressure injury related to mortality [120].

Pressure Injuries. Assessment There are specific procedures for the evaluation and treatment of pressure injuries that are detailed by the National Pressure Injury Advisory Panel [121] and the guidelines presented by the American College of Physicians based on best-quality evidence [122]. Of note is confirmation that a clinician's evaluation of a pressure injury is comparable to the results of a detailed assessment tool. High-risk patients benefit from "advanced static mattresses and overlays," and a multidisciplinary team provides the best treatment. The best outcomes rest with a team with a diversity of expertise [122].

Pressure Injuries. The Braden Scale The Braden Scale is a valued risk assessment tool for pressure sores [123]. It is one of the most commonly used tools because it "shows optimal validation, and best sensitivity and specificity compared to Norton Scale, Waterlow Scale and nurses' clinical judgment" [124]. The Braden scale inquires into six areas covering sensory perception (pressure discomfort to no impairment), moisture (constantly moist to barely moist), activity (bedfast to walks frequently), mobility (immobile to mobile), nutrition (rarely eats to good appetite), friction, and shear (needs help with repositioning to good muscle strength) with determinations of degree of change, maximal deterioration or harm to no impairment [123, 125].

MALNUTRITION Malnutrition/undernutrition is a GS that is tightly integrated with pressure injuries and eating/feeding problems. It is considered a major risk factor for the development and weakened response to wound healing [14]. Optimal nutrition enables requisite skin physiology to maintain collagen production, immunological protection and ample blood flow essential for health [117]. In contrast, malnutrition, a nutritional disorder, is a lack of consumption of nutrients induced by starvation, disease and/or older age, leading to weight loss (cell mass) and subsequent reduction in physical, mental and defense functions [126]. Thus, malnutrition may arise from multiple sources: disease with inflammation or without inflammation, socioeconomic/psychological, or hunger-related conditions [126].

Malnutrition. Prevalence Prevalence of malnutrition varies with the healthcare environment, with rates of 3.1–6.0% in community and outpatient settings, 17.5–22% in nursing homes and hospitals and 28.7–29.4% in long-term care and rehabilitation settings [127]. Whereas the identification of modifiable factors for malnutrition should be a prime research goal, a systematic analysis of 23 studies identified 30 potentially modifiable factors, but sadly, a majority of studies were considered of high bias and low quality [128]. The best evidence, albeit moderate, highlighted the following risk factors: "hospitalization, eating dependency, poor self-perceived health, poor physical function and poor appetite" [128].

Malnutrition. Assessment A nutritional care plan has been proposed to include specific steps: malnutrition risk screening, nutritional assessment and diagnostic procedures, nutritional care plan and its implementation, followed by supervision, evaluation, and documentation [126]. However, as noted by a recent review of screening and assessment tools available to identify malnutrition prior to emergency general surgery, consensus is lacking. Such variability in appropriate methods could potentially result in worse outcomes, longer stays and more healthcare expenditures [129]. Resolution of these issues is clearly needed.

PROBLEMS WITH EATING OR FEEDING A number of eating and feeding problems may arise with aging and comorbidities that decrease the QoL and worsen frailty. These are changes that reduce nutritional uptake, generally lead to a state of anorexia (extensive loss of body weight) and, importantly, are correctable. One such change is poor dentition, ill-fitting dentures, and oral pain that reduce the ability to chew, compromising the intake of fibers, vitamins, proteins and calcium and enhancing intake of fats and cholesterol [130–132]. Other physical factors relate to difficulty with ADLs (bathing, dressing, grooming in addition to self-feeding) and IADLS (handling finances, house chores, medication as well as shopping) and sensory reductions in sight and hearing, which hinder food shopping and food preparation [133]. Social isolation, whether eating alone or eating in a regimented atmosphere, often present in LTCFs, adds to eating difficulties [133]. Additional problems of dysphasia (difficulty in swallowing) and dry mouth are both conditions that aggravate frailty and contribute to eating problems [134].

Problems of Eating/Feeding. Assessment Several assessment tools of oral health have been validated for use in residential care facilities, e.g., Oral Health Assessment Tool (OHAT) [135] and in nursing homes, e.g., the Brief Oral Health Status Exam (BOHSE) [136]. Because of the tight association of poor oral health with diminished QoL, worsening of co-morbidities, and mortality, an inclusion of oral health assessment in the Comprehensive Geriatric Assessment (CGA) has been proposed for use in community-based personal health care [137]. This expanded CGA would query self-reported dental health, denture use, dental pain, saliva production, limitations on food due to oral issues and relevant oral symptoms [137]. It would also develop a plan to resolve presenting concerns [137].

UNINTENTIONAL WEIGHT/APPETITE LOSS Based on limited but comparable data, weight loss of 5% or more over a 6–12 period is associated with an increase in morbidity and mortality [138].

Unintentional Weight/Appetite Loss. Prevalence/Risk Factors Prevalence is estimated at 15–20% in the older population but may be more than double in nursing home facilities [139, 140]. Approximately 30% of unintentional weight loss is related to malignant disease, but the other 70% is attributed to a plethora of factors [138]. Likely inclusions are (1) *medical conditions* of CV, renal, endocrine, autoimmune, psychiatric, gastrointestinal (GI)-related and alcohol-related; (2) *medications* that alter taste/smell (e.g., allopurinol, angiotensin-converting enzyme (ACE) inhibitors, antibiotics, anticholinergics), cause dry mouth (e.g., anticholinergic, antihistamines, loop diuretics), difficulty in swallowing (e.g., bisphosphonates, doxycycline, NSAIDs), nausea/vomiting (e.g., amantadine, bisphosphonates, digoxin, dopamine agonists, metformin, selective serotonin reuptake inhibitor (SSRI)) and anorexia (similar to those producing nausea/vomiting plus opiates, tricyclic antidepressants) (3) *problems with eating/feeding* (discussed above), e.g., inability to feed oneself, impaired chewing, and social factors, e.g., isolation [138].

Unintentional Weight/Appetite Loss. Assessment Assessment of unintentional weight loss is challenging. It may involve laboratory/imaging tests to rule out the most common medical diseases of malignancies, GI conditions or psychiatric issues after which consideration for factors such as cachexia associated with organ failure, endocrinopathies (diabetes, hyperthyroidism), grave infections, e.g., TB, HIV, adverse drug reactions (ADRs), substance abuse, eating/feeding problems, and social factors, is required [141].

Unintentional Weight/Appetite Loss. Nonpharmacological Therapy To ameliorate unintentional weight loss, the cause(s) must be identified and addressed. Here a multipurpose team is required with the recommended inclusion of "dentists; dietitians; speech, occupational, or physical therapists; and social service workers" [138]. An updated systematic review of megestrol acetate use as an appetite stimulant in the treatment of anorexia-cachexia found that a drug-induced small increase in weight, albeit not clinically relevant, did not increase QoL [142]. Avoidance of appetite stimulants and high-calorie supplements is recommended due to lack of long-term efficacy and safety [138].

SLEEP DISORDERS It is estimated that half of those 65 years and older experience some type of sleeping issue such as insomnia (inability to fall asleep; inability to stay asleep), sleep-disordered breathing, e.g., sleep apnea (decreased or absent air flow during sleep), restless legs syndrome (uncomfortable feeling in legs mitigated by moving) and associated daytime sleepiness producing poor functioning while awake [143, 144]. These were initially considered unrelated to the aging process, which only slightly modifies the biological sleep/wake cycle (circadian rhythm) to reduce the time in deep sleep (and REM, rapid eye movement associated with quality sleep) and increase the duration of light sleep [145]. However, more recently, age changes have been implicated directly in the causation of insomnia, sleep apnea, and related changes, but the work requires confirmation [146].

Results of several studies show an independent relation between sleep problems and frailty [147–149]. In those ≥85 years of age, the greater the degree of frailty, the worse the sleep deterioration [147]. Conversely, in nonfrail older adults, the greater the sleep disturbance, the greater the risk of progression to frailty [144, 150, 151]. If, in fact, the frail individual responds poorly to stress, sleep perturbations serve to worsen frailty, making it even more important to identify sleep problems early and treat them [152].

Sleep Disorders. Assessment *Unresolved sleep issues have severe consequences.* They result in reduced physical and mental capacity during waking hours that may lead to accidents and falls, mood changes, e.g., irritability, chronic fatigue, and a worsening of morbidities, all leading to poor QoL, additional health care costs, and possible mortality [143]. It is proposed that an investigation of sleep health (*sleep duration continuity, timing, wakefulness/daytime sleepiness* and *sleep quality*) [153] be part of a Comprehensive Geriatric Assessment [143]. There are several validated questionnaires (Pittsburgh Sleep Quality Index (PSQI) [154], Insomnia Severity Index [155]; Stop-Bang Questionnaire [156] that supply a subjective view and clinical tests such as the in-laboratory polysomnography that provide objective measures of sleep disturbances.

Sleep Disorders. Nonpharmacological Therapy Cognitive behavior treatment of insomnia (CBTi) is considered the best therapy to treat sleep problems of the older adult and those with frailty because (a) it is evidenced based and (b) includes multiple effective methods, e.g., stimulus control (limiting the use of bed to sleep), sleep restriction (time in bed to equal time of sleep) along with psycho-education and cognitive therapy [143]. Sleep-disordered breathing is best treated with a highly effective device that provides continuous positive airway pressure (CPAP). However, it must be tailored to the patient for fit, comfort, and safety to achieve compliance [143]. The use of benzodiazepines, non-benzodiazepines (z-drugs) or sedating antidepressants is not advised as they produce "daytime sedation, falls and confusion," and any with anticholinergic activity (diphenhydramine) should be avoided in the older adult [143].

DEPRESSION "Depression is a common but serious mood disorder ...with symptoms of depressed mood or loss of interest, most of the time for at least 2 weeks, that interfere with daily activities" [157]. Depression is often confused with dementia, probably because there exists a purported relation between the two such that depression in the older adult is often aligned with cognitive impairment, and dementia is often associated with depression [13]. For a discussion of dementia, see Chap. 4.

Late-life depression (LLD) occurs in older adults without a prior history of depression [157]. According to the DSM-5, depression encompasses not only depressed mood but additional symptoms of "changes in appetite or weight (5% total body weight), sleep, energy, concentration, and psychomotor activity, feelings of inappropriate guilt or worthlessness and recurrent thoughts of death or suicide" [91].

Depression. Prevalence Estimates of prevalence range from 1% to 5% in community-dwelling older adults, 11.5% of hospitalized older adults and 13.5% in those requiring home health care [159].

Depression. Risk Factors LLD has been characterized as "common, recurrent and malignant" [160]. As with all GSs, multiple factors come together to foment depression. Known factors are: (1) various diseases such as CV, diabetes, and dementia that pathologically affect essential neurotransmitters, e.g., serotonin, norepinephrine, and dopamine, (2) psychological/sociological issues, e.g., childhood abuse, inactivity, and negative life events, and (3) genetics and personality traits, areas requiring more research [158]. Conditions such as cerebrovascular accident, Parkinson's disease, and status post-myocardial infarction increase the risk for depression, and conversely, depression increases the risk for these conditions [161]. Thus, there is a reciprocity between the effects of depression and medical health [162]. Exactly where and how vascular and brain network pathways cross is an area of intense research [162].

Depression. Diverse Therapies Depression is successfully treated with psychotherapy, especially the effective use of training in cognitive behavioral therapy [163]. Severe depression may require pharmacotherapy (selective serotonin reuptake inhibitor (SSRI), as the first choice, which, however, is counter to advice from Beers' Criteria® [100] and also advice on medications against GSs (MAGS) (see below). However, SSRIs (sertraline, paroxetine) and serotonin/norepinephrine reuptake inhibitor, SNRI (duloxetine), were found to be safe and effective in the treatment of LLD and did not increase mortality or elevate the risk of dementia or cognitive decline [164]. Atypical antipsychotics (quetiapine, aripiprazole) were also effective and safe, but in all cases, the dose needs to be as low as possible [164]. Early treatment is essential because LLD produces considerable disability and reduction in QoL, negatively affects the progression of many diseases, and creates a huge burden on family and healthcare providers and costs to society [158].

MEDICATION USE IN GERIATRIC SYNDROMES As emphasized in Chap. 3, the older adult is several-fold more sensitive to ADRs than a younger adult due to age-associated changes in pharmacokinetics (PK) and pharmacodynamics (PD), comorbidities (on average 9) and the need for multiple drugs leading to polypharmacy (at least ≥5) [21, 165]. This is particularly important to remember when confronted with the complexity of GSs. Drug use in GSs is especially challenging since study results show numerous classes of drugs can exacerbate GSs [10, 86, 100, 166] and/or increase the risk of hospitalizations [167, 168].

Medications Associated with Geriatric Syndromes (MAGS) Supplementing the defined potentially inappropriate medications (PIMs) of the Beers Criteria® (2015) [100] and the STOPP criteria [169], Saraf et al. (2016) [166] identified 153 medications associated with GSs (MAGS) and determined to what extent these medications were prescribed in older adults discharged from the hospital to a skilled nursing facility (SNF). These PIMs (given in Table 7.1) were associated with six GSs: falls, delirium, cognitive impairment, depression, urinary incontinence, and weight loss [166]. More than half of the MAGS had been previously identified as PIMs [100, 169] but 42% were not [166]. Of significance is the observation that on discharge to SNF, patients left with an average of 14 medications of which approximately 40% were MAGS, with many patients leaving with multiple MAGS [166]. In other settings, e.g., home health care, 98% of older adults used one MAGS and a total of 40% of drug use were MAGS, leading to an associated increase in hospitalizations [21].

As noted by Saraf et al. (2016) [166], there are many drugs that are inappropriate for the older adult, have questionable efficacy and lack clinical value. Depending on the country and operational criteria, the prevalence of PIMs in hospital settings may be as high as 79% [170]. This is especially worrisome for those with GSs. Table 7.1 indicates that antiepileptic drugs, mood stabilizers and barbiturates are inappropriate for all six GSs and drugs in four other categories: antipsychotics, antidepressants, antiparkinsonism and opioid agonists are linked to five GSs [166]. The GSs associated with the most MAGS is falls. Least MAGS were evident with the geriatric syndrome of weight loss [166]. Findings from other studies of inappropriate drug use in certain GSs provide confirmation for Saraf et al. (2016) [166]. Specifically, in hospital admission of older adults due to adverse drug events, approximately 25% experienced delirium associated with antidepressants, antipsychotics and antiseizure medications and a smaller number (~12%) are admitted due to falls related to drugs in categories of antidiabetic, antidepressant, antihypertensive and antipsychotic [167]. Results from a Malaysian teaching hospital study reported that opioid analgesics, vasodilator antihypertensives and beta-blockers were MAGS most commonly prescribed to older adults discharged from the hospital with GSs of falls, depression and delirium [171].

Relevant deprescribing is essential but difficult to achieve [168]. "Inappropriate prescribing can be reduced by adherence to prescribing guidelines, suitable monitoring and regular medication review" [172]. *Considering the multiplicity of age changes, presence of co-morbidities and polypharmacy, individualized care should be a top priority* [172].

COMPREHENSIVE GERIATRIC SYNDROME CARE "Comprehensive geriatric assessment is a systematic evaluation of frail older persons by a team of health professionals and consists of six core components: data gathering, team discussion, development of a treatment plan, and implementation of a treatment plan, with monitoring and revision as needed" [173]. Generally, regardless of the setting, hospital, home care or clinic, the comprehensive geriatric assessment (CGA) has benefitted patients with better outcomes [173]. The use of the CGA essentially

Table 7.1 Summary of medications associated with geriatric syndromes (MAGS) (reprinted with permission from Saraf et al., 2016 [166])

Major medication category	Delirium	Cognitive impairment	Falls	Unintentional weight and appetite loss	Urinary incontinence	Depression	Drug class/drug within each category
Antipsychotics		✓	✓		✓	✓	Atypical and typical antipsychotics and buspirone
Antidepressants	✓	✓	✓	✓	✓		Tricyclic and tetracyclic antidepressants, serotonin reuptake inhibitors, serotonin and norepinephrine reuptake inhibitors and aminoketone
Antiepileptics	✓	✓	✓	✓	✓	✓	Antiepileptics, mood stabilizers and barbiturates
Antiparkinsonism	✓	✓	✓		✓	✓	Aromatic amino acid decarboxylation inhibitor & catechol-O-methyltransferase inhibitor, catecholamine-depleting sympatholytic, catechol-O-methyltransferase inhibitor, dopaminergic agonist, ergot derivative, monoamine oxidase inhibitor, and non-ergot dopamine agonist
Benzodiazepines	✓	✓	✓				Benzodiazepines only
Non-benzodiazepine hypnotics	✓	✓	✓				Benzodiazepine analogs, non-benzodiazepine hypnotics, tranquilizers, gamma-aminobutyric acid A receptor agonist
Opioid agonists	✓	✓	✓		✓	✓	Full or partial opioid agonists, opiates, and opioids

Drug class							Examples
Non-opioid/non-steroidal antiinflammatory and/or analgesics		✓					Non-opioid analgesics, non-steroidal anti-inflammatory drugs (NSAIDs), COX-2 selective inhibitor NSAIDs
Antihypertensives		✓		✓		✓	Calcium channel blocker, beta adrenergic blocker, angiotensin-converting enzyme inhibitor, angiotensin 2 receptor blocker, alpha adrenergic blocker, diuretics (loop, potassium sparing, thiazide), nitrate vasodilators, and aldosterone blocker
Antiarrhythmic	✓		✓				Antiarrhythmics and cardiac glycosides
Antidiabetics		✓			✓		Insulin and insulin analogs, sulfonylureas, alpha-glucosidase inhibitor, amylin analog, biguanide, glinide, GLP-1 receptor agonist, and glucagon-like peptide-1 agonist
Anticholinergics and/or antihistamines	✓		✓		✓		Anticholinergics, histamine receptor antagonists, muscarinic antagonists, and combined anticholinergics and histamine receptor antagonists
Antiemetics	✓		✓		✓		Antiemetics, dopaminergic antagonists, and dopamine-2 receptor antagonist
Hormone replacement			✓			✓	Corticosteroids, progestin, estrogen, estrogen agonist/antagonist, and gonadotropin-releasing hormone receptor agonist
Muscle relaxers	✓		✓		✓		Muscle relaxers

(continued)

Table 7.1 (continued)

Major medication category	Delirium	Cognitive impairment	Falls	Unintentional weight and appetite loss	Urinary incontinence	Depression	Drug class/drug within each category
Immunosuppressants			✓				Calcineurin inhibitor immunosuppressant, folate analog metabolic inhibitor, and purine antimetabolite
Non-opioid cough suppressants & expectorants			✓				Expectorant, nonnarcotic antitussive, sigma-1 agonist, and uncompetitive N-methyl-D-aspartate receptor antagonist
Antimicrobiasl			✓	✓			Macrolide, cephalosporin, penicillin class, rifamycin, non-nucleoside analog reverse transcriptase inhibitor, and influenza A M2 protein inhibitor
Others	✓	✓	✓	✓	✓	✓	Beta3-adrenergic agonist, methylxanthine, cholinesterase inhibitor, interferon alpha and beta, partial cholinergic nicotinic agonist, tyrosine hydroxylase, retinoid, serotonin-1b and serotonin-1d receptor agonist, stimulant laxative, vitamin K antagonist, and platelet aggregation inhibitor

Associated syndrome checked if at least two or more medications within the wider class are associated with the syndrome extends care beyond traditional medicine to evaluate the multifactorial elements creating GSs that decrease QoL and increase mortality [173].

CGA is an intensive investigation into the health status of the older adult and can be accomplished over several office visits [173]. Table 7.2 covers the components of a Comprehensive Geriatric exam [174]. Practicing clinicians should be fully aware of the risk factors for GSs, as discussed above, as these factors are the first signs of a developing or developed GS. Many of the assessment tools in relation to specific GSs are also described above. Assessment forms are found online and on websites given in Tatum et al. [173].

Table 7.2 Components of the comprehensive geriatric assessment

Domain	Deficit	Interventions
Functional status	Limitations in basic activities of daily living or instrumental activities of daily living Timed Up and GO >13 s Falls history	Home safety evaluation Physiotherapy Occupational therapy Gait strengthening
Comorbidities	Comorbid conditions Hearing and visual impairments Pre-existing neuropathy	Co-management with primary care provider Referrals to subspecialty services
Cognition	Memory loss/impairment Confusion	Formal cognitive testing Delirium prevention Capacity assessment Involvement of caregivers
Nutrition	Weight loss >5% Iron deficiency or B12 deficiency anemia Problems with eating	Mini-Nutritional assessment Dietician involvement Supplementation Medications (mirtazapine or olanzapine are helpful in some circumstances) Speech and language pathologist for swallowing assessment
Psychological status	Feeling sad or depressed Anxiety	Geriatric Depression Scale Psychiatry referral Counseling Chaplaincy referral
Social circumstances	Patient lives alone Lack of social support Barriers to social activity	Social work referral Community resources Meal/transportation programs
Polypharmacy	≥5 Prescribed medications ≥1 Supplement	Pharmacy review of medications for interactions Discontinuation of unnecessary medications
Clinical symptoms	Pain Nausea Incontinence Diarrhea or constipation Neuropathy	Supportive care/pain management referral Single prescriber for opioids Educational interventions

Reproduced with permission from: O'Donnell et al. [174]

Essentials of a CGA include assessment of daily function with questions on ADLs and IADLs, assessment of falls with query as to past falls and a Timed-up-and-Go test, review of polypharmacy using the Beers Criteria® [100] and STOPP and START [169, 175], assessing recent weight loss, and possible screen for vision loss although not recommended, and screening for hearing loss and cognitive impairment only if complaints exist, assessment of urinary incontinence with direct questions on urine leakage and review of immunization record (see Chap. 6). Excellent guidance and pertinent resources for nurses in the assessment and treatment of GSs are found in Brown-O'Hara (2013) [2].

The CGA uses effective screening tools to identify GSs and to recommend validated interventions, preferably initiated in early stages, to prevent worsening and to improve QoL. Total geriatric care includes the CGA but additionally requires a team of health experts to provide more extensive coverage of the older adult with GSs. One example of total geriatric care is the comprehensive model of the Program of All-Inclusive Care of the Elderly (PACE), providing home care for the frail older adult [176], a system that has reduced hospital stays and improved QoL [176].

> *Alert:* Performing a Comprehensive Geriatric Assessment to identify geriatric syndromes early can lead to the application of best practices in the care of older adults to achieve the best outcomes possible.

RAPID GERIATRIC SYNDROME ASSESSMENT An important and easy-to-use geriatric assessment tool that proves helpful in all clinical settings, including hospitals and acute care, goes by the acronym of SPICES [177, 178]. SPICES stands for potentially serious geriatric conditions that may require immediate nursing assistance. They are identified as follows: *S*leep Disorders, *P*roblems with Eating or Feeding, *I*ncontinence, *C*onfusion, *E*vidence of Falls and *S*kin Breakdown [177]. This assessment tool is relevant for both healthy and frail older adults. "It provides a simple system for flagging areas in need of further assessment and provides a basis for standardizing the quality of care around certain parameters" [179].

Guidance

I. It is imperative that health providers for older adults appreciate the following concepts about geriatric syndromes (GSs):

A. GSs fall outside the understanding and practice of traditional medicine and hence require specific knowledge of identification and treatment.
   1. GSs develop from multiple interrelated factors to produce serious and costly conditions that rob the older adult of independence and QoL and increase the risk of mortality.
   2. Common GSs are frailty, sarcopenia, falls, pressure injuries, malnutrition, unintentional weight loss, delirium, cognitive decline, urinary incontinence, sleep disorders, problems with eating/feeding and depression.
B. Attention should focus on risk factors for GSs, of which the majority are known; similarly GSs can be identified by specific assessment tools.
   1. GSs benefit from the identification and correction of the cause(s).
   2. Some proven GS interventions are lifelong physical exercise (especially resistance exercise) for frailty, sarcopenia, falls, and cognitive decline. Optimal nutritional programs benefit pressure injuries, malnutrition, and unintentional weight loss. Insomnia and depression are helped with psychotherapy, and delirium requires physiotherapy and related aids. Urinary continence requires different strategies for different types.
   3. Comprehensive Geriatric Assessment followed by a comprehensive personalized care program yields the highest health outcomes and patient satisfaction; more rapid assessments (e.g., SPICES) identify GSs for immediate amelioration.
C. Drug use in GSs should be minimal and polypharmacy wisely reduced.
   1. Potentially inappropriate medications (PIMS) and medications associated with GSs (MAGS, Table 7.1) exacerbate GSs, and on medical review, unnecessary and ineffective drugs should be de-prescribed in consultation with the patient and a comprehensive health care team.
   2. Drug classes of the highest concern as PIMS and MAGS are antiepileptics, antidepressants, antiparkinson drugs, anticholinergics, antihistamines, opioid analgesics, and antipsychotics.
   3. Drug use in GSs should be limited to severe depression, extreme delirium and select cases of urinary incontinence.

References

1. Cruz-Jentoft AJ, Baeyens JP, Bauer JM, Boirie Y, Cederholm T, Landi F, et al. Sarcopenia: European consensus on definition and diagnosis. Age Ageing. 2010;39(4):412–23. https://doi.org/10.1093/ageing/afq034.
2. Brown-O'Hara T. Geriatric syndromes and their implications for nursing. Nursing. 2013;43(1):1–3. https://doi.org/10.1097/01.NURSE.0000423097.95416.50.
3. Flacker JM. What is a geriatric syndrome anyway? J Am Geriatr Soc. 2003;51(4):574–6. https://doi.org/10.1046/j.1532-5415.2003.51174.x.
4. Carlson C, Merel SE, Yukawa M. Geriatric syndromes and geriatric assessment for the generalist. Med Clin North Am. 2015;99(2):263–79. https://doi.org/10.1016/j.mcna.2014.11.003.
5. Morley JE, Vellas B, van Kan GA, Anker SD, Bauer JM, Bernabei R, et al. Frailty consensus: a call to action. J Am Med Dir Assoc. 2013;14(6):392–7. https://doi.org/10.1016/j.jamda.2013.03.022.
6. Gené Huguet L, Kostov B, Navarro González M, Hervás Docon A, Colungo Francia C, Vilaseca Llobet JM, et al. Long-term effects on preventing frailty and health care costs associated with a multifactorial intervention in the elderly: three-year follow-up data from the Pre-Frail 80 Study. Gerontology. 2022;68(10):1121–31. https://doi.org/10.1159/000521497.
7. Tuan SH, Chang LH, Sun SF, Li CH, Chen GB, Tsai YJ. Assessing the clinical effectiveness of an exergame-based exercise training program using ring fit adventure to prevent and postpone frailty and Sarcopenia among older adults in rural long-term care facilities: randomized controlled trial. J Med Internet Res. 2024;26:e59468. https://doi.org/10.2196/59468.
8. Sanford AM, Morley JE, Berg-Weger M, Lundy J, Little MO, Leonard K, et al. High prevalence of geriatric syndromes in older adults. PLoS One. 2020;15(6):e0233857. https://doi.org/10.1371/journal.pone.0233857.
9. Tuna F, Ustundag A, Basak CH, Tuna H. Rapid geriatric assessment, physical activity, and sleep quality in adults aged more than 65 years: a preliminary study. J Nutr Health Aging. 2019;23(7):617–22. https://doi.org/10.1007/s12603-019-1212-z.
10. Bell S, Vasilevskis E, Saraf A, Jacobsen JML, Kripalani S, Mixon AS, et al. Geriatric syndromes in hospitalized older adults discharged to skilled nursing facilities. J Am Geriatr Soc. 2016;64(4):715–22. https://doi.org/10.1111/jgs.14035.
11. Inouye SK, Studenski S, Tinetti ME, Kuchel GA. Geriatric syndromes: clinical, research, and policy implications of a core geriatric concept. J Am Geriatr Soc. 2007;55(5):780–91. https://doi.org/10.1111/j.1532-5415.2007.01156.x.
12. Mueller YK, Monod S, Locatelli I, Büla C, Cornuz J, Senn N. Performance of a brief geriatric evaluation compared to a comprehensive geriatric assessment for detection of geriatric syndromes in family medicine: a prospective diagnostic study. BMC Geriatr. 2018;18(1):72. https://doi.org/10.1186/s12877-018-0761-z.
13. Leyhe T, Reynolds CF 3rd, Melcher T, Linnemann C, Klöppel S, Blennow K, et al. A common challenge in older adults: classification, overlap, and therapy of depression and dementia. Alzheimers Dement. 2017;13(1):59–71. https://doi.org/10.1016/j.jalz.2016.08.007.
14. Saghaleini SH, Dehghan K, Shadvar K, Sanaie S, Mahmoodpoor A, Ostadi Z. Pressure ulcer and nutrition. Indian J Crit Care Med. 2018;22(4):283–9. https://doi.org/10.4103/ijccm.IJCCM_277_17.
15. Walston J, Buta B, Xue QL. Frailty screening and interventions: considerations for clinical practice. Clin Geriatr Med. 2018;34(1):25–38. https://doi.org/10.1016/j.cger.2017.09.004.
16. Fried LP. Conference on the physiologic basis of frailty. April 28, 1992, Baltimore, Maryland, U.S.A. Introduction Aging (Milano). 1992;4(3):251–2. PMID: 1420409.
17. Ferrucci L, Guralnik JM, Studenski S, Fried LP, Cutler GB Jr, Walston JD, et al. Designing randomized, controlled trials aimed at preventing or delaying functional decline and disability in frail, older persons: a consensus report. J Am Geriatr Soc. 2004;52(4):625–34. https://doi.org/10.1111/j.1532-5415.2004.52174.x.

18. O'Caoimh R, Sezgin D, O'Donovan MR, Molloy DW, Clegg A, Rockwood K, et al. Prevalence of frailty in 62 countries across the world: a systematic review and meta-analysis of population-level studies. Age Ageing. 2021;50(1):96–104. https://doi.org/10.1093/ageing/afaa219.
19. Theou O, Squires E, Mallery K, Lee JS, Fay S, Goldstein J, et al. What do we know about frailty in the acute care setting? A scoping review. BMC Geriatr. 2018;18:139. https://doi.org/10.1186/s12877-018-0823-2.
20. Ofori-Asenso R, Chin KL, Mazidi M, Zomer E, Ilomaki J, Zullo AR, et al. Global incidence of frailty and prefrailty among community-dwelling older adults: a systematic review and meta-analysis. JAMA Netw Open. 2019;2(8):e198398. https://doi.org/10.1001/jamanetworkopen.2019.8398.
21. Wang X, Hu J, Wu D. Risk factors for frailty in older adults. Medicine (Baltimore). 2022;101(34):e30169. https://doi.org/10.1097/MD.0000000000030169.
22. Tchalla A, Laubarie-Mouret C, Cardinaud N, Gayot C, Rebiere M, Dumoitier N, et al. Risk factors of frailty and functional disability in community-dwelling older adults: a cross-sectional analysis of the FREEDOM-LNA cohort study. BMC Geriatr. 2022;22(1):762. https://doi.org/10.1186/s12877-022-03447-z.
23. Searle SD, Mitnitski A, Gahbauer EA, Gill TM, Rockwood K. A standard procedure for creating a frailty index. BMC Geriatr. 2008;8:24. https://doi.org/10.1186/1471-2318-8-24.
24. Rockwood K, Mitnitski A. Frailty defined by deficit accumulation and geriatric medicine defined by frailty. Clin Geriatr Med. 2011;27(1):17–26. https://doi.org/10.1016/j.cger.2010.08.008.
25. Fried LP, Ferrucci L, Darer J, Williamson JD, Anderson G. Untangling the concepts of disability, frailty, and comorbidity: implications for improved targeting and care. J Gerontol A Biol Sci Med Sci. 2004;59(3):255–63. https://doi.org/10.1093/gerona/59.3.m255.
26. Little MO. The rapid geriatric assessment: a quick screen for geriatric syndromes. Mo Med. 2017;114(2):101–4. PMID: 30228554 PMCID: PMC6140035.
27. Abellan van Kan G, Rolland Y, Bergman H, Morley JE, Kritchevsky SB, Vellas B. The I.A.N.A Task Force on frailty assessment of older people in clinical practice. J Nutr Health Aging. 2008;12(1):29–37. https://doi.org/10.1007/BF02982161.
28. Subra J, Gillette-Guyonnet S, Cesari M, Oustric S, Vellas B, Platform T. The integration of frailty into clinical practice: preliminary results from the Gerontopole. J Nutr Health Aging. 2012;16(8):714–20. https://doi.org/10.1007/s12603-012-0391-7.
29. Turner G, Clegg A, British Geriatrics Society, Age UK, Royal College of General Practitioners. Best practice guidelines for the management of frailty: a British Geriatrics Society, Age UK and Royal College of General Practitioners report. Age Ageing. 2014;43(6):744–7. https://doi.org/10.1093/ageing/afu138.
30. Ravindrarajah R, Lee DM, Pye SR, Gielen E, Boonen S, Vanderschueren D, et al. The ability of three different models of frailty to predict all-cause mortality: results from the European Male Aging Study (EMAS). Arch Gerontol Geriatr. 2013;57(3):360–8. https://doi.org/10.1016/j.archger.2013.06.010.
31. Rockwood K, Mitnitski A. Frailty in relation to the accumulation of deficits. J Gerontol A Biol Sci Med Sci. 2007;62(7):722–7. https://doi.org/10.1093/gerona/62.7.722.
32. Lang PO, Michel JP, Zekry D. Frailty syndrome: a transitional state in a dynamic process. Gerontology. 2009;55(5):539–459. https://doi.org/10.1159/000211949.
33. Sun X, Liu W, Gao Y, Qin L, Feng H, Tan H, et al. Comparative effectiveness of non-pharmacological interventions for frailty: a systematic review and network meta-analysis. Age Ageing. 2023;52(2):afad004. https://doi.org/10.1093/ageing/afad004.
34. Lai CC, Tu YK, Wang TG, Huang YT, Chien KL. Effects of resistance training, endurance training and whole-body vibration on lean body mass, muscle strength and physical performance in older people: a systematic review and network meta-analysis. Age Ageing. 2018;47(3):367–73. https://doi.org/10.1093/ageing/afy009.
35. Fragala MS, Cadore EL, Dorgo S, Izquierdo M, Kraemer WJ, Peterson MD, et al. Resistance training for older adults: position statement from the National Strength and Conditioning

Association. J Strength Cond Res. 2019;33(8):2019–52. https://doi.org/10.1519/JSC.0000000000003230.
36. Bull FC, Al-Ansari SS, Biddle S, Borodulin K, Buman MP, Cardon G, et al. World Health Organization 2020 guidelines on physical activity and sedentary behaviour. Br J Sports Med. 2020;54(24):1451–62. https://doi.org/10.1136/bjsports-2020-102955.
37. Ni Lochlainn M, Cox NJ, Wilson T, Hayhoe RPG, Ramsay SE, Granic A, et al. Nutrition and frailty: opportunities for prevention and treatment. Nutrients. 2021;13(7):2349. https://doi.org/10.3390/nu13072349.
38. Lorenzo-López L, Maseda A, de Labra C, Regueiro-Folgueira L, Rodríguez-Villamil JL, Millán-Calenti JC. Nutritional determinants of frailty in older adults: a systematic review. BMC Geriatr. 2017;17(1):108. https://doi.org/10.1186/s12877-017-0496-2.
39. Silva R, Pizato N, da Mata F, Figueiredo A, Ito M, Pereira MG. Mediterranean diet and musculoskeletal-functional outcomes in community-dwelling older people: a systematic review and meta-analysis. J Nutr Health Aging. 2018;22:655–63. https://doi.org/10.1007/s12603-017-0993-1.
40. Kojima G, Avgerinou C, Iliffe S, Walters K. Adherence to Mediterranean diet reduces incident frailty risk: systematic review and meta-analysis. J Am Geriatr Soc. 2018;66(4):783–8. https://doi.org/10.1111/jgs.15251.
41. Lopez-Garcia E, Hagan KA, Fung TT, Hu FB, Rodríguez-Artalejo F. Mediterranean diet and risk of frailty syndrome among women with type 2 diabetes. Am J Clin Nutr. 2018;107(5):763–71. https://doi.org/10.1093/ajcn/nqy026.
42. Veronese N, Stubbs B, Noale M, Solmi M, Rizzoli R, Vaona A, et al. Adherence to a Mediterranean diet is associated with lower incidence of frailty: a longitudinal cohort study. Clin Nutr. 2018;37(5):1492–7. https://doi.org/10.1016/j.clnu.2017.08.028.
43. Coelho-Júnior HJ, Rodrigues B, Uchida M, Marzetti E. Low protein intake is associated with frailty in older adults: a systematic review and meta-analysis of observational studies. Nutrients. 2018;10(9):1334. https://doi.org/10.3390/nu10091334.
44. De Liao C, Lee PH, Hsiao DJ, Huang SW, Tsauo JY, Chen HC, Liou TH. Effects of protein supplementation combined with exercise intervention on frailty indices, body composition, and physical function in frail older adults. Nutrients. 2018;10(12):1916. https://doi.org/10.3390/nu10121916.
45. Marzetti E, Calvani R, Landi F, Hoogendijk EO, Fougère B, Vellas B, et al. Innovative medicines initiative: the SPRINTT project. J Frailty Aging. 2015;4(4):207–8. PMID: 2669316 PMCID: PMC4675469.
46. Azzolino D, Cesari M. Multicomponent interventions against frailty. JAR Life. 2021;10:17–8. https://doi.org/10.14283/jarlife.2021.3.
47. Fielding RA, Rejeski WJ, Blair S, Church T, Espeland MA, Gill TM, et al. LIFE Research Group. The lifestyle interventions and independence for elders study: design and methods. J Gerontol A Biol Sci Med Sci. 2011;66(11):1226–37. https://doi.org/10.1093/gerona/glr123.
48. Volkert D, Beck AM, Cederholm T, Cruz-Jentoft A, Goisser S, Hooper L, et al. ESPEN guideline on clinical nutrition and hydration in geriatrics. Clin Nutr. 2019;38:10–47. https://doi.org/10.1016/j.clnu.2018.05.024.
49. Bernabei R, Landi F, Calvani R, Cesari M, Del Signore S, Anker SD, et al. Multicomponent intervention to prevent mobility disability in frail older adults: randomised controlled trial (SPRINTT project). BMJ. 2022;377:e068788. https://doi.org/10.1136/bmj-2021-068788.
50. Guralnik JM, Simonsick EM, Ferrucci L, Glynn RJ, Berkman LF, Blazer DG, et al. A short physical performance battery assessing lower extremity function: association with self-reported disability and prediction of mortality and nursing home admission. J Gerontol. 1994;49(2):M85–94. https://doi.org/10.1093/geronj/49.2.m85.
51. Martin FC, Fanhoff AH, Falaschi P, Marsh D. Frailty and Sarcopenia. In: Orthogeriatrics: the management of older patients with fragility fractures [Internet]. 2nd edition. Cham (CH): Springer; 2021. Chapter 4.

52. Cruz-Jentoft AJ, Bahat G, Bauer J, Boirie Y, Bruyere O, Cederholm T, et al. Sarcopenia: revised European consensus on definition and diagnosis. Age Ageing. 2019;48(1):16–31. https://doi.org/10.1093/ageing/afy16.
53. Deschenes MR. Effects of aging on muscle fibre type and size. Sports Med. 2004;34(12):809–24. https://doi.org/10.2165/00007256-200434120-00002.
54. Janssen I, Heymsfield SB, Wang ZM, Ross R. Skeletal muscle mass and distribution in 468 men and women aged 18–88 yr. J Appl Physiol (1985). 2000;89(1):81–8. https://doi.org/10.1152/jappl.2000.89.1.81.
55. Petermann-Rocha F, Balntzi V, Gray SR, Lara J, Ho FK, Pell JP, et al. Global prevalence of sarcopenia and severe sarcopenia: a systematic review and meta-analysis. J Cachexia Sarcopenia Muscle. 2022;13(1):86–99. https://doi.org/10.1002/jcsm.12783.
56. Yuan S, Larsson SC. Epidemiology of sarcopenia: prevalence, risk factors, and consequences. Metabolism. 2023;144:155533. https://doi.org/10.1016/j.metabol.2023.155533.
57. Cruz-Jentoft AJ, Landi F, Schneider SM, Zuniga C, Arai H, Boirie Y, et al. Prevalence of and interventions for sarcopenia in ageing adults: a systematic review. Report of the International Sarcopenia Initiative (EWGSOP and IWGS). Age Ageing. 2014;43(6):748–59. https://doi.org/10.1093/ageing/afu115.
58. Skelton DA, Young A, Greig CA, Malbut KE. Effects of resistance training on strength, power, and selected functional abilities of women aged 75 and older. J Am GeriatrSoc. 1995;43(10):1081–7. https://doi.org/10.1111/j.1532-5415.1995.tb07004.x.
59. Vincent KR, Braith RW, Feldman RA, Magyari PM, Cutler RB, Persin SA, et al. Resistance exercise and physical performance in adults aged 60 to 83. J Am GeriatrSoc. 2002;50(6):1100–7. https://doi.org/10.1046/j.1532-5415.2002.50267.x.
60. Sayer AA, Syddall H, Martin H, Patel H, Baylis D, Cooper C. The developmental origins of sarcopenia. J Nutr Health Aging. 2008;12(7):427–32. https://doi.org/10.1007/BF02982703.
61. Taguchi CK, Menezes PL, Melo ACS, Santana LS, Conceição WRS, Souza GF. Frailty syndrome and risks for falling in the elderly community. Codas. 2022;34(6):e20210025. https://doi.org/10.1590/2317-1782/20212021025pt.
62. Ang GC, Low SL, How CH. Approach to falls among the elderly in the community. Singapore Med J. 2020;61(3):116–21. https://doi.org/10.11622/smedj.2020029.
63. National Safety Council. 2024. https://injuryfacts.nsc.org/home-and-community/safety-topics/older-adult-falls/#:~:text=Safety%20Topics,-Older%20Adult%20Falls&text=According%20to%20the%20Centers%20for,were%20treated%20in%20emergency%20departments
64. Keglovits M, Clemson L, Hu Y-L, Nguyen A, Neff AJ, Mandelbaum C, et al. A scoping review of fall hazards in the homes of older adults and development of a framework for assessment and intervention. Aust Occup Ther J. 2020;67(5):470–8. https://doi.org/10.1111/1440-1630.12682.
65. Shen Y, Shi Q, Nong K, Li S, Yue J, Huang J, et al. Exercise for sarcopenia in older people: a systematic review and network meta-analysis. J Cachexia Sarcopenia Muscle. 2023;14(3):1199–211. https://doi.org/10.1002/jcsm.13225.
66. Dautzenberg L, Beglinger S, Tsokani S, Zevgiti S, Raijmann RCMA, Rodondi N, et al. Interventions for preventing falls and fall-related fractures in community-dwelling older adults: a systematic review and network meta-analysis. J Am Geriatr Soc. 2021;69(10):2973–84. https://doi.org/10.1111/jgs.17375.
67. Hopewell S, Adedire O, Copsey BJ, Boniface GJ, Sherrington C, Clemson L, et al. Multifactorial and multiple component interventions for preventing falls in older people living in the community. Cochrane Database Syst Rev. 2018;7(7):CD012221. https://doi.org/10.1002/14651858.CD012221.pub2.
68. Haines TP, Hill AM, Hill KD, McPhail S, Oliver D, Brauer S, et al. Patient education to prevent falls among older hospital inpatients: a randomized controlled trial. Arch Intern Med. 2011;171(6):516–24. https://doi.org/10.1001/archinternmed.2010.444.

69. Hill A, McPhail S, Waldron N, et al. Fall rates in hospital rehabilitation units after individualised patient and staff education programmes: a pragmatic, stepped-wedge, cluster-randomised controlled trial. Lancet. 2015;385:2592–9.
70. Morris ME, Webster K, Jones C, Hill AM, Haines T, McPhail S, et al. Interventions to reduce falls in hospitals: a systematic review and meta-analysis. Age Ageing. 2022;51(5):afac077. https://doi.org/10.1093/ageing/afac077.
71. Cameron ID, Dyer SM, Panagoda CE, Murray GR, Hill KD, Cumming RG, et al. Interventions for preventing falls in older people in care facilities and hospitals. Cochrane Database Syst Rev. 2018;9(9):CD005465. https://doi.org/10.1002/14651858.CD005465.pub4.
72. Bilder GE. Human Biological. Aging from macromolecules to organ systems. Hoboken, New Jersey: John Wiley and Sons; 2016. p. 225–53.
73. Phillips C. Lifestyle modulators of neuroplasticity: how physical activity, mental engagement, and diet promote cognitive health during aging. Neural Plast. 2017;2017:3589271. https://doi.org/10.1155/2017/3589271.
74. Bai W, Chen P, Cai H, Zhang Q, Su Z, Cheung T, et al. Worldwide prevalence of mild cognitive impairment among community dwellers aged 50 years and older: a meta-analysis and systematic review of epidemiology studies. Age Ageing. 2022;51(8):afac173. https://doi.org/10.1093/ageing/afac173.
75. Jongsiriyanyong S, Limpawattana P. Mild cognitive impairment in clinical practice: a review article. Am J Alzheimers Dis Other Dement. 2018;33(8):500–7. https://doi.org/10.1177/1533317518791401.
76. Dominguez LJ, Veronese N, Vernuccio L, Catanese G, Inzerillo F, Salemi G, et al. Nutrition, physical activity, and other lifestyle factors in the prevention of cognitive decline and dementia. Nutrients. 2021;13(11):4080. https://doi.org/10.3390/nu13114080.
77. Richards M. The power of birth cohorts to study risk factors for cognitive impairment. Curr Neurol Neurosci Rep. 2022;22(12):847–54. https://doi.org/10.1007/s11910-022-01244-0.
78. Montreal Cognitive Assessment www.mocatest.org.
79. Borson S, Scanlan J, Brush M, Vitaliano P, Dokmak A. The mini-cog: a cognitive 'vital signs' measure for dementia screening in multi-lingual elderly. Int J Geriatr Psychiatry. 2000;15(11):1021–7. https://doi.org/10.1002/1099-1166(200011)15:11<1021::aid-gps234>3.0.co;2-6.
80. Ngandu T, Lehtisalo J, Solomon A, Levalahti E, Ahtiluoto S, Antikainen R, et al. A 2 year multidomain intervention of diet, exercise, cognitive training, and vascular risk monitoring versus control to prevent cognitive decline in at-risk elderly people (FINGER): a randomised controlled trial. Lancet. 2015;385(9984):2255–63. https://doi.org/10.1016/S0140-6736(15)60461-5.
81. Andrieu S, Guyonnet S, Coley N, Cantet C, Bonnefoy M, Bordes S, et al. Effect of long-term omega 3 polyunsaturated fatty acid supplementation with or without multidomain intervention on cognitive function in elderly adults with memory complaints (MAPT): a randomised, placebo-controlled trial. Lancet Neurol. 2017;16(5):377–89. https://doi.org/10.1016/S1474-4422(17)30040-6.
82. Langa KM. Levine DA The diagnosis and management of mild cognitive impairment: a clinical review. JAMA. 2014;312(23):2551–61. https://doi.org/10.1001/jama.2014.13806.
83. Wilson JE, Mart MF, Cunningham C, Shehabi Y, Girard TD, MacLullich AMJ, et al. Delirium. Nat Rev Dis Primers. 2020;6(1):90. https://doi.org/10.1038/s41572-020-00223-4.
84. Goldberg TE, Chen C, Wang Y, Jung E, Swanson A, Ing C, et al. Association of delirium with long-term cognitive decline: a meta-analysis. JAMA Neurol. 2020;77(11):1373–81. https://doi.org/10.1001/jamaneurol.2020.2273.
85. Inouye SK, Westendorp RG, Saczynski JS. Delirium in elderly people. Lancet. 2014;383(9920):911–22. https://doi.org/10.1016/S0140-6736(13)60688-1.
86. Clegg A, Young JB. Which medications to avoid in people at risk of delirium: a systematic review. Age Ageing. 2011;40(1):23–9. https://doi.org/10.1093/ageing/afq140.

References

87. Pandharipande PP, Girard TD, Jackson JC, Morandi A, Thompson JL, Pun BT, et al. Long-term cognitive impairment after critical illness. N Engl J Med. 2013;369(14):1306–16. https://doi.org/10.1056/NEJMoa1301372.
88. Cole MG, Bailey R, Bonnycastle M, McCusker J, Fung S, Ciampi A, et al. Partial and no recovery from delirium in older hospitalized adults: frequency and baseline risk factors. J Am Geriatr Soc. 2015;63(11):2340–8. https://doi.org/10.1111/jgs.13791.
89. Gibb K, Seeley A, Quinn T, Siddiqi N, Shenkin S, Rockwood K, et al. The consistent burden in published estimates of delirium occurrence in medical inpatients over four decades: a systematic review and meta-analysis study. Age Ageing. 2020;49(3):352–60. https://doi.org/10.1093/ageing/afaa040.
90. Morichi V, Fredecostante M, Morandi A, Di Santo SG, Mazzone A, Mossello E, et al. A point prevalence study of delirium in Italian nursing homes. Dement Geriatr Cogn Disord. 2018;46(1–2):27–41. https://doi.org/10.1159/000490722.
91. American Psychiatric Association. Diagnostic and statistical manual of mental disorders. 5th ed. 2013.
92. Trzepacz PT. A review of delirium assessment instruments. Gen Hosp Psychiatry. 1994;16(6):397–405. https://doi.org/10.1016/0163-8343(94)90115-5.
93. De J, Wand AP. Delirium screening: a systematic review of delirium screening tools in hospitalized patients. Gerontologist. 2015;55(6):1079–99. https://doi.org/10.1093/geront/gnv100.
94. Tieges Z, Maclullich AMJ, Anand A, Brookes C, Cassarino M, O'connor M, et al. Diagnostic accuracy of the 4AT for delirium detection in older adults: systematic review and meta-analysis. Age Ageing. 2021;50(3):733–43. https://doi.org/10.1093/ageing/afaa224.
95. https://www.merckmanuals.com/professional/multimedia/table/confusion-assessment-method-cam-for-diagnosing-delirium.
96. Bergeron N, Dubois MJ, Dumont M, Dial S, Skrobik Y. Intensive Care Delirium Screening Checklist: evaluation of a new screening tool. Intensive Care Med. 2001;27(5):859–64. https://doi.org/10.1007/s001340100909.
97. Scottish Intercollegiate Guidelines Network (SIGN). Risk Reduction and Management of Delirium. Edinburgh: SIGN; 2019. (SIGN publication; no.157). [March 2019]. Available from URL: http://www.sign.ac.uk. https://www.sign.ac.uk/media/1423/sign157.pdf. 2019.
98. Devlin J, Skrobik Y, Gelinas C, Needham D, Slooter AJC, Pandharipande PP, et al. Clinical practice guidelines for the prevention and management of pain, agitation/sedation, delirium, immobility, and sleep disruption in adult patients in the ICU. Crit Care Med. 2018;46(9):e825–73. https://doi.org/10.1097/CCM.0000000000003299.
99. Scottish Government Polypharmacy Model of Care Group. Polypharmacy Guidance, Realistic Prescribing, 3rd ed. Scottish Government 2018. Available from url: https://www.therapeutics.scot.nhs.uk/wp-content/uploads/2018/09/Polypharmacy-Guidance-2018.pdf.
100. By the 2023 American Geriatrics Society Beers Criteria® Update Expert Panel. American Geriatrics Society 2023 updated AGS Beers Criteria® for potentially inappropriate medication use in older adults. J Am Geriatr Soc. 2023;71(7):2052–81. https://doi.org/10.1111/jgs.18372.
101. Ng KT, Shubash CJ, Chong JS. The effect of dexmedetomidine on delirium and agitation in patients in intensive care: systematic review and meta-analysis with trial sequential analysis. Anaesthesia. 2019;74(3):380–92. https://doi.org/10.1111/anae.14472.
102. Rubin EB, Buehler AE, Halpern SD. States worse than death among hospitalized patients with serious illnesses. JAMA Int Med. 2016;176(10):1557–9. https://doi.org/10.1001/jamainternmed.2016.4362.
103. Gibbs CF, Johnson TM 2nd, Ouslander JG. Office management of geriatric urinary incontinence. Am J Med. 2007;120(3):211–20. https://doi.org/10.1016/j.amjmed.2006.03.044.
104. Batmani S, Jalali R, Mohammadi M, Bokaee S. Prevalence and factors related to urinary incontinence in older adults women worldwide: a comprehensive systematic review and meta-analysis of observational studies. BMC Geriatr. 2021;21(1):212. https://doi.org/10.1186/s12877-021-02135-8.

105. Diokno AC, Estanol MVC, Ibrahim IA, Balasubramaniam M. Prevalence of urinary incontinence in community dwelling men: a cross sectional nationwide epidemiological survey. Int Urol Nephrol. 2007;39(1):129–36. https://doi.org/10.1007/s11255-006-9127-0.
106. Vaughan CP, Markland AD, Smith PP, Burgio KL, Kuchel GA. American Geriatrics Society/National Institute on Aging Urinary Incontinence Conference Planning Committee and Faculty Report and Research Agenda of the American Geriatrics Society and National Institute on Aging Bedside-to-Bench Conference on Urinary Incontinence in Older Adults: a Translational Research Agenda for a Complex Geriatric Syndrome. J Am Geriatr Soc. 2018;66(4):773–82. https://doi.org/10.1111/jgs.15157.
107. Erekson EA, Ciarleglio MM, Hanissian PD, Strohbehn K, Bynum JP, Fried TR. Functional disability and compromised mobility among older women with urinary incontinence. Female Pelv Med Reconstruct Surg. 2015;21(3):170–5. https://doi.org/10.1097/SPV.0000000000000136.
108. Harvard Health, https://www.health.harvard.edu/bladder-and-bowel/medications-that-can-cause-urinary-incontinence.
109. Wei B, Zhao Y, Lin P, Qiu W, Wang S, Gu C, et al. The association between overactive bladder and systemic immunity-inflammation index: a cross-sectional study of NHANES 2005 to 2018. Sci Rep. 2024;14(1):12579. https://doi.org/10.1038/s41598-024-63448-3.
110. Haylen BT, de Ridder D, Freeman RM, Swift SE, Berghmans B, Lee J, et al. An International Urogynecological Association (IUGA)/International Continence Society (ICS) joint report on the terminology for female pelvic floor dysfunction. Neurourol Urodyn. 2010;29(1):4–20. https://doi.org/10.1002/nau.20798.
111. Aoki Y, Brown HW, Brubaker L, Cornu JN, Daly JO, Cartwright R. Urinary incontinence in women. Nat Rev Dis Primers. 2017;3:17042. https://doi.org/10.1038/nrdp.2017.42.
112. Brown JS, Bradley CS, Sebak LL, Richter HE, Kraus SR, Brubaker L, et al. The sensitivity and specificity of a simple test to distinguish between urge and stress urinary incontinence. Ann Intern Med. 2006;144(10):715–23. https://doi.org/10.7326/0003-4819-144-10-200605160-00005.
113. Vrijens DMJ, Spakman JI, van Koeveringe GA, Berghmans B. Patient-reported outcome after treatment of urinary incontinence in a multidisciplinary pelvic care clinic. Int J Urol. 2015;22(11):1051–7. https://doi.org/10.1111/iju.12885.
114. Weber MA, Kleijn MH, Langendam M, Limpes J, Heineman MJ, Roover JP. Local oestrogen for pelvic floor disorders: a systematic review. PLoS One. 2015;10(9):e0136265. https://doi.org/10.1371/journal.pone.0136265.
115. Dell'Atti L. Efficacy of Tadalafil once daily versus Fesoterodine in the treatment of overactive bladder in older patients. Eur Rev Med Pharmacol Sci. 2015;19(9):1559–63. PMID: 26004592.
116. Mondragon N, Zito PM. Pressure Injury. Treasure Island (FL): StatPearls Publishing; 2024.
117. Bilder GE. Human biological aging from macromolecules to organ systems. Hoboken, New Jersey: John Wiley and Sons; 2016. p. 101–22.
118. Anders J, Heinemann A, Leffmann C, Leutenegger M, Pröfener F, von Renteln-Kruse W. Decubitus ulcers: pathophysiology and primary prevention. Dtsch Arztebl Int. 2010;107(21):371–81; quiz 382. https://doi.org/10.3238/arztebl.2010.0371.
119. Lyder CH. Pressure ulcer prevention and management. JAMA. 2003;289(2):223–6. https://doi.org/10.1001/jama.289.2.223.
120. Labeau SO, Afonso E, Benbenishty J, Blackwood B, Boulanger C, Brett SJ, et al. Prevalence, associated factors and outcomes of pressure injuries in adult intensive care unit patients: the DecubICUs study. Intensive Care Med. 2021;47(2):160–9. https://doi.org/10.1007/s00134-020-06234-9.
121. Edsberg LE, Black JM, Goldberg M, McNichol L, Moore L, Sieggreen M. Revised national pressure ulcer advisory panel pressure injury staging system: revised pressure injury staging system. J Wound Ostomy Continence Nurs. 2016;43(6):585–97. https://doi.org/10.1097/WON.0000000000000281.

122. Qaseem A, Mir TP, Starkey M, Denberg TD, Clinical Guidelines Committee of the American College of Physicians. Risk assessment and prevention of pressure ulcers: a clinical practice guideline from the American College of Physicians. Ann Intern Med. 2015;162(5):359–69. https://doi.org/10.7326/M14-1567.
123. Bergstrom N, Braden BJ, Laguzza A, Holman V. The Braden scale for predicting pressure sore risk. Nurs Res. 1987;36(4):205–10. PMID: 3299278.
124. Pancorbo-Hidalgo PL, Garcia-Fernandez FP, Lopez-Medina IM, Alvarez-Nieto C. Risk assessment scales for pressure ulcer prevention: a systematic review. J Adv Nurs. 2006;54(1):94–110. https://doi.org/10.1111/j.1365-2648.2006.03794.x.
125. https://www.in.gov/health/files/Braden_Scale.pdf.
126. Cederholm T, Barazzoni R, Austin P, Ballmer P, Biolo G, Bischoff SC, et al. ESPEN guidelines on definitions and terminology of clinical nutrition. Clin Nutr. 2017;36(1):49–64. https://doi.org/10.1016/j.clnu.2016.09.004.
127. Cereda E, Pedrolli C, Klersy C, Bonardi C, Quarleri L, Cappello S, et al. Nutritional status in older persons according to healthcare setting: a systematic review and meta-analysis of prevalence data using MNA®. Clin Nutr. 2016;35(6):1282–90. https://doi.org/10.1016/j.clnu.2016.03.008.
128. O'Keeffe M, Kelly M, O'Herlihy E, O'Toole PW, Kearney PM, Timmons S, et al. Potentially modifiable determinants of malnutrition in older adults: a systematic review. Clin Nutr. 2019;38(6):2477–98. https://doi.org/10.1016/j.clnu.2018.12.007.
129. Ashmore DL, Rashid A, Wilson TR, Halliday V, Lee MJ. Identifying malnutrition in emergency general surgery: systematic review. BJS Open. 2023;7(5):zrad086. https://doi.org/10.1093/bjsopen/zrad086.
130. Landi F, Lattanzio F, Dell'Aquila G, Eusebi P, Gasperini B, Liperoti R, Belluigi A, Bernabei R, Cherubini A. Prevalence and potentially reversible factors associated with anorexia among older nursing home residents: results from the ULISSE project. J Am Med Dir Assoc. 2013;14:119–24. https://doi.org/10.1016/j.jamda.2012.10.022.
131. Kamdem B, Seematter-Bagnoud L, Botrugno F, Santos-Eggimann B. Relationship between oral health and Fried's frailty criteria in community-dwelling older persons. BMC Geriatr. 2017;17(1):174. https://doi.org/10.1186/s12877-017-0568-3.
132. Kimble R, Papacosta AO, Lennon LT, Whincup PH, Weyant RJ, et al. The relationships of dentition, use of dental prothesis and oral health problems with frailty, disability and diet quality: results from population-based studies of older adults from the UK and USA. J Nutr Health Aging. 2023;27(8):663–72. https://doi.org/10.1007/s12603-023-1951-8.
133. Landi F, Calvani R, Tosato M, Martone AM, Ortolani E, et al. Anorexia of aging: risk factors, consequences, and potential treatments. Nutrients. 2016;8(2):69. https://doi.org/10.3390/nu8020069.
134. Kang MG, Ji S, Park YK, Baek JY, Kwon YH, et al. The clinical frailty scale as a risk assessment tool for dysphagia in older inpatients: a cross-sectional study. Ann Geriatr Med Res. 2023;27(3):204–11. https://doi.org/10.4235/agmr.23.0053.
135. Chalmers JM, King PL, Spencer AJ, Wright FAC, Carter KD. The oral health assessment tool — validity and reliability. Aust Dent J. 2005;50(3):191–9. https://doi.org/10.1111/j.1834-7819.2005.tb00360.x.
136. Kayser-Jones J, Bird WF, Paul SM, Long L, Schell ES. An instrument to assess the oral health status of nursing home residents. Gerontologist. 1995;35(6):814–24. https://doi.org/10.1093/geront/35.6.814.
137. Aronoff-Spencer E, Asgari P, Finlayson TL, Gavin J, Forstey M, et al. A comprehensive assessment for community-based, person-centered care for older adults. BMC Geriatr. 2020;20:193. https://doi.org/10.1186/s12877-020-1502-7.
138. Gaddey HL, Holder KK. Unintentional weight loss in older adults. Am Fam Physician. 2021;104(1):34–40. PMID: 34264616.
139. Bouras EP, Lange SM, Scolapio JS. Rational approach to patients with unintentional weight loss. Mayo Clin Proc. 2001;76(9):923–9. https://doi.org/10.4065/76.9.923.

140. Alibhai SM, Greenwood C, Payette H. An approach to the management of unintentional weight loss in elderly people. CMAJ. 2005;172(6):773–80. https://doi.org/10.1503/cmaj.1031527.
141. https://bestpractice.bmj.com/topics/en-us/548#:~:text=In%20population%2Dbased%20 cohort%20studies,19%5D.
142. Ruiz-García V, López-Briz E, Carbonell-Sanchis R, Bort-Martí S, Gonzálvez-Perales JL. Megestrol acetate for cachexia-anorexia syndrome. A systematic review. J Cachexia Sarcopenia Muscle. 2018 Jun;9(3):444–52. https://doi.org/10.1002/jcsm.12292.
143. Rodriguez JC, Dzierzewski JM, Alessi CA. Sleep problems in the elderly. Med Clin North Am. 2015;99(2):431–9. https://doi.org/10.1016/j.mcna.2014.11.013.
144. Ribeiro BC, de Athayde CE, Silva A, de Souza LBR, de Araújo Moraes JB, Carneiro SR, et al. Risk stratification for frailty, impairment and assessment of sleep disorders in community-dwelling older adults. Exp Gerontol. 2024;187:112370. https://doi.org/10.1016/j.exger.2024.112370.
145. Vitiello MV, Moe KE, Prinz PN. Sleep complaints cosegregate with illness in older adults: clinical research informed by and informing epidemiological studies of sleep. J Psychosom Res. 2002;53:555–9. https://doi.org/10.1016/s0022-3999(02)00435-x.
146. Carvalhas-Almeida C, Cavadas C, Álvaro AR. The impact of insomnia on frailty and the hallmarks of aging. Aging Clin Exp Res. 2023;35(2):253–69. https://doi.org/10.1007/s40520-022-02310-w.
147. Çavuşoğlu Ç, Deniz O, Tuna Doğrul R, Çöteli S, Öncül A. Frailty is associated with poor sleep quality in the oldest old. Turk J Med Sci. 2021;51(2):540–6. https://doi.org/10.3906/sag-2001-168.
148. Wen Q, Yan X, Ren Z, Wang B, Liu Y, et al. Association between insomnia and frailty in older population: a meta-analytic evaluation of the observational studies. Brain Behav. 2023;13(1):e2793. https://doi.org/10.1002/brb3.2793.
149. Yan Z, Xu Y, Li K. Liu L The correlation between frailty index and incidence, mortality in obstructive sleep apnea: evidence from NHANES. Heliyon. 2024;10(12):e32514. https://doi.org/10.1016/j.heliyon.2024.e32514.
150. Ensrud KE, Blackwell TL, Redline S, Ancoli-Israel S, Paudel ML, et al. Sleep disturbances and frailty status in older community-dwelling men. J Am Geriatr Soc. 2009;57(11):2085–93. https://doi.org/10.1111/j.1532-5415.2009.02490.x.
151. Ensrud KE, Blackwell TL, Ancoli-Israel S, Redline S, Cawthon PM, et al. Sleep disturbances and risk of frailty and mortality in older men. Sleep Med. 2012;13(10):1217–25. https://doi.org/10.1016/j.sleep.2012.04.010.
152. Cochen V, Arbus C, Soto ME, Villars H, Tiberge M, et al. Sleep disorders and their impacts on healthy, dependent, and frail older adults. J Nutr Health Aging. 2009;13(4):322–9. https://doi.org/10.1007/s12603-009-0030-0.
153. Öberg S, Sandlund C, Westerlind B, Finkel D, Johansson L. The existing state of knowledge about sleep health in community-dwelling older persons – a scoping review. Ann Med. 2024;56(1):2353377. https://doi.org/10.1080/07853890.2024.2353377.
154. www.med.upenn.edu/cbti/assets/user-content/documents/Pittsburgh%20Sleep%20 Quality%20Index%20(PSQI).pdf.
155. www.ons.org/sites/default/files/InsomniaSeverityIndex_ISI.pdf.
156. www.sleepmedicine.com/files/files/StopBang_Questionnaire.pdf.
157. https://www.nimh.nih.gov/health/topics/depression.
158. Sekhon S, Patel J, Sapra A. Late-Onset Depression. In: StatPearls [Internet]. Treasure Island, FL: StatPearls Publishing; 2021. https://www.ncbi.nlm.nih.gov/books/NBK551507/.
159. NCOA. https://www.ncoa.org/article/how-common-is-depression-in-older-adults/.
160. Szymkowicz SM, Gerlach AR, Homiack D, Taylor WD. Biological factors influencing depression in later life: role of aging processes and treatment implications. Transl Psychiatry. 2023;13(1):160. https://doi.org/10.1038/s41398-023-02464-9.

161. Liebetrau M, Steen B, Skoog I. Depression as a risk factor for the incidence of first-ever stroke in 85-year-olds. Stroke. 2008;39(7):1960–5. https://doi.org/10.1161/STROKEAHA.107.490797.
162. Alexopoulos GS. Mechanisms and treatment of late-life depression. Transl Psychiatry. 2019;9(1):188. https://doi.org/10.1038/s41398-019-0514-6.
163. Johnco CJ, Zagic D, Rapee RM, Kangas M, Wuthrich VM. Long-term remission and relapse of anxiety and depression in older adults after Cognitive Behavioural Therapy (CBT): a 10-year follow-up of a randomised controlled trial. J Affect Disord. 2024;358:440–8. https://doi.org/10.1016/j.jad.2024.05.033.
164. Beyer JL, Johnson KG. Advances in pharmacotherapy of late-life depression. Curr Psychiatry Rep. 2018;20(5):34. https://doi.org/10.1007/s11920-018-0899-6.
165. Thomas EJ, Brennan TA. Incidence and types of preventable adverse events in elderly patients: population based review of medical records. BMJ. 2000;320(7237):741–4. https://doi.org/10.1136/bmj.320.7237.741.
166. Saraf AA, Petersen AW, Simmons SF, Schnelle JF, Bell SP, Kripalani S, et al. Medications associated with geriatric syndromes and their prevalence in older hospitalized adults discharged to skilled nursing facilities. J Hosp Med. 2016;11(10):694–700. https://doi.org/10.1002/jhm.2614. Epub 2016 June 3.
167. Wierenga PC, Buurman BM, Parlevliet JL, van Munster BC, Smorenburg SM, Inouye SK, et al. Association between acute geriatric syndromes and medication-related hospital admissions. Drugs Aging. 2012;29(8):691–9. https://doi.org/10.2165/11632510-000000000-00000.
168. Lund BC, Schroeder MC, Middendorff G, Brooks JM. Effect of hospitalization on inappropriate prescribing in elderly Medicare beneficiaries. J Am Geriatr Soc. 2015;63(4):699–707. https://doi.org/10.1111/jgs.13318.
169. Gallagher P, O'Mahony D. STOPP (Screening Tool of Older Persons' potentially inappropriate Prescriptions): application to acutely ill elderly patients and comparison with Beers' criteria. Age Ageing. 2008;37(6):673–9. https://doi.org/10.1093/ageing/afn197.
170. Hill-Taylor B, Sketris I, Hayden J, Byrne S, O'Sullivan D, Christie R. Application of the STOPP/START criteria: a systematic review of the prevalence of potentially inappropriate prescribing in older adults, and evidence of clinical, humanistic and economic impact. J Clin Pharm Ther. 2013;38(5):360–72. https://doi.org/10.1111/jcpt.12059.
171. Akkawi ME, Mohd Taufek NH, Abdul Hadi AD, Nik Lah NNNF. The prevalence of prescribing medications associated with geriatric syndromes among discharged elderly patients. J Pharm Bioallied Sci. 2020;12(Suppl 2):S747–51. https://doi.org/10.4103/jpbs.JPBS_305_19.
172. Davies EA, O'Mahony MS. Adverse drug reactions in special populations—the elderly. Br J Clin Pharmacol. 2015;80(4):796–807. https://doi.org/10.1111/bcp.12596.
173. Tatum PE III, Talebreza S, Ross JS. Geriatric assessment: an office-based approach. Am Fam Physician. 2018;97(12):776–84. PMID: 30216018.
174. O'Donnell CDJ, Hubbard J, Jin Z. Updates on the management of colorectal cancer in older adults. Cancers (Basel). 2024;16(10):1820. https://doi.org/10.3390/cancers16101820.
175. O'Mahony D, Cherubini A, Guiteras AR, Denkinger M, Beuscart JB, Onder G, et al. STOPP/START criteria for potentially inappropriate prescribing in older people: version 3. Eur Geriatr Med. 2023;14(4):625–32. https://doi.org/10.1007/s41999-023-00777-y.
176. Eng C, Pedulla J, Eleazer GP, McCann R, Fox N. Program of all-inclusive care for the elderly (PACE): an innovative model of integrated geriatric care and financing. J Am Geriatr Soc. 1997;45(2):223–32. https://doi.org/10.1111/j.1532-5415.1997.tb04513.x.
177. Fulmer T. How to try this: Fulmer SPICES. Am J Nurs. 2007;107(10):40–8; quiz 48–9. https://doi.org/10.1097/01.NAJ.0000292197.76076.e1.
178. Aronow HU, Borenstein J, Haus F, Braunstein GD, Bolton LB. Validating SPICES as a screening tool for frailty risks among hospitalized older adults. Nurs Res Pract. 2014;2014:1–5. https://doi.org/10.1155/2014/846759.
179. https://hign.org/consultgeri/try-this-series/fulmer-spices-overall-assessment-tool-older-adults.

Recreational Drugs: Alcohol, Marijuana, Nicotine

8

Abbreviations

ACh	Acetylcholine
ADH	Alcohol dehydrogenase
ADR	Adverse drug reaction
AEA	N-arachidonoyl-ethanolamine
ALDH	Acetaldehyde dehydrogenase
AUD	Alcohol use disorder
AUDIT	Alcohol Use Disorders Identification Test
BAC	Blood alcohol concentration
CAGE	Cut, Anger, Guilt, Eye (assessment)
CB1R	Cannabinoid receptor 1
CB2R	Cannabinoid receptor 2
CBD	Cannabidiol
CBN	Cannabinol
CNS	Central nervous system
COPD	Chronic obstructive pulmonary disease
CUD	Cannabis use disorder
CV	Cardiovascular
DDI	Drug-drug interaction
ED	Emergency department
GABA	Gamma-aminobutyric acid
gms/kg	Grams per kilogram
HDL-c	High density lipoprotein cholesterol
HPFS	Health professions follow-up study
IV	Intravenous
MC	Medicinal cannabis
MI	Myocardial infarction

© The Author(s), under exclusive license to Springer Nature Switzerland AG 2025
G. E. Bilder, P. Brown-O'Hara, *Drug Use in the Older Adult*,
https://doi.org/10.1007/978-3-031-84831-5_8

mM	Millimolar
nAChR	nicotine acetylcholine receptor
nAChR	nicotinic acetylcholine receptor
NHS	Nurses' health study
NNRT	Non-nucleoside reverse transcriptase inhibitor
OTC	Over-the-counter
PD	Pharmacodynamics
PK	Pharmacokinetics
RCT	Randomized controlled trial
SAMHSA	Substance Abuse and Mental Health Service Administration
SBIRT	Screening, Brief Intervention, and Referral to Treatment
T2DM	Type 2 diabetes mellitus
THC	Trans-delta- 9-tetrahydrocannabinol
TMREL	Theoretical minimum risk exposure level
TUB	Tobacco use disorder
USPSTF	U.S. Preventive Services Task Force
2-AG	2-arachidonoylglycerol
5HT3	5-hydroxytryptamine type 3
5HT3R	5-hyroxytryptamine 3 receptor

Introduction Wine, beer, spirits, marijuana and tobacco contain bioactive substances used by many older adults for the benefits of stress reduction, relaxation, pain relief, and/or increased alertness and focus. However, a plethora of study results have identified serious risk of harm with the use of these substances, especially when misused or abused in high amounts or for extended periods of time. In the older adult, these risks are compounded with age changes in pharmacokinetics (PK) and pharmacodynamics (PD) (see Chap. 2), comorbidities and associated medications (see Chaps. 3, 4, 5, 6, and 7) and age-related homeostatic changes in organs (see Chaps. 2 and 3). This chapter will discuss the purported benefits and confirmed risks of these recreational substances and their impact on the health of the older adult. Tables 8.1, 8.2, 8.3, and 8.4 provide additional support for the narrative.

Alcohol

Alcoholic Beverages. Introduction Based on data from a National Survey on Drug Use and Health (2021), the vast majority of older adults (82.1%) have consumed alcoholic beverages in their lifetime and 56.1% have consumed alcohol in the past year. Of those, a small percentage are binge or heavy drinkers (11.4% and 2.8%, respectively) [1]. The benefits/harms of alcohol use are dose-dependent. Light to modest use of alcohol (although actual amounts vary) provides protection against some diseases [2] and preserves cognition [3, 4], but the consumption of higher amounts increases the risks of falls and injuries [5], creates dependence and associated problems [6] and is the cause of certain cancers [7]. However, in addition to the amount of alcohol consumed, the effects of alcohol use are influenced by many factors to include the pattern of consumption and abstention throughout the lifespan, gender, genetic heterogeneity, socioeconomic/educational level, and race and ethnicity as well as age [8]. Hence, due to this complexity, some of the effects of alcohol use remain controversial [8].

Government Guidelines for Alcohol Consumption Older adults can choose not to drink, but because of the evidence (see below) that low levels of alcohol use offer some health benefits, the US Department of Agriculture and the Health and Human Services has established guidelines for alcohol consumption [9] (see Table 8.1). Table 8.1 guidelines are for US adults only and are not stratified by age. However, standard government drinking values differ among countries. Of the 37 countries with an established standard for low-risk drinking, the average drink contains 10 g (not 14 g alcohol as in the US) and low-risk drinking varies between 10 and 42 g per day for women and 10–56 g per day for men [10]. Furthermore, there is no consensus definition for bing and heavy drinking compounding public health research [10, 11].

Table 8.1 Dietary Guidelines for Americans 2020–2025 [9]. Recommended Guidelines For Alcohol Use

Gender/type of drinking	Amount (number of drinks)	Drink type	Gram (g)	Fluid ounce
Female	1	Regular beer (5% alcohol)	14	12
	1	Wine (12% alcohol)	14	5
	1	Distilled spirits (40% alcohol)	14	1.5
Male	2	Regular beer (5% alcohol)	28	24
	2	Wine (12% alcohol)	28	10
	2	Distilled spirits (40% alcohol)	28	3
Bing Drinking (within 2 hours period) BAC of 0.08% (or 0.08 g of alcohol per 100 milliliters)	≥4 drinks—female ≥5 drinks—male		56 70	
Heavy Drinking[a]	≥4 drinks—female or ≥8 drinks/week ≥5 drinks/day or ≥15/week—male			

[a] *NIAAA* National Institute of Alcohol Abuse and Alcoholism, *BAC* blood alcohol concentration

Alcohol. Pharmacokinetics The drug consumed in alcoholic drinks of beer, wine and spirits is ethanol (used interchangeably with alcohol), a product of yeast fermentation of sugars in grapes (wine) or malted barley or malted wheat (beer) and additional distillation (spirits) [12]. Ethanol is a "small" molecule, basically a two-carbon chemical entity. As a result, ethanol has limited binding capabilities, making it a very nonspecific/nonselective drug [13]. It is poorly fat-soluble and distributes solely in the water compartment of the body, i.e., blood and tissues [14]. Several factors, in addition to the volume of distribution, determine the blood alcohol concentration (BAC). These factors are the quantity of alcohol consumed, the rate of gastric emptying and the rate of alcohol oxidation [14].

The volume of distribution of ethanol is both gender and age-dependent [15, 16]. Thus, when equal amounts of ethanol are ingested (gms/kg), BAC is higher in women compared to men and higher in older adults compared to younger adults. This is because, with regard to gender, women have more fat and less muscle and water volume than men and hence higher alcohol concentrations [16]. With regard to age, age-related changes in body composition of reduced muscle mass and body water volume and gain of body fat result in higher blood levels of alcohol in older adults compared to younger adults [15].

Although a small amount of alcohol is metabolized in the stomach by the enzyme alcohol dehydrogenase (ADH), *the liver metabolizes most of the alcohol* [14]. In the empty stomach, alcohol readily enters the small intestine for absorption and passes to the liver for minor metabolism and recirculation in the blood and distribution to all organs. On return to the liver, two enzyme systems oxidize alcohol. Hepatic ADHs oxidize alcohol to acetaldehyde after which acetaldehyde is oxidized to acetate by acetaldehyde dehydrogenases (ALDHs). Alcohol is also, generally at higher concentrations, metabolized by CYP2E1, a hepatic cytochrome P450 enzyme and unlike ADHs and ALDHs, CYP2E1 is inducible, meaning the greater the alcohol consumption, the more enzyme is made, more or less keeping up with consumption. Alcohol-drug interactions largely occur here. Depending on the amount of alcohol consumed, increased or decreased clearance of prescribed medications may occur [14] (see drug interaction below).

Alcohol. Pharmacodynamics The effects of alcohol on the central nervous system (CNS) are dose-dependent. Generally, anxiolytic and euphoric effects occur at ~12 mM (0.049%), with legal intoxication at ~18 mM (0.075%) [13]. The latter is characterized by "slowed reaction times, motor incoordination, and cognitive impairment" and continues up to 50 mM (0.208%) [13]. *Thereafter, respiratory depression and death occur.* The acute effects of high amounts of alcohol cause injuries, accidents and fatalities [6]. Chronic effects of alcohol produce alcohol use disorder (AUD) and diseases (see below).

The mechanism of action of ethanol is complex because it affects multiple targets, neurotransmitters, receptors and signal pathways [13]. Ethanol is a sedative-depressant that enhances the activity of the two key inhibitory neurotransmitters: (1) gamma-aminobutyric acid (GABA-A) [17] and (2) glycine [18] and inhibits the excitatory effects of the neurotransmitter, glutamate [19]. Ethanol also influences the nicotinic acetylcholine receptor (nAChR) [20] and 5-hydroxytryptamine 3 receptors (5HT3R), members of the same super family as GABA-A [13]. Ethanol also affects many other receptors, directly and indirectly [13, 21].

Alcohol. Interaction with Age Changes Age effects influence the PK and PD of alcohol. Consequently, *age changes exacerbate the CNS depressant effects of alcohol, enhancing the risk of falls, increasing cognitive impairment and accelerating immunosenescence.*

Age effects on alcohol PK have been noted above. The change in body composition with age reduces body water volume and thus increases the blood concentration of alcohol relative to that experienced by younger adults consuming the same quantity of alcohol [15]. Age-related decreases in liver volume and hepatic blood flow also contribute to a reduction in alcohol oxidation and clearance [22]. This suggests that with age blood levels of alcohol may be higher and more prolonged and hence more sedating.

Many factors contribute to the increased risks of falls in the older adult. Some of these factors are reduced sensory perception (eyes, ears, proprioceptors in joints, ligaments, tendons), diminished muscle strength (dynapenia), lack of physical exercise, malnutrition, isolation, frailty, morbidities and polypharmacy [23]. To these factors, alcohol use has been added [23]. However, the relation between alcohol use and an increased risk of falls in the older adult is unclear and complicated by diverse methodologies such as alcohol levels and patterns of drinking measured prior to a fall [24]. To directly assess the role of alcohol use on injury-related falls, data from over 38,000 electronic emergency department (ED) records of injury-related falls in older adults were evaluated for evidence of alcohol use [24]. Approximately 1.9% of emergency visits for fall injuries were due to alcohol use. This relationship decreased with increasing age (4% for 65–74: 1.5% for 76–84; <1% for 85+) [24]. Head and facial injuries were more common in alcohol-related falls compared to non-alcohol-related falls [24]. Although not the main reason for a fall, alcohol use is a relevant and avoidable risk factor.

Immunosenescence describes the aging of the immune system in which some aspects of innate immunity (initial barriers, e.g., skin and cellular response to prevent pathogen invasion) and adaptive immunity (delayed, sophisticated T-cell defense and B-cell antibody production plus "memory" allowing a more rapid and stronger response on second encounter with the pathogen) become dysfunctional [25]. *Alcohol use worsens immunosenescence*, both innate immunity [26] and adaptive immunity [27], *resulting in a reduction in host defenses, especially to infections and injuries* [27, 28]. Specifically, alcohol use, both acute and chronic, modulates the function of innate cells such as neutrophils, phagocytes, and dendritic cells and alters the initial requisite inflammatory response to destroy pathogens and activate adaptive immunity [26, 28]. T and B-cell numbers are decreased and subset balance is perturbed, leading to dysfunction, especially evident with chronic heavy drinking [27]. Multiple alterations in immunity are clearly present with chronic heavy drinking, but aspects of immune dysfunction occur with acute alcohol use. Immunosenescence puts the older adult at a *higher risk of infections (Escherichia coli; Streptococcus pneumonia; Mycobacterium tuberculosis; Pseudomonas aeruginosa; herpes virus; gastroenteritis, bronchitis, influenza) and reduces the older adult's ability to recover from injuries* [25, 29]. *Both acute and chronic alcohol use elevates this risk even more.*

Alcohol. Effects on Cognition Whether light-moderate alcohol use benefits cognition remains controversial [2, 30, 31]. Results of a convincing study, albeit a small one, of 133 older adults were stratified into 3 groups: "never/minimal users (≤ 100 drinks in lifetime), former users (>100 drinks in lifetime and no alcohol in past 30 days), and current users (>100 drinks in lifetime and alcohol in past 30 days)" [32]. Participants took an extensive battery of cognitive tests, the result of which showed there was no relationship between alcohol and nonalcohol users after confounding variables (age, sex, education level, race and smoking amount) were removed [32]. Others have also reported that light-moderate use of alcohol does not negatively affect cognition [2, 30]. However, data from the A4 study (US, Canada, Australia, Japan) of over 4000 participants 65–85 years of age showed that light-moderate drinkers (1–2 drinks/day self-reported) compared to no drinks/day scored better on a battery of cognitive tests [31]. On the other hand, *chronic heavy use of alcohol over a lifetime is significantly associated with severe memory loss and increased risk of dementia* (see below).

Alcohol. Drug-Drug Interactions Alcohol interacts with a wealth of drugs, including prescription drugs, over-the-counter (OTC), and herbal remedies [33, 34] (see Table 8.2). Definite interactions have been verified with heavy consumption, but alcohol-drug interactions are also considered relevant with light-moderate alcohol use [35]. The prevalence of alcohol and alcohol-interactive drugs among current drinkers ≥ 65 years of age, according to findings from the National Health and Nutrition Examination Survey (NHANES 1999 to 2010) was 77.7% [36]. The most commonly used drugs among the older adult consuming alcohol are cardiovascular drugs, CNS psychoactive drugs and metabolic drugs [36]. An earlier survey of over 1000 older adults using at least one prescription medication reported that 63.6% used alcohol, supporting the conclusion that drug interactions with alcohol are common [37].

Alcohol and drugs interact at both the PK and PD levels (see Chap. 2). Adverse reactions range from nausea/vomiting, drowsiness and dizziness to loss of coordination, fainting, heart problems, internal bleeding, breathing difficulties, overdose and organ toxicity [33, 36]. Additionally, the efficacy of prescription medications may be reduced and organ toxicity may occur [33].

Alert: Alcohol interacts with a wealth of drugs, including prescription, OTC and herbal remedies. It should be avoided or consumed in moderation after consulting with your physician.

Table 8.2 Drugs (prescription, OTC, herbal remedies) that interact with alcohol [33, 34]

Symptom/disorder	Class/generic name		Type of interaction

Ulcers, indigestion, heartburn	H2 histamine receptor antagonists
	  Cimetidine
	  Nizatidine
	  Ranitidine
	Dopamine receptor antagonist
	  Metoclopramide
			↓ First pass by inhibiting stomach ADH-↑BAC
			↑ gastric emptying—↑BAC; sudden change in BP

Pain (muscle ache /minor arthritis), inflammation suppression/ fever	NSAIDs (OTC)
	  Aspirin
	  Ibuprofen
	  Naproxen
	  Ketoprfen (Rx)
	  Diclofenac (Rx)
	  Flurbiprofen (Rx)
	Antipyretic/analgesic
	  Acetaminophen
			↑ risk of bleeding; stomach upset; rapid heartbeat; ↑ gastric emptying (aspirin) to ↑BAC
			Liver damage—Alcohol ↑ metabolism of acetaminophen to toxic compound

Pain—severe (postoperative, oral surgery, migraines)	Opioids
	  Propoxyphene
	  Merepidine
	  Codeine
	  Oxycodone
	  Hydrocodone
	  Morphine
			↑ CNS effects—drowsiness, dizziness, sedation, ↓ motor coordination, slowed breathing, memory problems

Microbial infections	Antibiotics
	  Erythromycin
	  Isoniazide
	  Nitrofurantoin
	  Metronidazole
		Griseofulvin
		Ketoconazole
		Cycloserine
		Tinidazol
		Azithromycin
			↑ gastric emptying (erythromycin); ↑ risk of liver damage (isoniazid, ketoconazole)
			Stomach upset, vomiting, flushing, sudden change in BP

Anxiety/epilepsy	Benzodiazepines (sedatives)
	  Lorazepam
	  Buspirone
	  Clonazepam
	  Chlordiazepoxide
		Paroxetine
		Diazepam
		Midazolm
		Triazolam
		Temazepam
		Alprazolam
			↑ CNS effects—drowsiness, dizziness, sedation, ↓ motor coordination, ↑ risk of overdose, slowed breathing, behavioral and memory problems

(continued)

Table 8.2 (continued)

Symptom/disorder	Class/generic name		Type of interaction
Depression	Atypical antipsychotics Aripriprazone Ziprasidone Clozapine Ziprasidone Paliperidone Risperidone Quetiapine Olanzapine TCAs Clomipramine Amitriptyline Desipramine TeCA Mirtazapine Serotonin Modulator Nefazodone NDRI Bupropion	SSRIs Citalopram Escitalopram Fluvoxamine Paroxetine Fluoxetine Sertraline SNRIs Duloxetine Venlafaxine Desevenlafaxine SARI Trazodone MAOIs Phenelzine Tranylcypromine Herbal—St John's Wort	↑ sedation; sudden drop in BP (orthostatic hypotension) (TCAs); ↑ risk of overdose; feeling of depression; impaired motor control (quetiapine, mirtazapine) ↑alcohol effects (bupriopion) liver damage (duloxetine) ↑heart-related effects (MAOI)-↑BP when combined with tyramine-containing foods (cheese, red wine and beer products)
Diabetes	Sulfonylureas Tolazamide Chlorpropamide Glipizide Glipizide Tolbutamide Biguanide Metformin	GLP-1 agonists Liraglutide Exenatide Dulaglutide Semaglutide Tirzepatide	Hypoglycemia; disulfiram-like reaction (Chlorpropamide, glyburide, tolbutamide); nausea, weakness and ↑lactic acid in blood (metformin); ↑hepatic stress and reduced absorption and efficacy with alcohol (GLP-1 agonists)
High blood pressure	Calcium channel blockers Verapamil Amlodipine Diuretic TZD Hydrochlorothiazide Alpha agonist central Clonidine	ARB Losartan ACEIs Enalapril Quinapril Benzapril Lisinopril	Dizziness, fainting, possible arrhythmias
High cholesterol	Statins Lovastatin + Niacin Lovastatin Rosuvastatin	Atorvastatin Pravastatin Pravastatin + aspirin Simvastatin Ezetimibe + Simvastatin	Liver damage; ↑flushing/itching (niacin);↑ stomach bleeding (pravastatin + aspirin)

(continued)

Table 8.2 (continued)

Symptom/disorder	Class/generic name		Type of interaction
Seizures	Anticonvulsants Carbamazepine Oxcarbazepine Topiramate Lamotrigine Levetiracetam Pregabalin Gabapentin Phenytoin	Benzodiazepine Clonazepam Barbiturates Phenobarbital	↑ drowsiness, dizziness, risk of seizure (levetiracetam, phenytoin); behavioral change (suicidal thoughts—topiramate)
Blood clot prevention	Warfarin		Acute intake of alcohol ↓warfarin metabolism resulting in ↑ bleeding; chronic drinking-↑ warfarin metabolism decreasing efficacy
Sleeping problems	Sedative-hypnotics Zolpidem Eszopiclone Benzodiazepine Estazolam Temazepam	Antihistamines Diphenhydramine Doxylamine Herbal Chamomile Echinacea Valerian	↑ drowsiness, sleepiness, impaired motor control, slowed breathing, possible behavioral and memory problems
Allergies, colds	Antihistamines Diphenhydramine Chlorpheniramine Clemastine Hydroxyzine	Promethazine Loratadine Desloratadine Cyproheptadine	↓ First pass by inhibiting stomach ADH-↑BAL ↑ CNS effects—drowsiness, sedation, ↓ motor control;

ADH alcohol dehydrogenase, *BAC* blood alcohol concentration, *BP* blood pressure, ↑ increase, ↓ decrease, *OTC* over the counter, *TCAs* tricyclic antidepressants, *SSRIs* selective serotonin reuptake inhibitors, *SNRIs* serotonin & norepinephrine reuptake inhibitors, *NDRI* norepinephrine & dopamine reuptake inhibitors, *MAOIs* monoamine oxidase inhibitors, *TeCA* tetracyclic antidepressant, *SARI* serotonin-2 antagonist and reuptake inhibitor, *ACEIs* angiotensin converting enzyme inhibitors, *ARB* angiotensin receptor blocker, *TZD* thiazide, *NSAIDs* nonsteroidal antiinflammatory drugs, *CNS* central nervous system

Pharmacokinetic-Based Alcohol-Drug Interactions PK interactions occur at the site of metabolism of alcohol (see above): ADHs and ALDHs in the stomach and liver and the hepatic CYP enzymes, CYP2E1, but also CYP3A4 and CYP 1A2 [38]. Common interactions occur between alcohol, aspirin, and antihistamines. Aspirin and histamine antagonists (see Table 8.2, ulcer, allergy medications) compete with alcohol to reduce initial alcohol metabolism in the stomach, decreasing "first pass" and leading to slightly higher alcohol levels [39, 40]. Drugs that accelerate gastric emptying (metoclopramide and erythromycin) also raise alcohol levels [34]. *Disulfiram is one of several drugs used as an adjunct to help those addicted to alcohol* abstain [41]. It produces uncomfortable effects of flushing, nausea and vomiting because it blocks the metabolism of acetaldehyde to acetate, resulting in acetaldehyde toxicity. Importantly, there are a number of drugs (phenacetin, phenylbutazone, isoniazid, metronidazole, nitrofurantoin, sulfamethoxazole, sulfisoxazole, isosorbide dinitrate, nitroglycerin and sulfonylureas) that inhibit ALDH and when taken with alcohol produce the "disulfiram" reaction [34]. This creates a serious problem in patients with cardiovascular disease because flushing is the result of significant vasodilatation and a decrease in blood pressure, which would be especially harmful [34].

Pharmacodynamic-Based Alcohol-Drug Interactions Alcohol-drug interactions occur predominately in the CNS. Drugs that exert sedative effects add to or increase (synergistic) sedation produced by alcohol. Alcohol enhances the sedative and depressant effects of barbiturates, benzodiazepines, sedatives and hypnotics, opioids, antidepressants and antihistamines (see Table 8.2) [34]. Other interactions affect blood pressure by precipitating orthostatic hypotension (tricyclic antidepressants, TCAs) and abnormal heart rate (antihypertensive medications, nonsteroidal antiinflammatory drugs, NSAIDs) or have the potential to produce hypoglycemia (antidiabetic drugs).

Since alcohol use can induce CYP2E1 enzyme, the amount of consumed alcohol impacts the drug-alcohol interaction. For example, possible scenarios are: nondrinker, CYP metabolizes the drug, e.g., acetaminophen, isoniazid, phenobarbital normally; moderate alcohol consumption, alcohol and drug compete for metabolism, and the drug does not get metabolized, and drug concentration increases with possible adverse drug reaction (ADR); chronic heavy drinker (CYP induction) in a sober state, rapid metabolism of the drug occurs with loss of efficacy; chronic heavy drinker in state of intoxication, alcohol, and drug competes with a possible reduction in the metabolism of the drug, increased blood level, and ADRs [34].

ALCOHOL. LONG-TERM EFFECT ON HEALTH AND DISEASE The relation between alcohol use and health/disease risks is complicated [42]. On the one hand, light-moderate alcohol consumption decreases the risk for cardiovascular (CV) disease and Type 2 Diabetes Mellitus (T2DM) [2], but on the other hand, alcohol is classified as a Group 1 carcinogen (in the same group as asbestos and radiation) and "is causally linked to seven types of cancer, including esophagus, liver, colorectal, and breast cancers" [7]. This relation of alcohol to disease risk is represented by a J-shaped curve. This means that low alcohol consumption is associated with low disease risk or possible protection for some diseases but that higher alcohol use is associated with greater disease risks compared to nondrinkers [42–47].

POSSIBLE BENEFITS OF LIGHT ALCOHOL CONSUMPTION Results of numerous epidemiological studies show that the *relation between alcohol use and CV disease is dose (consumption) dependent* [48]. A review of the Nurses' Health Study (NHS) (1980–2012) and NHS II (1989–2011), a longitudinal survey (every 4 years) of self-reported alcohol drinking patterns, lifestyle choices and physicians diagnoses, found that moderate drinking (1 drink/day equal to 0.1–14.9 g/day) "is associated with a lower risk of hypertension, myocardial infarction, stroke, sudden cardiac death, gallstones, cognitive decline and all-cause mortality" [2]. Higher quantities (2–3 drinks/day) negate the beneficial effect of moderate drinking on the aforementioned conditions and all-cause mortality. Additionally, drinking small amounts throughout the week rather than the summation at one time produced even greater health benefits [2]. Others have found moderate drinking associated with reduced CV risk [42, 46, 49]. Meta-analyses reported that in a high-risk population of patients with MI, stroke or angina, there was a 22% risk reduction in CV mortality and 18% risk reduction in all-cause mortality with moderate drinking (7–8 g/day) [46]. Extending this analysis to include CV events in addition to cardiovascular mortality and all-cause mortality in a systematic and meta-analysis of over 14,000 CV patients in the UK, moderate drinking (105 grams/week) was associated with reduced risk for CV events as well as mortality and all-cause mortality [49]. (see Table 8.1 to compare to US guidelines).

The mechanism by which low alcohol intake lowers CV risk is poorly understood. Results of observational and interventional studies suggest that low dose alcohol (< 30 grams/day) reduces oxidative stress, increases HDL-c (high-density lipoprotein cholesterol) and in a variety of ways protects the endothelium from plaque formation [8, 50, 51]. However, there is considerable uncertainty around these findings due to confounding factors, e.g., patterns of consumption, definition of intake, and subjective study reports [8]. Whether low alcohol use affects hypertension, a risk factor for CV disease, is also debated. Results of a cross-sectional study of over 500 older adults at high risk for CV disease showed that consumption of 2–3 drinks/day elevates blood pressure but that light consumption is associated with reduced fluctuations of daytime blood pressure [52]. In a meta-analysis of 20 cohort studies (about a third included older adults) the risk for hypertension was elevated in men but not women compared to abstainers [53]. This is supported by many other studies [11]. Additional research on alcohol-CV relations is needed.

In a review of 4 observational studies, light-moderate alcohol consumption decreased the risk (35–53%) of T2DM in both men and women, with better results in those with healthy lifestyle adherence [8]. Similarly, results of the NHS I and II reported a 40% reduction in T2DM risk with low alcohol consumption (1–2 drinks/day) compared to lifetime abstainers [2]. In a 5 year prospective study of approximately 400 nondiabetic men and women (40–79 years), insulin sensitivity (as measured by fasting and post-glucose insulin) increased in those consuming light-moderate amounts of alcohol [54]. In contrast, an assessment of insulin sensitivity (euglycemic clamp) found that insulin sensitivity and secretion are not affected by 15, 50 or 158 grams/week of alcohol in over 800 nondiabetic men, 70 years of age, but heavier consumption was associated with abdominal adiposity, a serious risk factor for T2DM [55]. The evidence suggests that low consumption may be protective against T2DM, but the mechanism is obscure.

HARMFUL EFFECTS OF ALCOHOL USE Global prevalence estimates according to the Global Burden of Diseases, Injuries, and Risk Factors Study 2016 indicate that alcohol use is the seventh leading risk factor for death and disability-adjusted life years [56]. This study found that cancers accounted for 27% (female) and 18.9% (male) of the "total alcohol-attributable deaths among older adults" [56]. The GBD recommended amount of alcohol to reduce harm is zero standard drinks per day [56]. A more recent analysis updating relative risk curves and calculating the theoretical minimum risk exposure level (TMREL) by region, age, and gender reported a global TMREL of 0.534 drinks per day [57].

Alcohol. Cancer Risk It is clear that heavy alcohol consumption is associated with an increased risk of cancers of the mouth, pharynx/larynx, esophagus, liver, colorectum, and breast (postmenopausal) [58–60]. Heavy drinking is also associated with a possible increased risk of stomach cancer [61], lung cancer [62], pancreatic cancer [63], and gallbladder cancer [62].

Based on the results of the NHS and the Health professions follow-up study (HPFS), light-moderate drinking in men (intake of <30 grams/day) who have never smoked, cancer risk is minimal. However, the same is not true for women (non-smokers) because one drink/day (<15 g/day) increases the risk of breast cancer [64].

Alcohol. Cancer Pathology The mechanism by which alcohol (ethanol) causes cancers is not entirely understood, although many pathways are possible [60]. The first product of ethanol's metabolism is acetaldehyde, a chemical that is especially harmful to DNA, forming serious changes in its structure that may lead to mutations or perturb gene expression especially relevant to cancer-causing genes, e.g., oncogenes and tumor suppressor genes [60]. Additionally, acetaldehyde may damage protein structure and hence destroy function [65]. By inducing the CYP2E1 enzyme, ethanol generates oxygen radicals that also harm DNA and proteins [66] and adds to ethanol's ability to enhance inflammatory pathways [67]. Also, alcohol inhibits several key pathways such as one-carbon metabolism required for DNA methylation (gene expression) and DNA synthesis [65], oxidation of vitamin A to retinoic acid, lowering levels in blood and liver, linked to cancers and production of mediators that prevent liver fibrosis leading to hepatic cirrhosis, a precursor of liver cancer [60]. Estrogen levels and estrogen receptor activity increase with heavy alcohol consumption, a change associated with breast cancer development [68].

Alcohol. Tuberculosis Risk Results of several meta-analyses show that heavy alcohol consumption is a risk factor for tuberculosis [69–71]. Generally, greater than 40 grams per day is associated with a three to four fold higher risk of tuberculosis [69, 71]. Mechanistically, the function of macrophages that normally destroy mycobacteria, causative pathogens of tuberculosis, is hindered by alcohol, reducing phagocytosis (pathogen uptake and killing) and response to cytokines, inducing inflammation [72] and permitting the establishment of new tuberculosis and reemergence of latent infection [69, 70].

ALCOHOL. ALCOHOL USE DISORDER (AUD) According to the National Survey on Drug Use and Health (2023), a yearly face-face and web-based interview of civilian noninstitutionalized US residents, the percentage of older adults that engaged in bing alcohol use in the past month or heavy alcohol use is 9.7% and 2.4% respectively (roughly 5 + drinks/day for men and 4+ drinks/day for women) [73]. Although this is slightly reduced from 2019 (10.7% and 2.8%, respectively) [74] and significantly lower than in individuals 18–25 years of age, an extensive review of substance abuse disorders considers that the condition of alcohol use disorder (AUD), formerly alcoholism, in the older population, is underreported and underdiagnosed [75]. It is often *overlooked because AUD symptoms of depression and cognitive loss are considered age-related problems* and not AUD. Also, social restraints may prevent the older adult as well as the caretaker from confronting substance abuse.

Assessment Tools for Alcohol Use Disorder Recommendations from both the Substance Abuse and Mental Health Service Administration [76] Treatment Improvement Protocol (TIP) consensus panel and the U.S. Preventive Services Task Force [77] propose that the older adult be screened yearly in a primary care setting for alcohol misuse [76, 77]. The Alcohol Use Disorders Identification Test (AUDIT) [78] and the *CAGE questionnaire* [79] are considered helpful tools [74]. CAGE (Cut, Annoyed, Guilty, Eye) asks four questions about lifetime use of alcohol and a response to any one signals possible alcohol misuse [79]. (CAGE questionnaire may be found https://www.uspreventiveservicestaskforce.org. and AUDIT test may be found at https://nida.nih.gov/sites/default/files/files/AUDIT.pdfa).

Alcohol Use Disorder. Cognitive Decline Risk AUD is associated with cognitive impairment that may possibly lead to dementia [80]. One study of older adults enrolled in the Health and Retirement Study at an average age of 55 years found that AUD enhances age-related decline in cognition [81]. The AUD-related impairment affects all brain domains—verbal memory, working memory, verbal fluency, and attention [81]. In the Health and Retirement Study, participants were cognitively tested twice a year over a 19-year period. This study observed that severe memory loss was two times as likely in those with a history of AUD compared to those without a history of AUD [82]. Current heavy drinkers were excluded from this study. It was proposed that *AUD in early years influences cognitive activity later in life* [82, 83]. Others have reported excessive alcohol use accelerated the age-related loss of neuronal tissue [84]. This supports the "premature aging hypothesis" of alcohol dependence and aging in which early exposure to excessive alcohol use exerts effects later in life [84, 85]. The Framingham Offspring Study found that MRI-determined total cranial brain volume is inversely related to the amount of alcohol consumed [86]. Results of MRI brain scans of individuals from 20 to 69 years reveal neurobiological evidence that alcohol accelerated brain aging [84] and produced pathological damage [87]. One common pathway between the aging brain and alcohol use appears to be neuroinflammation that has been observed in preclinical studies [88]. It is debated as to whether morphological brain changes are due to direct alcohol-induced neurotoxicity or indirectly due to thiamine deficiency produced by AUD [89]. Abstinence as a correction to AUD suggests that restoration of some aspects of lost cognition is possible [89].

Alcohol Use Disorder. Non-pharmacological and Pharmacological Treatment Identification and treatment of AUD follows a plan of Screening, Brief Intervention, and Referral to Treatment (SBIRT) [90]. A positive screen result should be followed up with additional evaluation by the physician that would include a complete medical, mental, financial, and social history assessment, laboratory tests, and questions on sleep disorders and chronic pain. The brief intervention includes outpatient services for behavioral change and referral to substance abuse disorder treatment clinics that provide discussions of appropriate use, adverse effects of alcohol, e.g., falls, cognitive decline and motivational goals [74]. For the older adult requiring detoxification, inpatient treatment is recommended. If pharmacological treatment is required, naltrexone, acamprosate, and disulfiram are FDA-approved with the use of gabapentin and topiramate (off-label, anticonvulsant) [74, 91]. However, these medications are used cautiously in the elderly, at the lowest possible dose and with consideration of drug-drug interactions (see Chap. 3). Continued contact with caregivers and membership in social networks are successful nonpharmacological treatments.

Marijuana

Introduction According to the National Survey on Drug Use and Health (2022), of over 70,000 home and online interviews, 22% of the US population (12 and older) used marijuana in the past year. Thirty-eight percent of those were 18–25 years and 20.6% were 26 years and older [92]. An analysis of older adults showed an increasing trend of marijuana use from 2.4% (2015) to 4.2% (2018) [93]. This rising trend has continued to the near present. Results of a National Poll on Aging (2021) of 2000 individuals 50–80 years reveals that 12% of older adults used marijuana in the past year [94]. Of those using marijuana, 30% consumed it on 4 or more days per week [94].

Marijuana. Legal Status Marijuana (also called cannabis) is regulated in 3 different ways. Federally, marijuana is classified as a Schedule I drug according to Title II Comprehensive Drug Abuse Prevention and Control Act of 1970 (also known as the Controlled Substances Act (CSA)). The CSA established a "federal policy to regulate the manufacturing, distributing, importing/exporting, and use of regulated substances" [95]. With regard to marijuana, the CSA sorts drugs into one of five categories (Schedules) depending on verified medical use, abuse/addiction and harm [96]. Schedule I drugs or substances pose the greatest risk and are a drug or substance that (a) "has no currently accepted medical use in treatment in the United States, (b) has a high potential for abuse, and (c) there is a lack of accepted safety for use of the drug or other substance under medical supervision" (21 USC 812: Schedules of controlled substances). In addition to marijuana and synthetic analogs of the bioactive components, other members of Schedule I are diacetylmorphine (heroin), and psychedelic drugs, e.g., psilocybin, lysergic acid diethylamide (LSD) 3,4-methylenedioxymethamphetamine (MDMA) (ecstasy), methaqualone, and peyote [97]. Marijuana, if used early in life, is thought to lead to the use of other more potent and addicting drugs later in life [98]. Additionally, results of 9 cross-sectional studies with self-reported cannabis use found that substance abuse disorders were 2–3 times higher in the older adults who previously used cannabis [99].

The second and third legal designations of marijuana are state-dependent. As of Nov 13, 2023, 40 states and the District of Columbia have legalized the use of cannabis products for medical use and 24 states and the District of Columbia have legalized recreational or adult-use of cannabis [100]. So despite the federal law that defines marijuana as an illicit drug, nearly half of the states permit recreational use and 80% legally approve its use in medical practice. This has generated state-dispensaries that offer an abundance of cannabis products [101, 102] and has accelerated use in all age categories, as noted above.

However, marijuana is not a benign medicinal plant. At present, it has limited medical value and has confirmed adverse effects. In the older adult this adds negatively to biological aging and comorbidities and increases the risk of interaction with disease-appropriate medications. *Marijuana and its products should be used cautiously in the older adult.*

Marijuana. Chemistry of Phytocannabinoids The scientific name of the most commonly used marijuana plant is *Cannabis sativa L (family Cannabaceae)*, from which is derived psychoactive and other related substances. Several other strains of the marijuana plant are available in the US (C. indica, C. ruderalis, and C. afghanica) [103, 104]. The key chemical entities in marijuana are termed phytocannabinoids. They are derived from the nonfibrous part of the plant (mainly the flowers) and are chemically identified as (1) trans-delta-9-tetrahydrocannabinol (THC), the main psychoactive chemical in marijuana and (2) cannabidiol (CBD), the main non-psychoactive component in marijuana [102]. In addition to these two substances, the marijuana plant contains over 500 compounds, a fourth of which have been isolated and identified [105]. Also of note is the report that over the past 10 years (2009–2019), the THC content of herbal cannabis products increased by about 53% (from 9.75% to 14.88%), and the ratio of THC/CBD has varied significantly over the years [106]. Hemp, a cultivar of *Cannabis sativa L*, was legalized in 2018 by the USDA (Agriculture Improvement Act of 2018 (also known as the Farm Bill)) but may contain no more than 0.3% THC by dry weight. Although hemp is considered an excellent source of nutrients (essential amino acids, fats, minerals, vitamins and fiber), it is rich in CBD [107].

Chemically, the phytocannabinoids, THC and CBD, are large complex 21-carbon-containing molecules with poor water solubility and high lipid solubility. When consumed, they localize to adipose tissue. In isolated form, these compounds are unstable, light and temperature-sensitive, readily auto-oxidize and breakdown in solution [108].

In addition to phytocannabinoids derived from the marijuana plant, the body produces endogenous cannabinoids (endocannabinoids) [109]. Furthermore, synthetic cannabinoids have been created [110, 111], some of which, e.g., dronabinol, have been approved by the FDA for therapeutic use (see below).

MARIJUANA. ENDOCANNABINOID SYSTEM The advent of synthetic cannabinoid analogs allowed the discovery of the endocannabinoid system, receptors and endogenous agonists that mimic the biological effects of phytocannabinoids [112, 113]. Considerable research has identified two cannabinoid receptors, CB1R and CB2R, belonging to the G-protein-coupled receptor family [114]. CB1Rs predominate in brain tissue and skeletal muscle but are also expressed peripherally in the sympathetic nervous system, liver and pancreas, located on cell membranes and intracellularly [114, 115]. CB2Rs are found largely peripherally, prominently on immune cells with smaller amounts present in the CNS [116].

Marijuana. Endocannabinoid Receptors Two endogenous agonists of these receptors are N-arachidonoyl ethanolamine (AEA; anandamide) and 2-arachidonoyl glycerol (2-AG) [113, 117], with 2-AG considered the main endogenous agonist [114]. Stimulation of CB1Rs by endogenous cannabinoids produces retrograde nerve signaling such that their release postsynaptically reduces neurotransmitter release presynaptically and hence suppresses nerve transmission [114]. GABA-A and glycine are two of the many neurotransmitters modulated by endocannabinoids [118]. Activation of CB1Rs is associated with many functions (see Fig. 8.1). Activation of CB1Rs is thought to modulate many activities as well as many disorders of the CNS to include "appetite, learning and memory, anxiety, depression, schizophrenia, stroke, multiple sclerosis, neurodegeneration, epilepsy, and addiction" [114] and activities and disorders of the peripheral nervous system to include "pain, energy metabolism, cardiovascular and reproductive functions, inflammation, glaucoma, cancer, and liver and musculoskeletal disorders" [114].

Marijuana. Pharmacokinetics In a recent review on medical marijuana use in oncology, 11 routes of administration of marijuana were identified: oils and oral solutions, capsules, smoked, oromucosal sprays, edibles, vaporized (vaping), topical application, intramuscular, tablets, suppositories and percutaneous endoscopic gastrostomy [119]. Results of a national survey (2014–2016) focused on the older adult showed that the older adult preferred edibles, drinks and other oral formulations of cannabis, although those with frequent (daily/near daily) use preferred vaping [120].

Peak plasma levels of THC and onset of psychotropic effects, for example, depend on the route of administration [121, 122]. The pulmonary inhalation route (smoking or vaping) is the fastest and most effective, producing peak levels of THC within 3–10 minutes. Psychotropic effects occur within seconds to minutes, peak at 15–30 minutes and taper within 2–3 hours but lasting 4–12 hours depending on dose and desired effect [121, 122]. Unlike oral consumption, pulmonary inhalation as well as oromucal sprays avoid the first pass (metabolism by the liver) and are about 10–35% bioavailable compared to the oral route of approximately 6% bioavailability [122]. Thus, compared to inhalation, THC and CBD exposure from orally ingested marijuana is lower and takes about 2 hours to peak [122]. Although of considerable interest, the chemistry of THC and CBD (highly lipid soluble) limits

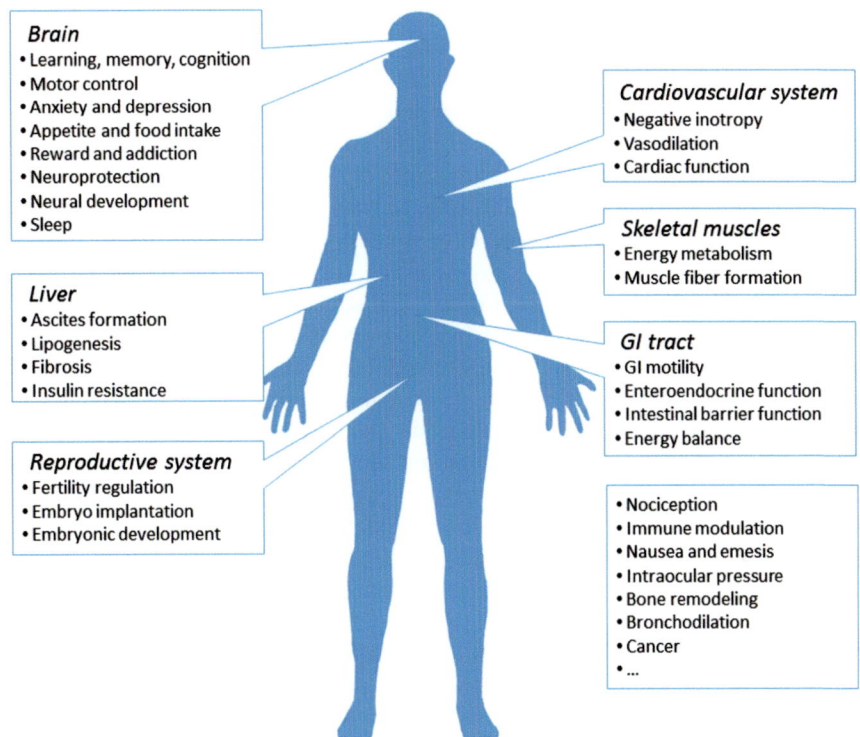

Fig. 8.1 Major localization sites and associated functions of the CB1R in the human body. (Reproduced with permission from Zou and Kumar (2018) [114])

transdermal delivery without some form of enhancement as with chemical gels, microneedles, encapsulation, and nanocarriers [123].

THC and CBD circulate tightly bound to lipoproteins [124] and distribute largely to adipose tissue, thereafter to liver and muscle tissue, as suggested by results of animal studies [125]. Distribution to the liver results in their metabolism. The P450 enzyme, CYP2C9, oxidizes THC to 11-OH-THC, a psychoactive metabolite and subsequently to an inactive metabolite [126]. The P450 CYP3A4 can also oxidize THC, but the metabolite is inactive [126]. THC, its 11-OH metabolite, and two naturally occurring phytocannabinoids, delta-8-tetrahydrocannabinol and cannabinol (CBN), are the only phytocannabinoids with psychoactive effects [127]. The contribution of psychoactivity is greatest from THC since its concentration in marijuana is the highest [127].

The metabolism of CBD yields numerous derivatives, of which the hydroxylated 7-COOH derivatives of CBD are the most prevalent [128]. There is considerable interest in these metabolites as they may be of therapeutic value and of which there are over 100. Many P450 enzymes oxidize CBD. They are CYP2C19, CYP1A1, CYP2D6, CYP3A4, CYP3A5, and to a small extent CYP2A9 [128].

Elimination of THC occurs via the urine and feces with the acidic metabolites both conjugated and nonconjugated, excreted in the urine (13–17% of total intravenous (IV) and oral dose, 72 hours) and nonconjugated metabolites in the feces (25–30% IV dose and 48–53% oral dose 72 hours) [129]. Limited information indicates that CBD and its metabolites are excreted intact or attached to glucuronic acid [128].

Marijuana. Pharmacodynamics Delta-9-THC and delta-8-THC bind similarly to CB1Rs as a partial agonist to produce psychotropic effects [130]. This is the "high" feeling or the intoxication that modifies mental activities of mood, awareness and thinking, changes sought with the recreational use of marijuana and related in part to THC-mediated blood flow changes in the brain [131]. THC also affects other receptors, e.g., 5-HT3A receptors (serotonin subtypes) [132]. THC produces antiemetic [133], analgesic [134, 135], appetite stimulation [136] and anti-glaucoma effects [137]. With chronic use, THC down-regulates the CBRs, resulting in reduced efficacy and tolerance [138].

CBD, the nonpsychotropic cannabinoid, produces a wide range of effects due to its allosteric (indirect) binding to CB1Rs and CB2Rs as well as binding to many other receptors, e.g., 5-HT and GABA-A receptors [139]. Although not completely understood, CBD modulates multiple receptors in addition to the endogenous cannabinoid system to produce anti-anxiolytic, anti-depressive, analgesic and sleep effects and is of purported therapeutic benefit in some diseases [139].

MARIJUANA. DRUG INTERACTIONS With MARIJUANA *The potential for adverse drug reactions (ADRs) due to DDIs with either THC or CBD is high* [138, 140]. DDIs may occur at the PK and/or at the PD level (see Tables 8.3 THC and 8.4 CBD).

Marijuana. Pharmacokinetic Interactions The P450 enzyme CYP3A4 metabolizes the vast majority of xenobiotics (foreign compounds, natural or synthetic) (see Chap. 3). Since THC and CBD are also metabolized by CYP3A4, numerous interactions are expected. THC and CBD will compete with drugs that are also metabolized by CYP3A4 and thus increase the bioavailability of the various drugs, e.g., immunosuppressants, antidepressants, benzodiazepines and may others shown in Tables 8.3 and 8.4. Drugs that inhibit CYP3A4 such as protease inhibitors and ketoconazole will increase the bioavailability of THC and CBD and in both cases elevate the risk for ADRs. Drugs such as phenytoin and carbamazepine induce CYP3A4 (increased enzyme concentration), resulting in enhanced metabolism of THC and CBD and decreased efficacy.

DDIs are actually even more complicated because THC is also metabolized by CYP2C9 and CYP2C19 and, in addition, inhibits carboxylesterase1, another drug metabolizing enzyme. Therefore, many other drugs are also affected and the effects

Table 8.3 THC Interaction with Drugs (reproduced with permission from Brown (2020) [138])

Cannabinoid	Pharmacokinetics		Pharmacodynamics	
THC	Enzyme	Outcome	Target effect	Outcome
	CYP3A4 substrates Immunosuppressants, antidepressants, antipsychotics, opioids, benzodiazepines, statins	↑ substrate bioavailability and ADRs	THC additive to antipsychotics, antihypertensive, opioids	↑ risk of depression, suicidal ideation
	CYP3A4 Inhibitors Protease inhibitors, ketoconazole, nefazodone, Amiodarone, verapamil, cimetidine, imatinib, tamoxifen	↑ THC bioavailability and ADRs		
	CYP3A4 inducers Phenytoin, carbamazepine topiramate, rifampicin pioglitazone	↓ THC bioavailability and efficacy		
	CYP2C9 substrates Antidepressants, antiepileptics, proton pump inhibitors, warfarin	↑ substrate bioavailability and ADRs	THC additive to sedative, hypnotics, antidepressants, antipsychotics	↑ risk of amnesia, impaired balance, disturbed attention, dizziness, lethargy, and somnolence
	CYP2C9 inhibitors Fluvoxmine, proton pump inhibitors, ketoconazole clopidogrel, fluconazole fluorouracil	↑ THC bioavailability and ADRs		
	CYP2C9 inducers Rifampin, phenytoin carbamazepine phenobarbital St John's Wort	↓ THC bioavailability and efficacy		
	CYP2C19 substrates Rosiglitazone, buprenorphine, montelukast, sulfonylureas, phenytoin warfarin	↑ substrate bioavailability and ADRs	THC additive to antihypertensive and anticholinergics	↑ risk of hypotension, syncope, and hypertension and tachycardia
	CES1 substrates/THC inhibitor Methylphenidate, cocaine meperidine prodrugs dabigatran clopidogrel, simvastatin	↑ substrate bioavailability and ADRs ↓ pro-drug availability	THC additive to immunosuppressants and immune-modulating drugs	↑ risk of infections

CES1 carboxylesterase 1, *THC* trans-delta-9-tetrahydrocannabinol, *ADR* adverse drug reaction, ↑ increase, ↓ decrease

Table 8.4 CBD interaction with Drugs (reproduced with permission from Brown and Winterstein (2019) [140])

Cannabinoid	Pharmacokinetics			Pharmacodynamics	
	Enzyme		Outcome	Target	Outcome
CBD	*CYP3A4 substrates* Immunosuppressants, chemotherapeutics, antidepressants, antipsychotics, opioids, benzodiazepines, z-hypnotics, statins, calcium channel blockers		↑ substrate bioavailability and ADRs	CBD additive with benzodiazepines, opioids, antidepressants, antiepileptics, antihistamines	Somnolence, sedation, lethargy, fatigue
	CYP3A4 inhibitors Strong: Protease inhibitors, ketoconazole, loperamide, nefazodone Moderate: Amiodarone, verapamil, cimetidine, aprepitant, imatinib		↑ CBD bioavailability, possible ↑ risk of ADRs	Additive with stimulants, antibiotics, chemotherapies, antiretrovirals, some antidepressants	↓ appetite
	CYP3A4 inducers Strong: Enzalutamide, phenytoin Moderate: Carbamazepine, topiramate, phenobarbital, rifampicin, efavirenz, pioglitazone		↓ CBD bioavailability ↓ efficacy	Additive with corticosteroids, tumor necrosis factor inhibitors, non-steroidal anti-inflammatory drugs, chemotherapy	↑ risk of bacterial and viral infections
	CYP2C19 substrates Antidepressants, antiepileptics, proton pump inhibitors, clopidogrel, propranolol, carisoprodol, cyclophosphamide, warfarin		↑ substrate bioavailability and ADRs	Additive with benzodiazepines, opioids, antidepressants, antiepileptics, antihistamines, antihypertensives, antiarrhythmics, sedatives/hypnotics, anticholinergics	Gait disturbances
	CYP2C19 inhibitors Strong: Fluvoxamine, fluoxetine Other: Proton pump inhibitors, cimetidine, ketoconazole, clopidogrel, fluconazole, efavirenz		↑ CBD bioavailability, possible ↑ risk of ADRs	Additive with alcohol, acetaminophen, sulfonamides, antifungals, ACE inhibitors, antipsychotics	↑ transaminase concentration (liver concern)
	CYP2C19 inducers Rifampin, carbamazepine, phenobarbital, phenytoin, St John's Wort		↓ CBD bioavailability ↓ efficacy		

CYP2C8/9 substrates Rosiglitazone, buprenorphine, Montelukast, celecoxib, sulfonylureas, losartan, naproxen, phenobarbital, phenytoin, rosuvastatin, valsartan, warfarin	↑ substrate bioavailability and ADRs
UGT1A9 substrates CBD inhibits Regorafenib, acetaminophen, canagliflozin, sorafenib, irinotecan, propofol, mycophenolate, valproic acid, haloperidol, ibuprofen, dabigatran, dapagliflozin	↑ substrate bioavailability and ADRs
UGT2B7 substrates, CBD inhibits Hydromorphone, losartan, ibuprofen, naproxen, ezetimibe, lovastatin, simvastatin, valproate, carbamazepine,	↑ substrate bioavailability and ADRs
BCRP, inhibition by CBD inactive metabolite Glyburide, imatinib, methotrexate, mitoxantrone, nitrofurantoin, prazosin, statins, dipyridamole	↑ substrate bioavailability and ADRs
BSEP inhibition by CBD inactive metabolite Paclitaxel, digoxin, statins, celecoxib, telmisartan, glyburide, ketoconazole, rosiglitazone,	↑ substrate bioavailability and ADRs

UGT uridine 5′-diphospho-glucoronosyltransferase, *BCRP* breast cancer resistance protein, *BSEP* bile salt export pump, *CBD* cannabidiol, *ADRs* adverse drug reactions, ↑ increase, ↓ decrease of THC may increase or decrease depending on the co-administered drug. Similarly but to a greater extent, CBD is metabolized not only by CYP3A4 but also CYP2C9, CYP2C8/9, and UGT1A9, UGT2B7. The latter 2 enzymes participate in phase II metabolism that adds glucuronic acid to drugs metabolized by P450 enzymes to accelerate excretion. CBD competes with many drugs at these sites (see Tables 8.3 and 8.4) to increase substrate and CBD bioavailability and risk of ADRs or decrease the efficacy of CBD [138, 140]. Complicating this further, a major inactive metabolite of CBD (7-COOH-CBD) inhibits two efflux transporters, BCRB (breast cancer resistance protein) and BSEP (bile salt export pump), that permits more substrate drug, e.g., glyburide, statins, and paclitaxal, to remain in circulation longer with potential for adverse effects [138, 140].

Marijuana. Pharmacodynamic Interactions Pharmacodynamically, THC and CBD-induced effects will add to similar effects of other drugs. With regard to THC, its psychotropic effects may enhance the depressive and suicidal ideation of antipsychotics, antihypertensives and opioids [138]. The sedative, somnolence, lethargy, and impaired balance produced by THC and CBD use sum with those of sedatives, hypnotics, antidepressants, and benzodiazepines. The orthostatic hypotensive effects of antihypertensive and anticholinergic drugs are additive to those of THC and elevate the risk of fainting and falls (Check Tables 8.3 and 8.4 for all interacting drug groups). Both THC and CBD increase the risk of infections, an effect that is worsened when co-administered with chemotherapy, NSAIDs, corticosteroids and immune-modulating therapies [138, 140].

MARIJUANA. MEDICAL ASSESSMENT Given the extensive interaction of THC and CBD with prescription and OTC drugs, initiation of THC or CBD use as medicinal cannabis, should proceed only after a compete medical assessment of patient health, current drug use (prescription and OTC), and comorbidities. The older adult with uncompromised health that uses marijuana for recreational or personal use needs to be aware of the potential of THC for psychotic effects and negative cardiovascular effects and in the case of THC and CBD, excessive sedation, increased risk of falls and increased risk of infections [138, 140] (see Fig. 8.2). Currently, clinicians are advised to avoid co-administration of drugs with the ability to interact with cannabis and are additionally recommended to "start low, go slow."

Echeverria-Villalobos et al. [141] also describe the harm that low and high doses of cannabis have on general and local anesthesia to include sympathetic activation (low doses) and parasympathetic activation (high doses) that adversely affect heart rate and blood pressure and that may progress to "malignant arrhythmias, coronary spasm, sudden death, cerebral hypoperfusion and stroke." Postoperative adverse effects of "hypothermia, shivering and increased platelet aggregation" have been reported [141]. It is recommended that *cannabis use should cease 72 hours prior to surgery* [141].

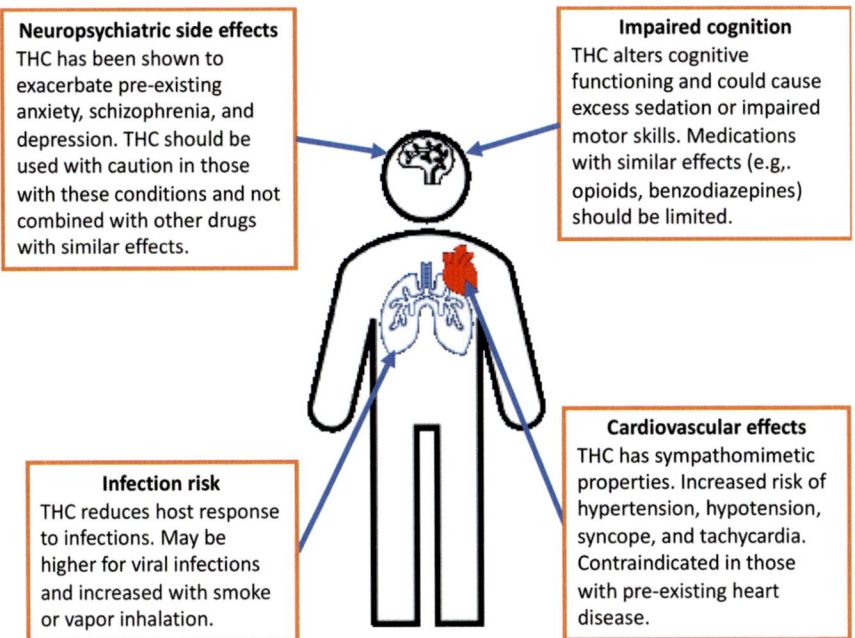

Fig. 8.2 Representation of the main adverse effects of tetrahydrocannabinol use that can be potentiated by other medications. (Reproduced with permission from Brown (2020) [138])

MARIJUANA. AGING Although there is a wealth of data from preclinical studies suggesting that low doses of THC are neuroprotective in the aging brain and chronic high doses of THC enhance the deteriorative aging effects on the structure and function of the brain, there are few studies on the effects of THC on the aging human body [142]. In a small study of 24 former long-term cannabis users (~ 30 years of abstinence) compared to nonusers (average age, 67 years), MRI scans showed a significant decrease in cortical thickness in hippocampal subregions in former heavy cannabis users compared to nonusers [143]. However, the parietal cortical thickness and location of some CBRs were unchanged in former cannabis users [143]. Results of a battery of neurological tests were lower in former cannabis users, but this did not reach significance, possibly due to the small number of participants [143]. Many studies of younger adults confirm these changes, reporting structural brain loss dependent on the first use of cannabis as a teenager [144]. A larger study that tracked heavy cannabis users from 18 to 45 years reported reduced hippocampal volume and cognitive defects [145] and further asked whether these changes may lead to future dementia. It is speculated that cannabis-induced brain changes are additive to age-dependent age changes and would worsen memory loss over time [142, 144].

MARIJUANA. USE IN DISEASES/DISORDERS Ideally it is important to understand the precise role of CB1Rs and CB2Rs in disease. However, this is complicated by the observed fluctuations of the receptors' presence even in the same disorder and, additionally, by the widespread presence of CBRs throughout the body. Hence, the development of specific cannabinoid agonists and antagonists is limited [146, 147].

Generally, as noted in a scoping review of over 160 publications in oncology but applicable to other diseases and disorders, the use of medical cannabis in those 18 years and older is for 3 reasons: pain management, treatment of refractory nausea and vomiting of chemotherapy and appetite stimulation [119]. To this is added seizure disorders and muscle spasticity [148]. Along these lines, the FDA has approved Epidiolex (purified CBD) for the treatment of drug-resistant seizures due to Lennox-Gastaut syndrome or Dravet syndrome (patients 2 years of age and older). Synthetic THC, dronabinol, in pill form (Marinol®), and solution (Syndros®) are approved for the treatment of nausea associated with cancer chemotherapy and anorexia associated with weight loss in AIDS patients. A synthetic analog of THC, nabilone (Cesamet®), is approved to stimulate appetite in AIDS patients and is approved as an anti-emetic in chemotherapy and pain suppressor in neuropathy [149].

Marijuana. Use in the Treatment of Pain Results of preclinical studies indicate that phytocannabinoids and endocannabinoids modulate (suppress) pain signaling [134]. Consequently, THC and CBD have been evaluated as a therapy for chronic pain (pain lasting 3–6 months, affecting quality of life). Several systemic and meta-analysis of these studies have been reported [135, 150–152]. A systemic analysis of 12 randomized controlled trials (RCTs), which differed in cannabis preparations, found that cannabis reduced neuropathic pain (pain due to nerve damage of multiple origins) in 5 studies but was without effect in 7 studies [151]. Another systematic review observed that the use of medicinal cannabis (MC) (various preparations and administration routes) for noncancer pain reduced the need for opioids by up to 75% and reduced emergency and hospital admissions in those using MC [150]. No optimal MC dose was established, and the authors recommended caution in MC use until more long-term health information is established [150]. In a meta-analysis of 33 studies of phytocannabinoids (inhaled, oral, and oromucosal) reported small but significant reduction in pain scores for both neuropathic and nonneuropathic pain [152]. When studies are stratified for the ratio of THC:CBD, a systemic analysis of 18 RCTs and 7 cohort studies (mean age 50–65) found that high THC:CBD ($\geq 2:1$) or comparable THC:CBD ratio produced moderate pain relief (neuropathic) but only the comparable THC:CBD preparations improve functionality. Dizziness and sedation were associated with these preparations which were oral or sublingual, synthetic or plant-extracted [135]. A review of several mostly "unadjusted" studies (mixed observational, cross-sectional, one RCT) that studied the older adult (≥50 yrs) who used MC for general non-cancer pain and, in one case, rheumatoid arthritis found beneficial effects on physical and mental health [153]. However, in an extensive review of 111 publications on the use of marijuana or cannabis-based drugs to treat chronic pain, Pantoja-Ruiz et al. (2022) [154] found a lack of high-quality evidence to support the use of cannabis for neuropathic pain, rheumatic diseases with chronic pain and headache and modest evidence to support the use of cannabis for multiple sclerosis-related pain and as an adjunct for cancer pain. Although it appears that MC provides some pain relief, the variability in preparation, the THC:CBD ratio, the route of administration, the origin of the pain, and the criteria of the studies prohibit, at present, a convincing understanding of the role of MC in pain suppression.

Marijuana Preparations, FDA-Approved and Others. Anti-emetic Effects In RCTs, nabilone and dronabinol successfully suppress nausea and vomiting induced by chemotherapy [155–157]. Results of other RCTs using THC extracts additionally show reduced nausea and antiemetic effects in patients receiving chemotherapy [158–160]. These trials also report side effects of THC to include reduced ability to concentrate, fewer social interactions and less activity as well as drowsiness, postural dizziness, lightheadedness, and, in a small percentage, euphoria. In a recent RCT of older adults (mean age 55 yrs), oral THC:CBD extract significantly reduced chemotherapy-induced nausea and vomiting when added to standard antiemetic therapy. Side effects of dizziness, sedation and disorientation were moderate [161].

Additional studies are needed to confirm the effect of cannabis on appetite stimulation in wasting syndromes. In a long-term (1-year) study, dronabinol improved appetite to allow patients with anorexia of AIDS to maintain a stable body weight [162]. Similarly, HIV-positive marijuana smokers increased caloric intake while taking high doses of dronabinol, although tolerance developed in some [163]. Other studies with dronabinol found it less effective than megestrol, an approved appetite stimulant for the wasting syndrome of HIV [164, 165]. Whether cannabis is an appetite stimulant in the anorexia-cachexia syndrome of cancer is not clear. Results of a phase III RCT found no effect of cannabis extract or THC compared to placebo to stimulate appetite [166], while results of a phase II study found oral THC enhanced appetite [167].

The use of CBD and CBD-containing products for self-medication of anxiety is on the rise [168]. Clinical trial results support this use, but these trials are small (10–60 participants) with an average dose of 300 mg [139, 148] and have been accused of CBD expectancy (placebo effect) [169]. The limited data on the use of CBD for anxiety has received a grade C recommendation [170]. *Products with THC are associated with increased anxiety* [148].

MARIJUANA. CANNABIS USE DISORDER (CUD) This refers to a serious dependent use of cannabis that produces impairment in control, physical addiction, social problems and use of cannabis in amounts larger than necessary or for longer periods than reasonable [171]. It is estimated that over a quarter of adults that use cannabis develop CUD [172]. Prevalence of CUD in the older adult is 0.3% (mean age 69) in a sample of inpatients [173], and in a study of US veterans, 65–75 years of age, CUD increased from ~0.35% in 2005 to 0.9–1.12% in 2019 [172]. This increase was only partially due to the medical and recreational legalization of marijuana [172]. Additional influence may come from the increase in potency of THC products [106] that lead to greater addiction [174]. Currently there are no approved pharmacotherapies for CUD, but psychosocial approaches such as cognitive behavioral therapy, motivational enhancement therapy and abstinence-based contingency management combined with the former two tend to reduce but not stop cannabis use [175].

Nicotine

Nicotine. Introduction Nicotine, the psychoactive substance in tobacco, is obtained mainly by combustion, that is, smoking tobacco (cigarettes, cigarillos, cigars, pipes). Nicotine may also be accessed via e-cigarettes (vapors), nicotine pouches, oronasal sprays, transdermal patches, inhalers, sublingual tablets, snuff, chewing tobacco, lozenges, and gum [176, 177]. Nicotine, whether experienced by smoking or by other means, heated solution, dissolved salt, or ground, offers no health benefits other than nicotine replacement therapy that mitigates nicotine dependence [178]. It is the nicotine that creates the smoking addiction that leads to tobacco use disorder (TUD) (DSM-5) and elevates the risk of cancers, diabetes, cardiovascular disease, and osteoporosis [179–184].

Chronic use of nicotine, alone, also accelerates aging and increases disease risk [185, 186]. Nicotine, whether from direct smoking or secondhand smoke, exerts negative effects across the lifespan from the fetus to the older adult [187]. Fortunately, smoking cessation, if maintained for years, reduces disease risk significantly and adds years to life expectancy [183, 188].

SMOKING PREVALENCE Although on the decline, the use of tobacco (commercial cigarette smoking) is still high and accounts for the "leading cause of preventable disease and death in the United States" [189]. Data from the National Health Interview Survey, 2021 reported that 11% of the older US population use any tobacco product daily or on some days, the lowest use of all age groups (highest use in 24–44 years of age). 9.8% use combustible tobacco products, 8.3% use cigarettes, 1.7% use e-cigarettes and 0.9% use smokeless tobacco. 81.9% of older adults quit smoking after smoking 100 cigarettes or more in their life time [189].

NICOTINE. PHARMACOLOGY Nicotine from the tobacco plant, *Nicotiana tabacum*, is considered a secondary metabolite evolving as a plant insecticide [190]. Chemically, nicotine is a large bicyclic compound generally termed an alkaloid and is present in up to 3% dry weight in tobacco leaves [191, 192]. Since nicotine is a weak base, absorption across body membranes is dependent on its ionization state (degree of positive charge) determined by the pH of the milieu.

Nicotine. Pharmacokinetics Since smoking releases nicotine in its ionized form, very little is absorbed by mouth. One puff allows nicotine to enter the small airways and alveolar sacs (site of gas exchange with a large surface area), where rapid absorption circulates nicotine to the brain within 10–20 seconds [176]. This extremely fast onset is considered the basis of behavioral addiction [193]. Nicotine from pipe smoking is mostly absorbed in the oral mucosa, as is nicotine from smokeless tobacco (snuff, chewing tobacco) [194]. Generally, although with considerable variability among smoked and smokeless tobacco products, the level of nicotine increases over 30 minutes and slowly declines over several hours [195]. The nicotine from products used to assuage nicotine withdrawal symptoms (gums, nasal sprays, sublingual tablets, transdermal patches, and lozenges) is absorbed more slowly and at lower levels [176]. Nasal sprays offer nicotine comparable to smoking [176]. In the blood, nicotine is poorly protein bound and equilibrates (unionized nicotine) not only with the brain but also the liver, kidney, lung, skeletal muscles, and spleen and less with adipose tissue [176].

With each pass through the liver, approximately 70% of the circulating nicotine is metabolized. Thus the clearance of nicotine is blood flow-dependent. Changes in hepatic blood flow caused by, for example, the normal physiology of meals, exercise, medications, or the pathology of disease, will alter nicotine metabolism. Nicotine is metabolized extensively in the liver to many metabolites, the main one of which is cotinine, devoid of pharmacological activity [191]. The hepatic P450 CYP2A6 enzyme handles most of the biotransformation with lesser contributions from CYP2B6 and CYP2E1. Cotinine is metabolized further to 3-hydroxycotinine and other metabolites. Both 3-hydroxycotinine and unchanged cotinine are excreted in the urine, although the former is in higher amounts [176]. Because cotinine has a longer half-life than nicotine, its presence in body fluids, plasma, saliva, and urine is considered evidence of smoking [176], exposure to second hand smoke [196, 197] and elevated lung cancer risk [198].

One small cross-sectional study found reduced nicotine clearance (higher nicotine levels) following intravenous infusion in older adults (20, 65–76 yrs) compared to young adults (20, 22–43 yrs). This was attributable to the expected age-influenced reduction in hepatic and renal clearance and smaller volume of distribution (reduced lean body mass) in older adults compared to younger adults [199].

Nicotine. Pharmacodynamics Nicotine binds to and stimulates nicotinic acetylcholine receptors (nAChRs), widely present in neuronal tissue throughout the brain [192] but also evident in nonneuronal tissue, e.g., epithelial cells, endothelial cells, immune cells, and mesenchymal fibroblasts [200]. nAChRs belong to the Cys-loop family of ligand-gated ion channels, to which GABA-A and 5HT3 receptors are also members [201]. nAChRs are composed of 5 subunits (pentimers) of either alpha or beta subtypes. The pentimers arrange themselves in variable fashion to facilitate channel transport of sodium, potassium and calcium [201, 202].

The physiological ligand for nAChRs is acetylcholine (ACh). Activation by ACh or nicotine generates depolarization and initiation of nerve activity. However, unlike nicotine, the actions of ACh are brief, due to rapid degradation by acetylcholine esterase [203]. Prolonged stimulation of nAChRs by nicotine leads to desensitization and altered sensitivities of other nAChR pentimers, possibly accounting for the addictive nature of nicotine [203].

Nicotine stimulation also leads to downstream effects that include the release of numerous neurotransmitters, chief of which is dopamine. Other neurotransmitters are released such as norepinephrine, serotonin, GABA, glutamate and endorphins that together possibly mediate the increase in mood, cognitive focus, and sensations of pleasure that smokers enjoy [192, 203]. Exactly what cognitive benefits are derived from nicotine is not clear, but results of numerous studies in humans suggest they are varied, depending on smoking history and state of nicotine withdrawal and may facilitate positive effects on mood [203]. Peripherally, nicotine acts as a sympathomimetic drug stimulating the sympathetic nervous system and adrenal catecholamine release to transiently increase heart rate and blood pressure [204].

NICOTINE. DRUG INTERACTIONS Since nicotine is metabolized by CYP2A6 and CYP2B6, drugs that also require these enzymes for metabolism will interact with nicotine clearance and vice versa. In particular, non-nucleoside reverse transcriptase inhibitors (NNRTs), e.g., nevirapine, used to treat HIV/AIDS, are metabolized by these enzymes, producing variable effects on NNRTs and nicotine, based on duration of smoking [205]. Unexpected changes in the efficacy of NNRTs are expected since there exists a high prevalence of smokers among HIV patients [206]. Using in vitro studies (human primary hepatic cell cultures, microsomes [cell components], and tissue biopsy), rifampin, and phenobarbital induce CYP2A6, CYP2B6, and CYP2E1 and accelerate nicotine metabolism [176, 207, 208]. Similarly, results of in vitro studies found that methoxsalen (8-methoxypsoralen), tranylcypromine, tryptamines and coumarin are inhibitors of CYP2A6 and hence reduce nicotine clearance [209]. The CYP2A6 inhibitory effect, albeit modest, by methoxsalen (8-methoxypsoralen) (used to treat psoriasis and vitiligo in which pigment is lost), and tranylcypromine, an antidepressant, is confirmed in humans [176, 210]. Interestingly, as these drugs inhibit the first pass of nicotine, thereby elevating nicotine levels, smokers consume fewer cigarettes [210].

Smoking itself decreases the metabolism of nicotine, and smoking cessation enhances it [211]. Additionally, smoking via the polycyclic *aromatic hydrocarbons generated in the combustion of tobacco enhances metabolism of drugs metabolized by CYP 1A2* [212]. This affects many drugs (check Chap. 3, Table 3.3) to include the following drug classes: antidepressants, antipsychotics, antiarrhythmics and many others. Although postulated some time ago, the impact of cigarette smoke on therapeutic medications needs continual assessment [212].

NICOTINE. DISEASES Smoking is causally related to lung cancer, the most common cancer-inducing death worldwide. In addition to lung cancer, an assessment of hundreds of epidemiological studies by the IARC [213, 214] found a causal relation between smoking and the following cancers: oral cavity, nasal cavity and nasal sinus, pharynx, larynx, esophagus (squamous-cell carcinoma, adenocarcinoma), pancreas, urinary bladder and renal pelvis, stomach, liver, kidney (renal-cell carcinoma), uterine cervix and bone marrow (myeloid leukemia). The relative risk varied with the cancer type, with a greater than 20-fold risk for lung cancer and a two- to three-fold risk for other cancers [214].

It was further established that cigarette smoke contains a wealth of carcinogens and toxins that are known to damage DNA in many ways and distort cell function and hence play a significant role in cancer development. The relation of cancers to smoking depends on the duration and intensity of smoking, factors which increase the exposure of the body to greater amounts of carcinogens and toxins. Examples of some powerful carcinogens and cytotoxins in smoke are polycyclic aromatic hydrocarbons (benzo[a]pyrene), N-nitrosamines, aromatic amines, aldehydes (acetaldehyde), volatile hydrocarbons (benzene), metals (arsenic, cadmium), and lead [214, 215]. These compounds readily bind to major biological molecules, DNA and proteins to mutate genes and alter protein function [216]. They also affect many P450 enzymes and influence the metabolism of therapeutic drugs (noted above).

Results of the 2020 Surgeon General's report added colorectal cancer to the above cancers caused by smoking. Additionally, morbidity and mortality of cardiovascular disease, stroke, and chronic obstructive pulmonary disease are causally related to smoking. Both nicotine and the plethora of components of combusted tobacco act through multiple pathways (endothelial damage, chronic inflammation, thrombus formation) to promote atherosclerosis and atherothrombosis and associated adverse events [217, 218]. Both active and passive smoking is involved in the initiation of these adverse changes [219].

Chronic obstructive pulmonary disease (COPD) is an irreversible lung disease that dramatically reduces respiratory function (see Chap. 5). COPD is attributed to many environmental pollutants, the chief of which is smoking and second hand smoke [220]. With similar pathological mechanisms as in cardiovascular disease, smoking is thought to produce chronic oxidative stress and inflammation in the airways that exceed repair mechanisms, leading to damaged alveolar sacs and hyper secretion [221] and may synergize with age changes in the lungs [222]. Alveolar macrophages are prime targets for the damaging effects of tobacco smoke-promoting lung disease [223].

Smoking has been long known to be involved in energy metabolism as an appetite suppressant. Weight maintenance is given as a common reason for smoking [224]. Due to the presence of nAChRs throughout the body, especially on metabolic tissue, e.g., pancreatic islets [225], adipose tissue [226], liver and skeletal muscle [227], nicotine is considered a major player in energy homeostasis [224]. However, epidemiological data link smoking to an elevated risk of Type 2 Diabetes Mellitus (T2DM) [227], indicating that nicotine and smoking eventually adversely affect energy homeostasis and body weight, especially fat distribution [228]. Small clinical trials in smokers show smoking acutely decreases glucose tolerance and insulin sensitivity and elevates serum cholesterol [229], and smokers with established T2DM exhibit reduced glucose utilization and decreased insulin activity compared to nonsmokers [230]. This data suggest that smoking should be added to the list of modifiable risk factors for T2DM [227].

NICOTINE. TOBACCO USE DISORDER There are numerous hypotheses as to why nicotine is extremely addicting. This could possibly be related to the rapidity in which nicotine enters the brain [193], to the ubiquitous presence of nAChRs, especially in the brain that releases dopamine [176], the upregulation of nAChRs by nicotine [231] and/or to the cognitive effects that enhance memory and focus [203]. Since the mortality rate of smokers is 3 times higher than nonsmokers, *it is imperative to stop smoking,* and adults who quit at age 45–54 gained an additional 6 years [183]. Quitting at any age reduces the risk of CV disease [232], secondary events of CV disease [233, 234], and cancer [235] and predicts better cancer outcomes [236], improves lung function in COPD [237], and ameliorates other diseases [238]. However, smoking cessation is difficult due to the withdrawal symptoms of dependence [239].

Tobacco Use Disorder. Pharmacotherapy Pharmacotherapy plans for smoking cessation are considered "mildly efficacious" [240]. "First line" therapies [239, 240] are (1) nicotine replacement therapy consisting of a transdermal patch, nasal spray, gum, inhaler, lozenges and e-cigarettes), (2) bupropion, an antidepressant that weakly inhibits the uptake of norepinephrine and dopamine [241] and (3) varenicline, a partial agonist at the nAChRs preventing nicotine binding [242]. Second-line therapies include nortriptyline, a tricyclic antidepressant agent, and clonidine, an antihypertensive drug. The potential adverse effects of these latter two drugs basically keep them as the last choice when other means fail [239]. First-line agents in clinical trials generally achieve 5–35% rates of smoking cessation [176].

Guidance
With a few exceptions, the scientific community does not recommend the use of recreational drugs: alcoholic beverages, marijuana (THC, CBD) and tobacco (nicotine, smoking) for the older adult.

This is based on the following data;

1. Use of each recreation substance has been documented to accelerate normal age changes and age changes alter the pharmacokinetics and pharmacodynamics of these substances, generally decreasing clearance, increasing blood levels and enhancing psychoactive effects.
2. The use of alcohol and marijuana produces sedative effects that, alone or additive with medications, increase the risk of accidents, falls, fractures and hospitalizations.
3. Use of each recreational substance elevates the risk of drug interactions with prescription medications, over-the-counter and herbal remedies that may (a) enhance the psychoactive effects of these substances and/or (b) generate adverse reactions of medications. Special note to use the lowest amount possible of medicinal or recreational marijuana in consideration of the extensive number of potential drug interactions.
4. Alcohol and smoking (toxins in smoke and nicotine) are carcinogens and chronic use is causally related to many types of cancers.
5. These recreational drugs also elevate the risk of other diseases: liver cirrhosis, tuberculosis (alcohol), infections (THC, CBD), cardiovascular disease, type 2 diabetes mellitus, chronic obstructive pulmonary disease, and osteoporosis (smoking, nicotine).
6. All three recreational drugs with chronic use produce substance use disorder, a psychosocial dependence with multiple symptoms, e.g., cognitive impairment, that decreases the quality of life. Cessation from these disorders is difficult but offers benefits of disease risk reduction.
7. The only valuable nicotine products are those used to aid smoking cessation.

Possible exceptions are (1) daily light consumption of alcohol ($\leq$ 14 gm, women; $\leq$ 28 gm, men) reduces the risk for cardiovascular disease, Type 2 diabetes mellitus but higher levels of use negate these benefits and (2) FDA-approved THC is efficacious in reducing nausea and vomiting of chemotherapy and stimulating appetite in cachexia.

A serious exercise program (running, jogging, walking, hiking), resistance (weights), and exercises for balance and stretch are recommended in place of recreational drug use to achieve relaxation and elevate mood.

References

1. National survey on drug use and health. 2021. (https://www.samhsa.gov/data/report/2021-nsduh-detailed-tables).
2. Mostofsky E, Mukamal KJ, Giovannucci EL, Stampfer MJ, Rimm EB. Key findings on alcohol consumption and a variety of health outcomes from the Nurses' Health Study. Am J Public Health. 2016;106(9):1586–91. https://doi.org/10.2105/AJPH.2016.303336.
3. Stampfer MJ, Kang JH, Chen J, Cherry R, Grosstein F. Effects of moderate alcohol consumption on cognitive function in women. N Engl J Med. 2005;352(3):245–53. https://doi.org/10.1056/NEJMoa041152.
4. Ganguli M, Vander Bilt J, Saxton JA, Shen C, Dodge HH. Alcohol consumption and cognitive function in late life: a longitudinal community study. Neurology. 2005;65(8):1210–7. https://doi.org/10.1212/01.wnl.0000180520.35181.24.
5. Taylor B, Irving HM, Kanteres F, Room R, Borges G, Cherpitel C, et al. The more you drink, the harder you fall: a systematic review and meta-analysis of how acute alcohol consumption and injury or collision risk increase together. Drug Alcohol Depend. 2010;110(1–2):108–16. https://doi.org/10.1016/j.drugalcdep.2010.02.011.
6. Satre DD, Hirschtritt ME, Silverberg MJ, Sterling SA. Addressing problems with alcohol and other substances among older adults during the COVID-19 pandemic. Am J Geriatr Psychiatry. 2020;28(7):780–3. https://doi.org/10.1016/j.jagp.2020.04.012.
7. Secretan B, Straif K, Baan R, Grosse Y, Ghissassi FE, Bouvard V, et al. A review of human carcinogens—part E: tobacco, areca nut, alcohol, coal smoke, and salted fish. Lancet. 2009;10(11):1033–4. https://doi.org/10.1016/s1470-2045(09)70326-2.
8. Minzer S, Losno RA, Casas R. The effect of alcohol on cardiovascular risk factors: is there new information? Nutrients. 2020;12(4):912. https://doi.org/10.3390/nu12040912.
9. Dietary Guidelines for Americans 2020–2025 USDA Publication #: USDA-FNS-2020-2025-DGA HHS Publication #: HHS-ODPHP-2020-2025-01-DGA-A.
10. Kalinowski A, Humphreys K. Governmental standard drink definitions and low-risk alcohol consumption guidelines in 37 countries. Addiction. 2016;111(7):1293–8. https://doi.org/10.1111/add.13341.
11. Roerecke M. Alcohol's impact on the cardiovascular system. Nutrients. 2021;13(10):3419. https://doi.org/10.3390/nu13103419.
12. Sicard D, Legras JL. Bread, beer and wine: yeast domestication in the Saccharomyces sensu stricto complex. C R Biol. 2011;334(3):229–36. https://doi.org/10.1016/j.crvi.2010.12.016.
13. Abrahao KP, Salinas AG, Lovinger DM. Alcohol and the brain: neuronal molecular targets, synapses, and circuits. Neuron. 2017;96(6):1223–38. https://doi.org/10.1016/j.neuron.2017.10.032.
14. Cederbaum AI. Alcohol metabolism. Clin Liver Dis. 2012;16(4):667–85. https://doi.org/10.1016/j.cld.2012.08.002.
15. Dufour MC, Archer L, Gordis E. Alcohol and the elderly. Clin Geriatr Med. 1992;8(1):127–41. https://doi.org/10.1111/add.13341.
16. Mumenthaler MS, Taylor JL, O'Hara R, Yesavage JA. Gender differences in moderate drinking effects. Alcohol Res Health. 1999;23(1):55–64. PMCID: PMC6761697.
17. Lobo IA, Harris RA. GABA(A) receptors and alcohol. Pharmacol Biochem Behav. 2008;90(1):90–4. https://doi.org/10.1016/j.pbb.2008.03.006.
18. Söderpalm B, Lidö HH, Ericson M. The glycine receptor: a functionally important primary brain target of ethanol. Alcohol Clin Exp Res. 2017;41(11):1816–30. https://doi.org/10.1111/acer.13483.
19. Lovinger DM, Roberto M. Synaptic effects induced by alcohol. Curr Top Behav Neurosci. 2023; https://doi.org/10.1007/7854_2022_412.
20. Rahman S, Engleman EA, Bell RL. Recent advances in nicotinic receptor signaling in alcohol abuse and alcoholism. Prog Mol Biol Transl Sci. 2016;137:183–201. https://doi.org/10.1016/bs.pmbts.2015.10.004.

21. Le Daré B, Lagente V, Gicquel T. Ethanol and its metabolites: update on toxicity, benefits, and focus on immunomodulatory effects. Drug Metab Rev. 2019;51(4):545–61. https://doi.org/10.1080/03602532.2019.1679169.
22. Kinirons MT, O'Mahony MS. Drug metabolism and ageing. Br J Clin Pharmacol. 2004;57(5):540–4. https://doi.org/10.1111/j.1365-2125.2004.02096.x.
23. Xu Q, Ou X, Li J. The risk of falls among the aging population: a systematic review and meta-analysis. Front Public Health. 2022;10:902599. https://doi.org/10.3389/fpubh.2022.902599.
24. Shakya I, Bergen G, Haddad YK, Kakara R, Moreland BL. Fall-related emergency department visits involving alcohol among older adults. J Saf Res. 2020;74:125–31. https://doi.org/10.1016/j.jsr.2020.06.001.
25. Wang Y, Dong C, Han Y, Gu Z, Sun C. Immunosenescence, aging and successful aging. Front Immunol. 2022;13:942796. https://doi.org/10.3389/fimmu.2022.942796.
26. Boule LA, Kovacs EJ. Alcohol, aging, and innate immunity. J Leukoc Biol. 2017;102(1):41–55. https://doi.org/10.1189/jlb.4RU1016-450R.
27. Pasala S, Barr T, Messaoudi I. Impact of alcohol abuse on the adaptive immune system. Alcohol Res. 2015;37(2):185–97. PMID: 26695744.
28. Szabo G, Mandrekar P. A recent perspective on alcohol, immunity and host defense. Alcohol Clin Exp Res. 2009;33(2):220–32. https://doi.org/10.1111/j.1530-0277.2008.00842.x.
29. McElhaney JE, Effros RB. Immunosenescence: what does it mean to health outcomes in older adults? Curr Opin Immunol. 2009;21(4):418–24. https://doi.org/10.1016/j.coi.2009.05.023.
30. Funk-White M, Moore AA, McEvoy LK, Bondi MW, Bergstrom J, Kaufmann CN. Alcohol use and cognitive performance: a comparison between Greece and the United States. Aging Ment Health. 2022;26(12):2440–6. https://doi.org/10.1080/13607863.2021.1998355.
31. Nallapu BT, Petersen KK, Lipton RB, Grober E, Sperling RA, Ezzati AJ. Association of alcohol consumption with cognition in older population: the A4 study. Alzheimers Dis. 2023;93(4):1381–93. https://doi.org/10.3233/JAD-221079.
32. Kalapatapu RK, Ventura MI, Barnes DE. Lifetime alcohol use and cognitive performance in older adults. J Addict Dis. 2017;36(1):38–47. https://doi.org/10.1080/10550887.2016.1245029.
33. https://www.niaaa.nih.gov/sites/default/files/publications/Harmful_Interactions.pdf.
34. Weathermon R, Crabb DW. Alcohol and medication interactions. Alcohol Res Health. 1999;23(1):40–54. PMID: 10890797 PMCID: PMC6761694.
35. Moore AA, Whiteman EJ, Ward KT. Risks of combined alcohol/medication use in older adults. Am J Geriatr Pharmacother. 2007;5(1):64–74. https://doi.org/10.1016/j.amjopharm.2007.03.006.
36. Breslow RA, Dong C, White A. Prevalence of alcohol-interactive prescription medication use among current drinkers: United States, 1999 to 2010. Alcoholism: Clin Exp Res. 2015;39(2):371–9. https://doi.org/10.1111/acer.12633.
37. Immonen S, Valvanne J, Pitkälä KH. The prevalence of potential alcohol-drug interactions in older adults. Scand J Prim Health Care. 2013;31(2):73–8. https://doi.org/10.3109/02813432.2013.788272.
38. Salmela KS, Kessova IG, Tsyrlov IB, Lieber CS. Respective roles of human cytochrome P-4502E1, 1A2, and 3A4 in the hepatic microsomal ethanol oxidizing system. Alcoholism: Clin Exp Res. 1998;22(9):2125–32. PMID: 9884161.
39. Roine R, Gentry RT, Hernandez-Munoz R, Baraona E, Lieber CS. Aspirin increases blood alcohol concentration in humans after ingestion of ethanol. JAMA. 1990;264:2406–8. PMID: 2231997.
40. Calleria J, Baraona E, Deulofeu R, Hernandez-Munoz R, Rodes J, Lieber CS. Effects of H-2 receptor antagonists on gastric alcohol dehydrogenase activity. Dig Dis Sci. 1991;36(12):1673–9. https://doi.org/10.1007/BF01296608.
41. Vallari RC, Pietruszko R. Human aldehyde dehydrogenase: mechanism of inhibition of disulfiram. Science. 1982;216(4546):637–9. https://doi.org/10.1126/science.7071604.
42. Li H, Xia N. Alcohol and the vasculature: a love-hate relationship? Pflugers Arch. 2023;475(7):867–75. https://doi.org/10.1007/s00424-023-02818-8.

43. O'Keefe EL, Di Nicolantonio JJ, O'Keefe JH, Lavie CJ. Alcohol and CV Health: Jekyll and Hyde J-Curves. Prog Cardiovasc Dis. 2018;61(1):68–75. https://doi.org/10.1016/j.pcad.2018.02.001.
44. Matsumoto C, Miedema MD, Ofman P, Gaziano JM, Sesso HD. An expanding knowledge of the mechanisms and effects of alcohol consumption on cardiovascular disease. J Cardiopulm Rehabil Prev. 2014;34(3):159–71. https://doi.org/10.1097/HCR.0000000000000042.
45. Fernández-Solà J. Cardiovascular risks and benefits of moderate and heavy alcohol consumption. Nat Rev Cardiol. 2015;12(10):576–87. https://doi.org/10.1038/nrcardio.2015.91.
46. Costanzo S, Di Castelnuovo A, Donati MB, Iacoviello L, De Gaetano G. Alcohol consumption and mortality in patients with cardiovascular disease. A meta-analysis. J Am Coll Cardiol. 2010;55(13):1339–47. https://doi.org/10.1016/j.jacc.2010.01.006.
47. Ronksley PE, Brien SE, Turner BJ, Mukamal KJ, Ghali WA. Association of alcohol consumption with selected cardiovascular disease outcomes: a systematic review and meta-analysis. BMJ. 2011;342:d671. https://doi.org/10.1136/bmj.d671.
48. Roerecke M, Rehm J. Alcohol consumption, drinking patterns, and ischemic heart disease: a narrative review of meta-analyses and a systematic review and meta-analysis of the impact of heavy drinking occasions on risk for moderate drinkers. BMC Med. 2014;12:182. https://doi.org/10.1186/s12916-014-0182-6.
49. Ding C, O'Neill D, Bell S, Stamatakis E, Britton A. Association of alcohol consumption with morbidity and mortality in patients with cardiovascular disease: original data and meta-analysis of 48,423 men and women. BMC Med. 2021;19(1):167. https://doi.org/10.1186/s12916-021-02040-2.
50. Brien SE, Ronksley PE, Turner BJ, Mukamal KJ, Ghali WA. Effect of alcohol consumption on biological markers associated with risk of coronary heart disease: systematic review and meta-analysis of interventional studies. BMJ. 2011;342:d636. https://doi.org/10.1136/bmj.d636.
51. Nova E, San Mauro-Martín I, Díaz-Prieto LE, Marcos A. Wine and beer within a moderate alcohol intake is associated with higher levels of HDL-c and adiponectin. Nutr Res. 2019;63:42–50. https://doi.org/10.1016/j.nutres.2018.12.007.
52. Jaubert MP, Jin Z, Russo C, Schwartz JE, Homma S, Elkind MSV, et al. Alcohol consumption and ambulatory blood pressure: a community-based study in an elderly cohort. Am J Hypertens. 2014;27(5):688–94. https://doi.org/10.1093/ajh/hpt235.
53. Roerecke M, Tobe SW, Kaczorowski J, Bacon S, Vafaei A, Hasan OSM, et al. Sex-specific associations between alcohol consumption and incidence of hypertension: a systematic review and meta-analysis of cohort studies. J Am Heart Assoc. 2018;7(13):e008202. https://doi.org/10.1161/JAHA.117.008202.
54. Kiechl S, Willeit J, Poewe W, Egger G, Oberhollenzer F, Muggeo M, et al. Insulin sensitivity and regular alcohol consumption: large, prospective, cross sectional population study (Bruneck study). BMJ. 1996;313(7064):1040–4. https://doi.org/10.1136/bmj.313.7064.1040.
55. Risérus U, Ingelsson E. Alcohol intake, insulin resistance, and abdominal obesity in elderly men. Obesity (Silver Spring). 2007;15(7):1766–73. https://doi.org/10.1038/oby.2007.210.
56. GBD 2016 Disease and Injury Incidence and Prevalence Collaborators. Global, regional, and national incidence, prevalence, and years lived with disability for 328 diseases and injuries for 195 countries, 1990–2016: A systematic analysis for the global burden of disease study 2016. Lancet. 2017;390(10100):1211–59. https://doi.org/10.1016/S0140-6736(17)32154-2.
57. GBD 2020 Alcohol Collaborators. Population-level risks of alcohol consumption by amount, geography, age, sex, and year: a systematic analysis for the Global Burden of Disease Study 2020. Lancet. 2022;400(10347):185–235. https://doi.org/10.1016/S0140-6736(22)00847-9.
58. Baan R, Straif K, Grosse Y, Secretan B, El Ghissassi F, Bouvard V, et al. Carcinogenicity of alcoholic beverages. Lancet Oncol. 2007;8(4):292–3. https://doi.org/10.1016/s1470-2045(07)70099-2.
59. Liu Y, Nguyen N, Colditz GA. Links between alcohol consumption and breast cancer: a look at the evidence. Womens Health. 2015;11:65–77. https://doi.org/10.2217/whe.14.62.

References

60. Rumgay H, Murphy N, Ferrari P, Soerjomataram I. Alcohol and cancer: epidemiology and Biological mechanisms. Nutrients. 2021;13(9):3173. https://doi.org/10.3390/nu13093173.
61. Morgan E, Arnold M, Camargo MC, Gini A, Kunzmann AT, Matsuda T et al. The current and future incidence and mortality of gastric cancer in 185 countries, 2020–40: a population-based modeling study. eClinicalMedicine, Published online 21 April 2022; https://doi.org/10.1016/j.eclinm.2022.101404.
62. Bagnardi V, Rota M, Botteri E, Tramacere I, Islami F, Fedirko V, et al. Alcohol consumption and site-specific cancer risk: a comprehensive dose-response meta-analysis. Br J Cancer. 2015;112(3):580–93. https://doi.org/10.1038/bjc.2014.579.
63. Tramacere I, Scotti L, Jenab M, Bagnardi V, Bellocco R, Rota M, et al. Alcohol drinking and pancreatic cancer risk: a meta-analysis of the dose-risk relation. Int J Cancer. 2010;126(6):1474–86. https://doi.org/10.1002/ijc.24936.
64. Cao Y, Willett WC, Rimm EB, Stampfer MJ, Giovannucci EL. Light to moderate intake of alcohol, drinking patterns, and risk of cancer: results from two prospective US cohort studies. BMJ. 2015;351:h4238. https://doi.org/10.1136/bmj.h4238.
65. Seitz HK, Stickel F. Molecular mechanisms of alcohol-mediated carcinogenesis. Nat Rev Cancer. 2007;7(8):599–612. https://doi.org/10.1038/nrc2191.
66. Millonig G, Wang Y, Homann N, Bernhardt F, Qin H, Mueller S, et al. Ethanol-mediated carcinogenesis in the human esophagus implicates CYP2E1 induction and the generation of carcinogenic DNA-lesions. Int J Cancer. 2011;128(3):533–40. https://doi.org/10.1002/ijc.25604.
67. Molina PE, Happel KI, Zhang P, Kolls JK, Nelson S. Focus on: alcohol and the immune system. Alcohol Res Health. 2010;33:97–108. PMID: 23579940 PMCID: PMC3887500.
68. Dumitrescu RG, Shields PG. The etiology of alcohol-induced breast cancer. Alcohol. 2005;35(3):213–25. https://doi.org/10.1016/j.alcohol.2005.04.005.
69. Lönnroth K, Williams B, Stadlin S, Jaramillo E, Dye C. Alcohol use as a risk factor for tuberculosis—a systematic review. BMC Public Health. 2008;8:289. https://doi.org/10.1186/1471-2458-8-289.
70. Rehm J, Samokhvalov AV, Neuman MG, Room R, Parry C, Lonnroth K, et al. The association between alcohol use, alcohol use disorders and tuberculosis (TB). A systematic review. BMC Public Health. 2009;9:450. https://doi.org/10.1186/1471-2458-9-450.
71. Imtiaz S, Shield KD, Roerecke M, Samokhvalov AV, Lönnroth K, Rehm J. Alcohol consumption as a risk factor for tuberculosis: meta-analyses and burden of disease. Eur Respir J. 2017;50(1):1700216. https://doi.org/10.1183/13993003.00216-2017.
72. Szabo G. Alcohol's contribution to compromised immunity. Alcohol Health Res World. 1997;21:39–41. PMID: 15706761.
73. National Survey on Drug Use and Health. 2023. https://www.hhs.gov/about/news/2023/11/13/hhs-samhsa-release-2022-national-survey-drug-use-health-data.html.
74. Joshi P, Duong KT, Trevisan LA, Wilkins KM. Evaluation and management of alcohol use disorder among older adults. Curr Geriatr Rep. 2021;10(3):82–90. https://doi.org/10.1007/s13670-021-00359-5.
75. Yarnell S, Li L, Mac Grory B, Trevisan L, Kirwin P. Substance use disorders in later life: a review and synthesis of the literature of an emerging public health concern. Am J Geriatr Psychiatry. 2020;28(2):226–36. https://doi.org/10.1016/j.jagp.2019.06.005.
76. Substance Abuse and Mental Health Services Administration, 2020; https://www.samhsa.gov/.
77. U.S. Preventive Services Task Force, 2023. https://www.uspreventiveservicestaskforce.org/uspstf/.
78. Berks J, McCormick R. Screening for alcohol misuse in elderly primary care patients: a systematic literature review. Int Psychogeriatr. 2008;20(6):1090–103. https://doi.org/10.1017/S1041610208007497.
79. Ewing JA. Detecting alcoholism. The CAGE questionnaire. JAMA. 1984;252(14):1905–7. https://doi.org/10.1001/jama.252.14.1905.

80. Sinforiani E, Zucchella C, Pasotti C, Casoni F, Bini P, Costa A. The effects of alcohol on cognition in the elderly: from protection to neurodegeneration. Funct Neurol. 2011;26(2):103–6. PMID: 21729592.
81. Kurihara K, Shiroma A, Koda M, Shinzato H, Takaesu Y, Kondo T. Age-related cognitive decline is accelerated in alcohol use disorder. Neuropsychopharmacol Rep. 2023;43(4):587–95. https://doi.org/10.1002/npr2.12395.
82. Kuzma E, Llewellyn DJ, Langa KM, Wallace RB, Lang IA. History of alcohol use disorders and risk of severe cognitive impairment: a 19-year prospective cohort study. Am J Geriatr Psychiatry. 2014;22(10):1047–54. https://doi.org/10.1016/j.jagp.2014.06.001.
83. Anttila T, Helkala E-L, Viitanen M, Kåreholt I, Fratiglioni L, Winblad B, et al. Alcohol drinking in middle age and subsequent risk of mild cognitive impairment and dementia in old age: a prospective population based study. BMJ. 2004;329(7465):539. https://doi.org/10.1136/bmj.38181.418958.BE.
84. Guggenmos M, Schmack K, Sekutowicz M, Garbusow M, Sebold M, Sommer C, et al. Quantitative neurobiological evidence for accelerated brain aging in alcohol dependence. Transl Psychiatry. 2017;7(12):1279. https://doi.org/10.1038/s41398-017-0037-y.
85. Zhao Q, Pfefferbaum A, Podhajsky S, Pohl KM, Sullivan EV. Accelerated aging and motor control deficits are related to regional deformation of central cerebellar white matter in alcohol use disorder. Addict Biol. 2020;25(3):e12746. https://doi.org/10.1111/adb.12746.
86. Paul CA, Au R, Fredman L, Massaro JM, Seshadri S, Decarli C, et al. Association of alcohol consumption with brain volume in the Framingham study. Arch Neurol. 2008;65(10):1363–7. https://doi.org/10.1001/archneur.65.10.1363.
87. Nunes PT, Kipp BT, Reitz NL, Savage LM. Aging with alcohol-related brain damage: Critical brain circuits associated with cognitive dysfunction. Int Rev Neurobiol. 2019;148:101–68. https://doi.org/10.1016/bs.irn.2019.09.002.
88. Carlson ER, Guerin SP, Nixon K, Fonken LK. The neuroimmune system – Where aging and excess alcohol intersect. Alcohol. 2023;107:153–67. https://doi.org/10.1016/j.alcohol.2022.08.009.
89. Topiwala A, Ebmeier KP. Effects of drinking on late-life brain and cognition. Evid Based Ment Health. 2018;21(1):12–5. https://doi.org/10.1136/eb-2017-102820.
90. Babor TF, McRee BG, Kassebaum PA, Grimaldi PL, Ahmed K, Bray J. Screening, brief intervention, and referral to treatment (SBIRT): toward a public health approach to the management of substance abuse. Subst Abus. 2007;28(3):7–30. https://doi.org/10.1300/J465v28n03_03.
91. Winslow BT, Onysko M, Hebert M. Medications for alcohol use disorder. Am Fam Physician. 2016;93(6):457–65. PMID: 26977830.
92. https://www.samhsa.gov/data/release/2022-national-survey-drug-use-and-health-nsduh-releases.
93. Han BH, Palamar JJ. Trends in cannabis use among older adults in the United States, 2015-2018. JAMA Intern Med. 2020;180(4):609–11. https://doi.org/10.1001/jamainternmed.2019.7517.
94. Fernandez AF, Coughlin L, Solway ES, Singer DC, Kullgren JT, Kirch M, et al. Prevalence and frequency of cannabis use among adults ages 50–80 in the United States. Cannabis Cannabinoid Res. 2024;9(1):59–64. https://doi.org/10.1089/can.2023.0056.
95. Gabay M. The federal controlled substances act: schedules and pharmacy registration. Hosp Pharm. 2013;48(6):473–4. https://doi.org/10.1310/hpj4806-473.
96. Ortiz NR, Preuss CV. Controlled substance act. In: StatPearls [Internet]. Treasure Island (FL): StatPearls Publishing; 2023.
97. https://www.dea.gov/drug-information/drug-scheduling.
98. https://nida.nih.gov/publications/research-reports/marijuana/marijuana-gateway-drug.
99. Vacaflor BE, Beauchet O, Jarvis GE, Schavietto A, Rej S. Mental health and cognition in older cannabis users: a review. Can Geriatr J. 2020;23(3):242–9. https://doi.org/10.5770/cgj.23.399.
100. https://mjbizdaily.com/map-of-us-marijuana-legalization-by-state.

101. Jikomes N, Zoorob M. Authors correction: the cannabinoid content of legal cannabis in Washington state varies systematically across testing facilities and popular consumer products. Sci Rep. 2020;10(1):14406. https://doi.org/10.1038/s41598-020-69680-x.
102. Cox EJ, Maharao N, Patilea-Vrana G, Unadkat JD, Rettie AE, McCune JS, et al. A marijuana-drug interaction primer: precipitants, pharmacology, and pharmacokinetics. Pharmacol Ther. 2019;201:25–38. https://doi.org/10.1016/j.pharmthera.2019.05.001.
103. Hillig KW, Mahlberg PG. A chemotaxonomic analysis of cannabinoid variation in cannabis (Cannabaceae). Am J Bot. 2004;91(6):966–75. https://doi.org/10.3732/ajb.91.6.966.
104. Welling M, Shapter T, Rose T, Liu L, Stanger R, King G. A belated green revolution for cannabis: virtual genetic resources for fast-track cultivar development. Front Plant Sci. 2016;7:1113. https://doi.org/10.3389/fpls.2016.01113.
105. Gonçalves J, Rosado T, Soares S, Simão AY, Caramelo D, Luís Â, et al. Cannabis and its secondary metabolites: their use as therapeutic drugs, toxicological aspects, and analytical determination. Medicines (Basel). 2019;6(1):31. https://doi.org/10.3390/medicines6010031.
106. ElSohly MA, Chandra S, Radwan M, Majumdar CG, Church JC. A comprehensive review of cannabis potency in the United States in the last decade. Biol Psychiatry Cogn Neurosci Neuroimaging. 2021;6(6):603–6. https://doi.org/10.1016/j.bpsc.2020.12.016.
107. Cerino P, Buonerba C, Cannazza G, D'Auria J, Ottoni E, Fulgione A, et al. A review of hemp as food and nutritional supplement. Cannabis Cannabinoid Res. 2021;6(1):19–27. https://doi.org/10.1089/can.2020.0001.
108. Fairbairn JW, Liebmann JA, Rowan MB. The stability of cannabis and its preparations on storage. J Pharm Pharmacol. 1976;28(1):1–7. https://doi.org/10.1111/j.2042-7158.1976.tb04014.x.
109. Martin BR, Mechoulam R, Razdan RK. Discovery and characterization of endogenous cannabinoids. Life Sci. 1999;65:573–95. https://doi.org/10.1016/s0024-3205(99)00281-7.
110. Ford BM, Tai S, Fantegrossi WE, Prather PL. Synthetic pot: not your grandfather's marijuana. Trends Pharmacol Sci. 2017;38(3):257–76. https://doi.org/10.1016/j.tips.2016.12.003.
111. Roque-Bravo R, Silva RS, Malheiro RF, Carmo H, Carvalho F, da Silva DD, et al. Synthetic cannabinoids: a pharmacological and toxicological overview. Annu Rev Pharmacol Toxicol. 2023;63:187–209. https://doi.org/10.1146/annurev-pharmtox-031122-113758.
112. Devane WA, Dysarz FA, Johnson MR, Melvin LS, Howlett AC. Determination and characterization of a cannabinoid receptor in rat brain. Mol Pharmacol. 1988;34(5):605–13. PMID: 2848184.
113. Devane WA, Hanus L, Breuer A, et al. Isolation and structure of a brain constituent that binds to the cannabinoid receptor. Science. 1992;258(5090):1946–9. https://doi.org/10.1126/science.1470919.
114. Zou S, Kumar U. Cannabinoid receptors and the endocannabinoid system: signaling and function in the central nervous system. Int J Mol Sci. 2018;19(3):833. https://doi.org/10.3390/ijms19030833.
115. Matsuda LA, Lolait SJ, Brownstein MJ, Young AC, Bonner TI. Structure of a cannabinoid receptorand functional expression of the cloned cDNA. Nature. 1990;346(6284):561–4. https://doi.org/10.1038/346561a0.
116. Liu QR, Pan CH, Hishimoto A, Li CY, Xi ZX, Llorente-Berzal A, et al. Species differences in cannabinoid receptor 2 (CNR2 gene): identification of novel human and rodent CB2 isoforms, differential tissue expression and regulation by cannabinoid receptor ligands. Genes Brain Behav. 2009;8(5):519–30. https://doi.org/10.1111/j.1601-183X.2009.00498.x.
117. Sugiura T, Kondo S, Sukagawa A, Nakane S, Shinoda A, Itoh K, et al. Arachidonoylgylcerol—a possible endogenous cannabinoid receptor-ligand in brain. Biochem BiophysRes Commun. 1995;215(1):89–97. https://doi.org/10.1006/bbrc.1995.2437.
118. Lu HC, Mackie K. Review of the endocannabinoid system. Biol Psychiatry Cogn Neurosci Neuroimaging. 2021;6(6):607–15. https://doi.org/10.1016/j.bpsc.2020.07.016.
119. Vinette B, Cote J, El-AKhas A, Mrad H, Chicoine G, Bilodear K. Routes of administration, reasons for use, and approved indications of medical cannabis in oncology: a scoping review. BMC Cancer. 2022;22(1):319. https://doi.org/10.1186/s12885-022-09378-7.

120. Subbaraman MS, Kerr WC. Cannabis use frequency, route of administration, and co-use with alcohol among older adults in Washington state. J Cannabis Res. 2021;3(1):17. https://doi.org/10.1186/s42238-021-00071-3.
121. Grotenhermen F. Pharmacokinetics and pharmacodynamics of cannabinoids. Clin Pharmacokinet. 2003;42(4):327–60. https://doi.org/10.2165/00003088-200342040-00003.
122. Lucas CJ, Galettis P, Schneider J. The pharmacokinetics and the pharmacodynamics of cannabinoids. Br J Clin Pharmacol. 2018;84(11):2477–82. https://doi.org/10.1111/bcp.13710.
123. Mahmoudinoodezh H, Teluktla SR, Bhangu SK, Bachari A, Cavalieri F, Mantri N. The transdermal delivery of therapeutic cannabinoids. Pharmaceutics. 2022;14(2):438. https://doi.org/10.3390/pharmaceutics14020438.
124. Klausner HA, Wilcox HG, Dingell JV. The use of zonal ultracentrifugation in the investigation of the binding of delta9-tetrahydrocannabinol by plasma lipoproteins. Drug Metab Dispos. 1975;3(4):314–9. PMID: 240663.
125. Child RB, Tallon MJ. Cannabidiol (CBD) Dosing: plasma pharmacokinetics and effects on accumulation in skeletal muscle, liver and adipose tissue. Nutrients. 2022;14(10):2101. https://doi.org/10.3390/nu14102101.
126. Bornheim LM, Lasker JM, Raucy JL. Human hepatic microsomal metabolism of delta 1-tetrahydrocannabinol. Drug Metab Dispos. 1992;20(2):241–6. PMID: 1352216.
127. Köguel CC, Loez-Pelayo H, Balcells-Olivdero MM, Colom J, Gual A. Psychoactive constituents of cannabis and their clinical implications: a systematic review. Adicciones. 2018;30(2):140–51. https://doi.org/10.20882/adicciones.858.
128. Ujváry I, Hanuš L. Human metabolites of cannabidiol: a review on their formation, biological activity, and relevance in therapy. Cannabis Cannabinoid Res. 2016;1(1):90–101. https://doi.org/10.1089/can.2015.0012.
129. Wall ME, Sadler BM, Brine D, Taylor H, Perez-Reyes M. Metabolism, disposition, and kinetics of delta-9-tetrahydrocannabinol in men and women. Clin Pharmacol Ther. 1983;34(3):352–63. https://doi.org/10.1038/clpt.1983.179.
130. Tagen M, Klumpers LE. Review of delta-8-tetrahydrocannabinol (delta(8) -THC): Comparative pharmacology with delta(9) -THC. Br J Pharmacol. 2022;179(15):3915–33. https://doi.org/10.1111/bph.15865.
131. van Hell HH, Bossong MG, Jager G, Kristo G, van Osch MJ, Zelaya F, et al. Evidence for involvement of the insula in the psychotropic effects of THC in humans: a double-blind, randomized pharmacological MRI study. Int J Neuropsychopharmacol. 2011;14(10):1377–88. https://doi.org/10.1017/S1461145711000526.
132. Morales P, Hurst DP, Reggio PH. Molecular targets of the Phytocannabinoids: a complex picture. ProgChem Org Nat Prod. 2017;103:103–31. https://doi.org/10.1007/978-3-319-45541-9_4.
133. Parker LA, Rock EM, Limebeer CL. Regulation of nausea and vomiting by cannabinoids. Br J Pharmacol. 2011;163(7):1411–22. https://doi.org/10.1111/j.1476-5381.2010.01176.x.
134. Finn DP, Haroutounian S, Hohmann AG, Krane E, Soliman N, Rice ASC. Cannabinoids, the endocannabinoid system, and pain: a review of preclinical studies. Pain. 2021;162:S5–S25. [PMID: 33729211]. https://doi.org/10.1097/j.pain.0000000000002268.
135. McDonagh MS, Morasc BJ, Wagner J, Ahmed AY, Fu R, Kansagara D, et al. Cannabis-based products for chronic pain: a systematic review. Ann Intern Med. 2022;175(8):1143–53. https://doi.org/10.7326/M21-4520.
136. Weltens N, Depoortere I, Tack J, Va Oudenhov L. Effect of acute Δ9-tetrahydrocannabinol administration on subjective and metabolic hormone responses to food stimuli and food intake in healthy humans: a randomized, placebo-controlled study. Am J Clin Nutr. 2019;109(4):1051–63. https://doi.org/10.1093/ajcn/nqz007.
137. Novack GD. Cannabinoids for treatment of glaucoma. Curr Opin Ophthalmol. 2016;27:146. https://doi.org/10.1097/ICU.0000000000000242.
138. Brown JD. Potential adverse drug events with Tetrahydrocannabinol (THC) due to drug-drug interactions. J Clin Med. 2020;9(4):919. https://doi.org/10.3390/jcm9040919.

139. Peng J, Fan M, An C, Ni F, Huang W, Luo J. A narrative review of molecular mechanism and therapeutic effect of cannabidiol (CBD). Basic Clin Pharmacol Toxicol. 2022;130(4):439–56. https://doi.org/10.1111/bcpt.13710.
140. Brown JD, Winterstein AG. Potential adverse drug events and drug-drug interactions with medical and consumer Cannabidiol (CBD) use. Clin Med. 2019;8(7):989. https://doi.org/10.3390/jcm8070989.
141. Echeverria-Villalobos M, Todeschini AB, Stoicea N, Fiorda-Diaz J, Weaver T, Bergese SD. Perioperative care of cannabis users: a comprehensive review of pharmacological and anesthetic considerations. J Clin Anesth. 2019;57:41–9. https://doi.org/10.1016/j.jclinane.2019.03.011.
142. Yoo HB, DiMuzio J, Filbey FM. Interaction of cannabis use and aging: from molecule to mind. J Dual Diagn. 2020;16(1):140–76. https://doi.org/10.1080/15504263.2019.166521.
143. Burggren AC, Siddarth P, Mahmood Z, London ED, Harrison TM, Merrill DA, et al. Subregional hippocampal thickness abnormalities in older adults with a history of heavy cannabis use. Cannabis Cannabinoid Res. 2018;3(1):242–51. https://doi.org/10.1089/can.2018.0035.
144. Orr JM, Paschall CJ, Banich MT. Recreational marijuana use impacts white matter integrity and subcortical (but not cortical) morphometry. Neuroimage Clin. 2016;12:47–56. https://doi.org/10.1016/j.nicl.2016.06.006.
145. Meier MH, Caspi A, Knodt R, Hall W, Ambler A, Harrington H, et al. Long-term cannabis use and cognitive reserves and hippocampal volume in midlife. Am J Psychiatry. 2022;179(5):362–74. https://doi.org/10.1176/appi.ajp.2021.21060664.
146. Miller LK, Devi LA. The highs and lows of cannabinoid receptor expression in disease: mechanisms and their therapeutic implications. Pharmacol Rev. 2011;63(3):461–70. https://doi.org/10.1124/pr.110.003491.
147. Di Marzo V. The endocannabinoid system: its general strategy of action, tools for its pharmacological manipulation and potential therapeutic exploitation. Pharmacol Res. 2009;60(2):77–84. https://doi.org/10.1016/j.phrs.2009.02.010.
148. Legare CA, Raup-Konsavage WM, Vrana KE. Therapeutic potential of cannabis, cannabidiol, and cannabinoid-based pharmaceuticals. Pharmacology. 2022;107(3–4):131–49. https://doi.org/10.1159/000521683.
149. https://www.fda.gov/news-events/public-health-focus/fda-and-cannabis-research-and-drug-approval-process.
150. Okusanya BO, Asaolu IO, Ehiri JE, Kimaru LJ, Okechukwu A, Rosales C. Medical cannabis for the reduction of opioid dosage in the treatment of non-cancer chronic pain: a systematic review. Syst Rev. 2020;9(1):167. https://doi.org/10.1186/s13643-020-01425-3.
151. Longo R, Oudshoorn A, Befus D. Cannabis for chronic pain: a rapid systematic review of randomized control trials. Pain Manag Nurs. 2021;22(2):141–9. https://doi.org/10.1016/j.pmn.2020.11.006.
152. Wong SSC, Chan WS, Cheung CW. Analgesic effects of cannabinoids for chronic non-cancer pain: a systematic review and meta-analysis with meta-regression. J Neuroimmune Pharmacol. 2020;15(4):801–29. https://doi.org/10.1007/s11481-020-09905-y.
153. Wolfe D, Corace K, Butler C, Rice D, Skidmore B, Patel Y, et al. Impacts of medical and non-medical cannabis on the health of older adults: findings from a scoping review of the literature. PLoS One. 2023;18(2):e0281826. https://doi.org/10.1371/journal.pone.0281826.
154. Pantoja-Ruiz C, Restrepo-Jimenez P, Castañeda-Cardona C, Ferreirós A, Rosselli D, Braz J. Cannabis and pain: a scoping review. Br J Anesthesiol. 2022;72(1):142–51. https://doi.org/10.1016/j.bjane.2021.06.018.
155. Ahmedzai S, Carlyle DL, Calder IT, Moran F. Anti-emetic efficacy and toxicity of nabilone, a synthetic cannabinoid, in lung cancer chemotherapy. Br J Cancer. 1983;48(5):657–63. https://doi.org/10.1038/bjc.1983.247.
156. Lane M, Vogel CL, Ferguson J, Krasnow S, Saiers JL, Hamm J, et al. Dronabinol and prochlorperazine in combination for treatment of cancer chemotherapy-induced nausea and vomiting. J Pain Symptom Manag. 1991;6(6):352–9. https://doi.org/10.1016/0885-3924(91)90026-z.

157. Meiri E, Jhangiani H, Vredenburgh JJ, Barbato LM, Carter FJ, Yang HM, et al. Efficacy of dronabinol alone and in combination with ondansetron versus ondansetron alone for delayed chemotherapy-induced nausea and vomiting. Curr Med Res Opin. 2007;23(3):533–43. https://doi.org/10.1185/030079907x167525.
158. Orr LE, McKernan JF, Bloome B. Antiemetic effect of tetrahydrocannabinol compared with placebo and prochlorperazine in chemotherapy-associated nausea and emesis. Arch Intern Med. 1980;140(11):1431–3. https://doi.org/10.1001/archinte.140.11.1431.
159. Chang AE, Shiling DJ, Stillman RC, Goldberg NH, Seipp CA, Barofsky I, et al. A prospective evaluation of delta-9-tetrahydrocannabinol as an antiemetic in patients receiving adriamycin and cytoxan chemotherapy. Cancer. 1981;47(7):1746–51. https://doi.org/10.1002/1097-0142(19810401)47:7<1746::aid-cncr2820470704>3.0.co;2-4.
160. Ungerleider JT, Andrysiak T, Fairbanks L, Goodnight J, Sarna G, Jamison K. Cannabis and cancer chemotherapy: a comparison of oral delta-9-THC and prochlorperazine. Cancer. 1982;50(4):636–45. https://doi.org/10.1002/1097-0142(19820815)50:4<636::aid-cncr2820500404>3.0.co;2-4.
161. Grimison P, Mersiades A, Kirby A, Lintzeris N, Morton R, Haber P, et al. Oral THC:CBD cannabis extract for refractory chemotherapy-induced nausea and vomiting: a randomised, placebo-controlled, phase II crossover trial. Ann Oncol. 2020;31(11):1553–60. https://doi.org/10.1016/j.annonc.2020.07.020.
162. Beal JE, Olson R, Lefkowitz L, Laubenstein L, Bellman P, Yangco B, et al. Long-term efficacy and safety of dronabinol for acquired immunodeficiency syndrome-associated anorexia. J Pain Symptom Manag. 1997;14(1):7–14. https://doi.org/10.1016/S0885-3924(97)00038-9.
163. Bedi G, Foltin RW, Gunderson EW, Rabkin J, Hart CL, Comer SD, et al. Efficacy and tolerability of high-dose dronabinol maintenance in HIV-positive marijuana smokers: a controlled laboratory study. Psychopharmacology. 2010;212(4):675–86. https://doi.org/10.1007/s00213-010-1995-4.
164. Timpone JG, Wright DJ, Li N, Egorin MJ, Enama ME, Mayers J, et al. The safety and pharmacokinetics of single-agent and combination therapy with megestrol acetate and dronabinol for the treatment of HIV wasting syndrome. The DATRI 004 Study Group. Division of AIDS Treatment Research Initiative. AIDS Res Hum Retroviruses. 1997;13(4):305–15. https://doi.org/10.1089/aid.1997.13.305.
165. Jatoi A, Windschitl HE, Loprinzi CL, Sloan JA, Dakhil SR, Mailliard JA, et al. Dronabinol versus megestrol acetate versus combination therapy for cancer-associated anorexia: a North Central Cancer Treatment Group study. Clin Oncol. 2002;20(2):567–73. https://doi.org/10.1200/JCO.2002.20.2.567.
166. Cannabis-In-Cachexia-Study-Group, Strasser F, Luftner D, Possinger K, Ernst G, Ruhstaller T, et al. Comparison of orally administered cannabis extract and delta-9-tetrahydrocannabinol in treating patients with cancer-related anorexia-cachexia syndrome: a multicenter, phase III, randomized, double-blind, placebo-controlled clinical trial from the Cannabis-In-Cachexia-Study-Group. J Clin Oncol. 2006;24(21):3394–400. https://doi.org/10.1200/JCO.2005.05.1847.
167. Nelson K, Walsh D, Deeter P, Sheehan F. A phase II study of delta-9-tetrahydrocannabinol for appetite stimulation in cancer-associated anorexia. J Palliat Care. 1994;10(1):14–8. PMID: 8035251.
168. Goodman S, Wadsworth E, Schauer G, Hammond D. Use and perceptions of cannabidiol products in Canada and in the United States. Cannabis Cannabinoid Res. 2022;7(3):355–64. https://doi.org/10.1089/can.2020.0093.
169. Spinella TC, Stewart SH, Naugler J, Yakovenko I, Barrett SP. Evaluating cannabidiol (CBD) expectancy effects on acute stress and anxiety in healthy adults: a randomized crossover study. Psychopharmacology. 2021;238(7):1965–77. https://doi.org/10.1007/s00213-021-05823-w.
170. Khan R, Naveed S, Mian N, Fida A, Raafey MA, Aedma KK. The therapeutic role of cannabidiol in mental health: a systematic review. J Cannabis Res. 2020;2(1):2. https://doi.org/10.1186/s42238-019-0012-y.

171. Gutkind S, Fink DS, Shmulewitz D, Stohl M, Hasin D. Psychosocial and health problems associated with alcohol use disorder and cannabis use disorder in U.S. adults. Drug Alcohol Depend. 2021;229(Pt B):109137. https://doi.org/10.1016/j.drugalcdep.2021.109137.
172. Hasin DS, Wall MM, Choi CJ, Alschuler DM, Malte C, Olfson M, et al. State cannabis legalization and cannabis use disorder in the US Veterans Health Administration, 2005 to 2019. JAMA Psychiatry. 2023;80(4):380–8. https://doi.org/10.1001/jamapsychiatry.2023.0019.
173. Mondal A, Dadana S, Parmar P, Mylavarapu M, Dong Q, Butt SR, et al. Association of cannabis use disorder with major adverse cardiac and cerebrovascular events in older non-tobacco users: a population-based analysis. Med Sci (Basel). 2024;12(1):13. https://doi.org/10.3390/medsci12010013.
174. Freeman TP, Craft S, Wilson J, Stylianou S, ElSohly M, Di Forti M, et al. Changes in delta-9-tetrahydrocannabinol (THC) and cannabidiol (CBD) concentrations in cannabis over time: systematic review and meta-analysis. Addiction. 2021;116(5):1000–10. https://doi.org/10.1111/add.15253.
175. Connor JP, Stjepanović D, Le Foll B, Hoch E, Budney AJ, Hall WD. Cannabis use and cannabis use disorder. Nat Rev Dis Primers. 2021;7(1):16. https://doi.org/10.1038/s41572-021-00247-4.
176. Benowitz NL, Hukkanen J, Jacob P 3rd. Nicotine chemistry, metabolism, kinetics and biomarkers. Handb Exp Pharmacol. 2009;192:29–60. https://doi.org/10.1007/978-3-540-69248-5_2.
177. Clarke E, Thompson K, Weaver S, Thompson J, O'Connell G. Snus: a compelling harm reduction alternative to cigarettes. Harm Reduct J. 2019;16(1):62. https://doi.org/10.1186/s12954-019-0335-1.DSM-5.
178. Hartmann-Boyce J, Chepkin SC, Ye W, Bullen C, Lancaster T. Nicotine replacement therapy versus control for smoking cessation. Cochrane Database Syst Rev. 2018;5(5):CD000146. https://doi.org/10.1002/14651858.CD000146.
179. Lu Y, Wang SS, Reynolds P, Chang ET, Ma H, Sullivan-Halley J, et al. Cigarette smoking, passive smoking, and non-Hodgkin lymphoma risk: evidence from the California Teachers Study. Am J Epidemiol. 2011;174(5):563–73. https://doi.org/10.1093/aje/kwr127.
180. Rastogi T, Girerd N, Lamiral Z, Bresso E, Bozec E, Boivin JM, et al. Impact of smoking on cardiovascular risk and premature ageing: findings from the STANISLAS cohort. Atherosclerosis. 2022;346:1–9. https://doi.org/10.1016/j.atherosclerosis.2022.02.017.
181. Chen D, Wu LT. Smoking cessation interventions for adults aged 50 or older: a systematic review and meta-analysis. Drug Alcohol Depend. 2015;154:14–24. https://doi.org/10.1016/j.drugalcdep.2015.06.004.
182. Hou W, Chen S, Zhu C, Gu Y, Zhu L, Zhou Z. Associations between smoke exposure and osteoporosis or osteopenia in a US NHANES population of elderly individuals. Front Endocrinol (Lausanne). 2023;14:1074574. https://doi.org/10.3389/fendo.2023.1074574.
183. Jha P, Ramasundarahettige C, Landsman V, Rostron B, Thun M, Anderson RN, et al. 21st-century hazards of smoking and benefits of cessation in the United States. N Engl J Med. 2013;368(4):341–50. https://doi.org/10.1056/NEJMsa1211128.
184. https://www.hhs.gov/sites/default/files/consequences-smoking-exec-summary.pdf.
185. Walters MS, De BP, Salit J, Buro-Auriemma LJ, Wilson T, Rogalski AM, et al. Smoking accelerates aging of the small airway epithelium. Respir Res. 2014;15(1):94. https://doi.org/10.1186/s12931-014-0094-1.
186. Huang Z, Sun S, Lee M, Maslov AY, Shi M, Waldman S, et al. Single-cell analysis of somatic mutations in human bronchial epithelial cells in relation to aging and smoking. J Nat Genet. 2022;54(4):492–8. https://doi.org/10.1038/s41588-022-01035-w.
187. Ren M, Lotfipour S, Leslie F. Unique effects of nicotine across the lifespan. Pharmacol Biochem Behav. 2022;214:173343. https://doi.org/10.1016/j.pbb.2022.173343.
188. 2020 Surgeon General' Report. https://www.hhs.gov/surgeongeneral/reports-and-publications/tobacco/2020-cessation-sgr-factsheet-key-findings/index.html.
189. Cornelius ME, Loretan CG, Jamal A, Lynn PCD, Mayer M, Alcantare IC, et al. Tobacco Product Use Among Adults – United States, 2021. MMWR Morb Mortal Wkly Rep. 2023;72(18):475–83. https://doi.org/10.15585/mmwr.mm7218a1.

190. Soloway SB. Naturally occurring insecticides. Environ Health Perspect. 1976;14:109–17. https://doi.org/10.1289/ehp.7614109.
191. https://pubchem.ncbi.nlm.nih.gov/compound/Nicotine.
192. Sansone L, Milani F, Fabrizi R, Belli M, Cristina M, Zaga V, et al. Nicotine: from discovery to biological effects. Int J Mol Sci. 2023;24(19):14570. https://doi.org/10.3390/ijms241914570.
193. Benowitz NL. Clinical pharmacology of inhaled drugs of abuse: implications in understanding nicotine dependence. NIDA Res Monogr. 1990;99:12–29. PMID: 2267009.
194. Tutka P, Mosiewicz J, Wielosz M. Pharmacokinetics and metabolism of nicotine. Pharmacol Rep. 2005;57(2):143–53. PMID: 15886412.
195. Benowitz NL, Porchet H, Sheiner L, Jacob P III. Nicotine absorption and cardiovascular effects with smokeless tobacco use: comparison with cigarettes and nicotine gum. Clin Pharmacol Ther. 1988;44(1):23–8. https://doi.org/10.1038/clpt.1988.107.
196. Lindsay RP, Tsoh JY, Sung HY, Max W. Secondhand smoke exposure and serum cotinine levels among current smokers in the USA. Tob Control. 2016;25(2):224–31. https://doi.org/10.1136/tobaccocontrol-2014-051782.
197. Kim J, Shim IK, Won SR, Ryu J, Lee J, Chung HM. Characterization of urinary cotinine concentrations among non-smoking adults in smoking and smoke-free homes in the Korean national environmental health survey (KoNEHS) cycle 3 (2015-2017). BMC Public Health. 2021;21(1):1324. https://doi.org/10.1186/s12889-021-11265-y.
198. Thomas CE, Wang R, Adams-Haduch J, Murphy SE, Ueland PM, Midttun Ø, et al. Urinary cotinine is as good a biomarker as serum cotinine for cigarette smoking exposure and lung cancer risk prediction. Cancer Epidemiol Biomarkers Prev. 2020;29(1):127–32. https://doi.org/10.1158/1055-9965.EPI-19-0653.
199. Molander L, Hansson A, Lunell E. Pharmacokinetics of nicotine in healthy elderly people. Clin Pharmacol Ther. 2001;69(1):57–65. PubMed: 11180039.
200. Wessler I, Kirkpatrick CJ. Acetylcholine beyond neurons: the non-neuronal cholinergic system in humans: non-neuronal cholinergic system in humans. Br J Pharmacol. 2008;154(8):1558–71. https://doi.org/10.1038/bjp.2008.185.
201. Alexander SP, Peters JA, Kelly E, Marrion NV, Faccenda E, Harding SD, et al. THE CONCISE GUIDE TO PHARMACOLOGY 2017/18: ligand-gated ion channels. Br J Pharmacol. 2017;174:S130–59. https://doi.org/10.1111/bph.13879.
202. Dani JA, Bertrand D. Nicotinic acetylcholine receptors and nicotinic cholinergic mechanisms of the central nervous system. Annu Rev Pharmacol Toxicol. 2007;47:699–729. https://doi.org/10.1146/annurev.pharmtox.47.120505.105214.
203. Valentine G, Sofuoglu M. Cognitive effects of nicotine: recent progress. Curr Neuropharmacol. 2018;16(4):403–14. https://doi.org/10.2174/1570159X15666171103152136.
204. Arastoo S, Haptonstall KP, Choroomi Y, Moheimani R, Nguyen K, Tran E, et al. Acute and chronic sympathomimetic effects of e-cigarette and tobacco cigarette smoking: role of nicotine and non-nicotine constituents. Am J Physiol Heart Circ Physiol. 2020;319(2):H262–H70. https://doi.org/10.1152/ajpheart.00192.2020.
205. Desai N, Burns L, Gong Y, Zhi K, Kumar A, Summers N, et al. An update on drug-drug interactions between antiretroviral therapies and drugs of abuse in HIV systems. J Expert Opin Drug Metab Toxicol. 2020;16(11):1005–18. https://doi.org/10.1080/17425255.2020.1814737.
206. Mdodo R, Frazier EL, Dube SR, Mattson CL, Sutton MY, Brooks JT, et al. Cigarette smoking prevalence among adults with HIV compared with the general adult population in the United States: cross-sectional surveys. Ann Intern Med. 2015;162(5):335–44. https://doi.org/10.7326/M14-0954.
207. Kyerematen GA, Morgan M, Warner G, Martin LF, Vesell ES. Metabolism of nicotine by hepatocytes. Biochem Pharmacol. 1990;40(8):1747–56. https://doi.org/10.1016/0006-2952(90)90351-k.
208. Madan A, Graham RA, Carroll KM, Mudra DR, Burton LA, Krueger LA, et al. Effects of prototypical microsomal enzyme inducers on cytochrome P450 expression in cultured human hepatocytes. Drug Metab Dispos. 2003;31(4):421–31. https://doi.org/10.1124/dmd.31.4.421.

209. Zhang W, Kilicarslan T, Tyndale RF, Sellers EM. Evaluation of methoxsalen, tranylcypromine, and tryptamine as specific and selective CYP2A6 inhibitors in vitro. Drug Metab Dispos. 2001;29(6):897–902. PMID: 11353760
210. Sellers EM, Kaplan HL, Tyndale RF. Inhibition of cytochrome P450 2A6 increases nicotine's oral bioavailability and decreases smoking. Clin Pharmacol Ther. 2000;68(1):35–43. https://doi.org/10.1067/mcp.2000.107651.
211. Benowitz NL, Jacob P 3rd. Effects of cigarette smoking and carbon monoxide on nicotine and cotinine metabolism. Clin Pharmacol Ther. 2000;67(6):653–9. https://doi.org/10.1067/mcp.2000.107086.
212. Zevin S, Benowitz NL. Drug interactions with tobacco smoking. An update. Clin Pharmacokinet. 1999;36(6):425–38. https://doi.org/10.2165/00003088-199936060-00004.
213. International Agency for Research on Cancer. IARC monographs on the evaluation of carcinogenic risks to humans. Lyon (France): IARC IARC; 1986.
214. International Agency for Research on Cancer. IARC monographs on the evaluation of carcinogenic risks to humans. Lyon (France): IARC; 2004.
215. https://www.fda.gov/tobacco-products/products-ingredients-components/chemicals-cigarettes-plant-product-puff.
216. Kier LD, Yamasaki E, Ames BN. Detection of mutagenic activity in cigarette smoke condensates. Proc Natl Acad Sci U S A. 1974;71(10):4159–63. https://doi.org/10.1073/pnas.71.10.4159.
217. Ambrose JA, Barua RS. The pathophysiology of cigarette smoking and cardiovascular disease: an update. J Am Coll Cardiol. 2004;43(10):1731–7. https://doi.org/10.1016/j.jacc.2003.12.047.
218. Ishida M, Sakai C, Kobayashi Y, Ishida TJ. Cigarette smoking and atherosclerotic cardiovascular disease. Atheroscler Thromb. 2024;31(3):189–200. https://doi.org/10.5551/jat.RV22015.
219. Dunbar A, Gotsis W, Frishman W. Second-hand tobacco smoke and cardiovascular disease risk: an epidemiological review. Cardiol Rev. 2013;21(2):94–100. https://doi.org/10.1097/CRD.0b013e31827362e4.
220. Huang X, Mu X, Deng L, Fu A, Pu E, Tang T, et al. The etiologic origins for chronic obstructive pulmonary disease. Int J Chron Obstruct Pulmon Dis. 2019;14:1139–58. https://doi.org/10.2147/COPD.S203215.
221. Kotlyarov S. The role of smoking in the mechanisms of development of chronic obstructive pulmonary disease and atherosclerosis. Int J Mol Sci. 2023;24(10):8725. https://doi.org/10.3390/ijms24108725.
222. Easter M, Bollenbecker S, Barnes JW, Krick S. Targeting aging pathways in chronic obstructive pulmonary disease. Int J Mol Sci. 2020;21(18):6924. https://doi.org/10.3390/ijms21186924.
223. Lugg ST, Scott A, Parekh D, Naidu B, Thickett DR. Cigarette smoke exposure and alveolar macrophages: mechanisms for lung disease. Thorax. 2022;77(1):94–101. https://doi.org/10.1136/thoraxjnl-2020-216296.
224. Zoli M, Picciotto MR. Nicotinic regulation of energy homeostasis. Nicotine Tob Res. 2012;14(11):1270–90. https://doi.org/10.1093/ntr/nts159.
225. Somm E. Nicotinic cholinergic signaling in adipose tissue and pancreatic islets biology: revisited function and therapeutic perspectives. Arch Immunol Ther Exp. 2014;62:87–101. https://doi.org/10.1007/s00005-013-0266-6.
226. Andersson K, Arner P. Systemic nicotine stimulates human adipose tissue lipolysis through local cholinergic and catecholaminergic receptors. Int J Obes Relat Metab Disord. 2001;25:1225–32. https://doi.org/10.1038/sj.ijo.0801654.
227. Maddatu J, Anderson-Baucum E, Evans-Molina C. Smoking and the risk of type 2 diabetes. Transl Res. 2017;184:101–7. https://doi.org/10.1016/j.trsl.2017.02.004.
228. Canoy D, Wareham N, Luben R, Welch A, Bingham S, Day N, et al. Cigarette smoking and fat distribution in 21,828 British men and women: a population-based study. Obes Res. 2005;13(8):1466–75. https://doi.org/10.1038/oby.2005.177.

229. Frati AC, Iniestra F, Ariza CR. Acute effect of cigarette smoking on glucose tolerance and other cardiovascular risk factors. Diabetes Care. 1996;19:112–8. https://doi.org/10.2337/diacare.19.2.112.
230. Targher G, Alberiche M, Zenere MB, Bonadonna RC, Muggeo M, Bonora E. Cigarette smoking and insulin resistance in patients with noninsulin-dependent diabetes mellitus. J Clin Endocrinol Metab. 1997;82:3619–24. https://doi.org/10.1210/jcem.82.11.4351.
231. Govind AP, Vezina P, Green WN. Nicotine-induced upregulation of nicotinic receptors: underlying mechanisms and relevance to nicotine addiction. Biochem Pharmacol. 2009;78(7):756–65. https://doi.org/10.1016/j.bcp.2009.06.011.
232. White WB. Smoking-related morbidity and mortality in the cardiovascular setting. Prev Cardiol. 2007;10(2 Suppl 1):1–4. https://doi.org/10.1111/j.1520-037x.2007.06050.x.
233. Wu AD, Lindson N, Hartmann-Boyce J, Wahedi A, Hajizadeh A, Theodoulou A, et al. Smoking cessation for secondary prevention of cardiovascular disease. Cochrane Database Syst Rev. 2022;8(8):CD014936. https://doi.org/10.1002/14651858.CD014936.pub2.
234. Okorare O, Evbayekha EO, Adabale OK, Daniel E, Ubokudum D, Olusiji SA, et al. Smoking cessation and benefits to cardiovascular health: a review of literature. Cureus. 2023;15(3):e35966. https://doi.org/10.7759/cureus.35966.
235. Yoo JE, Han K, Shin DW, Jung W, Kim D, Lee CM, et al. Effect of smoking reduction, cessation, and resumption on cancer risk: a nationwide cohort study. Cancer. 2022;128(11):2126–37. https://doi.org/10.1002/cncr.34172.
236. Florou AN, Gkiozos IC, Tsagouli SK, Souliotis KN, Syrigos KN. Clinical significance of smoking cessation in subjects with cancer: a 30-year review. Respir Care. 2014;59(12):1924–36. https://doi.org/10.4187/respcare.02559.
237. Tønnesen P. Smoking cessation and COPD. Eur Respir Rev. 2013;22(127):37–43. https://doi.org/10.1183/09059180.00007212.
238. Johnson GJ, Cosnes J, Mansfield JC. Review article: smoking cessation as primary therapy to modify the course of Crohn's disease. Aliment Pharmacol Ther. 2005;21(8):921–31. https://doi.org/10.1111/j.1365-2036.2005.02424.x.
239. Nides M. 2008. Update on pharmacologic options for smoking cessation treatment. Am J Med. 2008;121(4 Suppl 1):S20–31. https://doi.org/10.1016/j.amjmed.2008.01.016.
240. Fisher ML, Pauly JR, Froeliger B, Turner JR. Translational research in nicotine addiction. Cold Spring Harb Perspect Med. 2021;11(6):a039776. https://doi.org/10.1101/cshperspect.a039776.
241. Huecker MR, Smiley A, Saadabadi A. Bupropion StatPearls (internet) April 9, 2023. https://www.ncbi.nlm.nih.gov/books/NBK470212/.
242. Singh D, Saadabadi A. Varenicline StatPearls (internet) December 14, 2022. https://www.ncbi.nlm.nih.gov/books/NBK534846/.

Over-the-Counter Medications, Vitamins, Minerals, Biologicals, and Herbal Supplements

Abbreviations

AD	Alzheimer's Disease
ADAS-Cog	Alzheimer's Disease Assessment Scale-cognition
ADRs	Adverse drug reactions
AF	Atrial fibrillation
AG	American ginseng
ALA	Alpha linolenic acid
AMD	Age-related macular degeneration
AREDS	Age-Related Eye Disease Study
AREDS2	Follow-up to Age-Related Eye Disease Study
ASA	Acetylsalicylic acid, aspirin
CAC	Coronary artery calcium
COX1, COX2	Cyclooxygenase enzymes
CS	Chondroitin sulfate
CV	Cardiovascular
DHA	Docosahexaenoic acid
EPA	Eicosapentaenoic acid
FDA	Federal Drug Administration
g/dL	Grams per deciliter
GBE	*Gingko biloba* extract
GERD	Gastroesophageal reflux disease
GI	Gastrointestinal
GlcN	Glucosamine
GMP	Good Manufacturing Practice
GRASE	Generally recognized as safe and effective
H2RA	Histamine-2 receptor antagonists
Hb	Hemoglobin
ID	Iron deficiency

IDA	Iron deficiency anemia
IU	International units
KRG	Korean red ginseng
MCI	Mild cognitive impairment
mg/d	Milligrams/day
MI	Myocardial infarction
mmol/L	Millimoles per liter
MMSE	Mini mental state exam
MVM	Multivitamins/minerals
NDA	New drug application
ng/mL	Nanograms per milliliter
NHANES	National Health and Nutrition Examination Survey
nmol/L	Nanomoles per liter
NOAs	Non opioid analgesics
NSAIDs	Nonsteroidal antiinflammatory drugs
O3FAs	Omega-3 fatty acids
OA	Osteoarthritis
OTC	Over-the-counter
PHS II	Physicians' Health Study II
PIMs	Potentially inappropriate medications
PPIs	Proton pump inhibitors
PUD	Peptic ulcer disease
PUFA	Polyunsaturated fatty acids
RA	Rheumatoid arthritis
RCTs	Randomized clinical trials
RDA	Recommended daily allowance
ROS	Reactive oxygen species
SCN	Suprachiasmatic nucleus
SJW	St John's Wort
SKT	Syndrome-Kurztest
SSRIs	Selective serotonin reuptake inhibitors
T2DM	Type 2 Diabetes Mellitus

Introduction. Regulations The Food, Drug and Cosmetic Act of 1938 initiated the first attempt to distinguish between drugs requiring a prescription and those exempt and available for self-medication [1]. It was not until the Durham-Humphrey Amendment of 1951 that present-day distinction between prescription drugs and over-the-counter (OTC) drugs was clarified [2]. According to this amendment, drugs that are habit-forming, potentially toxic or may become unsafe if not properly supervised by a licensed practitioner must be obtained by a prescription and the drug must be labeled so. All others could be purchased without a prescription. Thus, two different pathways for positioning a drug on the market were established: new drug application (NDA) for prescription drugs and Over-the-Counter (OTC) Drug Review process (OTC drug monograph) process [3]. The latter was updated in 2020 [4]. Basically, sponsors of an OTC drug must obtain approval for an OTC monograph detailing "active ingredients, uses (indications), doses, routes of administration, labeling, and testing, under which an OTC drug in a given therapeutic category (e.g., sunscreen, antacid) is generally recognized as safe and effective (GRASE) for its intended use" [3] and the updated ancillary allows for additional oversight by both industry and the Federal Drug Administration (FDA) to "add, remove, or change a monograph" [3].

A dietary supplement is defined as a product supplementing the diet that contains any of the following components: vitamin, mineral, herb or botanical, amino acid, dietary substance that complements total food intake or concentrate, metabolite, extract or combination of the aforementioned [5]. A dietary supplement must be labeled as such and cannot contain an approved drug or biological. Dietary supplements marketed after 1994 are defined as "new dietary supplements."

Therefore, dietary supplements are not OTC drugs and are regulated loosely by the FDA [6]. The regulation covers the right to examine manufacturing facilities, handle complaints of adverse effects, and receive required notifications for new supplements not found in food. However, the FDA does not assess dietary supplements for safety or efficacy as required for a new drug prior to marketing. Essentially, *dietary supplements are regulated as a special category of foods*. Certain health claims are permitted as long as the supplement displays the FDA's disclaimer that the product has not been evaluated by the FDA and is not intended to diagnose, treat, cure or prevent disease. Thus, it is the manufacturer of the supplement that determines the quality and quantity of dietary supplements and is expected to follow the tenets of Good Manufacturing Practice (GMP) [7]. However, this loose regulation can neither assure safety nor efficacy [6].

The nonprescription availability of OTC medications, including analgesics, sleep and cold/allergy solution/tablets, gastrointestinal remedies, vitamins/minerals, food supplements and herbal remedies, allows individuals of all ages to self-medicate and to do so without the healthcare cost of seeing a physician or healthcare provider. Consequently, the OTC business from pharmacies, online sites and retail outlets in the USA registered 48 billion in sales in 2023 [8]. Ironically, it is especially lucrative in developed countries where there is an abundance of nutritious and fortified foods. The most popular dietary supplements in the USA are vitamin/mineral supplements, followed by vitamin D alone, then omega-3 fatty acids (O3FAs), calcium and vitamin B_{12} alone [9]. Although self-medication with OTC therapy allows for individual choice and reduced healthcare expenditure for the older adult with comorbidities, polypharmacy and age changes, it has a high potential for the creation of adverse drug reactions (ADRs) [10]. Additionally, many OTC remedies touting enhanced longevity or ameliorating effects of disease or age-related conditions have not been tested in randomized clinical trials (RCTs) and have unknown clinical validity.

Over-the-Counter Use of Medicinal Products. Prevalence The percentage of older adults who routinely use OTC medications/supplements and herbal remedies either alone or concurrently with prescription medications has been evaluated in a few studies. Two of the most quoted studies instituted home interviews of over 2000 multiethnic community dwellers, with an average age of 70–71 years, 5 years apart [11, 12]. In the 2005–2006 study, about 44% of this cohort used at least one OTC drug. This use declined to 37.7% 5 years later and the use of dietary supplements increased over this period from 51.8% to 63.7% [11, 12]. The use of at least one prescription drug increased from 84.1% to 87.7%. Significantly, there was an increased risk for serious ADRs with concurrent use of prescription drugs and OTC medications (in this case specifically dietary supplements) from 8.4% in 2005–2006 to 15.1% 5 years later [11, 12]. More recently (2020–2022) a survey of some 400 patients at a geriatric clinic, with an average age of 78.6 years, found that 15% experienced ADRs with concurrent use of prescription drugs and supplement use (primarily *Ginko biloba*, garlic and calcium). In this group, supplement and OTC drug use were 72.4% and 27.6% respectively [13].

This chapter will discuss the use of OTC drugs and dietary supplements (vitamins, minerals, herbal remedies) frequently used by the older adult. Among them are (1) sinus, cold and allergy drugs, (2) sleep remedies, (3) analgesics, (4) anti-inflammatory remedies, (5) relief aids for gastrointestinal diseases/conditions, (6) multivitamins and select minerals, (7) glucosamine/chondroitin, (8) omega-3 fatty acids, and (9) botanicals—*Gingko biloba*, ginseng, St. John's Wort, garlic. Summary information on the efficacy and safety of these products is presented in Table 9.1.

Over-the-Counter Drugs

SINUS, COLD, ALLERGY DRUGS A cross-sectional study that assessed brand names and generic OTC drugs marketed as nasal, sinus, cold and allergy remedies found considerable redundancy among 200 products and 14 brand names [14]. Eight different nonanalgesic drugs to include phenylephrine hydrochloride, dextromethorphan hydrobromide, pseudoephedrine hydrochloride, guaifenesin, chlorpheniramine maleate, brompheniramine maleate, diphenhydramine hydrochloride, and doxylamine succinate were identified as the active ingredient, with many OTC products containing several [2–4] of these drugs [14]. This study points out several important issues: (1) a brand name does not signify a single product, creating considerable confusion in drug selection and (2) over 75% of products have more than one drug, so the use of more than one OTC drug (common in severe illnesses) increases the risk of harm [14]. Furthermore, the efficacy of mucolytics (e.g., guaifenesin), antitussives (cough suppressants) (e.g., dextromethorphan), and decongestants (e.g., pseudoephedrine, phenylephrine) is suspect due to insufficient data of support, generally no better than placebo [15, 16].

The efficacy of OTC antihistamines in the treatment of colds (chlorpheniramine maleate, brompheniramine maleate, diphenhydramine hydrochloride, and doxylamine, first-generation antihistamines) has been evaluated in extensive reviews and deemed no better than placebo [17], no good evidence positive or negative [18] or effective only for the first 48 h of a cold [19]. Furthermore, antihistamine use for allergies or treatment of cold symptoms represents a serious problem for the older adult as discussed in Chap. 3. Beer's Criteria® (2023) [20] classified them as potentially inappropriate medications (PIMs) because they exert both sedative and anticholinergic effects (dry mouth, constipation, urinary retention, bowel obstruction, dilated pupils, blurred vision, increased heart rate, and decreased sweating) to which the older adult is particularly sensitive. Additionally, concurrent use of two or more drugs with anticholinergic actions promotes confusion, delirium and enhanced cognitive decline in addition to elevating the risk of accidents and falls [21–24].

On the other hand, second-generation antihistamines, available OTC, e.g., cetirizine, levocetirizine and loratadine are effective against allergic rhinitis (nasal mucous inflammation) and chronic urticaria (itchy rash) and are considered safe with less sedation than first-generation antihistamines [25]. However, there is no clinical trial data for the older adult. Whereas second-generation antihistamines are less sedating, they should not be used with those drugs on an extensive list of prescription medications A–Z [26]. If concurrent use is necessary, dose reduction of the OTC drug and/or the prescription drug is required.

SLEEP REMEDIES The sleep/wake cycle is one of many circadian activities regulated by the neural apparatus, the suprachiasmatic nucleus (SCN), located in the hypothalamus with extensive neuronal connections within the brain [27]. The hormone melatonin produced by the pineal gland contributes to the maintenance of our 24-h sleep/wake rhythm [28]. Light gathered through the eyes signals the SCN to inhibit melatonin production, producing the wake period of the day, but as the light declines, melatonin levels increase and activate sleep-promoting brain centers, thus acting as a nocturnal regulator of sleep [29].

With aging, the production and blood levels of melatonin gradually decline to fairly low amounts [30, 31]. This change is proposed as an explanation for insomnia, generally defined as having "difficulty either falling or staying asleep that is accompanied by daytime impairments to include fatigue, impaired memory and irritability" [32]. The use of OTC sleep remedies among the older adult with insomnia varies between 18% to approximately 36% [33, 34].

Melatonin. Efficacy Trials Therefore, replacement with exogenous melatonin, a popular OTC dietary supplement, should improve the perceived quality/quantity of sleep and, in fact, most RCTs show an improvement in some aspects of sleep with OTC melatonin products. Melatonin products are classified as dietary supplements, not OTC drugs, but are discussed here because of their physiological importance to sleep and sleep disturbances.

A scoping review of 17 RCTs with the older adult with and without comorbidities reported positive effects (15 out of 17 studies) on sleep with the use of extended or prolonged-release melatonin products as assessed with validated questionnaires before and after treatment. Most studies were small (<100 participants), ranging from 2 weeks to 1 year [29]. Of interest are the two studies that found melatonin to be ineffective with 4 weeks [35] and 2 months of use [36]. The latter used actigraphy, an external sensor that measures motor activity and provides an objective measure of sleep [36]. One small study of 80 patients with mild to moderate Alzheimer's Disease (AD) reported that prolonged release of melatonin improved cognitive function as well as sleep parameters over a 24-week period [37], although a larger study of 244 AD patients treated for 2 months with slow release melatonin showed no efficacy on "total sleep time, sleep efficiency, wake-time after sleep onset" [36].

Melatonin OTC products isolated from animals or microorganisms or chemically synthesized [38] and considered dietary supplements by the FDA are regulated differently than OTC drugs as noted above. Immediate-acting preparations have less sleep-inducing qualities [39] unlike the prolonged-release melatonin products discussed above, which are taken 1–2 h before bedtime. One study examined the pharmacokinetics of low (0.4 mg) and high dose (4 mg) "surge-sustained" preparations with 25% immediate release and 75% controlled release to mimic endogenous melatonin release in a small group of older adults experiencing insomnia [40]. Blood samples were collected before and on day 42 of treatment. Interestingly, plasma levels of both preparations were significantly elevated (seven-fold for low dose and 65-fold for high dose) above endogenous levels throughout the circadian cycle [40]. Serum levels of melatonin in the high-dose group postwaking hours exceeded endogenous levels (>50 pg/m verses 3–9 pg/mL), which may contribute to daytime drowsiness and increased risk of falls [40].

Melatonin. Pharmacokinetics Melatonin is metabolized by the liver and excreted by the kidneys [41] and according to in vitro hepatic culture assays, has no drug interactions except with CYP1A2 inhibitor, 5-methoxypsoralen (used in the treatment of skin diseases) [42]. However, although not studied, inducers of CYP1A2, e.g., rifampicin (antimicrobial) and omeprazole (proton pump inhibitor, PPI), if used concurrently with melatonin, may enhance its metabolism and negate its potential efficacy (see Chap. 3). Additionally, many prescription drugs are metabolized by CYP1A2, e.g., fluvoxamine (antidepressant), olanzapine (antipsychotic), naproxen (NSAID), propranolol (antihypertensive) and melatonin could compete with them and increase the risk for toxicity (Chap. 3).

Other Sleep Aids In addition to melatonin, there exist over 200 OTC drugs promoting sleep benefits and over half contain diphenhydramine and doxylamine, drugs with an avoidance recommendation for the older adult by the Beers Criteria® (2023) [20]. This is because these two drugs are first-generation antihistamines with all the issues discussed above. Unfortunately, many older adults use them to improve sleep quality/quantity and most are unaware of their potential harm. In a sample of 169 survey participants, 65 years and older, 59% used OTC sleeping products containing diphenhydramine and doxylamine within the last 30 days [43]. These drugs were marketed separately as sleep aids, e.g., Zzzzquil or in combination with an analgesic, e.g., Tylenol PM. Another product of concern is the highly marketed *Relaxium®*, for which there have been no clinical trials. *Relaxium®* contains 9 ingredients, 5 of which are herbal extracts plus magnesium, the amino acid, L-tryptophan, gamma-amino butyric acid and melatonin (5 mg). The interaction of these components and long-term safety are unknown. To minimize potentially harmful self-medication with sleep remedies containing undesired components, e.g., diphenhydramine and doxylamine or unknown components, requisite counseling with the pharmacist is a proposed intervention that has had success in other countries [43] and suggested for use here [33].

> Alert: There are over 200 OTC drugs that promote sleep and over ½ contain diphenhydramine and doxylamine, which are contraindicated in older adults.

ANALGESICS OTC pain-killers are termed analgesics or more specifically non-opioid analgesics (NOAs). Members of this group include aspirin (acetylsalicylic acid, ASA), ibuprofen, naproxen, acetaminophen (paracetamol), diclofenac and caffeine. Exactly how these drugs reduce pain is incompletely understood, but most of them inhibit one or both cyclo-oxygenase enzymes (COX1, COX2) to block the production of detrimental lipid mediators termed prostaglandins and thromboxane 2 [44, 45].

Generally, NOAs are used to relieve acute onset, short duration pain, for example, as with the removal of a tooth, other dental pain or after a soft tissue injury such as a strain or sprain. The efficacy of "21 different OTC analgesic drugs, doses, and formulations" was evaluated using information from 10 Cochrane reviews [46]. The summarized data indicated that efficacy ranged from 11% to 70% (that is OTC NOAs work in 1 out of 10 to 7 out of 10 patients) in reducing pain by 50% over a period of 6 h. Thus, the most efficacious OTC NOA was the combination of ibuprofen (400 mg) plus acetaminophen (1000 mg), followed by rapid-acting formulations of ibuprofen (200 and 400 mg), ibuprofen (200 mg) plus caffeine (100 mg), diclofenac potassium (50 mg) and acetaminophen and aspirin [46]. The authors note that taking NOAs with food slows absorption and delays the onset of pain relief. Adverse effects in this analysis were no different than placebo except for aspirin at 1000 mg dose (headache, nausea and dizziness) [46]. However, gastrointestinal adverse events may range from 37% for diclofenac, 7.2% for ibuprofen and 7.6% for acetaminophen [47]. Serious GI events (bleeding, ulcers) are rare when NOAs are taken correctly [47]. Use of higher than recommended doses or use for longer periods of time may cause liver toxicity and GI bleeding. In 2010, the FDA required that all OTC oral analgesics, antipyretics, and anti-rheumatic drugs carry a label warning consumers of this potential for adverse effects and to use these OTC drugs strictly as directed [48].

Although NOAs are the most commonly used OTC preparation among the older adult [49] with a preference for acetaminophen, aspirin and ibuprofen [50], the majority of RCTs included young adults, with an average age of 35–45 years. One meta-analysis and systemic review of RCTs with individuals 18–65 concluded that a 250 mg dose of aspirin was safe and effective in relieving the pain of a headache, tooth ache and cold [51]. Adverse event rates at 0–5.9% and mild-moderate dose-related dyspepsia (indigestion, GI pain) were noted [51]. However, the Beers Criteria® (2023) advises avoidance of aspirin and nonsteroidal anti-inflammatory drugs (NSAIDs) (the same drugs as NOAs) in the older adult with a history of gastric or duodenal ulcers since these drugs can antagonize former ulcers and create new ones [20].

Anti-inflammatory Drugs Because many of the NOAs (ibuprofen, naproxen, aspirin, diclofenac) inhibit one or both cyclooxygenases that produce inflammatory-inducing/promoting prostaglandins, they are also used to suppress inflammation in conditions such as rheumatoid arthritis (RA) and osteoarthritis (OA), the latter of which affects most older adults to some degree [52]. Thus, *NSAIDS are widely used by the older adult* [53].

Nonsteroidal Anti-inflammatory Drugs. Efficacy and Harm The anti-inflammatory effects of NSAIDs come with several serious adverse effects that include gastrointestinal (GI) ulcers/bleeding, serious cardiovascular (CV) adverse effects and nephrotoxicity evident with chronic use and high doses [54]. Efficacy and adverse effects stem from the inhibition of COX enzymes in that NSAID inhibition of COX2 suppresses inflammation but inhibits platelet function while NSAID inhibition of COX1 removes protective effects on the GI mucosa and kidneys and inhibits platelet aggregation, hence promoting bleeding and aggravation of kidney function [54, 55]. Prescription drugs originally included the selective COX2 inhibitors (rofecoxib and valdecoxib) that minimized GI bleeding but also elevated the risk for myocardial infarctions and were subsequently taken off the market [56]. However, nonselective COX inhibitors, such as OTC NSAIDs, also carry the risk of CV adverse effects and must be used with caution [55, 57]. An association between NSAID use and congestive heart failure (CHF) was observed in "matched case-control study of the relationship between recent use of NSAIDs and hospitalization with CHF" [58]. It was concluded that NSAIDs were responsible for 19% of hospital admissions with CHF [58].

Regarding nephrotoxicity, the Beers Criteria® [20] advises against the use of NSAIDs due to this risk. In a study of over 10,000 community-dwelling older adults followed for nearly 3 years, high-dose use of NSAID increased the risk for chronic kidney disease [59]. To minimize the risk of NSAID-induced GI ulcers, ibuprofen-phosphatidylcholine combination [60] and ibuprofen/famotidine [61] have been evaluated for GI ulcer protection in the older adult with OA or RA. Endoscopic results in both studies found gastroprotective effects with these products compared to ibuprofen alone [60, 61]. Famotidine is a histamine H2 receptor antagonist that may cause diarrhea, constipation, fatigue, and drowsiness [62].

NSAIDs. Drug-Drug Interactions The number of potential drug-drug interactions is high in the older population, where polypharmacy is common and where the prevalence of adverse effects with two or more drugs ranges from 26% [63, 64] to 85% [65], depending on the population and drug combinations. Concurrent use of

NSAIDs with a wide range of prescription medications leads to unwanted drug-drug interactions [54]. NSAIDs not only change the hepatic metabolism of prescription drugs (see Chap. 3) but can act to alter other aspects of PK and/or PD [54]. For example, simultaneous use of NSAIDs and aspirin and an antiplatelet drug leads to increased bleeding; antihypertensive drugs (angiotensin-converting enzyme inhibitors, angiotensin receptor blockers, beta-blockers, calcium channel blockers, diuretics) are less bioavailable in the presence of NSAIDs resulting in elevated blood pressure; NSAIDs plus warfarin, anticoagulants, corticosteroids or selective serotonin reuptake inhibitors lead to increase in GI bleeding; blood levels of digitalis glycosides or methotrexate increase with concurrent use of NSAIDs resulting in toxicities [54].

OTC REMEDIES FOR GASTROINTESTINAL DISEASES/ CONDITIONS *Gastroesophageal reflux disease (GERD) is considered the most common GI disease of the older person* [66]. Focused treatment is essential because although symptoms (regurgitation, heart burn) may be mild, complications (esophageal damage, atypical chest pain, throat and lung issues including chronic cough and pulmonary aspiration) in this age group may be severe [66, 67]. Another GI disease, peptic ulcer disease (PUD), exhibits symptoms similar to GERD and it is imperative to distinguish between them [67]. Prior to pharmacotherapy, lifestyle and dietary changes (weight loss, head-toe elevation for sleep, and cessation of tobacco, alcohol, caffeine, chocolate, and spicy foods) must be implemented [67].

Proton Pump Inhibitors Proton pump inhibitors (PPIs) act to decrease gastric acid production, which is the goal of GERD and PUD treatment, and are widely used [68]. Available OTC PPIs are omeprazole, esomaprazole and lansoprazole. Other treatment choices include the less potent antacids and histamine-2 receptor antagonists (H2RA) (famotidine, cimetidine) [67]. The preferred maintenance therapy is PPIs but efficacy onset requires 4–5 days of therapy [69]. Tolerance develops with H2Ras; hence; their use is preferred as an adjunct only, possibly at night. Antacids (e.g., aluminum hydroxide, calcium carbonate, sodium bicarbonate) bring only very short-term relief (minutes to an hour) and, therefore, are not preferred to treat GERDs or PUDs [67].

Proton Pump Inhibitors. Adverse Reactions Prolonged use of PPIs may lead to gastric changes (reactive elevation of the hormone gastrin and low or absent hydrochloride production) known as preconditions for gastric cancer [70]. Additionally, long-term use may affect calcium absorption and promote osteoporosis [70]. The Beers Criteria® also warns of the risk of pneumonia and *Clostridiun difficile* infections [20]. Results of PK/PD studies suggest that PPIs have the potential to interact with antiplatelet drugs and thus precipitate an adverse CV event, but clinical data does not support this concern [71]. H2RA use is considered inappropriate in patients with delirium [20]. Eliminated by the kidney, H2RAs require a dose adjustment in individuals with reduced kidney function [67].

Peptic Ulcer Therapy Recommendations for the treatment of PUD are to first identify the causative agent. The majority of gastric and intestinal ulcers are caused by *Helicobacter pylori* infection or inappropriate NSAID use [67]. With identification of the bacterial infection, one effective therapy includes antibiotics (clarithromycin plus amoxicillin or metronidazole) along with a PPI [72].

CONSTIPATION Constipation is a common condition in the older population that affects both health and quality of life. *Constipation is "a symptom-based disorder defined as unsatisfactory defecation and is characterized by infrequent stools, difficult stool passage, or both"* [73].

Constipation. Prevalence The global prevalence of chronic constipation is noted at 18.9% [74]. Many factors such as sedentary lifestyle, comorbidities (cardiovascular, metabolic, neurologic), polypharmacy (analgesics, calcium channel blockers, antipsychotics and others), age changes in colonic motility, sensitivity reduction in the rectum, malnutrition and abdominal and pelvic reduced muscle strength contribute to chronic constipation [75, 76]. There is a need to manage chronic constipation to not only improve quality of life but also to prevent anorectal complications (pain, fissures, hemorrhoids, bleeding) [76].

Constipation. OTC Therapy *Management of chronic constipation involves changes in lifestyle choices*, alteration of medications and use of laxatives. Lifestyle choices favor adding fiber to the diet, beginning low (5 g) and initiating a physical exercise program. Both are effective with moderate constipation but not with severe constipation [76]. All constipating-inducing drugs (e.g., opiates) should be stopped appropriately. The drug selection for the treatment of chronic constipation are numerous and include laxatives categorized as bulk-forming agents, stool softeners, osmotics, stimulants, suppositories/enemas, and prescription drugs such as prucalopride, linaclotide and lubiprostone [76, 77]. All but the prescription drugs are available OTC and are widely used as self-medication by the older adult [77].

Bulk-forming agents such as psyllium, calcium polycarbophil and methylcellulose are fiber preparations that absorb water to create stool bulk. The few studies to date show a benefit of fiber over placebo, particularly the use of soluble fiber (psyllium) [78]. Adverse events (bloating, flatulence, cramping) are evident with insoluble fiber, which requires a gradual introduction [78]. Stool softeners, docusate sodium and docusate calcium, are surfactants that change the tension of water and lipids on the stool surface, facilitating the uptake of water and thus softening the stool. Despite their wide use, numerous reviews and assessments of RCTs have found no efficacy [79]. Osmotics (e.g., Miralax), comprised of insoluble sugars (lactulose) or polyethylene glycol preparations, act by attracting water and electrolytes into the lower intestine, softening the stool and enhancing colonic motility [80]. Osmotics are considered safe and efficacious in controlling chronic constipation in the older adult but compositions with added sodium and potassium are of concern as they may disrupt electrolyte balance [76, 78]. Bisacodyl (e.g., Dulcolax®), sodium picosulfate and senna are stimulant laxatives that enhance intestinal muscle function and improve bowel motility. There is little data on safety and efficacy in the older adult, and since these preparations may contain sodium and/or magnesium, the need to start at the lowest possible dose after assessment of kidney function is important [76]. Water-based suppositories and enemas rather than potassium-based preparations (again with concern for electrolyte balance) are useful in the older adult who may have a disability [81].

Constipation. Prescription Therapy Among the prescription drugs of current use are prucalopride, a 5-hydroxytryptamine 4 receptor agonist; linaclotide, an agonist of the guanylate cyclase-C receptor; and lubiprostone, a chloride channel type-2 agonists. Prucalopride has been extensively studied. In cases where the aforementioned therapies of osmotics, stimulants and others have failed, prucalopride, as assessed by a meta-analysis of 16 RCTs (mostly European studies), is the drug of choice to treat chronic constipation as it is considered safe and effective [82]. The FDA approved prucalopride in 2018 for the treatment of chronic idiopathic constipation [83]. Common adverse effects include headache, nausea, abdominal pain and diarrhea [83]. It is excreted mostly by the kidneys [84]. Linaclotide and lubiprostone are considered pro-secretory agents, and both are considered efficacious and safe [77, 78]. Diarrhea is the main adverse effect of linaclotide, and diarrhea and nausea occur with lubiprostone [77]. Lubiprostone and linaclotide are poorly absorbed and thus are metabolized either in the stomach and middle intestine as is lubiprostone [85] or degraded in the intestine as is linaclotide [86].

Vitamins and Minerals—Dietary Supplements

Multivitamin/Mineral Multivitamins/minerals (MVM) are the most popular dietary supplements used among all ages but their use is highest in those 50 years and older [9, 87]. The main reason driving the use of MVM is the perception that these supplements improve and promote health, especially heart, bones, joints and eye health, prevent various diseases such as CV, cancer, and age-related macular degeneration [88, 89] and additionally moderate age-related functional loss [90].

Multivitamin/Mineral Efficacy. Cardiovascular Disease Clinical findings from individual trials and meta-analyses are clear that *MVM use does not protect against heart disease* but may offer a small benefit regarding cancer, although this result is inconsistent [91–94]. Results of the Physicians' Health Study II (PHS II), an RCT of more than 14 thousand male physicians (average age at the start was 64 years) who took MVM (Centrum Silver®) for more than a decade, found that MVM did not prevent CV disease (myocardial infarction (MI), stroke or CV mortality) [91]. These findings were reinforced with additional systematic reviews and meta-analyses of RCTs and prospective cohort studies of MVM use and CV events that showed chronic use of MVM provided no benefit in preventing CV disease and death [92, 93]. In a recent large-scale RCT (Cocoa Supplement and Multivitamin

Outcomes Study (COSMOS)) of men 60 years and older and women 65 years and older, daily MVM use for over 3.5 years had no preventive effect on CV disease [94].

Multivitamin and Mineral Efficacy. Cancer However, this same study examined the incidence of cancers and found no effect of MVM on the incidence of total invasive cancers but did find a significant reduction in lung cancer but not breast, colorectal, prostate or melanoma [94]. The PHS II reported an 8% decrease in total cancers with MVM use [89]. O'Connor et al. [93], in a large systematic review, noted that MVM use may produce a small decrease in risk of cancer but considered the data suboptimal. Earlier findings from the PHS I (male physicians 40–85 years at study start) reported that long-term use (12 years) of beta-carotene (provitamin A, 50 mg every other day) had no protective effects on the incidence of cancers [95]. Results of the PHS II studied the effect of specific vitamins, E (400 IU synthetic α-tocopherol) or C (500 mg synthetic ascorbic acid) use in male physicians and found that neither protected against prostate or any other cancer [96]. The large prospective NIH-AARP Diet and Health Study cohort with 11 years of follow-up reported that daily multivitamin use (all types, e.g., one-a-day, stress tabs, therapeutic type) had no preventive effect on 4 serious and fatal upper GI cancers (esophageal squamous cell carcinoma, esophageal adenocarcinoma, gastric cardia adenocarcinoma, or gastric noncardia adenocarcinoma cancer) [97]. The use of a single vitamin/mineral (vitamin C, iron) was associated with a lower risk of one cancer and a higher risk for another [97]. Additionally, there is evidence, albeit weak, that vitamins exert adverse effects: vitamin A contributes to hip fractures, vitamin E contributes to hemorrhage stroke and calcium contributes to kidney stones [93].

Multivitamin/Mineral Efficacy. Age-Related Macular Degeneration The use of some vitamins may have efficacy in slowing the progression of age-related macular degeneration (AMD), a deteriorative condition of the eye (sight loss in the central region of the retina) purportedly facilitated by free radicals induced by light [98]. Results of 8 years of vitamin E or C every other day reported no benefit from these vitamins on the prevention of AMD [99]. In contrast, a review of 26 RCTs, including over 11,000 participants, 65–75 years of age, that evaluated the use of MVM on the progression of early and intermediary AMD observed that the use of antioxidant vitamins (vitamin C, E, beta-carotene) and zinc slowed progression to late AMD [100]. This review included two USA RCTs, the Age-Related Eye Disease Study (AREDS) and a follow-on study, AREDS2. *Interestingly, the currently recommended OTC ocular supplements (vitamin C 500 mg, vitamin E 500 IU, copper 2 mg, zinc 80 mg, lutein 10 mg, zeaxanthin 2 mg) by the ARDS2 exceed the Food and Drug Administration's guidelines for these substances* [101, 102]. Beta-carotene, in the original OTC ocular supplement, was subsequently omitted due to the risk of lung cancer in current and former smokers [103, 104]. Another concern is that the concurrent use of ocular ARDS2-recommended supplements with general MVM supplements may achieve harmful levels of vitamins/minerals in older adults [101].

Multivitamin/Mineral Efficacy. Osteoporosis Regarding bone health and the prevention of fractures, the literature is mixed. Vitamin D is an important player in maintaining bone density and, hence, optimizing bone strength to prevent breakage from a fall. However, the body receives vitamin D from many sources such as sunshine-dependent synthesis in the skin and kidney, from a number of foods (tofu, seafood) and with consumption of fortified cereals and juices. A recent review [105] published a consensus statement that, after reviewing the best studies to date, found that *with the exception of house-bound or nursing home residents, the older adult receives a sufficient amount of vitamin D from diverse sources mentioned above and hence does not need vitamin D supplements.* However, if in doubt, a simple blood test can determine whether the vitamin D level is adequate (established range 30–50 nmol/L; 12–20 ng/mL). Furthermore, high amounts of vitamin D (60,000 IU) in the older adult for 5 years elevated fracture risk [106].

Multivitamin/Mineral Efficacy. Cognition Whether MVM use improves mental acuity in older adults is controversial. Two studies [107, 108] examined the effect of daily use of a commercially available MVM. The first of the two, a large 6000 male participants (PHS II), measured cognitive function with validated cognitive tests 4 times over a 12-year period by phone and found no effect of supplements on cognitive test scores [107]. The second study (COMOS-mind) was somewhat smaller (~2000 participants), 73 years of age, included both men and women and assessed cognitive function annually over a 3-year period, also by phone. This study concluded that global cognitive, episodic memory, and executive function scores were improved with supplementation and those with a history of CV disease benefited the most [108]. There was a significant "practice" effect at 3 years compared to the baseline for episodic memory but not for executive function [108]. Additionally, results of the COSMOS-Web ancillary study (similar to COSMOS-mind but separate) assessed cognition with a battery of internet-based computerized cognitive tests. The use of Centrum Silver® daily for 3 years in over 3000 participants, with an average age of 71 years, improved immediate recall above the practice effect but not memory retention, executive function, or novel object recognition [109].

Smaller and shorter duration studies that used computerized tests found conceptual recognition memory improved within 8 weeks in men (50–74 years of age) with sedentary life style taking MVM plus herbal supplements (Swisse Men's Ultivite®) [110]. Similarly, a small group of older women with complaints of memory loss tested with a computerized battery of cognitive tests after 16 weeks of MVM (Swisse Women's 50+ Ultivite®) showed improvement in "speed of response on a measure of spatial working memory" [111]. One additional study using the above men's MVM and women's MVM for small groups of men and women (55–65 years), respectively, for 16 weeks observed no effect on various computerized tests [112], although, in all three preceding studies, blood levels of B_6 and B_{12} were elevated with MVM use. It appears that *MVM use may benefit those with deficiencies in cognition* [112]. However, how well improvement on a cognitive test score translates to the activities of daily living is unknown.

Until MVM use is definitively demonstrated to benefit a decline in cognition, onset of cancers and prevent the progression of AMD, the *only scientifically convincing reason for taking MVM is to treat a known vitamin/mineral deficiency arising from disease, frailty, chemotherapy or an incredibly poor diet* [113]. The Food and Nutrition Board of the National Research Council determines the recommended dietary allowance (RDA) of essential nutrients, including vitamins and minerals [114]. This board defines RDAs as "the levels of intake of essential nutrients that, on the basis of scientific knowledge, are judged by the Food and Nutrition Board to be adequate to meet the known nutrient needs of practically all healthy persons." They also indicate that consumption of a varied diet ("variety of foods from diverse food groups") achieves the RDA for vitamins and minerals for most adults. In addition, the availability of fortified foods further assures attainment of the RDA. Nutritional deficiencies are defined as "intake of nutrients that is lower than the estimated average requirement" [113]. Nutritional deficiencies are likely in situations of poor appetite due to medications, frailty syndromes and metabolic diseases, and disorders of limited nutrient absorption. Symptoms and low blood concentrations of vitamins and minerals alert the physician to a possible deficiency. Uncorrected vitamin/mineral deficiencies definitely lead to serious debilitating conditions such as goiter (iodine), rickets (and osteomalacia) (vitamin D), beriberi (thiamine, B_1), pellagra (niacin, B_3), and pernicious anemia (B_{12}). Correcting vitamin/mineral deficiencies under physician supervision is necessary.

Calcium Supplements. Age-Related Bone Changes Daily use of calcium supplements with or without added vitamin D is widespread among middle-aged and postmenopausal women and continues on into later years. As of 2022, this activity supports a 3.8 billion dollar industry that is projected to double in 2023 [115].

Beginning in the 1980s, with very little human data, the medical and pharmaceutical industry promoted the consumption of calcium supplements for optimal bone health based on studies of calcium balance, not bone density or fracture risk. Support for calcium supplements and reduced fracture risk came from the original study that evaluated calcium supplements plus vitamin D and fractures in frail older women who resided in a nursing home and who were also severely vitamin D deficient [116]. Currently, this study group is considered to have had osteomalacia and is not representative of community-dwelling older adults [117]. Therefore, the early recommendations are indeed questionable.

It is known that both men and women lose bone calcium with age, with greater loss in women than men due to the serious decline in estrogen production (bone-forming hormone) with menopause, and lesser lifetime muscle mass with reduced physical activity [118, 119]. This loss largely impacts women because their bone mass is initially smaller than in men, and the menopause-related loss is greater than in men, elevating the lifetime risk of fractures [120]. Whereas the calcium-deficient individual benefits from calcium plus vitamin D supplements in the treatment of serious bone loss disease (osteoporosis, osteomalacia) with its very high risk of fractures as with the Chapuy et al. [116] study, individuals without calcium deficiency and no bone disease were similarly assumed to benefit from calcium supplements, purported to create stronger bones, and hence fewer fractures.

Blood calcium levels are tightly regulated by two hormones, the parathyroid hormone and calcitonin. It has been shown that consumption of a calcium supplement decreases the production and secretion of the parathyroid hormone and reduces biomarkers of bone resorption and transiently increases bone mineral density (~0.5–1%) but has no long-term cumulative effect [117]. *Ingestion of excess calcium (via supplements) does not, in the long run, benefit bone density* because of the tight homeostatic regulation of blood calcium, essential for optimal function of the nervous and CV systems [121].

Calcium Supplements. Current Use Recommendations The data from several large systematic reviews and meta-analyses of RCTs conclude that *calcium supplements do not strengthen bones or reduce the risk of fractures* [122, 123]. Zhao et al. [123] analyzed 33 RCTs that included the older adult of both genders in most of the trials. Trial size ranged from 50 to over 2000 participants consuming calcium (0.48–1.6 g/d), calcium plus vitamin D (0.5 g/d + 700 IU vitamin D to 1.2 g/d + 4000 IU vitamin D) or vitamin D alone (400–4000 IU/d) compared to placebo or no treatment for 4 months to 7 years. There was no evidence that either calcium or vitamin D alone or in combination were related to fracture risk in the hip or elsewhere [123]. Another assessment of 26 RCTs of calcium supplement use found no benefit on fracture risk in the largest studies with the least bias [122]. Based on "adequate evidence," the *US Preventive Task Force (USPTF)* "*recommends against daily supplementation with 400 IU or less of vitamin D and 1000 mg or less of calcium for the primary prevention of fractures in community-dwelling, postmenopausal women*" [124]. *Based on insufficient evidence, higher amounts of vitamin D and calcium are not recommended. A diagnosis of osteoporosis is treated by a practicing clinician.*

Calcium Supplements. Adverse Effects The use of calcium supplements is associated with serious adverse effects involving the function of the GI and CV systems [117]. GI effects range from constipation and flatulence to severe abdominal symptoms requiring hospitalizations [125]. An increase incidence of MI is associated with calcium/vitamin D use as observed in an RCT of older women [126] and in a meta-analysis of 15 RCTs [127]. Additionally, the risk of coronary artery calcium (CAC) deposits, an established biomarker of CV disease [128], increased in long-term use of calcium supplements but not in those who obtained calcium at various levels from their diets [129]. This was a large multiethnic prospective cohort study that measured CAC at baseline and 10 years later in men and women, with an average age of 62 years [129]. Calcium intake ranged from <400 mg calcium to >1435 mg daily obtained in the diet and/or in 42% who used supplements [129].

There is controversial evidence that calcium supplements plus vitamin D may contribute to the formation of kidney stones [130]. Vitamin D is associated with hypercalciuria (urinary excretion of calcium) in some individuals, forming kidney stones [131]. Studies evaluating the use of supplemental vitamin D alone report evidence of an increased risk of hypercalciuria but no appearance of kidney stones [132], although the risk is higher in "stone formers" (those with a history of kidney stones) [130].

Magnesium Supplements Magnesium, like calcium, is a mineral essential for nerve, muscle, bone and metabolic activities [133–135]. Hypomagnesemia, a deficiency of this mineral below acceptable levels of 0.76–1.15 mmol/L, is associated with numerous diseases such as Type 2 diabetes mellitus (T2DM), AD, and CV disease [136]. Despite the fact that serum levels of magnesium do not reflect the totality of magnesium in the body, this measurement remains in use [136]. Magnesium levels decline with age, possibly related to bone and muscle mass loss (also like calcium, these are storage sites of magnesium), diseases, e.g., poorly controlled diabetes, certain medications and dietary selections [136]. The RDA suggests daily dietary magnesium ingestion should be 420 mg for older men and 320 mg for older women [137]. However, according to the National Health and Nutrition Examination Survey (NHANES) [138] 2017–2020, using validated survey questionnaires, sampling over 1000 men and women, found diet alone did not achieve the RDA. A third of those over 60 years of age use magnesium supplements, which surprisingly enable women to achieve the RDA but not men [139].

Magnesium Supplements. Efficacy Whether magnesium supplements in the older adult have any additional benefit beyond correcting a deficiency is not clear [140]. Results of the InCHIANTI (aging in the Chianti area) study reported a direct association with serum magnesium level and degree of muscle strength (grip, ankle, knee torque, lower leg power) in community-dwelling older adults (67 years of age) [141]. The higher the magnesium level, the better the physical performance, with the best performance at magnesium levels greater than the normal range. Use of the supplement was not assessed [141]. In middle-aged overweight women, 8 weeks of daily magnesium supplement (250 mg magnesium oxide, poorly bioavailable) failed to significantly improve functional mobility and muscle strength [142]. In a similar 8-week study with overweight women (71 years of age), daily magnesium supplements (300 mg/d bioavailable magnesium) still had no effect on a battery of physical function tests that included hand-grip, knee strength, walking speed and balance [143].

Other effects of magnesium supplements have been studied. Magnesium supplements (citrate, oxide, sulfate) for 24 weeks in older adults (63 years) did not alter aortic stiffness as measured by the validated carotid-to-femoral pulse wave velocity test [144]. One study of community-dwelling older adults (65 years) found that daily magnesium (520 mg elemental magnesium) for 4 weeks did not prevent nocturnal leg cramps [145]. Results from a cross-sectional study of older adults (age 69 years) of the NHANES 2011–2014 found several nutrients in food associated with higher cognitive function, one of which was magnesium [146]. However, there are no data on the effects of magnesium supplement use on cognitive function. As noted by Barbagallo et al. [147], "while it is advisable to maintain a satisfactory magnesium balance with a sufficient dietary intake of magnesium, the possible role of magnesium supplements is still unclear."

Magnesium. Adverse Effects The use of magnesium supplements may cause GI symptoms such as diarrhea, nausea and vomiting, although the above studies consider these adverse effects mostly comparable to placebo. As reviewed by Gröber et al. [136], concomitant use of magnesium supplements and several classes of drugs (aminoglycosides, bisphosphonates, calcium channel blockers, fluoroquinolones, skeletal muscle relaxants and tetracyclines) may affect absorption and reduce efficacy [136]. More recently, studies have shown that minerals such as magnesium chelate antiretroviral inhibitors and decrease their absorption [148]. Additionally, drugs influencing renal function, e.g., potassium-sparing diuretics, may elevate magnesium levels, possibly to toxic levels [136].

Iron Supplements. Treatment of Iron Deficiency Iron deficiency (ID) defined as inadequate absorption and/or excessive loss leading to iron-deficiency anemia (IDA) is common worldwide, affecting nearly 2 billion people as of 2021 [149]. Prevalence in community-dwelling older adults in about 12% but can climb to 47% in residential homes [150]. Although iron is found throughout the body, approximately 70% of it is located in the hemoglobin (Hb) of red blood cells and the myoglobin in the muscle, where it plays an essential role in oxygen transport and storage [151]. Iron also plays key roles in metabolism, oxygen sensing, synthesis of hormones and neurotransmitters, inflammation and microbial defense and storage and transport of itself [152]. ID leads to reduced functionality in all of these activities [153].

There are countless causes of ID. In general terms, iron intake is poorly bioavailable or the need is high. Specifically, to focus on a few causative factors, ID stems from a poor quality diet, absorption or appetite suppression [154], medications (e.g., aspirin) [155], and chronic diseases, some with known mechanisms, e.g., systemic inflammation of CV disease, elevated iron regulator, hepcidin, in kidney disease, impaired Hb synthesis in AD and others with complex or unknown mechanisms, e.g., frailty (see Chap. 7), and osteoporosis [153].

A major difficulty with studies of ID in all age groups is the lack of consensus on the legitimate "normal" value and, additionally, the most relevant biomarker (serum ferritin, transferrin saturation, serum iron) for ID [153]. Cut-off Hb values (Hb < 12 g/dL in women and Hb < 13 g/dL in men) were established by the WHO in 1968 independent of older adults who are presently still without age-associated relevant Hb cut-off values and definitive interpretation of biomarkers [153].

Iron levels, as determined by Hb measurements in an 18-year longitudinal study of healthy 70-year-old adults, declined with age during this time period [156]. Thus, *iron deficiency anemia increases with age* [150, 153, 157].

Iron Supplements. Iron Deficiency Anemia Therapy Oral iron supplements, intravenous iron and blood transfusions are possible treatments for IDA. The use of these treatments should be considered only after the cause of the ID has been determined by a practicing clinician [158]. Due to the complexity of IDA in the older adult, oral iron supplements may benefit only some individuals [153]. Also, iron absorption is low in many older adults due to acidic reduction with the use of PPIs [159] or hypochlorhydria [160]. The data are sparse regarding the successful treatment of IDA with oral iron supplements in the older adult [161]. Several studies reported that 4–6 weeks of oral iron supplement (200 mg/d) increased Hb by only 0.35 g/dL, an amount of unknown clinical significance. On the other hand, small quantities (15 mg) are considered less toxic (avoidance of GI issues of constipation, nausea, diarrhea, abdominal pain, and heartburn) [162] and produce similar increases in Hb compared to higher doses [163]. Higher doses, regardless of age, are considered inappropriate due to the efficient homeostatic mechanisms regulating endogenous iron [164].

There is only one study on disease prevention with iron supplementation. The use of iron supplements (5 mg iron fumarate) for 11 years was associated with a decreased risk of one cancer, esophageal carcinoma, but an increased risk for another, noncardia adenocarcinoma [97].

Iron Supplement Guidelines for Treatment of Iron Deficiency Wawer et al. [153] suggest the need for the development of the following guidelines for clinicians treating IDA in the older adult: (1) define the relevant ID biomarkers indicative of the condition, (2) define the appropriate dose of iron for ID of chronic diseases, e.g., kidney disease, irritable bowel disease and (3) determine the possible influence on iron status with changes in diet and exercise.

Biologicals

Glucosamine/Chondroitin Supplements OTC glucosamine and/or chondroitin are supplements popular with the older adult for the treatment of joint arthritis [165]; some also use calcium, magnesium and vitamin D [166]. The two main types of joint arthritis are OA and RA. OA is a degenerative joint condition of the knees, hips, hands and/or shoulders that worsens with age and obesity and is responsible for significant disability and reduced mobility for the older adult [167]. RA, on the other hand, is an autoimmune disease that can occur at any age and is aggressively treated with prescription drugs [168]. Both, however, lead to joint pain, remodeled joints and limits on function and mobility [167, 168].

Chondroitin sulfate (CS) plays an important role in the connective tissue of humans, participating in many functions, especially in maintaining the integrity of articular cartilage of joints, as well as exerting anti-inflammatory effects [169, 170]. Similarly, glucosamine (GlcN) is an essential component of cartilage, optimizing the health of joints [171]. Numerous RCTs have evaluated GlcN (HCl or sulfate) and CS alone or together primarily for the prevention of pain and structural changes in knee osteoarthritis [172, 173].

Glucosamine/Chondroitin Supplements. Osteoarthritis Therapy OA is assessed in several ways: (1) validated questionnaires, e.g., Western Ontario and McMaster osteoarthritis index (WOMAC), rating pain, stiffness, and physical function with a scale of 0–4, none to extreme [174]; (2) visual analog scale (VAS) rating pain intensity from mild to very severe (0–10) [175]; (3) Lequesne's index rates pain or discomfort, walking distance and activities of daily living [176]; (4) radiographic analysis of joints. A meta-analysis of 48 RCTs of CS use for 6 months or more concluded that a small benefit on reduction of pain (pain questionnaires), joint structure (x-rays) and quality of life (Lequesne's index) was evident and adverse effects were no different than placebo [172]. A later meta-analysis of 30 RCTs overlapping with several RCTs included in the Singh et al. [172] analysis agreed that CS use was better than placebo in relieving pain and improving mobility and added that GlcN-HCl use reduced stiffness [173]. In contract, an extensive systemic and meta-analysis by the European Alliance of Association of Rheumatology (EULAR) found considerable inconsistencies among study results and concluded that the small benefit from CS and/or GlcN-HCl on OA was not clinically relevant [177]. Regrettably, the average age of participants in most of the included RCTs noted above was less than 60 years of age.

Results of RCTs with individuals 65 years and older with OA using CS and/or GlcN are also inconsistent. A 6-month study found that degenerative changes in knee OA were reduced with CS (800 mg daily) [178]. Another RCT observed that the combination of CS (800 mg) plus GlcN-HCl (1000 mg) plus manganese (76 mg) daily for 6 months reduced pain as determined by the Lequesne's index [179] and CS (1200 mg) plus GlcN-HCl (1500 mg) daily for 6 months was comparable to the anti-inflammatory drug, celecoxib (200 mg) daily in suppressing pain and functional limitations and joint deterioration [180]. RCTs of longer duration report CS and GlcN-HCl reduced joint narrowing but no difference in pain reduction compared to placebo at 2 years [181]. Purified GlcN-sulfate use for 3 years improved function and reduced the need for prescription drugs [182, 183]. In contrast, Messier et al. [184] reported that CS (1200 mg) plus GlcN-HCl (1500 mg) and exercise (aerobic and resistance) were no better than exercise alone. Roman-Blas et al. [185] also found CS and GlcN-HCl in the same amounts for 6 months were ineffective in reducing pain and improving function in knee OA. Several studies reported adverse effects, primarily abdominal pain and dyspepsia [181, 183]. *CS and GlcN-HCl supplements appear to benefit some older adults with OA.*

Glucosamine/Chondroitin Supplements. Preparations and Concerns There is concern about the extensive variability of CS preparations on the market [186]. Commercial chondroitin may be extracted with various methods from any one or all of the following: "from bovine, porcine, and chicken, or marine sources such as cartilaginous fish, sharks and skate, but also bony fishes" and may also contain proteins with allergic potential, microbes (bacteria, viruses, prions), and intentional adulterating substances (surfactants, lactose) [186]. These products not only lack efficacy but may produce adverse effects. Commercial glucosamine may be prepared by either hydrolytic or enzymatic cleavage of chitin or chitosan (exoskeleton of shell fish) or by fermentation with engineered microbes and can be prepared as an acid (HCl), sulfate or acetylated product [187]. Commercial preparation of glucosamine carries the same concerns as chondroitin.

OMEGA-3 FATTY ACIDS Omega-3 fatty acids (O3FA) are long-chain polyunsaturated fatty acids (PUFA). The three main ones are eicosapentaenoic acid (EPA) and docosahexaenoic acid (DHA) found in fish and alpha linolenic acid (ALA) found in plants [188]. The first two have become popular OTC dietary supplements thought to preserve brain and heart health. Physiologically, ingested O3FAs are incorporated into cell membranes where they exert a wealth of anti-inflammatory effects [189]. In humans, the level of O3FAs is mainly determined by the extraction of lipids from the membranes of red blood cells (RBCs) and expressed relative to total extracted fats. An 8–12% level of EPA and DHA is considered normal, although this may vary with different nonstandardized assays [190].

Omega-3 Fatty Acids. Cognitive Effects Regarding O3FAs and cognition, results of observational studies indicate that (1) a low dietary intake of O3FAs increases the risks of dementia, (2) AD patients have a lower brain level of O3FAs and (3) higher dietary intake of O3FAs lowers the risk of cognitive decline [191]. However, this fails to establish causality, and the results of interventional RCTs reach a different conclusion. Numerous studies with the healthy older adult (200–1680 participants), with an average age of 70–75 years, who consumed daily amounts of EPA and DHA ranging from 500 to 800 mg DHA, 200–360 mg EPA or totals up to 1800 mg for 6 months to 5 years found no benefit of O3FA supplements on a battery of cognitive tests [192–196]. A small study (30 participants in test and control group) of high doses of O3FA (2200 mg/d) for 26 weeks reported a 26% increase in the score on an executive function test, enhanced MRI-defined brain connectivity, increased level of brain-derived neurotrophic factor and reduced fasting insulin levels [197]. In older adults with memory complaints, O3FA use was without effect [198] or only improved test scores on verbal fluency [199]. A systematic meta-analysis of 25 RCTs concluded that O3FAs had no effect on global cognitive function but "might have a mild effect on memory in healthy individuals" [200]. Additionally, Canhada et al. [201] *recommend against the use of O3FA in the treatment of AD as the data at present does not support its use.*

Omega-3 Fatty Acids. Cardiovascular Effects Results of observational and epidemiological studies indicate that a diet high in fatty fish or O3FAs is associated with a lower risk of CV disease events [202, 203]. In contrast, one multinational study with over 13,000 statin-treated participants with elevated CV risk observed that 4 g (combined DHA and EPA) daily for 1 year (study stopped early) provided no beneficial effect on CV events [204]. Another large study (25,000) of older adults, average age, 67 years, taking 460 mg EPA and 380 mg DHA for over 5 years with significantly elevated O3FA levels had no effect on major CV events, e.g., MI, stroke, CV mortality or cancer incidence [205]. Furthermore, a comprehensive systematic review of 79 RCTs assessing the effects of O3FAs mainly as supplements concluded that moderate and high-quality evidence shows there is no effect on mortality or CV health [206]. However, it gets more complicated. An extensive review of multiple meta-analyses of RCTs examining the effect of O3FAs on CV risk (2013–2023) pointed to mixed results. In some meta-analyses, O3FAs lowered CV risk by 7–14%, with higher daily doses (>3 g) more efficacious [189]. The data, or at least results of certain trials, were sufficient for the American Heart Association (AHA) to recommend "EPA+DHA or EPA-only, at a dose of 4 g/d, are clinically useful for reducing triglycerides, after any underlying causes are addressed and diet and lifestyle strategies are implemented" [207]. Similar organizations in Europe recommended O3FAs (specifically prescription icosapent ethyl, 4 g/d) for patients with hyper triglyceride levels (135–499 mg/dl) [208]. The AHA has also extended the use of O3FA supplements to individuals with a recent MI and heart failure without preserved left ventricular function based on RCT results showing mortality and hospitalization reduction, respectively [209].

Omega-3 Fatty Acids. Adverse Reactions There are several concerns about the potential adverse effects of O3FAs [210]. Firstly, O3FAs are sensitive to oxidation (temperature, light, water) and peroxides, which may have biological effects but most likely are toxic [211]. Unless chemically analyzed, there is no way to determine the degree of oxidation and possible loss of efficacy in purchased products [211]. Secondly, there is a serious concern that the use of O3FAs increases the risk of atrial fibrillation (AF) (rapid and irregular heartbeats predisposing to a stroke). Djuricic and Calder [210] concluded that "individual trials and meta-analyses of mostly recent trials indicate that long-chain omega-3 PUFAs increase the risk of AF, especially when used at high doses." In fact, the risk is dose-related in a U-shaped manner, with low doses (<1 g/d) and high doses (>1 g/d) increasing the risk for AF [212]. Thirdly, although reported infrequently, adverse effects depending on the dose may also include GI disturbances such as diarrhea, nausea, dyspepsia, and abdominal discomfort [204]. Finally, O3FAs integrate into the platelet membrane, compete with a normal substrate (arachidonic acid) of key enzymes, cyclooxygenase and lipoxygenase and disrupt platelet aggregation, leading to unwanted bleeding, occurring at doses >2 g/d [213]. Fortunately, data from numerous clinical trials indicate so far that this is not a real-world concern but merely a theoretical one [210].

Table 9.1 Over-the-counter drugs and dietary supplements used by the older adult

Over-the-counter medications/category	Drugs	Efficacy	Adverse drug reactions; concerns
Cold/sinus/allergy	Mucolytic—guaifenesin Cough suppressant—dextromethorphan hydrobromide Decongestant—phenylephrine HCl, pseudoephedrine hydrochloride First-generation antihistamine/allergy—chlorpheniramine maleate, brompheniramine maleate, diphenhydramine HCl, doxylamine succinate Second-generation antihistamines—cetirizine, levocetirizine and loratadine nasal steroids—fluticasone and triamcinolone	Efficacy of mucolytics, decongestants and cough suppressants is questionable Inconsistent efficacy for first-generation antihistamines Second-generation antihistamines efficacious with less sedation—no data for the older adult	Antihistamines are PIMs (Beers' Criteria®) due to sedation and anticholinergic effects Concurrent use of 2 or more leads to delirium, cognitive impairment, accidents and falls Significant drug interactions with all antihistamines
Sleep aids	Melatonin (considered a dietary supplement, not a drug) Multiple sleep aids with diphenhydramine and doxylamine *Relaxium®*	Subjective data indicate efficacy of prolonged-release melatonin used 2 weeks to 1 year; objective data show no efficacy. Inconsistent findings with AD patients; immediate release formulation ineffective. No efficacy data on *Relaxium®*	High-dose prolonged-release melatonin may cause daytime drowsiness and increase the risk of falls; possible interaction with drugs metabolized by CYP1A2 Many OTC sleep aids contain antihistamines considered PIMs

(continued)

Table 9.1 (continued)

Over-the-counter medications/ category	Drugs	Efficacy	Adverse drug reactions; concerns
Pain	Acetaminophen, NSAIDs (aspirin, ibuprofen, naproxen, diclofenac) caffeine	Generally all have some degree of efficacy; various preparations of ibuprofen are the best for acute pain of soft tissue, dental pain	Acetaminophen hepatotoxicity with high-dose use NSAIDs—use short term to avoid GI toxicity of dyspepsia, peptic ulcer disease, and bleeding. Complete avoidance if history of gastric or duodenal ulcers; high-dose/long-term evidence of elevated risk of CV events and progression to kidney disease NSAIDs and acetaminophen have extensive interaction with prescription medications
Nonsteroidal anti-inflammatory drugs (NSAIDs)	Aspirin Ibuprofen Naproxen Diclofenac	Efficacious in the treatment of osteoarthritis (OA)	High doses long term use increase the risk of adverse CV events (exacerbation of CHF), nephrotoxicity and GI bleeding. Beers criteria® considers NSAIDs as PIMs. Numerous DDIs with NSAIDs and prescription drugs
GI disorders—gastroesophageal reflux disease (GERDs); peptic ulcer disease (PUD)	Proton pump inhibitors—omeprazole, esomaprazole, lansoprazole, Histamine 2 receptor antagonists (H2RA) —amotidine, cimetidine Antacids	PPIs—preferred therapy for GERDs and PUDs. H2RA less efficacious than PPIs Antacids—very short term for symptom relief	Prolonged use of PPIs—development of precancerous conditions in the stomach, osteoporosis, pneumonia and *C. difficile* infection as per Beers' Criteria® H2RA is contraindicated in delirium; dose adjustment in kidney disease

(continued)

Table 9.1 (continued)

Over-the-counter medications/category	Drugs	Efficacy	Adverse drug reactions; concerns
Chronic constipation	Laxatives—bulk-forming agents—psyllium, calcium polycarbophil and methylcellulose Stool softeners—docusate sodium and docusate calcium Osmotics—lactulose, polyethylene glycol Stimulants—bisacodyl, sodium picosulfate and senna Suppositories/enemas—glycerin with and without stimulants	BFA—efficacious, especially soluble fiber Stool softeners—not efficacious Osmotics/stimulants—considered efficacious but evidence low to moderate; use products without added electrolytes Suppositories/enemas—useful in special settings	Possible bloating, cramping, flatulence with some, e.g., BFA. Laxative with sodium, potassium and/or magnesium used cautiously with reduced kidney function
Dietary supplements			
Vitamins/minerals (MVM)	Centrum silver AREDS2®	No efficacy in prevention of CV events or mortality; small cancer preventive effect but data subpar; no anti-cancer effects with individual use of vitamins A, E, C; Vitamin D supplement not needed for bone health; Inconsistent effects of MVM on cognition Progression to late AMD slowed with use of vitamins (C, E, beta-carotene) and zinc	Possible adverse effects of hip fractures (vitamin A), kidney stones (calcium), and bleeding (vitamin E). High vitamin D (60,000 IU) long term increases of the risk of fractures AREDS2®-recommended supplements for AMD contain an amount > RDA and additive with MVM is harmful. MVM recommended only for deficiencies

(continued)

Table 9.1 (continued)

Over-the-counter medications/ category	Drugs	Efficacy	Adverse drug reactions; concerns
Minerals	Calcium (Ca) Magnesium (Mg) Iron (Fe)	Ca/Vitamin D no longer recommended for the prevention of fractures in community-dwelling postmenopausal women; ineffective in lowering fracture risk	Ca may produce GI adverse effects (constipation, flatulence, severe abdominal pain). Ca accumulates in coronary arteries on long-term use. Vitamin D may cause the initiation of kidney stones in those with a history of stones
		Mg has no efficacy on the enhancement of muscle function; use only to correct deficiency	Mg decreases absorption of amino-glycosides, bisphosphonates, calcium channel blockers, fluoroquinolones, skeletal muscle relaxants, tetracyclines, antiretroviral inhibitors; co-used with potassium-sparing diuretics, Mg levels ↑ to toxic level.
		Fe supplements—few studies but generally ineffective; identification of the cause of anemia with physician's advice	Long-term treatment of Fe deficient anemia with oral Fe sulfate is associated with GI adverse effects (constipation, nausea, diarrhea, abdominal pain, heartburn)
Osteoarthritis supplements	Glucosamine HCl/ sulfate Chondroitin sulfate (CS)	Inconsistent efficacy results for OA in older adults. Modest evidence for a small benefit.	Reports of abdominal pain and dyspepsia; Concern for unwanted contaminants in CS and GlcN-HCl preparations
Omega-3-fatty acids (O3FAs)	Eicosapentaenoic acid (EPA) Docosahexaenoic acid (DHA)	Very modest beneficial effect on memory AHA and European health associations recommend EPA or EPA+ DHA to treat elevated triglycerides, recent MI and heart failure without preserved LV function along with standard therapy	Oxidation to peroxides may reduce efficacy and create toxicities Low and high doses of O3FAs increase the risk of AF GI adverse effects of diarrhea, nausea, dyspepsia, and abdominal discomfort have been reported

(continued)

Table 9.1 (continued)

Over-the-counter medications/category	Drugs	Efficacy	Adverse drug reactions; concerns
Ginkgo Biloba	Standardized extract (EGb761®)	Possible benefit on cognition in early dementia. No CV or cancer protection	Supplements are not standardized, so quality and quantity are in doubt. Drug interaction expected since GBE induces CYP2C19 and can ↓ efficacy of PPIs, anti-seizure drugs and others
St John's Wort	Standardized preparations	Anti-depressant efficacy but little data in the older adult	Commercial preparations are not standardized; Inducer of CYP3A4 and other CYPs and P-gp with high potential for prescription drug interaction. Potential to interact with SSRIs to precipitate the serotonin syndrome
Ginseng	Korean/American proprietary preparations	Modest evidence for glycemic control in T2DM; insufficient evidence on stroke recovery and memory improvement needs confirmation	Prolonged use/high doses—adverse effects of diarrhea, skin rash, nervousness, euphoria, insomnia, headaches, edema, variable BP changes
Garlic	Proprietary preparations—Allicor (timed release garlic powder), aged black garlic.	Promising effects to reduce dyslipidemia, hypertension, and reduce risks of CV disease but effects need confirmation in large trials	Cessation of use 1–2 weeks prior to elective surgery to avoid bleeding and hypoglycemic adverse effects. Lowers drug level of saquinavir by an unknown mechanism. Substrates of CYP1A2 and CYP2C19 so will compete with drugs using these enzymes

PIMs Potentially inappropriate medications, *AMD* age-related macular degeneration, *AD* Alzheimer's Disease, *DDIs* drug-drug interactions, *CV* cardiovascular, *CHF* congestive heart failure, *H2RA* histamine 2 receptor antagonist, *BFA* bulk forming agents, *Ca* calcium, *Mg* magnesium, *Fe* iron, *GlcN* glucosamine, *CS* chondroitin sulfate, *AHA* American Heart Association, *T2DM* Type 2 Diabetes Mellitus, *P-gp* P-glycoprotein, multidrug transporter, *GI* gastrointestinal, ↓ decrease, *LV* left ventricle, *MI* myocardial infarction, *AREDS2* Age-Related Eye Disease Study 2, *RDA* recommended daily allowance, *MVM* multivitamins and minerals, *AF* atrial fibrillation, *GBE Gingko biloba* extract, PPIs proton pump inhibitors, BP blood pressure

Botanicals (Herbal Extracts)

Gingko Biloba Extracts of the leaves of the *Gingko biloba* tree, the oldest tree on the planet, have been used medicinally for centuries in Asia [214]. The components of the *Gingko biloba* extracts (GBE) are predominately flavonoids (quercetin, kaempferol, and others), smaller amounts of terpenoids (ginkgolides A, B, C, and J, bilobalides), and organic acids. The first two components are bioactive [215]. Extensive investigations in animal models treated with GBE support a neuroprotective role for GBE [215]. GBE in these studies exerts effects ranging from anti-inflammatory, improved blood flow, neuronal protection, reduction of amyloid beta plaques and neurofibrillar tangle accumulation, and suppression of oxidation [216].

Gingko Biloba. Cognitive Effects in Alzheimer's Disease In most RCTs, the majority of participants ingested EGb761®, a stable, standardized GBE product developed by Schwabe Pharmaceuticals, Karlsruhe, Germany. Investigations focused on (1) slowing the progression of AD, (2) slowing the progression of mild cognitive impairment (MCI) and (3) slowing age-related cognitive decline. A variety of cognitive tests were employed, such as Alzheimer's Disease Assessment Scale-cognition (ADAS-Cog) (11 tests, e.g., word recall, naming objects) [217] or Syndrom-Kurztest (SKT) (9 subtests, some for memory and other relevant to speed of information processing) [218], and/or the mini-mental state exam (MMSE)(basically a screening test for MCI) [219].

A meta-analysis of 20 RCTs assessing EGb761® in slowing the progression of AD found 14 of the 20 trials showed improved cognition in AD patients who consumed EGb 761®, common dose was 204 mg with a duration of 20 weeks to 20 years and 13 of the 14 included older adults [216]. Results of 6 trials showed no benefit, and 4 of these trials included those over 60 years of age [216]. In another meta-analysis, 8 out of 9 RCTs of MCI and EGb761®used for a minimum of 8 weeks report positive effects over placebo either on reduction of neuropsychiatric symptoms, geriatric rating scale or global rating change [220]. Although many studies were in a foreign language, those in English included participants with an average age of 63–65 years [221, 222]. Thus, *standardized GBE at high doses for at least 2 months may benefit brain function in early dementia.*

Gingko Biloba. Cognition in Healthy Older Adults In *healthy community-dwelling older adults, results of RCTs have generally shown that ingestion of EGb761® does not improve cognition* [223–226]. These trials included 200–3000 older adults treated for 6 weeks to 6 years, with either 120 mg or 240 mg EGb761® daily and tested for memory, attention, visuospatial, executive function, language, and global cognition. In contrast, a 6-week study of participants 60 years and older consuming 180 mg EGb761® did better on tests of delayed recall and recognition of audio-verbal material than those taking placebo [227]. A European 20-year follow-up population study (retrospective analysis) reported that older adults (>500) who used EGb761® did better on cognitive tests (MMSE, visual memory test, verbal fluency assessed every 2–3 years) than those who did not use the GBE [228]. It is argued that age-associated changes in cognition are a slow process; hence, long-term investigations are required to determine the effects of GBE on cognition in the healthy older adult [228].

Gingko Biloba. Other Effects Regarding other possible benefits of GBE, the secondary outcome from a large RCT of over 3000 older adults (Ginko Evaluation of Memory, GEM) found that EGb761 (120 mg twice daily) for over 6 years did not reduce the risk of cancer [229], lower blood pressure or decrease the incidence of hypertension [230] or reduce the risk of CV events or mortality [231].

Gingko Biloba. Preparations and Concerns A pertinent cautionary note emphasizes the fact that clinical trials were conducted with GBE that is stable and standardized so that the same dose is consumed throughout the study regardless of duration. This is not the case for OTC GBEs. The consumer has no assurance of the content on any one purchase [232, 233]. In a comparison of labels of 17 pharmaceutical grade GBE preparations with 46 OTC GBE supplements, all pharmaceutical grade GBEs met compliance requirements on individual chemical components (see above), but only 1% of dietary supplements met this criteria, and the remainder provided no information [232]. Information on safe duration of use, potential drug interactions, and adverse effects were also lacking on OTC supplements, and doses ranged from 0.45 to 510 mg compared to the 120 or 240 mg standard dose of pharmaceutical products [232]. Chemical analysis of the content of OTC GBE found convincing evidence of adulteration (added compounds) or mismatch between content and label [234–236].

Gingko Biloba. Adverse Effects Another concern is the potential adverse effects of GBEs. GBE induces the hepatic drug-metabolizing enzyme CYP2C19, causing an acceleration in the breakdown of drugs metabolized by this enzyme [237] (see Chap. 3). In particular, the PPI, omeprazole [238], antiseizure drugs, valproate and phenytoin [239], and antidiabetic drug, tolbutamide [240] were metabolized rapidly in the presence of GBE; and consequently, effects of these drugs were reduced. Based on statistical analysis of medical data, concurrent use of GBE and warfarin may increase the risk of bleeding [241].

ST JOHN'S WORT St John's Wort (SJW) is a preparation from the plant *Hypericum perforatum*, a yellow flowering herb, considered in the USA as an agricultural weed harmful to livestock. There exist a large number of relevant medicinal compounds in SJW, with the two most important bioactive ones, hypericin and hyperforin [242]. Other components include flavonoids, e.g., quercetin, essential oils, tannins, acids and alcohols [242]. In Europe, standardized preparations are produced, but no such regulations exist in the USA, so the quality of SJW preparations is highly variable [243].

St John's Work. Antidepressant Effects Similar to GBE, SJW has been used for medicinal purposes for centuries. Unlike GBE, SJW is primarily of value as an antidepressant. The most recent Cochran meta-analysis of RCTs using *Hypericum* extracts compared to placebo (18 trials) or compared to a standard antidepressant (17 trials) to treat mild-moderate depression concluded that *Hypericum* extracts "are superior to placebo in patients with major depression ..." and "are similarly effective as standard antidepressants" [243]. Only one of the included trials studied the older adult. In the lone study of less than 200 participants, with an average age of 69 years, the SJW extract, LoHyp-57, compared to fluoxetine (selective serotonin reuptake inhibitor, SSRI) for 6 weeks, was as effective as the antidepressant in ameliorating mild-moderate major depression (Hamilton Depression Scale) [244]. Results of later trials are mixed with SJW reducing severity in major depression compared to paroxetine (SSRI) [245], one trial with two different preparations of SJW showing antidepressive effects [246] and a report of no effect of SJW compared to sertraline (SSRI) or placebo in major depression [247] or no effect of SJW compared to citalopram (SSRI) or placebo in minor depression [248]. Again, all of these recent trials excluded the older adult.

St John's Work. Adverse Effects Adverse effects of standardized SJW extracts are comparable to placebo and infrequent and milder than those of prescription antidepressants [244]. However, the main concern with SJW is the evidence that it is an inducer of CYP3A4 [249, 250] and the efflux transporter, P-gp [251]. Other CYP isotypes, e.g., CYP1A2, CYP2C9, CYP2C19, CYP2D6, and CYP2E1, have also been identified as targets of SJW induction [242]. This means *SJW has the potential to interact with a large number of medications* (see Chap. 3), *leading to altered drug levels and adverse effects* [242].

Studies show that concurrent use of SJW for 10 days or more decreases the bioavailability of many drugs, e.g., the second-generation antihistamine fexofenadine [252], cardiac digoxin and related glycosides [253], anticancer drug imatinib mesylate [254], immunosuppressant cyclosporin [255], antihypertensive drugs, e.g., verapamil, nifedipine [256], sulfonylurea, gliclazide [257] and anticoagulant, warfarin [258]. Additionally with an unexplained mechanism, SJW can add to the effects of SSRIs and cause serotonin syndrome, a life-threatening whole-body reaction of tachycardia, hypertension and hyperthermia [242]. It is clear that the use of SJW has a super high potential for drug interactions, and the use of this OTC dietary supplement should be discussed with a practicing physician before use.

GINSENG Ginseng used medicinally is a root extract of the plant, most commonly *Panax ginseng* C.A. Meyer (Korean origin). There exist over ten other Panax species [259]. As with other botanicals, extraction yields numerous diverse chemical components, many with different biological effects. The components of ginseng are particularly diverse, possibly accounting for the multiplicity of its physiological effects, at least in animal and cell culture models [260]. One of the main biologically active components is the ginsenosides, steroid-like structures with sugar attachments, termed saponins, of which these is a large assortment. Other biologically active compounds in ginseng are "essential oils, antioxidants, polyacetylenic alcohols, peptides, amino acids, polysaccharides, and vitamins" [260].

Ginseng. Multiplicity of Effects Ginseng has been studied in numerous RCTs throughout the world. Most studies are small (group size 20–300), exclude the older adult and test different preparations of ginseng from Korean red ginseng (*Panax ginseng*) (KRG), American ginseng (*Panax quinquefolius L*) (AG), and fractionated and proprietary preparations of ginsenosides for different indications. To focus on the older adult (55 and older), KRG and AG use for 12 and 8 weeks, respectively, improved glycemic control in T2DM patients [261, 262], lowered HbA1C [262] and, in another study of T2DM patients, lowered systolic blood pressure [263]. These findings suggest ginseng may be a beneficial adjunct to traditional therapy [262]. Several studies showed that KRG [264] and AG [265] ameliorated cancer-related fatigue. A large study of nearly 2000 participants per group reported a small but significantly increased rate of recovery following a stroke in those treated with a proprietary Chinese ginseng product (Panax notoginseng Saponins) for 3 months [266]. In 40 older adults with subjective memory complaints, taking a Korean proprietary preparation of Panax sprouts (ThinkGIN™) containing higher amounts of ginsenosides than those used in the above studies improved their scores on several memory and cognitive tests and lowered the level of plasma acetylcholinesterase, suggesting a potential elevation in the neurotransmitter, acetylcholine assisted with memory improvement [267]. In contrast, ginseng (Panax ginseng G115 capsules) for 1 year had no effect on the reduction of acute exacerbation of COPD [268].

Ginseng. Adverse Effects Clearly, proprietary preparations of ginseng, generally at large doses, have some legitimate biological effects that will likely be evaluated in larger trials in the future. Unlike SJW, ginseng does not have any clinically relevant effects on the CYP enzymes [269]. Although it is generally considered safe, adverse effects of ginseng use, such as diarrhea, skin rash, nervousness, euphoria, insomnia, edema, blood pressure increase or decrease, have been reported, generally with high doses for prolonged periods [270]. Cautionary use is advised with oral hypoglycemic drugs, caffeine, phenelzine (monoamine oxidase inhibitor) and warfarin [270].

GARLIC EXTRACT Garlic is the well-known bulb of the plant *Allium sativum*, consumed in foods but also used for centuries in the herbal treatment of disease [271]. Allicin, a sulfur-containing chemical, is the component with the greatest biological effect, also giving garlic its flavor and scent [272]. Sulfur-containing compounds predominate in garlic. S-allyl-L-cysteine sulfoxide (alliin) appears in the highest concentration in garlic and is the precursor of allicin [271]. Damage to the garlic converts alliin to allicin via the enzyme allinase, providing the plant with an antimicrobial defense molecule [273]. The sulfur reactivity of allicin and another similar compound, e.g., ajoene, enable extracts of garlic to exert a multiplicity of beneficial outcomes, including antimicrobial and anticancer effects [273].

Garlic Extract. Diverse Effects in Experimental Models There is convincing evidence from studies with cell cultures and animal models that garlic and/or isolated allicin inhibit proliferation and survival of cancer cells, exert antioxidant effects possibly by stimulating antioxidative enzyme activity or influencing level of reactive oxygen species (ROS), express anti-inflammatory activity via multiple mechanisms, are neuroprotective with the enhancement of memory and inhibition of acetylcholinesterase activity in mice and reduce total cholesterol, low-density lipoproteins and triglycerides in rabbits [271]. These are a few of the many effects of garlic extracts in experimental studies [271].

Garlic Extract. Cardiovascular Effects In RCTs that include some older adults with average age of 55 years and older, the following effects of garlic have been observed: 12 month treatment with proprietary Allicor (timed release garlic powder) in 51 patients with coronary heart disease reduced LDL cholesterol and lowered projected future risk of heart attack and death [274]; 12 month treatment with aged garlic extract (2.4 g/d) reduced percentage of vulnerable plaques (computerized tomography) in 27 patients with metabolic syndrome [275], reduced CAC, glucose and blood pressure in 46 patients at high risk of CV disease [276] and increased microvascular circulation in 61patients at high risk of CV disease [277]; 12 weeks of aged black garlic (250 mg proprietary black garlic extract) reduced blood pressure several mmHg in 39 Grade 1(systolic pressure 130–139 mmHg) hypertensive patients [278]; higher doses of aged black garlic (480 and 960 mg/d) for 12 weeks lowered systolic blood pressure similarly by more than 11 mm Hg in 17 and 15 patients, respectively, with uncontrolled systolic hypertension [279]; 3 months of large amounts of garlic (1 g extracted garlic/capsule, 2 capsules twice daily) lowered total cholesterol and triglycerides, and increased high density lipoprotein-cholesterol and fibrinolytic activity (favoring anti-clotting mechanisms) in 30 patients with coronary artery disease [280]. Although these RCTs with various preparations of garlic show several health benefits, these studies are small and need confirmation with significantly larger studies. Additionally, they were done with proprietary preparations whose strict formulation would not be present in OTC garlic extracts.

Garlic Extract. Adverse Effects Garlic extracts have antiplatelet activity capable of inhibiting platelet aggregation, as shown in vitro [281]. Although this effect in humans is controversial [282], a cautionary recommendation by the American Society of Anesthesiologists and the American Association of Nurse Anesthetists warns patients to stop the use of garlic extracts 1–2 weeks prior to elective surgery to avoid the risk of bleeding [283]. Based on results of the hypoglycemic and insulin-sensitizing effects of alliin, (considerably more stable than allicin and highly likely to be found in OTC preparations) in a study with diet-induced obese mice [284], the potential adverse effect of hypoglycemia is also considered as a reason to avoid garlic use 1–2 weeks prior to elective surgery [283]. Garlic use, simultaneous with a protease inhibitor, significantly reduces the bioavailability of saquinavir [285]. Adverse interactions of concomitant use of garlic extracts with prescription drugs metabolized by CYP3A4 (amlodipine, atorvastatin, simvastatin, verapamil) have been reported [286]; the explanation for these interactions remains poorly understood since garlic extract is only known as a substrate of CYP1A2 and CYP2C19 [287].

MISUSE/ABUSE OF OTC DRUGS/VITAMINS/MINERALS/BIOLOGICALS/ HERBAL SUPPLEMENTS It is clear that the use of OTC drugs, vitamins/minerals, biologicals and herbal supplements is high in the population of older adults [6, 11, 12]. Associated with this is an elevated risk of adverse reactions due to any of the following: (1) inappropriate concurrent use of OTC products and prescription drugs [288], (2) use at incorrect dose and/or duration of OTC products leading to organ damage and hospitalizations [289], (3) lack of candor with prescribing clinician as to OTC product use leading to duplication, and overdosing [290], (4) belief that all OTC products are safe and effective [291], and (5) lack of accurate and complete labeling on OTC products [232].

A recent study "sought to explore how older adults select and would hypothetically use (dosing and duration) OTC pain and sleep medications and if the selected medications would be considered safe use" [292]. Results of interviews with community-dwelling older adults consisting of a "walking interview" through a pharmacy's OTC aisles soliciting selections on analgesic and sleep aids and a follow-up interview inquiring of knowledge on use (dose, duration, side effects) revealed four types of OTC misuse—"drug-drug interaction, drug-disease interaction, drug-age interaction, and usage that exceeds product labeling recommendations" [292]. Although a small study (20 participants, average age 75.7 years), 90% committed at least one type of misuse with the most common type of drug-drug interactions, especially pain medications (OTC with prescription drug). "In total, 87 potential instances of misuse in nineteen participants were documented" [292].

To use OTC drugs, vitamins/minerals, biologicals and herbal remedies appropriately and to avoid adverse effects, self-medication needs to be linked to accessible, understandable information to support an informed decision [292]. Safari et al. [6] summarize three ideas to achieve this: *(1) educate the consumer by clear product labeling, encourage ready access to the pharmacist to answer questions and provide accurate updates and education with web-linked health technology and/or through a healthcare provider; (2) improve the communication between the patient and the healthcare provider such that the healthcare provider knows the identity of OTC products used by the older adult and can provide appropriate guidance with education and/or dose adjustments; continuing education of healthcare provider is also important and the interaction with the pharmacist is essential* [33]*; and (3) regulate herbal/dietary supplements, specifically, to bring the GMP for supplements in line with rules required for OTC drugs to establish reproducible quantity and quality* [6, 293].

Guidance
I. The use of OTC products by the older adult represents a serious challenge for the healthcare provider because
   A. Those of every age harbor the mistaken believe that all OTC drugs, vitamins/minerals, biologicals, and herbal remedies are safe and effective
   B. The older adult is reluctant to reveal their use of OTC medicinal products, and they, more than any other age group, use the most
   C. In the process of self-medication, the older adult fails to seek information on reasonable dose, duration, possible interaction with prescription medications or age changes and reproducible quality of the OTC product. This lack of information leads to potential adverse and toxic effects.
II. To address these issues, the healthcare provider should
   A. Develop a positive and open dialogue with the older adult as to their use of OTC products and seek to identify all of them
   B. Educate oneself on the efficacy/safety of the most widely used OTC products by the older adult as set forth in this chapter and summarized in Table 9.1
   C. Provide guidance that emphasizes the use of OTC products for short periods of time at the lowest dose, identify OTC drugs/supplements that interact with prescription drugs or age changes, and emphasize the absence of efficacy of certain OTC products as well as the lack of quality control on dietary/herbal supplements.
III. Key points of emphasis
   A. Cold, sinus, allergy remedies and sleep aids should be avoided because they contain first-generation antihistamines that cause sedation and anticholinergic effects; decongestants, mucolytics, and cough suppressants are ineffective.
   B. Pain and anti-inflammatory drugs should be used short term as high doses/long-term use produce organ toxicity; high potential for interaction with prescription medications.
   C. Proton pump inhibitors are efficacious for gastroesophageal reflux disease and peptic ulcer disease and preferred over histamine 2 receptor antagonists and antacids but have serious long-term adverse effects; correction of disease cause is best; stool softeners are ineffective laxatives, but others, not containing salts, aid in relief of mild-moderate constipation.
   D. Some dietary supplements have very modest benefits in select conditions. These include prolonged-release melatonin (sleep aid), chondroitin sulfate/glucosamine (osteoarthritis), omega-3 fatty acids (hypertriglyceridemia), *Gingko biloba* extracts (memory improvement in early dementia), ginseng extracts (glycemic control in Type 2 diabetes mellitus). The major issue is that efficacy was determined

(continued)

with purified and standardized products that would not be available to the average older adult.
E. Dietary/herbal supplements that are not efficacious are multivitamins and minerals (do not protect against cardiovascular disease, cancers), vitamin D plus calcium (no reduction in fracture risk), magnesium (no enhanced muscle function), and iron (little benefit in iron deficiency). Most of these are valuable only if there is a proven vitamin/mineral deficiency.
F. Dietary/herbal supplements have the potential for adverse effects. Many produce GI adverse effects. Most interact negatively with prescription drugs (most notorious, St John's Wort), and some slow recovery from elective surgery if not terminated several weeks prior (garlic extracts). There is also the risk of toxicity due to contaminants in extracts.

References

1. https://www.fda.gov/about-fda/changes-science-law-and-regulatory-authorities/part-ii-1938-food-drug-cosmetic-act
2. https://www.fda.gov/about-fda/changes-science-law-and-regulatory-authorities/part-iii-drugs-and-foods-under-1938-act-and-its-amendments
3. https://www.fda.gov/drugs/otc-drug-review-process-otc-drug-monographs
4. Federal Food, Drug and Cosmetic (FD&C) Act. Section 505G reforms.
5. Dietary Supplement Health and Education Act (DSHEA) of 1994 accessed: https://ods.od.nih.gov/About/DSHEA_Wording.aspx
6. Safari D, DeMarco EC, Scanion L, Grossberg GT. Over-the-counter remedies in older adults patterns of use, potential pitfalls, and proposed solutions. Clin Geriatr Med. 2022;38(1):99–118. https://doi.org/10.1016/j.cger.2021.07.005.
7. https://www.fda.gov/food/information-consumers-using-dietary-supplements/questions-and-answers
8. Mikulic M. OTC medication retail sales in the U.S. 1965–2023. https://www.statista.com/statistics/307237/otc-sales-in-theus/. May 24, 2024.
9. Mishra S, Stierman B, Gahche JJ, Potischman N. Dietary supplement use among adults: United States, 2017–2018. NCHS Data Brief, no 399. Hyattsville, MD: National Center for Health Statistics; 2021. https://doi.org/10.15620/cdc:1011.
10. Ylä-Rautio H, Siissalo S, Leikola S. Drug-related problems and pharmacy interventions in non-prescription medication, with a focus on high-risk over-the-counter medications. Int J Clin Pharm. 2020;42(2):786–95. https://doi.org/10.1007/s11096-020-00984-8.
11. Qato DM, Alexander GC, Conti RM, Johnson M, Schumm P, Lindau ST. Use of prescription and over-the-counter medications and dietary supplements among older adults in the United States. JAMA. 2008;300(24):2867–78. https://doi.org/10.1001/jama.2008.892.
12. Qato DM, Wilder J, Schumm LP, Gillet V, Alexander GC. Changes in prescription and over-the-counter medication and dietary supplement use among older adults in the United States, 2005 vs 2011. JAMA Intern Med. 2016;176(4):473–82. https://doi.org/10.1001/jamainternmed.2015.8581.

References

13. Jaqua EE, Gonzalez J, Bahjri K, Erickson S, Garcia C, Santhavachart M, et al. Analyzing potential interactions between complementary and alternative therapies, over-the-counter, and prescription medications in the older population. Perm J. 2024;28(2):70–7. https://doi.org/10.7812/TPP/23.183.
14. McCoul ED. Assessment of pharmacologic ingredients in common over-the-counter Sinonasal medications. JAMA Otolaryngol Head Neck Surg. 2020;146(9):810–5. https://doi.org/10.1001/jamaoto.2020.1836.
15. Hoffer-Schaefer A, Rozycki HJ, Yopp MA, Rubin BK. Guaifenesin has no effect on sputum volume or sputum properties in adolescents and adults with acute respiratory tract infections. Respir Care. 2014;59(5):631–6. https://doi.org/10.4187/respcare.02640.
16. Weinberger M, Hendeles L. Nonprescription medications for respiratory symptoms: facts and marketing fictions. Allergy Asthma Proc. 2018;39(3):169–76. https://doi.org/10.2500/aap.2018.39.4117.
17. Kim SY, Chang YJ, Cho HM, Hwang Y-W, Moon YS. Non-steroidal anti-inflammatory drugs for the common cold. Cochrane Database Syst Rev. 2015;2015(9):CD006362.
18. Smith SM, Schroeder K, Fahey T. Over-the-counter (OTC) medications for acute cough in children and adults in community settings. Cochrane Database Syst Rev. 2014;2014(11):CD001831.
19. De Sutter AI, Saraswat A, van Driel ML. Antihistamines for the common cold. Cochrane Database Syst Rev. 2015;2015(11):CD009345. https://doi.org/10.1002/14651858.CD009345.pub2.
20. By the 2023 American Geriatrics Society Beers Criteria® Update Expert Panel. American Geriatrics Society 2023 updated AGS Beers Criteria® for potentially inappropriate medication use in older adults. J Am Geriatr Soc. 2023;71(7):2052–81. https://doi.org/10.1111/jgs.18372.
21. Tune LE. Anticholinergic effects of medication in elderly patients. J Clin Psychiatry. 2001;62(Suppl 21):11–4.
22. Araklitis G, Robinson D, Cardozo L. Cognitive effects of anticholinergic load in women with overactive bladder. Clin Interv Aging. 2020;15:1493–503. https://doi.org/10.2147/CIA.S252852.
23. Egberts A, Moreno-Gonzalez R, Alan H, Ziere G, Mattace-Raso FUS. Anticholinergic drug burden and delirium: A systematic review. J Am Med Dir Assoc. 2021;22(1):65–73.e4. https://doi.org/10.1016/j.jamda.2020.04.019.
24. Naseri A, Sadigh-Eteghad S, Seyedi-Sahebari S, Hosseini M-S, Hajebrahimi S, Salehi-Pourmehr H. Cognitive effects of individual anticholinergic drugs: a systematic review and meta-analysis. Neuropsychol. 2023;17:e20220053. https://doi.org/10.1590/1980-5764-DN-2022-0053.
25. Naqvi A, Patel P, Gerriets V. Cetirizine. 2024 May 6. In: StatPearls [Internet]. Treasure Island (FL): StatPearls Publishing; 2024.
26. https://www.mayoclinic.org/drugs-supplements/levocetirizine-oral-route/precautions/drg-20071083?p=1
27. Herzog ED. Neurons and networks in daily rhythms. Nat Rev Neurosci. 2007;8(10):790–802. https://doi.org/10.1038/nrn2215.
28. Tricoire H, Moller M, Chemineau P, Malpaux B. Origin of cerebrospinal fluid melatonin and possible function in the integration of photoperiod. Reprod Suppl. 2003;61:311–21.
29. Frost R, Mathew S, Thomas V, Uddin S, Salame A, Vial C, et al. A scoping review of over-the-counter products for depression, anxiety and insomnia in older people. BMC Complement Med Ther. 2024;24(1):275. https://doi.org/10.1186/s12906-024-04585-0.
30. Waldhauser F, Kovacs J, Reiter E. Age-related changes in melatonin levels in humans and its potential consequences for sleep disorders. Exp Gerontol. 1998;33(7–8):759–72. https://doi.org/10.1016/s0531-5565(98)00054-0.
31. Kunz D, Schmitz S, Mahlberg R, Mohr A, Stoter C, Wolf KJ, et al. A new concept for melatonin deficit: on pineal calcification and melatonin excretion. Neuropsychopharmacology. 1999;21(6):765–72. https://doi.org/10.1016/S0893-133X(99)00069-X.

32. https://www.sleepfoundation.org/insomnia
33. Albert SM, Roth T, Toscani M, Vitiello MV, Zee P. Sleep health and appropriate use of OTC sleep aids in older adults-recommendations of a gerontological society of America workgroup. Gerontologist. 2017;57(2):163–70. https://doi.org/10.1093/geront/gnv139.
34. Maust DT, Solway E, Clark SJ, Kirch M, Singer DC, Malani P. Prescription and nonprescription sleep product use among older adults in the United States. Am J Geriatr Psychiatry. 2019;27(1):32–41. https://doi.org/10.1016/j.jagp.2018.09.004.
35. Baskett JJ, Broad JB, Wood PC, Duncan JR, Pledger MJ, English J, et al. Does melatonin improve sleep in older people? A randomised crossover trial. Age Ageing. 2003;32:164–70. https://doi.org/10.1093/ageing/32.2.164.
36. Singer C, Tractenberg RE, Kaye J, Schafer K, Gamst A, Grundman M, et al. A multicenter, placebo-controlled trial of melatonin for sleep disturbance in Alzheimer's disease. Sleep. 2003;26(7):893–901. https://doi.org/10.1093/sleep/26.7.893.
37. Wade AG, Farmer M, Harari G, Fund N, Laudon M, Nir T, et al. Add-on prolonged-release melatonin for cognitive function and sleep in mild to moderate Alzheimer's disease: A 6-month, randomized, placebo-controlled, multicenter trial. Clin Interv Aging. 2014;9:947–61. https://doi.org/10.2147/CIA.S65625.
38. https://www.nccih.nih.gov/health/melatonin-what-you-need-to-know
39. Mun JG, Wang D, Doerflein Fulk DL, Fakhary M, Gualco SJ, et al. A randomized, double-blind, crossover study to investigate the pharmacokinetics of extended-release melatonin compared to immediate-release melatonin in healthy adults. J Diet Suppl. 2024;21(2):182–94. https://doi.org/10.1080/19390211.2023.2206475.
40. Gooneratne NS, Edwards AYZ, Zhou C, Cuellar N, Grandner MA, Barrett JS. Melatonin pharmacokinetics following two different oral surge-sustained release doses in older adults. J Pineal Res. 2012;52(4):437–45. https://doi.org/10.1111/j.1600-079X.2011.00958.x.
41. Brzezinski A. Melatonin in humans. N Engl J Med. 1997;336(3):186–95. https://doi.org/10.1056/NEJM199701163360306.
42. Papagiannidou E, Skene DJ, Ioannides C. Potential drug interactions with melatonin. Physiol Behav. 2015;2014(131):17–24. https://doi.org/10.1016/j.physbeh.2014.04.016.
43. Abraham O, Schleiden L, Albert SM. Over-the-counter medications containing diphenhydramine and doxylamine used by older adults to improve sleep. Int J Clin Pharm. 2017;39(4):808–17. https://doi.org/10.1007/s11096-017-0467-x.
44. FitzGerald GA, Patrono C. The coxibs, selective inhibitors of cyclooxygenase-2. N Eng J Med. 2001;345(6):433–42. https://doi.org/10.1056/NEJM200108093450607.
45. Graham GG, Davies MJ, Day RO, Mohamudally A, Scott KF. The modern pharmacology of paracetamol: therapeutic actions, mechanism of action, metabolism, toxicity and recent pharmacological findings. Immunopharmacology. 2013;21(3):201–32. https://doi.org/10.1007/s10787-013-0172-x.
46. Moore RA, Wiffen PJ, Derry S, Maguire T, Roy YM, Tyrrell L. Non-prescription (OTC) oral analgesics for acute pain – an overview of Cochrane reviews. Cochrane Database Syst Rev. 2015;2015(11):CD010794. https://doi.org/10.1002/14651858.CD010794.pub2.
47. Moore N, Scheiman JM. Gastrointestinal safety and tolerability of oral non-aspirin over-the-counter analgesics. Postgrad Med. 2018;130(2):188–99. https://doi.org/10.1080/00325481.2018.1429793.
48. https://www.govinfo.gov/content/pkg/FR-2009-04-29/pdf/E9-9684.pdf
49. Jerez-Roig J, Medeiros LF, Silva VA, Bezerra CL, Cavalcante LA, Piuvezam G, et al. Prevalence of self-medication and associated factors in an elderly population: a systematic review. Drugs Aging. 2014;31(12):883–96. https://doi.org/10.1007/s40266-014-0217-x.
50. Karłowicz-Bodalska K, Sauer N, Jonderko L, Wiela-Hojeńska A. Over the counter pain medications used by adults: a need for pharmacist intervention. Int J Environ Res Public Health. 2023;20(5):4505. https://doi.org/10.3390/ijerph20054505.

51. McCarthy DM. Efficacy and gastrointestinal risk of aspirin used for the treatment of pain and cold. Best Pract Res Clin Gastroenterol. 2012;26(2):101–12. https://doi.org/10.1016/j.bpg.2012.01.008.
52. Cai Y, Han Z, Cheng H, Li H, Wang K, Chen J, et al. The impact of ageing mechanisms on musculoskeletal system diseases in the elderly. Front Immunol. 2024;15:1405621. https://doi.org/10.3389/fimmu.2024.140562.
53. Pilotto A, Franceschi M, Leandro G, Di Mario F. NSAID and aspirin use by the elderly in general practice: effect on gastrointestinal symptoms and therapies. Drugs Aging. 2003;20(9):701–10. https://doi.org/10.2165/00002512-200320090-00006.
54. Wongrakpanich S, Wongrakpanich A, Melhado K, Rangaswami J. A comprehensive review of non-steroidal anti-inflammatory drug use in the elderly. Aging Dis. 2018;9:143–50. https://doi.org/10.14336/AD.2017.0306.
55. Garcia Rodriguez LA, Tacconelli S, Patrignani P. Role of dose potency in the prediction of risk of myocardial infarction associated with nonsteroidal anti-inflammatory drugs in the general population. J Am Coll Cardiol. 2008;52(20):1628–36. https://doi.org/10.1016/j.jacc.2008.08.041.
56. https://www.sciencenews.org/article/cox-2-inhibitor-pulled-market
57. Kearney PM, Baigent C, Godwin J, Halls H, Emberson JR, Patrono C. Do selective cyclo-oxygenase-2 inhibitors and traditional nonsteroidal anti-inflammatory drugs increase the risk of atherothrombosis? Meta-analysis of randomised trials. BMJ. 2006;332(7553):1302–8. https://doi.org/10.1136/bmj.332.7553.1302.
58. Page J, Henry D. Consumption of NSAIDs and the development of congestive heart failure in elderly patients: an underrecognized public health problem. Arch Intern Med. 2000;160(6):777–84. https://doi.org/10.1001/archinte.160.6.777.
59. Gooch K, Culleton BF, Manns BJ, Zhang J, Alfonso H, Tonelli M, et al. NSAID use and progression of chronic kidney disease. Am J Med. 2007;120(3):280.e1–7. https://doi.org/10.1016/j.amjmed.2006.02.015.
60. Lanza FL, Marathi UK, Anand BS, Lichtenberger LM. Clinical trial: comparison of ibuprofen-phosphatidylcholine and ibuprofen on the gastrointestinal safety and analgesic efficacy in osteoarthritic patients. Aliment Pharmacol Ther. 2008;28(4):431–42. https://doi.org/10.1111/j.1365-2036.2008.03765.x.
61. Bello AE, Kent JD, Holt RJ. Gastroprotective efficacy and safety of single-tablet ibuprofen/famotidine vs ibuprofen in older persons. Phys Sportsmed. 2015;43(3):193–9. https://doi.org/10.1080/00913847.2015.1066229.
62. No authors listed. Histamine Type-2 receptor antagonists (H2 blockers, 2018). In: LiverTox: clinical and research information on drug-induced liver injury [internet]. Bethesda, MD: National Institute of Diabetes and Digestive and Kidney Diseases; 2012. 2018. Bookshelf ID: NBK547929.
63. Johnell K, Klarin I. The relationship between number of drugs and potential drug-drug interactions in the elderly: a study of over 600,000 elderly patients from the Swedish prescribed drug register. Drug Saf. 2007;30(10):911–8. https://doi.org/10.2165/00002018-200730100-00009.
64. Tulner LR, Frankfort SV, Gijsen GJ, van Campen JP, Koks CH, Beijnen JH. Drug-drug interactions in a geriatric outpatient cohort: prevalence and relevance. Drugs Aging. 2008;25(4):343–55. https://doi.org/10.2165/00002512-200825040-00007.
65. Schneider KL, Kastenmüller K, Weckbecker K, Bleckwenn M, Böhme M, Stingl JC. Potential drug-drug interactions in a cohort of elderly, polymedicated primary care patients on antithrombotic treatment. Drugs Aging. 2018;35(6):559–68. https://doi.org/10.1007/s40266-018-0550-6.
66. Chait M. Gastroesophageal reflux disease: important considerations for the older patients. World J Gastrointest Endosc. 2010;2(12):388–96. https://doi.org/10.4253/wjge.v2.i12.388.
67. Fox RK, Muniraj T. Pharmacologic therapies in gastrointestinal diseases. Med Clin N Am. 2016;100(4):827–50. https://doi.org/10.1016/j.mcna.2016.03.009.

68. Kanno T, Moayyedi P. Proton pump inhibitors in the elderly, balancing risk and benefit: an age-old problem. Curr Gastroenterol Rep. 2019;21(12):65. https://doi.org/10.1007/s11894-019-0732-3.
69. Stedman CA, Barclay ML. Review article: comparison of the pharmacokinetics, acid suppression and efficacy of proton pump inhibitors. Aliment Pharmacol Ther. 2000;14(8):963–78. https://doi.org/10.1046/j.1365-2036.2000.00788.x.
70. Lodato F, Azzaroli F, Turco L, Mazzella N, Buonfiglioli F, Zoli M, et al. Adverse effects of proton pump inhibitors. Best Pract Res Clin Gastroenterol. 2010;24(2):193–201. https://doi.org/10.1016/j.bpg.2009.11.004.
71. Jourdi G, Hulot JS, Gaussem P. An update on oral antiplatelet drug interactions with proton pump inhibitors: what are the risks? Expert Opin Drug Metab Toxicol. 2024;20:749. https://doi.org/10.1080/17425255.2024.2378888.
72. Chey WD, Wong BC. American College of Gastroenterology guideline on the management of Helicobacter pylori infection. Am J Gastroenterol. 2007;102(8):1808–25. https://doi.org/10.1111/j.1572-0241.2007.01393.x.
73. Brandt LJ, Prather CM, Quigley EM, Schiller LR, Schoenfeld P, Talley NJ. Systematic review on the management of chronic constipation in North America. Am J Gastroenterol. 2005;100(Suppl 1):S5–S21. https://doi.org/10.1111/j.1572-0241.2005.50613_2.x.
74. Salari N, Ghasemianrad M, Ammari-Allahyari M, Rasoulpoor S, Shohaimi S, Mohammadi M. Global prevalence of constipation in older adults: a systematic review and meta-analysis. Wien Klin Wochenschr. 2023;135(15–16):389–98. https://doi.org/10.1007/s00508-023-02156-w.
75. Gallagher P, O'Mahony D. Constipation in old age. Best Pract Res Clin Gastroenterol. 2009;23(6):875–87. https://doi.org/10.1016/j.bpg.2009.09.001.
76. Mari A, Hahamid M, Amara H, Baker FA, Yaccob A. Chronic constipation in the elderly patient: updates in evaluation and management. Korean J Fam Med. 2020;41(3):139–45. https://doi.org/10.4082/kjfm.18.0182.
77. Gras-Miralles B, Cremonini F. A critical appraisal of lubiprostone in the treatment of chronic constipation in the elderly. Clin Interv Aging. 2013;8:191–200. https://doi.org/10.2147/CIA.S30729.
78. Ford AC, Moayyedi P, Lacy B, Lembo A, Saio Y, Schiller L, et al. Task force on the management of functional bowel disorders. Am J Gastroenterol. 2014;109 Suppl 1:S2–26; quiz S27. https://doi.org/10.1038/ajg.2014.187.
79. Hannoodee S, Patel P, Annamaraju P. Docusate. Treasure Island (FL): StatPearls Publishing; 2024.
80. Spinzi G, Amato A, Imperiali G, Lenoci N, Mandelli G, Paggi S, et al. Constipation in the elderly: management strategies. Drugs Aging. 2009;26(6):469–74. https://doi.org/10.2165/00002512-200926060-00003.
81. Rao SSC, Go JT. Update on the management of constipation in the elderly: new treatment options. Clin Interv Aging. 2010;5:163–71. https://doi.org/10.2147/cia.s8100.
82. Sajid MS, Hebbar M, Baig MK, Li A, Philipose Z. Use of prucalopride for chronic constipation: A systematic review and meta-analysis of published randomized, controlled trials. J Neurogastroenterol Motil. 2016;22(3):412–22. https://doi.org/10.5056/jnm16004.
83. Mahajan R. Prucalopride: A recently approved drug by the Food and Drug Administration for chronic idiopathic constipation. Int J Appl Basic Med Res. 2019;9(1):1–2. https://doi.org/10.4103/ijabmr.IJABMR_412_18.
84. Flach S, Scarfe G, Dragone J, Ding J, Seymur M, Pennick M, et al. A phase I study to investigate the absorption, pharmacokinetics, and excretion of [(14)C]prucalopride after a single oral dose in healthy volunteers. Clin Ther. 2016;38(9):2106–15. https://doi.org/10.1016/j.clinthera.2016.08.003.
85. Rivkin A, Chagan. Lubiprostone: chloride channel activator for chronic constipation. Clin Ther. 2006;28(12):2008–21. https://doi.org/10.1016/j.clinthera.2006.12.013.

86. Busby RW, Kessler MM, Bartolini WP, Byrant AP, Hannig G, Higgins CS, et al. Pharmacologic properties, metabolism, and disposition of linaclotide, a novel therapeutic peptide approved for the treatment of irritable bowel syndrome with constipation and chronic idiopathic constipation. J Pharmacol Exp Ther. 2013;344(1):196–206. https://doi.org/10.1124/jpet.112.199430.
87. Tan ECK, Eshetie TC, Gray SL, Marcum ZA. Dietary supplement use in middle-aged and older adults. J Nutr Health Aging. 2022;26(2):133–8. https://doi.org/10.1007/s12603-022-1732-9.
88. Bailey RL, Gahche JJ, Miller PE, Thomas PR, Dwyer JT. Why US adults use dietary supplements. JAMA Intern Med. 2013;173(5):355–61. https://doi.org/10.1001/jamainternmed.2013.2299.
89. Hardy ML, Duvall K. Multivitamin/multimineral supplements for cancer prevention: implications for primary care practice. Postgrad Med. 2015;127(1):107–16. https://doi.org/10.1080/00325481.2015.993284.
90. Walrand S. Dietary supplement intake among the elderly: hazards and benefits. Curr Opin Clin Nutr Metab Care. 2018;21(6):465–70. https://doi.org/10.1097/MCO.0000000000000512.
91. Sesso HD, Christen WG, Bubes V, Smith JP, MacFadyen J, Schvartz M, et al. Multivitamins in the prevention of cardiovascular disease in men: the Physicians' Health Study II randomized controlled trial. JAMA. 2012;308(17):1751–60. https://doi.org/10.1001/jama.2012.14805.
92. Kim J, Choi J, Kwon SY, McEvoy JW, Blaha MJ, Blumenthal RS, et al. Association of multivitamin and mineral supplementation and risk of cardiovascular disease: A systematic review and meta-analysis. Circ Cardiovasc Qual Outcomes. 2018;11(7):e004224. https://doi.org/10.1161/CIRCOUTCOMES.117.004224.
93. O'Connor EA, Evans CV, Ivlev I, Rushkin MC, Thomas RG, Martin A, et al. Vitamin, mineral, and multivitamin supplementation for the primary prevention of cardiovascular disease and cancer: a systematic evidence review for the U.S. Preventive Services Task Force Evidence Synthesis, No. 209 Agency for Healthcare Research and Quality (US); Jun Report No: 21-05278-EF-1; 2021. Bookshelf ID: NBK581642.
94. Sesso HD, Rist PM, Aragaki AK, Rautiainen S, Johnson LG, Friedenberg G, et al. Multivitamins in the prevention of cancer and cardiovascular disease: the COcoa supplement and Multivitamin Outcomes Study (COSMOS) randomized clinical trial. Am J Clin Nutr. 2022;115(6):1501–10. https://doi.org/10.1093/ajcn/nqac056.
95. Hennekens CH, Buring JE, Manson JE, Stampfer M, Rosner B, Cook NR, et al. Lack of effect of long-term supplementation with beta carotene on the incidence of malignant neoplasms and cardiovascular disease. N Engl J Med. 1996;334(18):1145–9. https://doi.org/10.1056/NEJM199605023341801.
96. Gaziano JM, Glynn RJ, Christen WG, Kurth T, Belanger C, MacFadyen J, et al. Vitamins E and C in the prevention of prostate and total cancer in men: the Physicians' Health Study II randomized controlled trial. JAMA. 2009;301(1):52–62. https://doi.org/10.1001/jama.2008.862.
97. Dawsey SP, Hollenbeck A, Schatzkin A, Abnet CC. A prospective study of vitamin and mineral supplement use and the risk of upper gastrointestinal cancers. PLoS One. 2014;9(2):e88774. https://doi.org/10.1371/journal.pone.0088774.
98. https://www.nei.nih.gov/learn-about-eye-health/eye-conditions-and-diseases/age-related-macular-degeneration
99. Christen WG, Glynn RJ, Sesso HD, Curth T, Macfadyen J, Bubes V, et al. Vitamins E and C and medical record-confirmed age-related macular degeneration in a randomized trial of male physicians. Ophthalmology. 2012;119(8):1642–9. https://doi.org/10.1016/j.ophtha.2012.01.053.
100. Evans JR, Lawrenson JG. Antioxidant vitamin and mineral supplements for slowing the progression of age-related macular degeneration. Cochrane Database Syst Rev. 2023;9(9):CD000254. https://doi.org/10.1002/14651858.CD000254.

101. Vellos K, Highland J, Yousefzai R, Stoddard A, Johnson E, Gaynes BI. Dosage considerations in the combined use of ocular-specific vitamins and nutrients and multivitamin products: A systemic review and analysis. J Am Pharm Assoc (2003). 2019;59(3):423–31. https://doi.org/10.1016/j.japh.2019.01.013.
102. https://www.fda.gov/food/nutrition-facts-label/daily-value-nutrition-and-supplement-facts-labels
103. Chew EY, Clemons TE, Agrón E, Domalpally A, Keenan TDL, Vitale S, et al. Long-term outcomes of adding lutein/zeaxanthin and ω-3 fatty acids to the AREDS supplements on age-related macular degeneration progression: AREDS2 report 28. JAMA Ophthalmol. 2022;140(7):692–8. https://doi.org/10.1001/jamaophthalmol.2022.1640.
104. Zhang Y, Yang J, Na X, Zhao A. Association between beta-carotene supplementation and risk of cancer: a meta-analysis of randomized controlled trials. Nutr Rev. 2023;81(9):1118–30. https://doi.org/10.1093/nutrit/nuac110.
105. Giustina A, Bouillon R, Dawson-Hughes B, Ebeling PR, Lazaretti-Castro M, Lips P, et al. Vitamin D in the older population: a consensus statement. Endocrine. 2023;79(1):31–44. https://doi.org/10.1007/s12020-022-03208-3.
106. Waterhouse M, Ebeling PR, McLeod DSA, English D, Romero BD, Baxter C, et al. The effect of monthly vitamin D supplementation on fractures: a tertiary outcome from the population-based, double-blind, randomised, placebo-controlled D-Health trial. Lancet Diabetes Endocrinol. 2023;11(5):324–32. https://doi.org/10.1016/S2213-8587(23)00063-3.
107. Grodstein F, O'Brien J, Kang JH, Dushkes R, Cook NR, Okereke O, et al. A randomized trial of long-term multivitamin supplementation and cognitive function in men: the physicians' health study II. Ann Intern Med. 2013;159(12):806–14. https://doi.org/10.7326/0003-4819-159-12-201312170-00006.
108. Baker LD, Manson JE, Rapp SR, Sesso HD, Gaussoin SA, Shumaker SA, et al. Effects of cocoa extract and a multivitamin on cognitive function: a randomized clinical trial. Alzheimers Dement. 2023;19(4):1308–19. https://doi.org/10.1002/alz.12767.
109. Yeung LK, Alschuler DM, Wall M, Luttmann-Gibson H, Copeland T, Hale C, et al. Multivitamin supplementation improves memory in older adults: a randomized clinical trial. Am J Clin Nutr. 2023;118(1):273–82. https://doi.org/10.1016/j.ajcnut.2023.05.011.
110. Harris E, Macpherson H, Vitetta L, Kirk J, Sali A, Pipingas A. Effects of a multivitamin, mineral and herbal supplement on cognition and blood biomarkers in older men: a randomised, placebo-controlled trial. Hum Psychopharmacol. 2012;27(4):370–7. https://doi.org/10.1002/hup.2236.
111. MacPherson H, Ellis KA, Sali A, Pipingas A. Memory improvements in elderly women following 16 weeks treatment with a combined multivitamin, mineral and herbal supplement a randomized controlled trial. Psychopharmacology. 2012;220:351–65. https://doi.org/10.1007/s00213-011-2481-3.
112. Harris E, Macpherson H, Pipingas A. Improved blood biomarkers but no cognitive effects from 16 weeks of multivitamin supplementation in healthy older adults. Nutrients. 2015;7(5):3796–812. https://doi.org/10.3390/nu7053796.
113. Kiani AK, Dhuli K, Donaato K, Aquilanti B, Velluti V, Matera G, et al. Main nutritional deficiencies. J Prev Med Hyg. 2022;63(2 Suppl 3):E93–E101. https://doi.org/10.15167/2421-4248/jpmh2022.63.2S3.2752.
114. https://www.ncbi.nlm.nih.gov/books/NBK234926
115. https://www.futuremarketinsights.com/reports/calcium-supplements-market
116. Chapuy MC, Arlot ME, Duboeuf F, Brun J, Crouzet B, Arnaud S, et al. Vitamin-D3 and calcium to prevent hip fractures in elderly women. N Engl J Med. 1992;327(23):1637–42. https://doi.org/10.1056/NEJM199212033272305.
117. Reid IR, Bristow SM, Bolland MJ. Calcium supplements: benefits and risks. J Intern Med. 2015;278(4):354–68. https://doi.org/10.1111/joim.12394.
118. Bilder GE. Human biological aging: from macromolecules to organ systems. Hoboken, NJ: Wiley; 2016. Chapter 8. p. 3–62.

119. Rogmark C, Fedorowski A, Hamrefors V. Physical activity and psychosocial factors associated with risk of future fractures in middle-aged men and women. J Bone Miner Res. 2021;36(5):852–60. https://doi.org/10.1002/jbmr.4249.
120. McPhee C, Aninye IO, Horan LJ. Recommendations for improving women's bone health throughout the lifespan. Womens Health (Larchmt). 2022;31(12):1671–6. https://doi.org/10.1089/jwh.2022.0361.
121. Dawale K, Agrawal A. Parathyroid hormone secretion and related syndromes. Cureus. 2022;14(10):e30251. https://doi.org/10.7759/cureus.30251.
122. Bolland MJ, Leung W, Tai V, Bastin S, Gamble GD, Grey A, et al. Calcium intake and risk of fracture: systematic review. BMJ. 2015;351:h4580. https://doi.org/10.1136/bmj.h4580.
123. Zhao JG, Zeng XT, Wang J, Liu L. Association between calcium or vitamin D supplementation and fracture incidence in community-dwelling older adults: a systematic review and meta-analysis. JAMA. 2017;318(24):2466–82. https://doi.org/10.1001/jama.2017.19344.
124. US Preventive Services Task Force, Grossman DC, Curry SJ, Owens DK, Barry MJ, Caughey AB, Davidson KW, Doubeni CA, Epling JW Jr, Kemper AR, Krist AH, Kubik M, Landefeld S, Mangione CM, Silverstein M, Simon MA, Tseng C-W. Vitamin D, calcium, or combined supplementation for the primary prevention of fractures in community-dwelling adults: US Preventive Services Task Force Recommendation Statement. JAMA. 2018;319(15):1592–9. https://doi.org/10.1001/jama.2018.3185.
125. Lewis JR, Zhu K, Prince RL. Adverse events from calcium supplementation: relationship to errors in myocardial infarction self-reporting in randomized controlled trials of calcium supplementation. J Bone Miner Res. 2012;27(3):719–22. https://doi.org/10.1002/jbmr.1484.
126. Bolland MJ, Barber PA, Doughty RN, Mason B, Horne A, Ames R, et al. Vascular events in healthy older women receiving calcium supplementation: randomised controlled trial. BMJ. 2008;336(7638):262–6. https://doi.org/10.1136/bmj.39440.525752.BE.
127. Bolland MJ, Avenell A, Baron JA, Grey A, MacLennan GS, Gamble GD, et al. Effect of calcium supplements on risk of myocardial infarction and cardiovascular events: meta-analysis. BMJ. 2010;341:c3691. https://doi.org/10.1136/bmj.c3691.
128. Blaha MJ, Blumenthal RS, Budoff MJ, Nasir K. Understanding the utility of zero coronary calcium as a prognostic test: a Bayesian approach. Circ Cardiovasc Qual Outcomes. 2011;4(2):253–6. https://doi.org/10.1161/CIRCOUTCOMES.110.958496.
129. Anderson JJB, Kruszka B, Delaney JAC, He K, Burke GL, Alonso A, et al. Calcium intake from diet and supplements and the risk of coronary artery calcification and its progression among older adults: 10-year follow-up of the multi-ethnic study of atherosclerosis (MESA). J Am Heart Assoc. 2016;5(10):e003815. https://doi.org/10.1161/JAHA.116.003815.
130. Letavernier E, Daudon M, Vitamin D. Hypercalciuria and kidney stones. Nutrients. 2018;10(3):366. https://doi.org/10.3390/nu10030366.
131. Taylor EN, Hoofnagle AN, Curhan GC. Calcium and phosphorus regulatory hormones and risk of incident symptomatic kidney stones. Clin J Am Soc Nephrol CJASN. 2015;10:667–75. https://doi.org/10.2215/CJN.07060714.
132. Malihi Z, Wu Z, Stewart AW, Lawes CM, Scragg R. Hypercalcemia, hypercalciuria, and kidney stones in long-term studies of vitamin D supplementation: a systematic review and meta-analysis. Am J Clin Nutr. 2016;104:1039–51. https://doi.org/10.3945/ajcn.116.134981.
133. Romani AM. Cellular magnesium homeostasis. Arch Biochem Biophys. 2011;512(1):1–23. https://doi.org/10.1016/j.abb.2011.05.010.
134. Kirkland AE, Sarlo GL, Holton KF. The role of magnesium in neurological disorders. Nutrients. 2018;10(6):730. https://doi.org/10.3390/nu10060730.
135. Ciosek Ż, Kot K, Kosik-Bogacka D, Łanocha-Arendarczyk N, Rotter I. The effects of calcium, magnesium, phosphorus, fluoride, and lead on bone tissue. Biomol Ther. 2021;11(4):506. https://doi.org/10.3390/biom11040506.
136. Gröber U, Schmidt J, Kisters K. Magnesium in prevention and therapy. Nutrients. 2015;7(9):8199–226. https://doi.org/10.3390/nu7095388.

137. https://ods.od.nih.gov/factsheets/Magnesium-HealthProfessional
138. https://www.cdc.gov/nchs/nhanes/index.htm
139. https://www.ars.usda.gov/ARSUserFiles/80400530/pdf/1720/Table_37_SUP_GEN_1720.pdf
140. Wang R, Chen C, Liu W, Zhou T, Xun P, He K, et al. The effect of magnesium supplementation on muscle fitness: a meta-analysis and systematic review. Magnes Res. 2017;30(4):120–32. https://doi.org/10.1684/mrh.2018.0430.
141. Dominguez LJ, Barbagallo M, Lauretani F, Bandinelli S, Bos A, Corsi AM, et al. Magnesium and muscle performance in older persons: the InCHIANTI study. Am J Clin Nutr. 2006;84(2):419–26. https://doi.org/10.1093/ajcn/84.1.419.
142. Moslehi N, Vafa M, Sarrafzadeh J, Rahimi-Foroushani A. Does magnesium supplementation improve body composition and muscle strength in middle-aged overweight women? A double-blind, placebo-controlled, randomized clinical trial. Biol Trace Elem Res. 2013;153:111–8. https://doi.org/10.1007/s12011-013-9672-1.
143. Veronese N, Berton L, Carraro S, Bolzetta F, De Rui M, Perissinotto E, et al. Effect of oral magnesium supplementation on physical performance in healthy elderly women involved in a weekly exercise program: a randomized controlled trial. Am J Clin Nutr. 2014;100(3):974–81. https://doi.org/10.3945/ajcn.113.080168.
144. Schutten JC, Joris PJ, Groendijk I, Eelderink C, Groothof D, van der Veen Y, et al. Effects of magnesium citrate, magnesium oxide, and magnesium sulfate supplementation on arterial stiffness: a randomized, double-blind, placebo-controlled intervention trial. J Am Heart Assoc. 2022;11(6):e021783. https://doi.org/10.1161/JAHA.121.021783.
145. Roguin Maor N, Alperin M, Shturman E, Khairaldeen H, Friedman M, Karkabi K, et al. Effect of magnesium oxide supplementation on nocturnal leg cramps: a randomized clinical trial. JAMA Intern Med. 2017;177(5):617–23. https://doi.org/10.1001/jamainternmed.2016.9261.
146. Devarshi PP, Gustafson K, Grant RW, Mitmesser SH. Higher intake of certain nutrients among older adults is associated with better cognitive function: an analysis of NHANES 2011-2014. BMC Nutr. 2023;9(1):142. https://doi.org/10.1186/s40795-023-00802-0.
147. Barbagallo M, Veronese N, Dominguez LJ. Magnesium in aging, health and diseases. Nutrients. 2021;13(2):463. https://doi.org/10.3390/nu13020463.
148. Bordes C, Leguelinel-Blache G, Lavigne JP, Mauboussin JM, Laureillard D, Faure H, et al. Interactions between antiretroviral therapy and complementary and alternative medicine: a narrative review. Clin Microbiol Infect. 2020;26(9):1161–70. https://doi.org/10.1016/j.cmi.2020.04.019.
149. GBD 2021 Anaemia Collaborators. Prevalence, years lived with disability, and trends in anaemia burden by severity and cause, 1990–2021: findings from the Global Burden of Disease Study 2021. Lancet Haematol. 2023;10(9):e713–34. https://doi.org/10.1016/S2352-3026(23)00160-6.
150. Stauder R, Thein SL. Anemia in the elderly: clinical implications and new therapeutic concepts. Haematologica. 2014;99(7):1127–30. https://doi.org/10.3324/haematol.2014.109967.
151. Wallace DF. The regulation of iron absorption and homeostasis. Clin Biochem Rev. 2016;37(2):51–62. PMCID: PMC5198508
152. Ganz T, Nemeth E. Iron homeostasis in host defence and inflammation. Nat Rev Immunol. 2015;15(8):500–10. https://doi.org/10.1038/nri3863.
153. Wawer AA, Jennings A, Fairweather-Tait SJ. Iron status in the elderly: a review of recent evidence. Mech Ageing Dev. 2018;175:55–73. https://doi.org/10.1016/j.mad.2018.07.003.
154. Lopez-Contreras MJ, Zamora-Porero S, Lopez MA, Marin JF, Zamora S, Perez-Llaas FP. Dietary intake and iron status of institutionalized elderly people: relationship with different factors. J Nutr Health Aging. 2010;14(10):816–21. https://doi.org/10.1007/s12603-010-0118-6.
155. Fleming DJ, Jacques PF, Massaro JM, D'Agostino RB, Wilson PW, Wood RJ. Aspirin intake and the use of serum ferritin as a measure of iron status. Am J Clin Nutr. 2001;74(2):219–26. https://doi.org/10.1093/ajcn/74.2.219.

156. Nilsson-Ehle H, Jagenburg R, Landahl S, Svanborg A. Blood haemoglobin declines in the elderly: implications for reference intervals from age 60 to 88. Eur J Haematol. 2000;65(5):297–305. https://doi.org/10.1034/j.1600-0609.2000.065005297.x.
157. Migone De Amicis M, Poggiali E, Mtta I, Minonzio F, Fabio G, Hu C, et al. Anemia in elderly hospitalized patients: prevalence and clinical impact. Intern Emerg Med. 2015;10(5):581–6. https://doi.org/10.1007/s11739-015-1197-5.
158. Fairweather-Tait SJ, Wawer AA, Gillings R, Jennings A, Myint PK. Iron status in the elderly. Mech Ageing Dev. 2014;136–137:22–8. https://doi.org/10.1016/j.mad.2013.11.005.
159. Hamzat H, Sun H, Ford JC, Macleod J, Soiza RL, Mangoni AA. Inappropriate prescribing of proton pump inhibitors in older patients. Drugs Aging. 2012;29(8):681–90. https://doi.org/10.1007/BF03262283.
160. Britton E, McLaughlin JT. Ageing and the gut. Proc Nutr Soc. 2013;72(1):173–7. https://doi.org/10.1017/S0029665112002807.
161. Tay HS, Soiza RL. Systematic review and meta-analysis: what is the evidence for oral iron supplementation in treating anaemia in elderly people? Drugs Aging. 2015;32(2):149–58. https://doi.org/10.1007/s40266-015-0241-5.
162. Tolkien Z, Stecher L, Mander AP, Pereira DI, Powell JJ. Ferrous sulfate supplementation causes significant gastrointestinal side-effects in adults: a systematic review and meta-analysis. PLoS One. 2015;10(2):e0117383. https://doi.org/10.1371/journal.pone.0117383.
163. Lindblad AJ, Cotton C, Allan GM. Tools for practice iron deficiency anemia in the elderly. Can Fam Phys. 2015;61(2):159.
164. Prentice AM, Mendoza YA, Pereira D, Cerami C, Wegmuller R, Constable A, et al. Dietary strategies for improving iron status: balancing safety and efficacy. Nutr Rev. 2017;75(1):49–60. https://doi.org/10.1093/nutrit/nuw055.
165. Wilson PB. Dietary supplementation is more prevalent among adults with arthritis in the United States population. Complement Ther Med. 2016;29:152–7. https://doi.org/10.1016/j.ctim.2016.10.004.
166. Olivera EJ, Palacios C. Use of supplements in Puerto Rican older adults residing in an elderly project. P R Health Sci J. 2012;31(4):213–9.
167. Di Nicola V. Degenerative osteoarthritis a reversible chronic disease. Regen Ther. 2020;15:149–60. https://doi.org/10.1016/j.reth.2020.07.007.
168. Radu AF, Bungau SG. Management of rheumatoid arthritis: an overview. Cells. 2021;10(11):2857. https://doi.org/10.3390/cells10112857.
169. Nandini CD, Sugahara K. Role of the sulfation pattern of chondroitin sulfate in its biological activities and in the binding of growth factors. Adv Pharmacol. 2006;53:253–79. https://doi.org/10.1016/S1054-3589(05)53012-6.
170. du Souich P, García AG, Vergés J, Montell E. Immunomodulatory and anti-inflammatory effects of chondroitin sulphate. J Cell Mol Med. 2009;13:1451–63. https://doi.org/10.1111/j.1582-4934.2009.00826.x.
171. Block JA, Oegema TR, Sandy JD, Plaas A. The effects of oral glucosamine on joint health: is a change in research approach needed? Osteoarthr Cartil. 2010;18(1):5–11. https://doi.org/10.1016/j.joca.2009.07.005.
172. Singh JA, Noorbaloochi S, MacDonald R, Maxwell LJ. Chondroitin for osteoarthritis. Cochrane Database Syst Rev. 2015;1:CD005614. https://doi.org/10.1002/14651858.CD005614.pub2.
173. Zhu X, Sang L, Wu D, Rong J, Jiang L. Effectiveness and safety of glucosamine and chondroitin for the treatment of osteoarthritis: a meta-analysis of randomized controlled trials. J Orthop Surg Res. 2018;13(1):170. https://doi.org/10.1186/s13018-018-0871-5.
174. https://www.princetonhcs.org/-/media/files/forms/princeton-rehabilitation/womac.pdf
175. Haefeli M, Elfering A. Pain Assessment. Eur Spine J. 2006;15(Suppl 1):S17–24. https://doi.org/10.1007/s00586-005-1044-x.
176. https://oarsi.org/sites/oarsi/files/docs/2013/lequesne_eng_ndex.pdf

177. Gwinnutt JM, Wieczorek M, Rodríguez-Carrio J, Balanescu A, Bischoff-Ferrari HA, Boonen A, et al. Effects of diet on the outcomes of rheumatic and musculoskeletal diseases (RMDs): systematic review and meta-analyses informing the 2021 EULAR recommendations for lifestyle improvements in people with RMDs. RMD Open. 2022;8(2):e002167. https://doi.org/10.1136/rmdopen-2021-002167.
178. Wildi LM, Raynauld J-P, Martel-Pelletier J, Beaulieu A, Bessette L, Morin F, et al. Chondroitin sulfate reduces both cartilage volume loss and bone marrow lesions in knee osteoarthritis patients starting as early as 6 months after initiation of therapy: a randomized, double-blind, placebo-controlled pilot study using MRI. Ann Rheum Dis. 2011;70(6):982–9. https://doi.org/10.1136/ard.2010.140848.
179. Das A Jr, Hammad TA. Efficacy of a combination of FCHG49 glucosamine hydrochloride, TRH122 low molecular weight sodium chondroitin sulfate and manganese ascorbate in the management of knee osteoarthritis. Osteoarthr Cartil. 2000;8(5):343–50. https://doi.org/10.1053/joca.1999.0308.
180. Hochberg MC, Martel-Pelletier J, Monfort J, Möller I, Castillo JR, Arden N, et al. Combined chondroitin sulfate and glucosamine for painful knee osteoarthritis: a multicentre, randomised, double-blind, non-inferiority trial versus celecoxib. Ann Rheum Dis. 2016;75(1):37–44. https://doi.org/10.1136/annrheumdis-2014-206792.
181. Fransen M, Agaliotis M, Nairn L, Votrubec M, Bridgett L, Su S, et al. Glucosamine and chondroitin for knee osteoarthritis: a double-blind randomised placebo-controlled clinical trial evaluating single and combination regimens. Ann Rheum Dis. 2015;74(5):851–8. https://doi.org/10.1136/annrheumdis-2013-203954.
182. Reginster JY, Deroisy R, Rovati LC, Lee RL, Lejeune E, Bruyere O, et al. Long-term effects of glucosamine sulphate on osteoarthritis progression: a randomised, placebo-controlled clinical trial. Lancet. 2001;357(9252):251–6. https://doi.org/10.1016/S0140-6736(00)03610-2.
183. Pavelka K, Gatterova J, Olejarova M, Machacek S, Giacovelli G, Rovati LC. Glucosamine sulfate use and delay of progression of knee osteoarthritis: a 3-year, randomized, placebo-controlled, double-blind studyArch Intern Med. 2002;162(18):2113–23. https://doi.org/10.1001/archinte.162.18.2113.
184. Messier SP, Mihalko S, Loeser RF, Legault C, Jolla J, Pfruender J, et al. Glucosamine/chondroitin combined with exercise for the treatment of knee osteoarthritis: a preliminary study. Osteoarthr Cartil. 2007;15(11):1256–66. https://doi.org/10.1016/j.joca.2007.04.016.
185. Roman-Blas JA, Castañeda S, Sánchez-Pernaute O, Largo R, Herrero-Beaumont G. Combined treatment with chondroitin sulfate and glucosamine sulfate shows no superiority over placebo for reduction of joint pain and functional impairment in patients with knee osteoarthritis: a six-month multicenter, randomized, double-blind, Placebo-Controlled Clinical Trial. Arthritis Rheumatol. 2017;69(1):77–85. https://doi.org/10.1002/art.39819.
186. Volpi N. Chondroitin sulfate safety and quality. Molecules. 2019;24(8):1447. https://doi.org/10.3390/molecules24081447.
187. Pan S-K, Wu S-J, Kim J-M. Preparation of glucosamine by hydrolysis of chitosan with commercial α-amylase and glucoamylase. J Zhejiang Univ Sci B. 2011;12(11):931–4. https://doi.org/10.1631/jzus.B1100065.
188. https://ods.od.nih.gov/factsheets/Omega3FattyAcids
189. Djuricic I, Calder PC. Beneficial outcomes of omega-6 and omega-3 polyunsaturated fatty acids on human health: an update for 2021. Nutrients. 2021;13(7):2421. https://doi.org/10.3390/nu13072421.
190. Tribulova N, Szeiffova Bacova B, Egan Benova T, Knezl V, Barancik M, et al. Omega-3 index and anti-arrhythmic potential of Omega-3 PUFAs. Nutrients. 2017;9(11):1191. https://doi.org/10.3390/nu9111191.
191. Troesch B, Eggersdorfer M, Laviano A, Rolland Y, Smith AD, Warnke I, et al. Expert opinion on benefits of long-chain Omega-3 fatty acids (DHA and EPA) in aging and clinical nutrition. Nutrients. 2020;12(9):2555. https://doi.org/10.3390/nu12092555.

192. van de Rest O, Geleijnse JM, Kok FJ, van Staveren WA, Dullemeijer C, Olderikkert MGM, et al. Effect of fish oil on cognitive performance in older subjects: a randomized, controlled trial. Neurology. 2008;71(6):430–8. https://doi.org/10.1212/01.wnl.0000324268.45138.86.
193. Dangour AD, Allen E, Elbourne D, Fasey N, Fletcher AE, Hardy P, et al. Effect of 2-y n-3 long-chain polyunsaturated fatty acid supplementation on cognitive function in older people: A randomized, double-blind, controlled trial. Am J Clin Nutr. 2010;91:1725–32. https://doi.org/10.3945/ajcn.2009.29121.
194. Mahmoudi MJ, Hedayat M, Sharifi F, Mirarefin M, Nazari N, Mehrdad N, et al. Effect of low dose x-3 poly unsaturated fatty acids on cognitive status among older people: a double-blind randomized placebo-controlled study. J Diabetes Metab Disord. 2014;13(1):34. https://doi.org/10.1186/2251-6581-13-34.
195. Chew EY, Clemons TE, Agron E, Launer LJ, Grodstein F, Bernstein PS, et al. Effect of omega-3 fatty acids, lutein/zeaxanthin, or other nutrient supplementation on cognitive function: the areds2 randomized clinical trial. JAMA. 2015;314(8):791–801. https://doi.org/10.1001/jama.2015.9677.
196. Andrieu S, Guyonnet S, Coley N, Cantet C, Bonnefoy M, Bordes S, et al. Effect of long-term omega 3 polyunsaturated fatty acid supplementation with or without multidomain intervention on cognitive function in elderly adults with memory complaints (MAPT): a randomised, placebo-controlled trial. Lancet Neurol. 2017;16:377–89. https://doi.org/10.1016/S1474-4422(17)30040-6.
197. Witte AV, Kerti L, Hermannstädter HM, Fiebach JB, Schreiber SJ, Schuchardt JP, et al. Long-chain omega-3 fatty acids improve brain function and structure in older adults. Cereb Cortex. 2014;24:3059–68. https://doi.org/10.1093/cercor/bht163.
198. Phillips M, Childs C, Calder P, Roges PJ. No effect of omega-3 fatty acid supplementation on cognition and mood in individuals with cognitive impairment and probable Alzheimer's disease: a randomised controlled trial. Int J Mol Sci. 2015;16(10):24600–13. https://doi.org/10.3390/ijms161024600.
199. Sinn N, Milte CM, Street SJ, Buckley JD, Coates AM, Pekov J, et al. Effects of n-3 fatty acids, EPA v. DHA, on depressive symptoms, quality of life, memory and executive function in older adults with mild cognitive impairment: a 6-month randomised controlled trial. Br J Nutr. 2012;107(11):1682–93. https://doi.org/10.1017/S0007114511004788.
200. Alex A, Abbott KA, McEvoy M, Schofield PW, Garg ML. Long-chain omega-3 polyunsaturated fatty acids and cognitie decline in non-demented adults: a systematic review and meta-analysis. Nutr Rev. 2019;78:563–78. https://doi.org/10.1093/nutrit/nuz073.
201. Canhada S, Castro K, Schweigert Perry I, Luft VC. Omega-3 fatty acids' supplementation in Alzheimer's disease: a systematic review. Nutr Neurosci. 2018;21:529–38. https://doi.org/10.1080/1028415X.2017.1321813.
202. Mozaffarian D, Lemaitre RN, King IB, Song X, Huang H, Sacks FM, et al. Plasma phospholipid long-chain ω-3 fatty acids and total and cause-specific mortality in older adults: a cohort study. Ann Intern Med. 2013;158(7):515–25. https://doi.org/10.7326/0003-4819-158-7-201304020-00003.
203. Del Gobbo LC, Imamura F, Aslibekyan S, Marklund M, Virtanen JK, Wennberg M, et al. Cohorts for heart and aging research in genomic epidemiology (CHARGE) fatty acids and outcomes research consortium (FORCe). ω-3 polyunsaturated fatty acid biomarkers and coronary heart disease: pooling project of 19 cohort studies. JAMA Intern Med. 2016;176(8):1155–66. https://doi.org/10.1001/jamainternmed.2016.2925.
204. Nicholls SJ, Lincoff AM, Garcia M, Bash D, Ballantyne CM, Barter PJ, et al. Effect of high-dose Omega-3 fatty acids vs corn oil on major adverse cardiovascular events in patients at high cardiovascular risk: the STRENGTH randomized clinical trial. JAMA. 2020;324(22):2268–80. https://doi.org/10.1001/jama.2020.22258.
205. Manson JE, Cook NR, Lee IM, Christen W, Bassuk SS, Mora S, et al. Marine n-3 fatty acids and prevention of cardiovascular disease and cancer. N Engl J Med. 2019;380(1):23–32. https://doi.org/10.1056/NEJMoa1811403.

206. Abdelhamid AS, Brown TJ, Brainard JS, Biswas P, Thorpe GC, Moore HJ, et al. Omega-3 fatty acids for the primary and secondary prevention of cardiovascular disease. Cochrane Database Syst Rev. 2018;7(7):CD003177. https://doi.org/10.1002/14651858.CD003177.pub3.
207. Skulas-Ray AC, Wilson PW, Harris WS, Brinton EA, Kris-Etherton PM, et al. Omega-3 fatty acids for the management of hypertriglyceridemia: a science advisory from the American Heart Association. Circulation. 2019;140(12):e673–91. https://doi.org/10.1161/CIR.0000000000000709.
208. Mach F, Baigent C, Catapano AL, Koskinas KC, Casula M, Batimon L, et al. 2019ESC/EAS guidelines for the management of dyslipidaemias: lipid modification to reduce cardiovascular risk. Eur Heart J. 2020;41(1):111–88. https://doi.org/10.1093/eurheartj/ehz455.
209. Siscovick DS, Barringer TA, Fretts AM, Wu JH, Lichtenstein AH, Costello RB, et al. Omega-3 polyunsaturated fatty acid (fish oil) supplementation and the prevention of clinical cardiovascular disease: a science advisory from the American Heart Association. Circulation. 2017;135(15):e867–e84. https://doi.org/10.1161/CIR.0000000000000482.
210. Djuricic I, Calder PC. Pros and cons of long-chain Omega-3 polyunsaturated fatty acids in cardiovascular health. Annu Rev Pharmacol Toxicol. 2023;63:383–406. https://doi.org/10.1146/annurev-pharmtox-051921-090208.
211. Albert BB, Cameron-Smith D, Hofman PL, Cutfield WS. Oxidation of marine omega-3 supplements and human health. Biomed Res Int. 2013;2013:464921. https://doi.org/10.1155/2013/464921.
212. Fatkin D, Cox CD, Martinac B. Fishing for links between omega-3 fatty acids and atrial fibrillation. Circulation. 2022;145(14):1037–9. https://doi.org/10.1161/CIRCULATIONAHA.121.058596.
213. Woodman RJ, Mori TA, Burke V, Puddey IB, Barden A, Watts GF, et al. Effects of purified eicosapentaenoic acid and docosahexaenoic acid on platelet, fibrinolytic and vascular function in hypertensive type 2 diabetic patients. Atherosclerosis. 2003;166(1):85–93. https://doi.org/10.1016/s0021-9150(02)00307-6.
214. Isah T. Rethinking Ginkgo biloba L. Medicinal uses and conservation. Pharmacogn Rev. 2015;9(18):140–8. https://doi.org/10.4103/0973-7847.162137.
215. Singh SK, Srivastav S, Castellani RJ, Plascencia-Villa G, Perry G. Neuroprotective and antioxidant effect of Ginkgo biloba extract against AD and other neurological disorders. Neurotherapeutics. 2019;16(3):666–74. https://doi.org/10.1007/s13311-019-00767-8.
216. Xie L, Zhu Q, Lu J. Can we use Ginkgo biloba extract to treat Alzheimer's disease? Lessons from preclinical and clinical studies. Cells. 2022;11(3):479. https://doi.org/10.3390/cells11030479.
217. Kueper JK, Speechley M, Montero-Odasso M. The Alzheimer's Disease Assessment Scale–Cognitive Subscale (ADAS-Cog): modifications and responsiveness in pre-dementia populations. A narrative review. J Alzheimers Dis. 2018;63(2):423–44. https://doi.org/10.3233/JAD-170991.
218. Lehfeld H, Stemmler M. The newly normed SKT reveals differences in neuropsychological profiles of patients with MCI, mild dementia and depression. Diagnostics (Basel). 2019;9(4):163. https://doi.org/10.3390/diagnostics9040163.
219. Folstein MF, Folstein SE, McHugh PR. "Mini-mental state." A practical method for grading the cognitive state of patients for the clinician. J Psychiatr Res. 1975;12(3):189–98. https://doi.org/10.1016/0022-3956(75)90026-6.
220. Hort J, Duning T, Hoerr R. Ginkgo biloba extract EGb 761 in the treatment of patients with mild neurocognitive impairment: a systematic review. Neuropsychiatr Dis Treat. 2023;19:647–60. https://doi.org/10.2147/NDT.S401231.
221. Gavrilova SI, Preuss UW, Wong JW, Hoerr R, Kaschel R, Bachinskaya N, et al. Efficacy and safety of Ginkgo biloba extract EGb 761® in mild cognitive impairment with neuropsychiatric symptoms: a randomized, placebo-controlled, double-blind, multi-center trial. Int J Geriatr Psychiatry. 2014;29(10):1087–95. https://doi.org/10.1002/gps.4103.

222. Tian J, Shi J, Wei M, Ni J, Fang Z, Gao J, et al. Chinese herbal medicine Qinggongshoutao for the treatment of amnestic mild cognitive impairment: a 52-week randomized controlled trial. Alzheimers Dement. 2019;5(1):441–9. https://doi.org/10.1016/j.trci.2019.03.001.
223. Solomon PR, Adams F, Silver A, Zimmer J, DeVeaux R. Ginkgo for memory enhancement: a randomized controlled trial. JAMA. 2002;288(7):835–40. https://doi.org/10.1001/jama.288.7.835.
224. DeKosky ST, Williamson JD, Fitzpatrick AL, Kronmal RA, Ives DG, Saxton JA, et al. Ginkgo biloba for prevention of dementia: a randomized controlled trial. JAMA. 2008;300(19):2253–62. https://doi.org/10.1001/jama.2008.683.
225. Snitz BE, O'Meara ES, Carlson MC, Arnold AM, Ives DG, Rapp SR, et al. Ginkgo biloba for preventing cognitive decline in older adults: a randomized trial. JAMA. 2009;302(24):2663–70. https://doi.org/10.1001/jama.2009.1913.
226. Vellas B, Coley N, Ousset P-J, Berrut G, Dartigues J-F, Dubois B, et al. Long-term use of standardised ginkgo biloba extract for the prevention of Alzheimer's disease (GuidAge): a randomised placebo-controlled trial. Lancet Neurol. 2012;11:851–9. https://doi.org/10.1016/S1474-4422(12)70206-5.
227. Mix JA, Crews WD Jr. A double-blind, placebo-controlled, randomized trial of Ginkgo biloba extract EGb 761 in a sample of cognitively intact older adults: neuropsychological findings. Hum Psychopharmacol. 2002;17(6):267–77. https://doi.org/10.1002/hup.412.
228. Amieva H, Meillon C, Helmer C, Barberger-Gateau P, Dartigues JF. Ginkgo biloba extract and long-term cognitive decline: a 20-year follow-up population-based study. PLoS One. 2013;8:e52755. https://doi.org/10.1371/journal.pone.0052755.
229. Biggs ML, Sorkin BC, Nahin RL, Kuller LH, Fitzpatrick AL. Ginkgo biloba and risk of cancer: secondary analysis of the Ginkgo Evaluation of Memory (GEM) study. Pharmacoepidemiol Drug Saf. 2010;19(7):694–8. https://doi.org/10.1002/pds.1979.
230. Brinkley TE, Lovato JF, Arnold AM, Furberg CD, Kuller LH, Burke GL, et al. Effect of Ginkgo biloba on blood pressure and incidence of hypertension in elderly men and women. Am J Hypertens. 2010;23(5):528–33. https://doi.org/10.1038/ajh.2010.14.
231. Kuller LH, Ives DG, Fitzpatrick AL, Carlson MC, Mercado C, Lopez OL, et al. Does Ginkgo biloba reduce the risk of cardiovascular events? Circ Cardiovasc Qual Outcomes. 2010;3(1):41–7. https://doi.org/10.1161/CIRCOUTCOMES.109.871640.
232. Tabert M, Seifert R. Critical analysis of ginkgo preparations: comparison of approved drugs and dietary supplements marketed in Germany. Naunyn Schmiedebergs Arch Pharmacol. 2024;397(1):451–61. https://doi.org/10.1007/s00210-023-02602-6.
233. Crawford C, Boyd C, Deuster PA. Dietary supplement ingredients for optimizing cognitive performance among healthy adults: a systematic review. J Altern Complement Med. 2021;27(11):940–58. https://doi.org/10.1089/acm.2021.0135.
234. Harnly JM, Luthria D, Chen P. Detection of adulterated Ginkgo biloba supplements using chromatographic and spectral fingerprints. JAOAC Int. 2012;95(6):1579–87. https://doi.org/10.5740/jaoacint.12-096.
235. Gafner S. Ginkgo extract adulteration in the global market: A brief review. HerbalGram. 2016;109:58–9. American Botanical Council Found on http://cms.herbalgram.org/herbalgram/issue109/hg109-qualcontrol-ginkgo.html
236. Fransen HP, Pelgrom SM, Stewart-Knox B, de Kaste D, Verhagen H. Assessment of health claims, content, and safety of herbal supplements containing Ginkgo biloba. Food Nutr Res. 2010;30:54. https://doi.org/10.3402/fnr.v54i0.5221
237. Mei N, Guo X, Ren Z, Kobayashi D, Wada K, Guo L. Review of Ginkgo biloba-induced toxicity, from experimental studies to human case reports. J Environ Sci Health C Environ Carcinog Ecotoxicol Rev. 2017;35:1–28. https://doi.org/10.1080/10590501.2016.1278298.
238. Yin OQ, Tomlinson B, Waye MM, Chow AH, Chow MS. Pharmacogenetics and herb-drug interactions: experience with Ginkgo biloba and omeprazole. Pharmacogenetics. 2004;14(12):841–50. https://doi.org/10.1097/00008571-200412000-00007.

239. Samuels N, Finkelstein Y, Singer SR, Oberbaum M. Herbal medicine and epilepsy: proconvulsive effects and interactions with antiepileptic drugs. Epilepsia. 2008;49(3):373–80. https://doi.org/10.1111/j.1528-1167.2007.01379.x.
240. Uchida S, Yamada H, Li XD, Maruyama S, Ohmori Y, Oki T, et al. Effects of Ginkgo biloba extract on pharmacokinetics and pharmacodynamics of tolbutamide and midazolam in healthy volunteers. J Clin Pharmacol. 2006;46(11):1290–8. https://doi.org/10.1177/0091270006292628.
241. Stoddard GJ, Archer M, Shane-McWhorter L, Bray BE, Redd DF, Proulx J, et al. Ginkgo and warfarin interaction in a large veterans administration population. AMIA Annu Symp Proc. 2015;2015:1174–83. eCollection 2015
242. Klemow KM, Bartlow A, Crawford J, Kocher N, Shah H, Ritsick M, et al. Medical attributes of St. John's Wort (Hypericum perforatum). In: Benzie IFF, Wachtel-Galor S, editors. Herbal medicine: biomolecular and clinical aspects. 2nd ed. Boca Raton (FL): CRC Press/Taylor & Francis; 2011. Chapter 11.
243. Linde K, Berner M, Kriston L. St John's wort for major depression. Cochrane Database Syst Rev. 2008;2008(4):CD000448. https://doi.org/10.1002/14651858.CD000448.pub3.
244. Hamilton M. A rating scale for depression. J Neurol Neurosurg Psychiatry. 1960;23(1):56–62. https://doi.org/10.1136/jnnp.23.1.56.
245. Seifritz E, Hatzinger M, Holsboer-Trachsler E. Efficacy of Hypericum extract WS() 5570 compared with paroxetine in patients with a moderate major depressive episode – a subgroup analysis. Int J Psychiatry Clin Pract. 2016;20(3):126–32. https://doi.org/10.1080/13651501.2016.1179765.
246. Di Pierro F, Risso P, Settembre R. Role in depression of a multi-fractionated versus a conventional Hypericum perforatum extract. Panminerva Med. 2018;60(4):156–60. https://doi.org/10.23736/S0031-0808.18.03518-8.
247. Sarris J, Fava M, Schweitzer I, Mischoulon D. St John's wort (Hypericum perforatum) versus sertraline and placebo in major depressive disorder: continuation data from a 26-week RCT. Pharmacopsychiatry. 2012;45(7):275–8. https://doi.org/10.1055/s-0032-1306348.
248. Rapaport MH, Nierenberg AA, Howland R, Dording C, Schettler PJ, Mischoulon D. The treatment of minor depression with St. John's Wort or citalopram: failure to show benefit over placebo. J Psychiatr Res. 2011;45(7):931–41. https://doi.org/10.1016/j.jpsychires.2011.05.001.
249. Roby CA, Anderson GD, Kantor E, Dryer DA, Burstein AH. St John's Wort: effect on CYP3A4 activity. Clin Pharmacol Ther. 2000;67(5):451–7. https://doi.org/10.1067/mcp.2000.106793.
250. Whitten DL, Myers SP, Hawrelak JA, Wohlmuth H. The effect of St John's wort extracts on CYP3A: a systematic review of prospective clinical trials. Br J Clin Pharmacol. 2006;62(5):512–26. https://doi.org/10.1111/j.1365-2125.2006.02755.x.
251. Hennessy M, Kelleher D, Spiers JP, Barry M, Kavanagh P, Mulcahy F, et al. St Johns wort increases expression of P-glycoprotein: implications for drug interactions. Br J Clin Pharmacol. 2002;53(1):75–82. https://doi.org/10.1046/j.0306-5251.2001.01516.x.
252. Wang ZQ, Hamman MA, Huang SM, Lesko LJ, Hall SD. Effect of St John's wort on the pharmacokinetics of fexofenadine. Clin Pharmacol Ther. 2002;71(6):414–20. https://doi.org/10.1067/mcp.2002.124080.
253. Johne A, Brockmoller J, Bauer S, Maurer A, Langheinrich M, Roots I. Pharmacokinetic interaction of digoxin with an herbal extract from St John's wort (Hypericumperforatum). Clin Pharmacol Ther. 1999;66(4):338–45. https://doi.org/10.1053/cp.1999.v66.a101944.
254. Frye RF, Fitzgerald SM, Lagattuta TF, Hruska MW, Egorin MJ. Effect of St John's wort on imatinib mesylate pharmacokinetics. Clin Pharmacol Ther. 2004;76(4):323–9. https://doi.org/10.1016/j.clpt.2004.06.007.
255. Breidenbach T, Kliem V, Burg M, Radermacher J, Hoffmann MW, Klempnauer J. Profound drop of cyclosporin A whole blood trough levels caused by St. John's wort (Hypericum perforatum). Transplantation. 2000;69(10):2229–30. https://doi.org/10.1097/00007890-200005270-00052.

256. Tannergren C, Engman H, Knutson L, Hedeland M, Bondesson U, Lennernas H. St John's wort decreases the bioavailability of R- and S-verapamil through induction of the first-pass metabolism. Clin Pharmacol Ther. 2004;75(4):298–309. https://doi.org/10.1016/j.clpt.2003.12.012.
257. Xu H, Williams KM, Liauw WS, Murray M, Day RO, McLachlan AJ. Effects of St John's wort and CYP2C9 genotype on the pharmacokinetics and pharmacodynamics of gliclazide. Br J Pharmacol. 2008;153(7):1579–86. https://doi.org/10.1038/sj.bjp.0707685.
258. Jiang X, Blair EY, McLachlan AJ. Investigation of the effects of herbal medicines on warfarin response in healthy subjects: a population pharmacokinetic-pharmacodynamic modeling approach. J Clin Pharmacol. 2006;46(11):1370–8. https://doi.org/10.1177/0091270006292124.
259. Yun T-K. Brief introduction of Panax ginseng C.A. Meyer. J Korean Med Sci. 2001;16(Suppl):S3–5. https://doi.org/10.3346/jkms.2001.16.S.S3.1011-8934.
260. Wee JJ, Park KM, Chung A-S. Biological activities of ginseng and its application to human health. In: Benzie IFF, Wachtel-Galor S, editors. Herbal medicine: biomolecular and clinical aspects. 2nd ed. Boca Raton (FL): CRC Press/Taylor & Francis; 2011. Chapter 8.
261. Vuksan V, Sung MK, Sievenpiper JL, Stavro PM, Jenkins AL, Di Buono M, et al. Korean red ginseng (Panax ginseng) improves glucose and insulin regulation in well-controlled, type 2 diabetes: results of a randomized, double-blind, placebo-controlled study of efficacy and safety. Nutr Metab Cardiovasc Dis. 2008;18(1):46–56. https://doi.org/10.1016/j.numecd.2006.04.003.
262. Vuksan V, Xu ZZ, Jovanovski E, Jenkins AL, Beljan-Zdravkovic U, Sievenpiper JL, et al. Efficacy and safety of American ginseng (Panax quinquefolius L.) extract on glycemic control and cardiovascular risk factors in individuals with type 2 diabetes: a double-blind, randomized, cross-over clinical trial. Eur J Nutr. 2019;58(3):1237–45. https://doi.org/10.1007/s00394-018-1642-0.
263. Mucalo I, Jovanovski E, Rahelić D, Božikov V, Romić Z, Vuksan V. Effect of American ginseng (Panax quinquefolius L.) on arterial stiffness in subjects with type-2 diabetes and concomitant hypertension. J Ethnopharmacol. 2013;150(1):148–53. https://doi.org/10.1016/j.jep.2013.08.015.
264. Kim JW, Han SW, Cho JY, Chung IJ, Kim JG, Lee KH, et al. Korean red ginseng for cancer-related fatigue in colorectal cancer patients with chemotherapy: a randomised phase III trial. Eur J Cancer. 2020;130:51–62. https://doi.org/10.1016/j.ejca.2020.02.018.
265. Barton DL, Liu H, Dakhil SR, Linquist B, Sloan JA, Nichols CR, et al. Wisconsin Ginseng (Panax quinquefolius) to improve cancer-related fatigue: a randomized, double-blind trial, N07C2. J Natl Cancer Inst. 2013;105(16):1230–8. https://doi.org/10.1093/jnci/djt181.
266. Wu L, Song H, Zhang C, Wang A, Zhang B, Xiong C, et al. Efficacy and safety of Panaz notoginseng Saponins in the treatment of adults with ischemic stroke in China: a randomized clinical trial. JAMA Netw Open. 2023;6(6):e2317574. https://doi.org/10.1001/jamanetworkopen.2023.17574.
267. Baek HI, Ha KC, Park YK, Kim TY, Park SJ. Efficacy and safety of Panax ginseng sprout extract in subjective memory impairment: a randomized, double-blind, placebo-controlled clinical trial. Nutrients. 2024;16(12):1952. https://doi.org/10.3390/nu16121952.
268. Chen Y, Lin L, Wu L, Xu Y, Shergis JL, Zhang AL, et al. Effect of Panax Ginseng (G115) capsules versus placebo on acute exacerbations in patients with moderate to very severe COPD: a randomized controlled trial. Int J Chron Obstruct Pulmon Dis. 2020;15:671–80. https://doi.org/10.2147/COPD.S236425.
269. Gurley BJ, Gardner SF, Hubbard MA, Williams DK, Gentry WB, Cui Y, et al. Clinical assessment of effects of botanical supplementation on cytochrome P450 phenotypes in the elderly: St John's wort, garlic oil, Panax ginseng and Ginkgo biloba. Drugs Aging. 2005;22(6):525–39. https://doi.org/10.2165/00002512-200522060-00006.
270. Kiefer D, Pantuso T. Panax ginseng. Am Fam Phys. 2003;68(8):1539–42.

271. El-Saber Batiha G, Magdy Beshbishy A, Wasef LG, Elewa YHA, Al-Sagan AA, Abd El-Hack ME. Chemical constituents and pharmacological activities of garlic (Allium sativum L.): a review. Nutrients. 2020;12(3):872. https://doi.org/10.3390/nu12030872.
272. Rahman MS. Allicin and other functional active components in garlic: health benefits and bioavailability. Int J Food Prop. 2007;10:245–68. https://doi.org/10.1080/10942910601113327.
273. Borlinghaus, Albrecht F, MCH G, Nwachukwu ID, Slusarenko AJ. Allicin: chemistry and biological properties. Molecules. 2014;19(8):12591–618. https://doi.org/10.3390/molecules190812591.
274. Sobenin IA, Pryanishnikov VV, Kunnova LM, Rabinovich YA, Martirosyan DM, Orekhov AN. The effects of time-released garlic powder tablets on multifunctional cardiovascular risk in patients with coronary artery disease. Lipids Health Dis. 2010;9:119. https://doi.org/10.1186/1476-511X-9-119.
275. Matsumoto S, Nakanishi R, Li D, Alani A, Rezaeian P, Prabhu S, Abraham J, et al. Aged garlic extract reduces low attenuation plaque in coronary arteries of patients with metabolic syndrome in a prospective randomized double-blind study. J Nutr. 2016;146(2):427S–32S. https://doi.org/10.3945/jn.114.202424.
276. Wlosinska M, Nilsson AC, Hlebowicz J, Hauggaard A, Kjellin M, Fakhro M, et al. The effect of aged garlic extract on the atherosclerotic process – a randomized double-blind placebo-controlled trial. BMC Complement Med Ther. 2020;20(1):132. https://doi.org/10.1186/s12906-020-02932-5.
277. Wlosinska M, Nilsson AC, Hlebowicz J, Malmsjö M, Fakhro M, Lindstedt S. Aged garlic extract preserves cutaneous microcirculation in patients with increased risk for cardiovascular diseases: a double-blinded placebo-controlled study. Int Wound J. 2019;16(6):1487–93. https://doi.org/10.1111/iwj.13220.
278. Serrano JCE, Castro-Boqué E, García-Carrasco A, Morán-Valero MI, González-Hedström D, Bermúdez-López M, et al. Antihypertensive effects of an optimized aged garlic extract in subjects with grade I hypertension and antihypertensive drug therapy: a randomized, triple-blind controlled trial. Nutrients. 2023;15(17):3691. https://doi.org/10.3390/nu15173691.
279. Ried K, Frank OR, Stocks NP. Aged garlic extract reduces blood pressure in hypertensives: a dose-response trial. Eur J Clin Nutr. 2013;67(1):64–70. https://doi.org/10.1038/ejcn.2012.178.
280. Bordia A, Verma SK, Srivastava KC. Effect of garlic (Allium sativum) on blood lipids, blood sugar, fibrinogen and fibrinolytic activity in patients with coronary artery disease. Prostaglandins Leukot Essent Fatty Acids. 1998;58(4):257–63. https://doi.org/10.1016/s0952-3278(98)90034-5.
281. Srivastava K. Evidence for the mechanism by which garlic inhibits platelet aggregation. Prostaglandins Leukot Med. 1986;22(3):313–21. https://doi.org/10.1016/0262-1746(86)90142-3.
282. Macan H, Uykimpang R, Alconcel M, Takasu J, Razon R, Amagase H, et al. Aged garlic extract may be safe for patients on warfarin therapy. J Nutr. 2006;136(3 Suppl):793S–5S. https://doi.org/10.1093/jn/136.3.793S.
283. Elvir Lazo OL, White PF, Lee C, Cruz Eng H, Matin JM, Lin C, et al. Use of herbal medication in the perioperative period: potential adverse drug interactions. J Clin Anesth. 2024;95:111473. https://doi.org/10.1016/j.jclinane.2024.111473.
284. Zhai B, Zhang C, Sheng Y, Zhao C, He X, Xu W, et al. Hypoglycemic and hypolipidemic effect of S-allyl-cysteine sulfoxide (alliin) in DIO mice. Sci Rep. 18(8, 1):3527. https://doi.org/10.1038/s41598-018-21421-x.
285. Piscitelli SC, Burstein AH, Welden N, Gallicano KD, Falloon J. The effect of garlic supplements on the pharmacokinetics of saquinavir. Clin Infect Dis. 2002;34:234–8. https://doi.org/10.1086/324351.
286. Blalock SJ, Gregory PJ, Patel RA, Norton LL, Callahan LF, Jordan JM. Factors associated with potential medication-herb/natural product interactions in a rural community. Altern Ther Health Med. 2009;15(5):26–34.

287. Matura JM, Shea LA, Bankes VA. Dietary supplements, cytochrome metabolism, and pharmacogenetic considerations. Ir J Med Sci. 2022;191(5):2357–65. https://doi.org/10.1007/s11845-021-02828-4.
288. Ryff CD, Seeman T, Weinstein M. National survey of midlife development in the United States (MIDUS II): biomarker project, 2004–2009: inter-university consortium for political and social research 2012; 2013. https://doi.org/10.3886/ICPSR29282.v2.
289. Kaufman DW, Kelly JP, Rosenberg L, Anderson TE, Mitchell AA. Recent patterns of medication use in the ambulatory adult population of the United States: the Slone survey. JAMA. 2002;287(3):337–44. https://doi.org/10.1001/jama.287.3.337.
290. Serper M, McCarthy DM, Patzer RE, King JP, Bailey SC, Smith SG, et al. What patients think doctors know: beliefs about provider knowledge as barriers to safe medication use. Patient Educ Couns. 2013;93(2):306–11. https://doi.org/10.1016/j.pec.2013.06.030.
291. Fielding S, Slovic P, Johnston M, Lee AJ, Bond CM, Watson MC, et al. Public risk perception of non-prescription medicines and information disclosure during consultations: a suitable target for intervention? Int J Pharm Pract. 2018;26(5):423–32. https://doi.org/10.1111/ijpp.12433.
292. Stone JA, Lester CA, Aboneh EA, Phelan CH, Welch LL, Chui MA. A preliminary examination of over the counter medication misuse rates in older adults. Res Social Adm Pharm. 2017;13(1):187–92. https://doi.org/10.1016/j.sapharm.2016.01.004.
293. Sarma N, Giancaspro G, Venema J. Dietary supplements quality analysis tools from the United States Pharmacopeia. Drug Test Anal. 2016;8(3–4):418–23. https://doi.org/10.1002/dta.1940.

Anti-aging Drugs

Abbreviations

AD	Alzheimer's disease
AMPK	AMP protein kinase
CV	Cardiovascular
D	Dasatinib
DNA	Deoxyribonucleic acid
F	Fisetin
FDA	Food and Drug Administration
GLP-1	Glucagon like peptide-1
mTOR	Mechanistic target of rapamycin
mTORC1	mTOR complex 1
mTORC2	mTOR complex 2
NAD+	Nicotinamide adenine dinucleotide
PK	Pharmacokinetics
Q	Quercetin
RCT	Randomized controlled trial
SASP	Senescent-associated secretory phenotype
STACs	Sirtuin Activating Compounds
T2DM	Type 2 diabetes mellitus
µM	Micromolar

INTRODUCTION. THERAPEUTIC EXPECTATION OF ANTI-AGING DRUGS The older adult is defined demographically with population statistics (see Chap. 1) and individually as a biological phenotype. By definition, the phenotype encompasses the entirety of an individual's physiology (generally structure, function, and interrelations of the two) influenced by the interaction of an individual's genes with the environment. The inherited genes, the actual DNA sequence (popularly, the blueprint for the human body), is termed the genotype. The phenotype and genotype of each individual are now readily accessible with a plethora of probes: measurement of biomarkers, internal assessments with imaging techniques, physiological analysis of conditions of rest, stress and disease, whole genome sequencing and epigenetic analyses [1]. However, the *phenotype that represents healthy aging and longevity is considered the most complex of all phenotypes* [2] and this is one that future pharmacotherapy seeks to improve and prolong.

Of significance to the development of anti-aging drugs is the knowledge that *aging is the premier risk factor for major diseases* [3]. Therefore, it is reasoned that preventing or forestalling key aspects of aging should also prevent or forestall the onset of principal chronic diseases, e.g., cardiovascular, cancer and neurodegenerative diseases [4] (illustrated in Fig. 10.1). This hypothesis, originating from a rapidly growing research sector of aging called Geroscience [6], is expected to increase the number of diseases and disability-free years referred to as the health span and decrease the number of years managing diseases and disabilities referred to as the senescent span [4] (see Fig. 10.2).

Extension of the health span and, additionally, the lifespan has already been achieved in several animal models (fruit fly, roundworm, mouse, nonhuman primate) with one of three approaches: caloric restriction [7–9], genetic manipulations [10] and use of select anti-aging drugs [11, 12]. A fourth intervention that increases the health span, though absent data on the life span effect in humans, is adherence

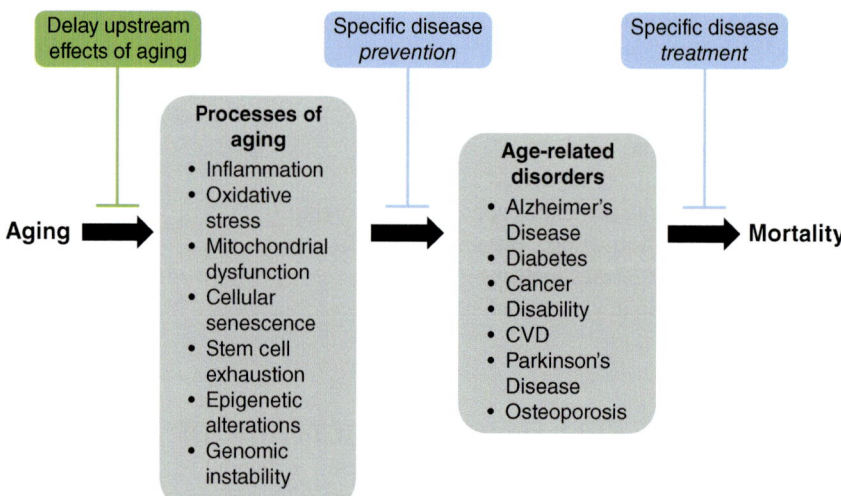

Fig. 10.1 Compressing morbidity by slowing the processes of aging. Slowing the fundamental biological processes of aging as a tactic for delaying the age of onset of multiple co-morbidities, as opposed to preventing or treating individual age-associated clinical disorders. (Reproduced with permission from Seals and Melov [5])

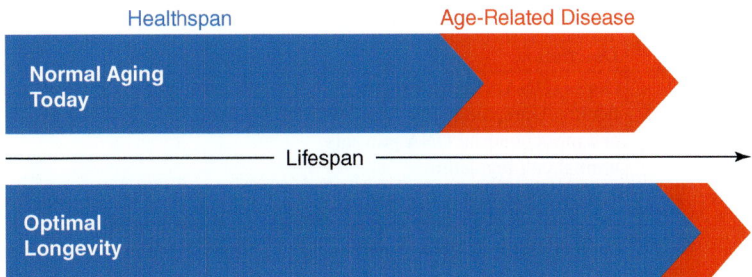

Fig. 10.2 Increasing healthspan and optimal longevity. Comparision of current vs. ideal healthspan. Extending healthspan is a critical component of achieving optimal longevity, defined as living long, but with good health, function, productivity and independence. (Reproduced with permission from Seals and Melov [5])

to a program of lifelong aerobic and resistance exercise [13, 14]. Physical exercise is mentioned repeatedly as an effective nonpharmacological prevention and co-therapy for primary diseases (see Chaps. 4 and 5). The focus of this chapter is the current development of pharmacotherapy with anti-aging drugs, which could be used in conjunction with exercise. Tables 10.1 and 10.2 supplement the narrative.

HALLMARKS OF AGING It was proposed approximately 10 years ago that the aging phenotype is largely dependent on specific physiological mechanisms termed the hallmarks of aging [4]. At that time 9 hallmarks of aging were observed. Those initially identified were (1) DNA instability, (2) telomere attrition (shortening of the ends of chromosomes), (3) epigenetic alterations (changes in gene expression), (4) loss of proteostasis (aberrant protein metabolism), (5) deregulated nutrient-sensing (altered general metabolism of sugars, fats, etc.), (6) mitochondrial dysfunction (loss of energy), (7) cellular senescence (cell aging), (8) stem cell exhaustion (inability to replace missing cells), and (9) altered intercellular communication (reduced interaction between cells) [4].

Recently, five additional age changes were added as hallmarks of aging: (1) disabled macroautophagy (inability to recycle harmful proteins), (2) chronic inflammation, (3) microbiome disturbances (bacterial imbalance in gastrointestinal (GI) tract), (4) altered mechanical properties, and (5) splicing dysregulation (abnormal gene rearrangement) [15, 16]. The hallmarks of aging are explained in detail in Table 10.1. Thus far, anti-aging therapy in clinical trials has investigated (a) deregulated nutrient-sensing, (b) cell senescence, (c) epigenetic alterations, (d) chronic inflammation and (e) microbiome disturbances. Clinical results are discussed in more detail below. Notably, many of the clinical trials, with some exceptions, enrolled the older adult (see Table 10.2).

Table 10.1 Hallmarks of aging and impact on aging

Hallmark	Description	Impact on aging
1. Genetic instability	Genes (DNA) require structural fidelity. Unrepaired damage of nuclear and mitochondrial DNA prevents normal cell regulation.	Reduced organ function creates vulnerability to stress and disease
2. Telomere attrition	Telomeres are the noncoding protective ends of chromosomes. With the replication of DNA during each cell division, the telomeres shorten. Critical shortening inhibits future cell division	Cells that no longer can divide, accumulate toxic material. Cell renewal (replacement) is essential for optimal organ function
3. Epigenetic alterations	Genes are highly regulated by processes such as DNA methylation, histone acetylation, chromosome remodeling and noncoding RNA. Changes in these processes influence which genes are expressed and which become silent.	Impaired gene expression suppresses and corrupts normal cell function
4. Loss of proteostasis	Proteostasis is a network that supports the proper folding of proteins and appropriate disposal when proteins are no longer needed. The disappearance of this network promotes the accumulation of aberrant, nonfunctional proteins	The presence of abnormal and unwanted proteins results in a buildup of aggregates of misfolded proteins that contributes to pathologies of AD and Parkinson's disease.
5. Deregulated nutrient-sensing	Extensive complex of ligands, enzyme pathways, and gene regulators that sense nutrients, e.g., sugars and stress levels. Largely driven by the mTOR complex and highly interactive with other hallmarks.	Deregulation in the form of overstimulation depresses processes of autophagy, anti-oxidation and DNA repair, changes that accelerate aging.
6. Disabled macroautophagy	Macroautophagy is a "recycling" process that dismantles damaged proteins and lipids to re-utilize essential components. Loss of macroautophagy allows unwanted macromolecules to accumulate.	The buildup of unwanted proteins and lipids reduces the availability of essential molecules and produces a toxic environment that harms the cell.
7. Mitochondrial dysfunction	Mitochondria are organelles that assist with the metabolism of nutrients and produce the energy molecule ATP. Mitochondria also cross-talk with the nucleus and, when needed, issue the command for a cell to disappear (apoptosis, cell suicide).	Dysfunctional mitochondria fail to produce an adequate amount of energy for the cell, produce harmful reactive oxygen species and cause the cell to disappear, leading to organ atrophy.
8. Cell senescence	Aging of normal cells characterized by an increase in size, secretion of pro-inflammatory factors, pro-aging factors and enzymes destructive to surroundings and resisting apoptosis	The presence of senescent cells decreases organ function, promotes low-grade inflammation and initiates diseases

(continued)

Table 10.1 (continued)

Hallmark	Description	Impact on aging
9. Stem cell exhaustion	A stem cell is pluripotent (replacing itself or becoming any other cell type). Stem cell niches occur in most tissues to replace lost cells and are subject to hallmarks of aging as other cell types.	Stem cell exhaustion decreases organ renewal and repair following injury. Organ function declines and is more vulnerable to future insults.
10. Altered intercellular communication	Communication between cells depends on components of multiple systems, e.g., CNS, RAAS, HPA and many circulating pro and anti-aging factors. These systems decline with age.	Intercellular communication facilitates optimal responses to internal and external stresses. Deterioration in intercellular communication weakens the organism.
11. Chronic inflammation	Chronic systemic inflammation (inflammaging) exerts negative effects throughout the body and adds to age changes in the immune system. This hallmark is highly integrated with all other hallmarks.	Chronic inflammation primes the body for pathologies, e.g., atherosclerosis, cancers, osteoarthritis, vertebral degeneration
12. Dysbiosis	The diverse bacteria in the intestinal tract (collectively the microbiota) serve multiple functions: nutrient processing, production of essential compounds: vitamins, bile acids, fatty acids, amino acids, and cross-talk with the CNS and PNS. Disruption of this network between the microbiota and organ systems creates dysbiosis.	The change in the bacterial profile of microbiota with aging is associated with immunosenescence, cognitive decline and pathologies, e.g., obesity and T2DM
13. Dysregulation of RNA processing	Genes (DNA) transcribe (code for) RNA, which translates this information into specific amino acid sequences unique to each protein. Proteins serve as enzymes, antibodies, structural components, channels, transporters and hormones. Perturbation of this intermediate stage will adversely impact the formation of proteins	Disruption of RNA processing produces defective proteins or abnormal levels of protein with wide repercussions on many other hallmarks of aging.
14. Altered mechanical properties	Many cells are highly mobile depending on the flexibility of fibrous and collageneous proteins; internally the cytoskeleton and nuclear structures allow the flow of essential molecules. Altered external and internal structural proteins prevent normal cell behavior.	Cells need to move or change shape in response to stress; Cross-linking of structural proteins or replacement with mechanically deficient proteins produces organ stiffness and contributes to pathologies, e.g., hypertension and heart failure.

Refs. [4, 15–17]

AD Alzheimer's disease, *CNS* central nervous system, *PNS* peripheral nervous system, *RAAS* renin-angiotensin-aldosterone-system, *HPA* hypothalamic-pituitary axis, *mTOR* mechanistic target of rapamycin, named because rapamycin acts by inhibiting this complex, *T2DM* Type 2 diabetes mellitus

Anti-aging Drugs

RAPAMYCIN AND RAPALOGUES Rapamycin is an FDA-approved macrolide antibiotic and organ transplant immunosuppressant. Structural analogs of rapamycin termed rapalogues, such as everolimus, are also FDA approved and are used as a stent coating to prevent restenosis (reclosure of an artery). Additionally, rapamycin, a well-studied inhibitor of mTOR (discussed below), is the first pharmacological agent to consistently extend the maximal lifespan in all species tested thus far: yeast [50], roundworm [51], fruit fly [52], and mouse [11, 53]. Prior to these spectacular results, life-long caloric restriction (generally a 35% daily calorie reduction) was the only intervention that increased the maximal lifespan of all species studied [54, 55]. Of particular importance with rapamycin is the observation that administration of rapamycin to mice late in life (at 19 months) also extended the life span and did so in both sexes [11], and furthermore, the positive effects lasted long after the termination of rapamycin therapy [56]. This signaled the utility of rapamycin and rapalogues as anti-aging compounds that diminish established age changes. Additionally, it spotlighted the advent of a novel ant-aging therapy with effects persisting beyond the drug's presence [57]. Since these seminal findings, rapamycin has been evaluated in many genetic models of disease and as expected from its lifespan extension effects, rapamycin also retards disease progression in cancers, neurodegenerative diseases (Alzheimer's disease, AD models, Parkinson's disease, Parkinson's disease models), and cardiovascular pathologies [57]. Furthermore, rapamycin treatment in mice slowed age-associated cognitive decline, improved immune function and suppressed negative effects of cell senescence (characteristic aging at the cell level) [57].

Rapamycin and Rapalogues. Mechanism of Action Rapamycin and rapalogues inhibit the enzyme, mTOR (named derived from **m**echanistic **t**arget **o**f **r**apamycin) [58–60]. mTOR is a serine/threonine kinase that is strongly instrumental in regulating metabolism, cell growth and proliferation, aging and disease and is considered "one of the most important signaling networks in biology" [61]. Its overexpression is clearly a hallmark of aging (see Table 10.1). Two multi-compound complexes, mTORC1 and mTORC2 have been identified with distinct but overlapping functions [61]. mTORC1 (of which the most is known), activates many pathways to achieve cell growth and proliferation and does so only in the presence of an abundance of nutrients, e.g., proteins, fats, nucleotides, and ATP [61]. To achieve this, mTORC1 regulates an incredible array of enzymes, transcriptional factors, binding proteins, receptors, metabolic mediators, hormones, e.g., insulin and organelles, e.g., mitochondria and lysosomes [61]. In starvation, as with caloric restriction without malnutrition, the limited amount of nutrients inhibits mTORC1, permitting other less harmful metabolic pathways to be activated [61]. *Pharmacological inhibition of mTORC1 by rapamycin or caloric restriction-nutrient-based inhibition of mTOR optimizes metabolic pathways with less oxidative stress, reduced insulin use and efficient recycling to preserve tissue function and thereby extend the healthspan and lifespan.*

Rapamycin and Rapalogues. Clinical Evidence In humans, rapamycin has been evaluated in older adults in 4 clinical trials (see Table 10.2). These were mostly small studies with older adults, 3 of which evaluated orally administered rapamycin for 1–3 months and found rapamycin to be relatively safe [43], able to prevent immune suppression induced by cancer surgery [45] and to reduce some senescent biomarkers in patients undergoing cardiac rehabilitation [46]. In the fourth study, rapamycin, applied topically for 6–8 months, produced anti-aging skin effects by reducing senescent cell number and enhancing normal collagen synthesis [44]. A larger randomized clinical trial (RCT) with over 200 healthy older adults treated for 6 weeks with the rapalogue, everolimus, demonstrated enhanced immunity to influenza vaccination [42], suggesting enhancement of one aspect of immunosenescence (aging of the immune system).

METFORMIN One of the first drugs considered to have anti-aging therapeutic potential is metformin. Approved by the FDA in 1995 for the treatment of Type 2 diabetes mellitus (T2DM), it is currently the "first-line therapy for newly diagnosed individuals with T2DM" [62, 63] (see Chap. 4).

Metformin. Mechanism of Action Metformin exerts multiple effects. Glucose lowering and increased insulin sensitivity of metformin are due to effects on both the liver and intestine [64], largely but not solely from activation of the energy sensor, adenosine monophosphate-activated protein kinase (AMPK) [65]. In addition to the activation of AMPK in the enterocytes of the intestine, metformin enhances glucagon-like peptide-1 (GLP-1) release and wields beneficial effects on the metabolism of the microbiota (intestinal bacteria) [64]. Other effects of metformin include inhibition of monocyte-macrophage conversion necessary for the progression of the atherosclerotic plaque [66], suppression of antiinflammatory mediators in cell cultures, animals and nondiabetic humans [19], inhibition of the nutrient-sensing protein complex, mTORC1, that links nutrients with the synthesis of macromolecules when sufficient ATP is available [67] and endothelium protection (safeguarding lining of blood vessels) [68].

Metformin. Anti-aging Effects In consideration of the many effects whereby metformin might interfere with pro-aging pathways, metformin is proposed as a "geroprotector," that is, a drug that could extend the healthspan and possibly the lifespan of humans [69] (see Fig. 10.1). However, metformin-induced extension of healthspan and lifespan in animal models of aging (roundworm, rodents) has been confirmed in some studies [69–72] but not in others [73–75]. Furthermore, studies showing an increase in lifespan have been criticized for the use of metformin concentrations (as with roundworms) or plasma levels (as in rodents) manyfold higher than the average acceptable metformin level of 20 μM in man [76].
Nevertheless, a retrospective observational analysis of 2000 subjects taking metformin or sulfonylurea monotherapy compared with case-matched patients without diabetes concluded that diabetic patients taking metformin lived longer than non-diabetic controls and those taking sulfonylureas [77]. A systematic meta-analysis of

Table 10.2 Anti-aging pharmacological therapies

Drug class	Relevant drug/compound	Aging target(s)	Clinical trials
Metabolic modulator	Metformin, approved first-line therapy for T2DM	Multiple pathways: Activation of energy sensor, AMP protein kinase that influences many downstream pathways, e.g., inhibition of nutrient sensor, mTOR complex, ↓ Oxidative stress and pro-inflammatory mediators Removes senescent cells Effects on glucose/insulin control/fatty acid metabolism in both hepatic and extrahepatic (microbiota) domains Protective effects on vascular endothelial cells (blood vessels)	(1) 6 wks, 14 glucose intolerant pts, crossover study shows differential expression of genes in skeletal muscle and subcutaneous fat that support anti-aging effects (enhancing DNA repair, metabolism, collagen and mitochondria) MILES (Metformin In Longevity Study [23]) (2) 2 wks pretreatment with metformin/placebo, 20 glucose tolerant volunteers ~70 years (+ 5 days bed rest prevents disuse-muscle atrophy by preserving muscle fibers, decreasing inflammation and preventing matrix remodeling [18] (3) Subset analysis of NCT00473876 measures plasma cytokines after 4 months of metformin in 33 nondiabetic CV pts (63 years) and shows ↓ presence of proinflammatory cytokines, especially aging-associated cytokine CCL11 (C-C motif chemokine ligand 11) [19]. 4.1 year metformin treatment of 80 pts with MCI, overweight/obese with untreated diabetes show improvement on one of two cognitive tests; ave. age 65 years [20] *Ongoing Trials* (4) >7000 prediabetic with CV disease, ≥ 18 years, metformin or placebo 4.5 years; primary outcome—time to death, CV event, hospitalization. CSP #2002—Investigation of Metformin in Pre-Diabetes on Atherosclerotic Cardiovascular OuTcomes (VA-IMPACT) NCT02915198 ongoing (5) Phase II- 145 pts. ≥65 years metformin/placebo for 2 years, frailty scale as primary endpoint expected improvement due to antiinflammatory and ↓ insulin resistance with metformin (Metformin for Preventing Frailty in High-risk older adults NCT02570672 ongoing) (6) 6 years, 14 centers, 3000 volunteers (65–79) metformin or placebo to determine the ability of metformin to forestall age-associated diseases: CV, cancer, dementia, and decrease mortality, functional age changes and biomarkers. Proposed trial TAME (*Targeting Aging with Metformin*) [24, 35]

Sirtuin activating compounds (STACs)	Resveratrol, SRT2104	STACs activate sirtuins. Sirtuins (SIRT1, SIRT6 and SIRT7) deacetylate histones surrounding DNA, exerting epigenetic effects and changing gene expression. Sirtuins influence energy metabolism, cell survival, DNA repair, tissue regeneration, and ↓ inflammation and ROS. Sirtuins are activated by caloric restriction in mice, resulting in ↑ healthspan and lifespan.	(1) SRT2104 (2 g/d) 28 days, small crossover study—producing favorable lipid profile, no anti-aging effects on vascular or platelet function, ave. age 38 years [36]. (2) SRT2104 @ 4 doses 0.25–2 g/d, 28 days in T2DM does not improve glycemic control but did improve lipid profile; PK not dose related and variable [37]. (3) SRT2104 @ 0.5–1 g/d, 39 moderate-severe psoriasis pts., 84 days show improvement in skin biopsies of psoriasis; ↓ responsive genes for IL-17 and TNFα, ave. age 40–50 year range; GI adverse effects [38]. (4) SRT2104 chronic (1 wk) and acute 2 g/d ↓ inflammatory response to LPS-injection in health volunteers (18–35 years) [39]. (5) SRT2104 at 50 or 500 mg/d, 8 wks in 26 mild-moderate UC pt. is without ameliorative effects due to study faults, but UC biomarker, calprotectin, significantly reduced [40]. (6) SRT2104 in 15 T2DM pts., 28 days 2 g/d show significant weight loss but no effect on glucose control or endothelial or platelet function, ave. age 58 years [41].
Rapamycin and rapalogs	Rapamycin (sirolimus), RAD001(everolimus)	Inhibits mTORC1, chief regulator of metabolism and inhibitor of autophagy. With mTOR inhibition, other more efficient metabolic pathways are utilized, with reduced oxidative stress and the need for insulin.	(1) Everolimus for 6 wks, 3 doses in 218 healthy ≥65 years ↑ antibody titers to influenza vaccine given 2 wks post dosing and 4 wks post vaccination. Mouth ulcers are the most common adverse effect [42]. (2) Rapamycin 11 healthy adults (70–95 years) 1 mg 8 wks is safe but no effect on cognition, inflammatory markers, physical activities, or glycemic control; ↓ RBC parameters [43]. (3) Rapamycin, topically 6–8 months, improves aging skin in 11/13 older adults by decreasing biomarkers of senescent cells and stimulating collagen VII production [44]. (4) Rapamycin low dose, 28 d prior to bladder cancer surgery reduces surgery-induced immune dysfunction, ave. age 70 [45]. (5) Rapamycin low dose to cardiac rehabilitation pts., 12 wks ↓ senescent cells in fat and inflammatory markers but no effect on frailty, ave. age 74 years [46].

(continued)

Table 10.2 (continued)

Drug class	Relevant drug/compound	Aging target (s)	Clinical trials
Senolytics	Dasatinib + quercetin (D + Q); fisetin (F); (ABT-263, A1331852, A1155463—only animal studies thus far)	Death of senescent cells. This results in the permanent removal of these harmful aged cells that were chronic producers of inflammatory mediators and destructive enzymes.	(1) Pilot feasibility study of D + Q, 3 doses/wk., 3 wks, treatment of 14 idiopathic pulmonary fibrosis (IPF) pts—improved general physical function but no effect on pulmonary function; mild-moderate adverse effects, ave. age 71 years [47] (2) Pilot feasibility study of D + Q to 5 AD pts. for 12 wks—no effect on cognition or neuroimaging but trending decrease in SASP factors, only D entered brain, ave. age 76 years [48] (3) D + Q for 3 days to 9 diabetic CKD pts. ↓senescent cells in adipose tissue but not in skin, ↓ secretory factors in plasma [49] *Ongoing Trials* NCT03675724 Alleviation by Fisetin of Frailty, Inflammation, and Related Measures in Older Adults NCT03430037 Alleviation by Fisetin of Frailty, Inflammation, and Related Measures in Older Women NCT06113016 Prevention of Frailty With Fisetin and Exercise (PROFFi) in Breast Cancer Survivors NCT04815902 Use of Senolytic and Anti-Fibrotic Agents to Improve the Beneficial Effect of Bone Marrow Stem Cells for Osteoarthritis NCT04210986 completed Senolytic Drugs Attenuate Osteoarthritis-Related Articular Cartilage Degeneration: A Clinical Trial
Senomorphics	Rapamycin, metformin, resveratrol, aspirin, NF-kβ inhibitors (SR12343) p38MAPK inhibitors (BIRB 796,UR-13756), JAK/STAT inhibitors (ruxolitinib), statins, ATM inhibitors	Inhibitors of different pathways used by the senescent cell to produce harmful secretory factors.	See above for metformin/rapamycin. Others not selectively studied in humans to date.

T2DM type II diabetes mellitus, *wks* weeks, *pts* patients, *g/d* grams per day, *ave* average; *LPS* lipopolysaccharide (inflammatory initiator), *UC* ulcerative colitis, *CV* cardiovascular, *MCI* mild cognitive impairment, *ROS* reactive oxygen species, *AD* Alzheimer's Disease, *SASP* senescent-associated secretory phenotype, *CKD* chronic kidney disease, ↓ decrease, ↑ increase, *ATM* Ataxia Telangiectasia Mutated kinase, *PK* pharmacokinetics

53 studies reported that all-cause mortality in diabetics taking metformin was lower than nondiabetics and diabetics taking other antidiabetic drugs or insulin. Additionally, cancer and cardiovascular rates were lower in diabetics taking metformin compared to diabetics on other antidiabetic therapies [78]. A substudy of a RCT to treat anemia in patients with kidney failure and diabetes showed that those taking metformin had a reduced risk of all-cause mortality, CV death and combined endpoints compared to nonusers of metformin [79]. Together these findings suggest that *metformin offers additional benefits beyond control of the symptoms of diabetes*. Several clinical trials have and/or are engaged in obtaining data to that effect (see Table 10.2).

Metformin. Clinical Evidence Results of a large study showed metformin not only controls hyperglycemia in obese diabetics [62] but also decreases cardiovascular mortality, all-cause mortality and CV events in diabetic patients with CV disease but not in CV patients without diabetes [80]. In addition to its anti-hyperglycemic and CV protective effects and its efficacy in the treatment of polycystic ovarian syndrome [81], there is suggestive evidence that metformin may be beneficial in several other diseases [82]. For example, several studies report a reduced risk of cancer in those taking metformin [83, 84], and a modest protective effect against cancer risk [85]. However, two analyses found no support for a cancer risk reduction with metformin treatment [86, 87].

As with cancer therapy, the role of metformin in the treatment of neurodegenerative disease is not fully understood. Several studies indicate that short- and long-term (4–5 years) use of metformin prevents cognitive decline in older adults with diabetes [88, 89]. Similarly, according to a meta-analysis of population-based cohort studies, long-term use (≥4 years) of metformin reduces the risk of neurodegeneration [90]. In contrast, results of a meta-analysis of other observational studies concluded that metformin had no preventive effect on any type of neurodegenerative disease [91] and may even increase the risk of neurodegenerative disease [21, 22]. A comprehensive review of the many studies that have used metformin to treat diseases other than T2DM is found in Triggle et al. [82].

Briefly, several trials with metformin for anti-aging benefit in men have been completed. The Miles (Metformin in Longevity Study) measured gene expression in select tissues, skeletal muscle and fat [23]. Although a small study, metformin-induced the expression of a number of significant age-retarding genes, e.g., DNA repair genes and affected multiple metabolic pathways exerting positive effects on mitochondria and extracellular matrix [23]. A second study of slightly over 2 weeks of treatment with metformin was sufficient to prevent disuse muscle atrophy and cellular senescence in nondiabetics [18]. Several studies are ongoing (Investigation of Metformin in Pre-Diabetes on Atherosclerotic Cardiovascular Outcomes; Metformin for Preventing Frailty in High-Risk Older Adults) or in the planning stages (Targeting Aging with Metformin, TAME). Among these, the TAME trial has received considerable attention (https://www.afar.org tame trial). The TAME trial, distinguished as the first clinical trial to target aging per se, is a double-blinded placebo-controlled large (3000 nondiabetic volunteers 65–80 years, multiple centers) study of 6 years with a 3.5-year follow-up [24]. The hypothesis is that metformin will reduce the onset of non-diabetic diseases, reduce age-related decline in measured parameters (gait speed, cognition) and reduce hallmarks of aging, e.g., cell senescence and hence increase the healthspan and extend the lifespan.

SIRTUINS Sirtuins are a family (genes SIRT1–7) of nicotinamide adenine dinucleotide (NAD^+)-dependent histone deacetylase enzymes [25]. These enzymes are capable of changing the structure of other proteins, especially those surrounding DNA (the histones), to influence gene expression. They are homologous (similar) to histone deacetylase enzymes originally discovered in yeast and causally related via upregulation (increase in amount and activity) to lifespan extension [26]. Similar to yeast enzymes, sirtuins are major players in forestalling aging and improving responses to stress [27]. Sirtuins are epigenetic modulators (affecting gene expression, not DNA sequence). Epigenetic alteration is a hallmark of aging (see Table 10.1). Additionally, sirtuins also deacetylase proteins other than histones and hence are involved in an abundance of protective activities throughout the cell, e.g., cell survival, DNA repair, stress response, mitochondrial biogenesis (dividing to increase number), energy sensing and metabolism [28].

Sirtuins. Anti-aging Effects Sirtuins, present throughout the cell, rely heavily on the small molecule NAD^+. NAD^+, a key coenzyme in many metabolic reactions and a substrate for sirtuins, declines with age in mice [29] and humans [30], thereby diminishing the anti-aging effects of sirtuins [31]. In mice, caloric restriction and exercise upregulate (enhance) sirtuins and NAD^+ and increase the healthspan and lifespan [32]; removal of SIRT genes negates the health benefits of caloric restriction and exercise [33, 34]. These observations prompted a search for *SirTuin Activating Compounds* (STACs) that could be geroprotectors in humans to extend the healthspan.

Sirtuins. Sirtuin-Activating Compounds The most famous STAC is resveratrol, a naturally occurring STAC compound extracted from grapes and wine and commercially available as an over-the-counter supplement. Resveratrol has been tested in over 20 clinical trials to treat cancers, CV disease, diabetes, neurological disease and nonalcoholic fat liver [92]. Although these trials were small (9–66 participants, one study of 119 participants), variable durations (8 days to 6 months, one at 31 months) and variable doses (10 mg–5 grams, two with micronized resveratrol), most (16 trials) reported benefits such as improved glycemic control in diabetes, decreased inflammation and reduced pro-aging biomarkers in neurological and cardiovascular disease [92]. However, resveratrol is poorly bioavailable due to its rapid metabolism and excretion [93], hence the discovery of synthetic STACs: SRT2104, SRT2379, SRT3025 with better pharmacokinetics (PK). Synthetic STACs have been successful in ameliorating CV and metabolic diseases in numerous animal models [94]. As reviewed by Dai et al. [95], one of these STACs, SRT2104, has undergone clinical testing (see Table 10.2). Although SRT2104 exerts some antiinflammatory effects (ulcerative colitis, psoriasis) and some lipid-lowering (diabetics, smokers, healthy volunteers), the variable PK, although improved over resveratrol, hinders expected efficacy seen in animal studies [95]. As yet, STACs have not been evaluated in the older adult.

SENOTHERAPY. SENOLYTICS The therapeutic target of senolytics is the senescent cell. Cell senescence is a hallmark of aging (see Table 10.1). Briefly, in response to molecular stress, e.g., DNA damage, oxidative stress, telomere attrition (loss of protective ends on chromosomes), a cell experiences growth arrest and converts to a highly secretory state, termed the senescent-associated secretory phenotype (SASP), that produces and secretes an array of pro-inflammatory factors, destructive enzymes and cancer-inducing substances [96–98]. Senescent cells are anti-aging targets for several reason. Firstly, the secretory products from senescent cells are harmful to surrounding healthy cells and tissue structures and account for the low-grade chronic inflammation called inflammaging, an underpinning of most diseases, and secondly, these cells resist apoptosis (biological mechanism of cell suicide) and thus persist to continue to undermine organ function, thereby promoting aging and elevating the risk for diseases [99, 100].

Senolytics. Mechanism of Action Senolytics include a variety of drugs that act by one of several pathways to drive the senescent cell into oblivion, i.e., to commit apoptosis (cell suicide) [101]. It is reasoned that since senescent cells are a major cause of pathological changes leading to disease, their removal will forestall the onset of disease. Furthermore, senescent cells promote other hallmarks of aging in addition to inflammaging such as oxidative stress and fibrosis that would also disappear in their absence and thereby retard aging.

Senolytics. Repurposed Drugs Many of the senolytics are known drugs, now repurposed because of their ability to limit the survival of senescent cells. The most notable at present are dasatinib (D), quercetin (Q) and fisetin (F). Dasatinib is a tyrosine kinase inhibitor and an FDA-approved chemotherapeutic drug [102]. Q and F are polyphenolic flavonols found in a variety of fruits and vegetables but with biological activities overlapping that of D [101]. Many other drugs exhibit senolytic activity, generally observed at the in vitro (cell culture) level but with a mechanism of action different from D, Q and F and include geldanamycin, an antitumor drug, curcumin, a plant extract, several antibiotics (e.g., azithromycin) and the investigational anticancer drug, e.g., navitoclax (ABT-263) [101].

The results of animal research with senolytics are spectacular. D + Q treatment in a variety of animal models reduces the senescent cell population and, therefore, improves age-related decline in cardiac, pulmonary, and metabolic function and exercise capacity, as well as decreases disease progression of atherosclerosis and osteoporosis [103]. A reduction in age-related pathology and lifespan extension is evident with F treatment of mice, even in late life [104].

Senolytics. Clinical Evidence Three small pilot trials in humans have been completed with D + Q therapy (see Table 10.2). Results suggest that larger studies are reasonable. One study administered D + Q intermittently (3 days for 3 weeks) to 14 patients with idiopathic pulmonary fibrosis. Whereas pulmonary function was not changed, physical activities of walk distance, gait speed, and chair-stand times were significantly improved with senolytic therapy [47]. The second pilot study administered D + Q for 3 days to 9 patients with diabetic kidney disease. Eleven days post treatment, there was a reduction in senescent cells in tissue biopsies of fat and a decrease in SASP factors in the blood [49]. The third 12-week study of D + Q treatment of early symptomatic AD patients found a reduction in SASP inflammatory factors but no effect on cognition or neuroimaging [48]. As reviewed by Chaib et al. (2022), many trials are currently in progress (phase II with F) with objectives to (1) improve frailty in adult survivors of childhood cancer, (2) prevent premature aging in hematopoietic stem cell survivors, (3) improve skeletal muscle health, (4) improve benefits of bone marrow stem cell treatment, reduce cartilage degradation and decrease pain in osteoarthritis, (5) alleviate frailty and inflammation in older women, and (6) decrease complications of COVID-19. It is not clear why all future trials will test F when the initial feasibility and tolerability studies used D + Q therapy.

SENOTHERAPY. SENOMORPHICS Another means to suppress the destructive effects of senescent cells is to block the cellular pathways that produce the harmful secretory products. Drugs that accomplish this are termed senomorphics. Because the senescent cells produce and secrete an abundance of injurious substances, a variety of drugs with different mechanisms of action are effective in blocking this destructive activity. It is not surprising that drugs such as rapamycin, metformin, and resveratrol discussed have this ability since they inhibit in different ways the master commander of metabolism, mTOR. Other drugs that block the secretory activity of senescent cells target specific pathways. For example, SR12343, a recently developed chemical entity, inhibits the transcriptional factor NF-kβ to block the secretory activity of senescent fibroblasts in culture [105] and retards senescence changes in mice [106]. Another target involved in the abnormal secretory function of senescent cells is the mitogen-activated protein kinases (MAPKs) that include several subfamilies of kinases converting extracellular stresses to intracellular effects on metabolism, growth, proliferation and mobility [107]. Several second-generation MAPK inhibitors (BIRB 796 and UR-13756) are senomorphics in culture [108]. A different pathway, the Janus kinase/signal transducer and activator of transcription (JAK/STAT), is upregulated in senescent cells, and a JAK inhibitor, ruxolitinib, is approved to treat myelofibrosis (a type of cancer of the bone marrow) prevents secretion of inflammatory mediators both in vitro in human preadipocytes and in vivo in mice [109]. Additionally, well-known drugs, aspirin and statins, have the potential to block the secretory activity of the senescent cell [106]. Both drugs are protective of endothelial senescence by enhancing the production of nitric oxide, an antioxidant and vasodilator [110, 111].

ANTI-AGING DRUGS. CHALLENGES The field of geroscience is in its early stages. It faces many challenges [112]. The hypothesis that inhibition of the drivers of aging will prevent the onset of age-associated diseases and syndromes and thereby lengthen the healthspan is amply supported by results of preclinical animal studies. However, translation to humans faces several issues. One of the most serious is how to convince the FDA to approve a drug that inhibits one or several hallmarks of aging since the FDA mandate requires RCT results to show drug safety and efficacy for a specific disease. Despite the fact that aging is the major risk factor for disease, nevertheless, aging is not a disease. Thus, it is proposed that future clinical trials with anti-aging drugs target a single disease or disease-related function and rigorously demonstrate effects on validated biomarkers of aging [112].

Another challenge is that studies to date (see Table 10.2) are small, of short duration, and with administration of a single dose with a focus on safety and tolerability. Although some have yielded promising beneficial anti-aging effects, larger trials, longer durations and dose-responses are the essential next steps. Presently, there is considerable interest in the TAME trial, a large 6-year study to track the ability of daily dosing of metformin to prevent the onset of multiple diseases [24]. As discussed below, several anti-aging drugs possess the potential for adverse effects. These will need to be addressed for long-term use.

Anti-aging Drugs. Safety Although present data indicate that the anti-aging drugs are safe, they are not without potentially adverse effects, especially on long-term use. For example, metformin causes adverse GI effects, leading to intolerance for many [113] and possible vitamin B_{12} deficiency [114]. Although controversial, metformin may prevent the positive effects of exercise [115, 116]. Another concern relates to the use of contrast medium in patients taking metformin. Established guidelines require that metformin be discontinued prior to the use of contrast medium in diabetic patients with seriously reduced kidney function to prevent contrast medium-induced acute kidney injury [117]. However, the degree of kidney impairment for this requirement was not defined [117]. More recently, several meta-analyses of clinical trials concluded that in cases of kidney function greater than the estimated glomerular filtration rate of 30 (eGFR $\geq$30 mL/min/1.73 m^2), abstention of metformin is not necessary, and its presence did not cause contrast medium-induced acute kidney injury or lactic acidosis [118, 119].

Ulcers of the oral cavity are common with rapamycin therapy [120], an adverse effect that may be minimized with intermittent use of rapamycin. A potentially serious adverse outcome with senolytics is delayed and abnormal wound healing. This is expected since senescent cells perform this essential function and with senolytic therapy, senescent cell numbers would decline dramatically [121, 122].

Although new investigational anti-aging drugs are on the horizon, considerable work remains to evaluate these compounds in large RCTs spanning years. There is the need for proof of concept that negating one or more hallmarks of aging will, in fact, prevent the onset of disease and extend the healthspan.

> **Guidance**
> I. Geroscientists hypothesize that essential age changes, the hallmarks of aging, can be retarded with select drugs, and since aging is the major risk factor for disease, this approach would produce many disease-free years for the older adult. In other words, it would expand the healthspan and compress the senescent span.
> II. Drugs currently of interest that show some beneficial "anti-aging" effects in clinical trials are:
>
>   A. Rapamycin and rapalogues—inhibiting mTOR, a key nutrient sensor
>   B. Senolytics/senomorphs—inducing cell death in senescent cells/blocking harmful secretory factors
>   C. Metformin—exhibiting inhibitory effects on energy and nutrient sensors and other pathways
>   D. Sirtuins-activating compounds—influencing epigenetic expression to modify gene effects
>
> III. It is reasonable to continue this approach with larger, longer and more detailed clinical trials. Current anti-aging drugs have adverse effects that may be limiting on prolonged use. Prophylactic drug use in the healthy older adult requires absolute long-term safety.
> IV. Supplemental to the pharmacotherapy of the future is engagement in a program of lifelong physical exercise. The data overwhelmingly support this approach as essential for healthspan maintenance.

References

1. Slavkin HC. From phenotype to genotype. J Dent Res. 2014;93(7 Suppl):3S–6S. https://doi.org/10.1177/0022034514533569.
2. Brooks-Wilson AR. Genetics of healthy aging and longevity. Hum Genet. 2013;132(12):1323–38. https://doi.org/10.1007/s00439-013-1342-z.
3. Niccoli T, Partridge L. Ageing as a risk factor for disease. Curr Biol. 2012;22(17):R741–52. https://doi.org/10.1016/j.cub.2012.07.024.
4. López-Otín C, Blasco MA, Partridge L, Serrano M, Kroemer G. The hallmarks of aging. Cell. 2013;153(6):1194–217. https://doi.org/10.1016/j.cell.2013.05.039.
5. Seals DR, Melov S. Translational geroscience: emphasizing function to achieve optimal longevity. Aging (Albany NY). 2014;6(9):718–30. https://doi.org/10.18632/aging.100694.
6. Burch JB, Augustine AD, Frieden LA, Hadley E, Howcroft TK, Johnson R, et al. Advances in geroscience: impact on healthspan and chronic disease. J Gerontol A Biol Sci Med Sci. 2014;69(Suppl 1):S1–3. https://doi.org/10.1093/gerona/glu041.
7. McCay CM. Effect of restricted feeding upon aging and chronic diseases in rats and dogs. Am J Public Health Nations Health. 1947;37(5):521–8. PMID: 20297444
8. Colman RJ, Beasley TM, Kemnitz JW, Johnson SC, Weindruch R, Anderson RM. Caloric restriction reduces age-related and all-cause mortality in rhesus monkeys. Nat Commun. 2014;5:3557. https://doi.org/10.1038/ncomms4557.

9. Ros M, Carrascosa JM. Current nutritional and pharmacological anti-aging interventions. Biochim Biophys Acta Mol basis Dis. 2020;1866(3):165612. https://doi.org/10.1016/j.bbadis.2019.165612.
10. Parrella E, Longo VD. Insulin/IGF-I and related signaling pathways regulate aging in nondividing cells: from yeast to the mammalian brain. ScientificWorldJournal. 2010;10:161–77. https://doi.org/10.1100/tsw.2010.8.
11. Harrison DE, Strong R, Sharp ZD, Nelson JF, Astle CM, Flurkey K, et al. Rapamycin fed late in life extends lifespan in genetically heterogeneous mice. Nature. 2009;460(7253):392–5. https://doi.org/10.1038/nature08221.
12. Zhang Y, Zhang J, Wang S. The role of rapamycin in healthspan extension via the delay of organ aging. Ageing Res Rev. 2021;70:101376. https://doi.org/10.1016/j.arr.2021.101376.
13. Groessl EJ, Kaplan RM, Rejeski WJ, Katula JA, Glynn NW, King AC, et al. Physical activity and performance impact long-term quality of life in older adults at risk for major mobility disability. Am J Prev Med. 2019;56(1):141–6. https://doi.org/10.1016/j.amepre.2018.09.006.
14. Gries KJ, Baue U, Perkins RK, Lavin KM, Overstreet BS, D'Acquisto LJ, et al. Cardiovascular and skeletal muscle health with lifelong exercise. J Appl Physiol. 2018;125(5):1636–45. https://doi.org/10.1152/japplphysiol.00174.2018.
15. Schmauck-Medina T, Molière A, Lautrup S, Zhang J, Chlopicki S, Madsen HB, et al. New hallmarks of ageing: a 2022 Copenhagen ageing meeting summary. Aging (Albany NY). 2022;14(16):6829–39. https://doi.org/10.18632/aging.204248.
16. López-Otín C, Blasco MA, Partridge L, Serrano M, Kroemer G. Hallmarks of aging: an expanding universe. Cell. 2023;186(2):243–78. https://doi.org/10.1016/j.cell.2022.11.001.
17. Tchkonia T, Palmer AK, Kirkland JL. New horizons: novel approaches to enhance healthspan through targeting cellular senescence and related aging mechanisms. J Clin Endocrinol Metab. 2021;106(3):e1481–7. https://doi.org/10.1210/clinem/dgaa728.
18. Petrocelli J, McKenzie AI, deHart NMMP, Reidy PT, Mahmassani ZS, Keeble AR, et al. Disuse-induced muscle fibrosis, cellular senescence, and senescence-associated secretory phenotype in older adults are alleviated during re-ambulation with metformin pre-treatment. Aging Cell. 2023;22(11):e13936. https://doi.org/10.1111/acel.13936.
19. Cameron AR, Morrison VL, Levin D, Mohan M, Forteath C, Beall C, et al. Antiinflammatory effects of metformin irrespective of diabetes status. Circ Res. 2016;119(5):652–65. https://doi.org/10.1161/CIRCRESAHA.116.308445.
20. Luchsinger JA, Perez T, Chang H, Mehta P, Steffener J, Pradabhan G, et al. Metformin in amnestic mild cognitive impairment: results of a pilot randomized placebo controlled clinical trial. J Alzheimers Dis. 2016;51(2):501–14. https://doi.org/10.3233/JAD-150493.
21. Imfeld P, Bodmer M, Jick SS, Meier CR. Metformin, other antidiabetic drugs, and risk of Alzheimer's disease: a population-based case–control study. J Am Geriatr Soc. 2012;60(5):916–21. https://doi.org/10.1111/j.1532-5415.2012.03916.x.
22. Kuan Y-C, Huang K-W, Lin C-L, Hu C-J, Kao C-H. Effects of metformin exposure on neurodegenerative diseases in elderly patients with type 2 diabetes mellitus. Prog Neuro-Psychopharmacol Biol Psychiatry. 2017;79:77–83. https://doi.org/10.1016/j.pnpbp.2017.06.002.
23. Kulkarni AS, Brutsaert EF, Anghel V, Zhang K, Bloomgarden N, Pollak M, et al. Metformin regulates metabolic and nonmetabolic pathways in skeletal muscle and subcutaneous adipose tissues of older adults. Aging Cell. 2018;17(2):e12723. https://doi.org/10.1111/acel.12723.
24. Barzilai N, Crandall JP, Kritchevsky SB, Espeland MA. Metformin as a tool to target aging. Cell Metab. 2016;23(6):1060–5. https://doi.org/10.1016/j.cmet.2016.05.011.
25. Landry J, Sutton A, Tafrov S, Heller R, Stebbins J, Pillus L, et al. The silencing protein SIR2 and its homologs are NAD-dependent protein deacetylases. Proc Natl Acad Sci USA. 2000;97(11):5807–11. https://doi.org/10.1073/pnas.110148297.
26. Imai S, Armstrong CM, Kaeberlein M, Guarente L. Transcriptional silencing and longevity protein Sir2 is an NAD-dependent histone deacetylase. Nature. 2000;403(6771):795–800. https://doi.org/10.1038/35001622.

27. Bonkowski MS, Sinclair DA. Slowing ageing by design: the rise of NAD+ and sirtuin-activating compounds. Nat Rev Mol Cell Biol. 2016;17(11):679–90. https://doi.org/10.1038/nrm.2016.93.
28. Chang HC, Guarente L. SIRT1 and other sirtuins in metabolism. Trends Endocrinol Metab. 2014;25(3):138–45. https://doi.org/10.1016/j.tem.2013.12.001.
29. Camacho-Pereira J, Tarragó MG, Chini CCS, Nin V, Escande C, Warner GM, et al. CD38 dictates age-related NAD decline and mitochondrial dysfunction through an SIRT3-dependent mechanism. Cell Metab. 2016;23:1127–39. https://doi.org/10.1016/j.cmet.2016.05.006.
30. Zhu X-H, Lu M, Lee B-Y, Ugurbil K, Chen W. In vivo NAD assay reveals the intracellular NAD contents and redox state in healthy human brain and their age dependences. Proc Natl Acad Sci. 2015;112(9):2876–81. https://doi.org/10.1073/pnas.1417921112.
31. Imai S-I, Guarente L. NAD+ and sirtuins in aging and disease. Trends Cell Biol. 2014;24(8):464–71. https://doi.org/10.1016/j.tcb.2014.04.002.
32. Radak Z, Koltai E, Taylor AW, Higuchi M, Kumagai S, Ohno H, et al. Redox-regulating sirtuins in aging, caloric restriction, and exercise. Free Radic Biol Med. 2013;58:87–97. https://doi.org/10.1016/j.freeradbiomed.2013.01.004.
33. Mostoslavsky R, Chua KF, Lombard DB, Pang WW, Fischer MR, Gellon L, et al. Genomic instability and aging-like phenotype in the absence of mammalian SIRT6. Cell. 2006;124(2):315–29. https://doi.org/10.1016/j.cell.2005.11.044.
34. Kanfi Y, Naiman S, Amir G, Peshti V, Zinman G, Nahum L, et al. The sirtuin SIRT6 regulates lifespan in male mice. Nature. 2012;483(7388):218–21. https://doi.org/10.1038/nature10815.
35. Justice JN, Niedernhofer L, Robbins PD, Aroda VR, Espeland MA, Kritchevsky SB. Development of clinical trials to extend healthy lifespan. Cardiovasc Endocrinol Metab. 2018;7(4):80–3. https://doi.org/10.1097/XCE.0000000000000159.
36. Venkatasubramanian S, Noh RM, Daga S, Langrish JP, Joshi NV, Mills NL, et al. Cardiovascular effects of a novel SIRT1 activator, SRT2104, in otherwise healthy cigarette smokers. J Am Heart Assoc. 2013;2(3):e000042. https://doi.org/10.1161/JAHA.113.000042.
37. Baksi A, Kraydashenko O, Zalevkaya A, Stets R, Elliott P, Haddad J, et al. A phase II, randomized, placebo-controlled, double-blind, multi-dose study of SRT2104, a SIRT1 activator, in subjects with type 2 diabetes. Br J Clin Pharmacol. 2014;78(1):69–77. https://doi.org/10.1111/bcp.12327.
38. Krueger JG, Suárez-Fariñas M, Cueto I, Khacherian A, Matheson R, Parish LC, et al. A randomized, placebo-controlled study of SRT2104, a SIRT1 activator, in patients with moderate to severe psoriasis. PLoS One. 2015;10(11):e0142081. https://doi.org/10.1371/journal.pone.0142081.
39. van der Meer AJ, Scicluna BP, Moerland PD, Lin J, Jacobson EW, Vlasuk GP, et al. The selective Sirtuin 1 activator SRT2104 reduces endotoxin-induced cytokine release and coagulation activation in humans. Crit Care Med. 2015;43(6):e199–202. https://doi.org/10.1097/CCM.0000000000000949.
40. Sands BE, Joshi S, Haddad J, Freudenberg JM, Oommen DE, Hoffmann E, et al. Assessing colonic exposure, safety, and clinical activity of SRT2104, a novel oral SIRT1 activator, in patients with mild to moderate ulcerative colitis. Inflamm Bowel Dis. 2016;22(3):607–14. https://doi.org/10.1097/MIB.0000000000000597.
41. Noh RM, Venkatasubramanian S, Daga S, Langrish J, Mills NL, Lang NN, et al. Cardiometabolic effects of a novel SIRT1 activator, SRT2104, in people with type 2 diabetes mellitus. Open Heart. 2017;4(2):e000647. https://doi.org/10.1136/openhrt-2017-000647.
42. Mannick JB, Morris M, Hockey HUP, Roma G, Beibel M, Kulatycki K, et al. TORC1 inhibition enhances immune function and reduces infections in the elderly. Sci Transl Med. 2018;10(449):eaaq1564. https://doi.org/10.1126/scitranslmed.aaq1564.
43. Kraig E, Linehan LA, Liang H, Romo TQ, Liu Q, Wu Y, et al. A randomized control trial to establish the feasibility and safety of rapamycin treatment in an older human cohort: immunological, physical performance, and cognitive effects. Exp Gerontol. 2018;105:53–69. https://doi.org/10.1016/j.exger.2017.12.026.

44. Chung CL, Lawrence I, Hoffman M, Elgindi D, Nadhan K, Potnis M, et al. Topical rapamycin reduces markers of senescence and aging in human skin: an exploratory, prospective, randomized trial. Geroscience. 2019;41(6):861–9. https://doi.org/10.1007/s11357-019-00113-y.
45. Svatek RS, Ji N, de Leon E, Mukherjee NZ, Kabra A, Hurez V, et al. Rapamycin prevents surgery-induced immune dysfunction in patients with bladder cancer. Cancer Immunol Res. 2019;7(3):466–75. https://doi.org/10.1158/2326-6066.CIR-18-0336.
46. Singh M, Jensen MD, Lerman A, Kushwaha S, Rihal CS, Gersh BJ, et al. Effect of low-dose rapamycin on senescence markers and physical functioning in older adults with coronary artery disease: results of a pilot study. J Frailty Aging. 2016;5(4):204–7. https://doi.org/10.14283/jfa.2016.112.
47. Justice JN, Nambiar AM, Tchkonia T, LeBrasseur NK, Pascual R, Hashmi SK, et al. Senolytics in idiopathic pulmonary fibrosis: results from a first-in-human, open-label, pilot study. EBioMedicine. 2019;40:554–63. https://doi.org/10.1016/j.ebiom.2018.12.052.
48. Gonzales MM, Garbarino VR, Kautz TF, Palavicini JP, Lopez-Cruzan M, Dehkordi SK, et al. Senolytic therapy in mild Alzheimer's disease: a phase 1 feasibility trial. Nat Med. 2023;29(10):2481–8. https://doi.org/10.1038/s41591-023-02543-w.
49. Hickson LJ, Langhi Prata LGP, Bobart SA, Evans TK, Giorgadze N, Hashmi SK, et al. Senolytics decrease senescent cells in humans: preliminary report from a clinical trial of Dasatinib plus Quercetin in individuals with diabetic kidney disease. EBioMedicine. 2019;47:446–56. https://doi.org/10.1016/j.ebiom.2019.08.069.
50. Kaeberlein M, Powers RW 3rd, Steffen KK, Westman EA, Hu D, Dang N, et al. Regulation of yeast replicative life span by TOR and Sch9 in response to nutrients. Science. 2005;310(5751):1193–6. https://doi.org/10.1126/science.1115535.
51. Vellai T, Takacs-Vellai K, Kovacs ZY, AL, Orosz L, Muller F. Genetics: influence of TOR kinase on lifespan in C. elegans. Nature. 2003;426(6967):620. https://doi.org/10.1038/426620a.
52. Kapahi P, Zid BM, Harper T, Koslover D, Sapin V, Benzer S. Regulation of lifespan in Drosophila by modulation of genes in the TOR signaling pathway. Curr Biol. 2004;14(10):885–90. https://doi.org/10.1016/j.cub.2004.03.059.
53. Wu JJ, Liu J, Chen EB, Wang JJ, Cao L, Narayan N, et al. Increased mammalian lifespan and a segmental and tissue-specific slowing of aging after genetic reduction of mTOR expression. Cell Rep. 2013;4(5):913–20. https://doi.org/10.1016/j.celrep.2013.07.030.
54. McCay CM, Crowell MF, Maynard LA. The effect of retarded growth upon the length of life span and upon the ultimate body size. 1935. Nutrition. 1989;5(3):155–71. discussion 172
55. Anderson RM, Weindruch R. The caloric restriction paradigm: implications for healthy human aging. Am J Hum Biol. 2012;24:101–6. https://doi.org/10.1002/ajhb.22243.
56. Bitto A, Ito TK, Pineda VV, LeTexier NJ, Huang HZ, Sutlief E, et al. Transient rapamycin treatment can increase lifespan and healthspan in middle-aged mice. eLife. 2016;5:e16351. https://doi.org/10.7554/eLife.16351.
57. Selvarani R, Mohammed S, Richardson A. Effect of rapamycin on aging and age-related diseases-past and future. Geroscience. 2021;43(3):1135–58. https://doi.org/10.1007/s11357-020-00274-1.
58. Brown EJ, Albers MW, Shin TB, Ichikawa K, Lane KCT, WS. A mammalian protein targeted by G1-arresting rapamycin–receptor complex. Nature. 1994;369(6483):756–8. https://doi.org/10.1038/369756a0.
59. Sabatini DM, Erdjument-Bromage H, Lui M, Tempst P, Snyder SH. RAFT1: a mammalian protein that binds to FKBP12 in a rapamycin-dependent fashion and is homologous to yeast TORs. Cell. 1994;78(1):35–43. https://doi.org/10.1016/0092-8674(94)90570-3.
60. Sabers CJ, Martin MM, Brunn GJ, Williams JM, Duont FJ, Wiederrcht G, et al. Isolation of a protein target of the FKBP12–rapamycin complex in mammalian cells. J Biol Chem. 1995;270(2):815–22. https://doi.org/10.1074/jbc.270.2.815.
61. Liu GY, Sabatini DM. mTOR at the nexus of nutrition, growth, ageing and disease. Nat Rev Mol Cell Biol. 2020;21(4):183–203. https://doi.org/10.1038/s41580-019-0199-y.

62. Group UKPDS. Effect of intensive blood-glucose control with metformin on complications in overweight patients with type 2 diabetes (UKPDS 34). Lancet. 1998;352(9131):854–65. https://doi.org/10.1016/S0140-6736(98)07037-8.
63. Ahmad E, Sargeant JA, Zaccardi F, Khunti K, Webb DR, Davies MJ. Where does metformin stand in modern day management of type 2 diabetes? Pharmaceuticals. 2020;13(12):427. https://doi.org/10.3390/ph13120427.
64. Rena G, Hardie DG, Person ER. The mechanisms of action of metformin. Diabetologia. 2017;60(9):1577–85. https://doi.org/10.1007/s00125-017-4342-z.
65. Hardie DG, Ross FA, Hawley SA. AMPK: a nutrient and energy sensor that maintains energy homeostasis. Nat Rev Mol Cell Biol. 2012;13(4):251–62. https://doi.org/10.1038/nrm3311.
66. Vasamsetti SB, Karnewar S, Kanugula AK, Thatipalli AR, Kumar JM, Kotamraju S. Metformin inhibits monocyte-tomacrophage differentiation via AMPK-mediated inhibition of STAT3 activation: potential role in atherosclerosis. Diabetes. 2015;64(6):2028–41. https://doi.org/10.2337/db14-1225.
67. Howell JJ, Hellberg K, Turner M, Talbott G, Kolar MJ, Ross DS, et al. Metformin inhibits hepatic mTORC1 signaling via dose-dependent mechanisms involving AMPK and the TSC complex. Cell Metab. 2017;25(2):463–71. https://doi.org/10.1016/j.cmet.2016.12.009.
68. Mather KJ, Verma S, Anderson TJ. Improved endothelial function with metformin in type 2 diabetes mellitus. J Am Coll Cardiol. 2001;37(5):1344–50. https://doi.org/10.1016/s0735-1097(01)01129-9.
69. Onken B, Driscoll M. Metformin induces a dietary restriction-like state and the oxidative stress response to extend C. elegans healthspan via AMPK, LKB1 and SKN-1. PLoS One. 2010;5(1):e8758. https://doi.org/10.1371/journal.pone.0008758.
70. Anisimov VN, Berstein LM, Popovich IG, Zabezhinski MA, Egormin PA, Piskunova TS, et al. If started early in life, metformin treatment increases life span and postpones tumors in female SHR mice. Aging (Albany NY). 2011;3(2):148–57. https://doi.org/10.18632/aging.100273.
71. Martin-Montalvo A, Mercken EM, Mitchell SJ, Palacios HH, Mote PL, Scheibye-Knudsen M, et al. Metformin improves healthspan and lifespan in mice. Nat Commun. 2013;4:2192. https://doi.org/10.1038/ncomms3192.
72. Cabreiro F, Au C, Leung KY, Vergara-Irigaray N, Cocheme HM, Noori T, et al. Metformin retards aging in C. elegans by altering microbial folate and methionine metabolism. Cell. 2013;153(1):228–39. https://doi.org/10.1016/j.cell.2013.02.035.
73. Smith DL, Elam CF, Mattison JA, Lane MA, Roth GS, Ingram DK. Metformin supplementation and life span in Fischer-344 rats. J Gerontol A Biol Sci Med Sci. 2010;65(5):468–74. https://doi.org/10.1093/gerona/glq033.
74. Strong R, Miller RA, Antebi A, Astle CM, Bogue M, Denzel MS, et al. Longer lifespan in male mice treated with a weakly estrogenic agonist, an antioxidant, an a-glucosidase inhibitor or a Nrf2-inducer. Aging Cell. 2016;15(5):872–84. https://doi.org/10.1111/acel.12496.
75. Espada L, Dakhovnik A, Chaudhari P, Martirosyan A, Miek L, Poliezhaieva T, et al. Loss of metabolic plasticity underlies metformin toxicity in aged Caenorhabditis elegans. Nat Metab. 2020;2(11):1316–31. https://doi.org/10.1038/s42255-020-00307-1.
76. Mohammed I, Hollenberg MD, Ding H, Triggle CR. A critical review of the evidence that metformin is a putative anti-aging drug that enhances healthspan and extends lifespan. Front Endocrinol. 2021;12 https://doi.org/10.3389/fendo.2021.718942.
77. Bannister CA, Holden S, Jenkins-Jones S, Morgan CL, Halcox J, Schernthaner G, et al. Can people with type 2 diabetes live longer than those without? A comparison of mortality in people initiated with metformin or sulphonylurea monotherapy and matched, non-diabetic controls. Diabetes Obes Metab. 2014;16(11):1165–73. https://doi.org/10.1111/dom.12354.
78. Campbell JM, Bellman SM, Stephenson MD, Lisy K. Metformin reduces all-cause mortality and diseases of ageing independent of its effect on diabetes control: a systematic review and meta-analysis. Ageing Res Rev. 2017;40:31–44. https://doi.org/10.1016/j.arr.2017.08.003.

79. Charytan DM, Solomon SD, Ivanovich P, Remuzzi G, Cooper ME, McGill JB, et al. Metformin use and cardiovascular events in patients with type 2 diabetes and chronic kidney disease. Diabetes Obes Metab. 2019;21(5):1199–208. https://doi.org/10.1111/dom.13642.
80. Han Y, Xie H, Liu Y, Gao P, Yang X, Shen Z. Effect of metformin on all-cause and cardiovascular mortality in patients with coronary artery diseases: a systematic review and an updated meta-analysis. Cardiovasc Diabetol. 2019;18(1):1–16. https://doi.org/10.1186/s12933-019-0900-7.
81. Velazquez EM, Mendoza S, Hamer T, Sosa F, Glueck CJ. Metformin therapy in polycystic ovary syndrome reduces hyperinsulinemia, insulin resistance, hyperandrogenemia, and systolic blood pressure, while facilitating normal menses and pregnancy. Metabolism. 1994;43:647–54. https://doi.org/10.1016/0026-0495(94)90209-7.
82. Triggle CR, Mohammed I, Bshesh K, Marei I, Ye K, Ding H, MacDonald R, et al. Metformin: is it a drug for all reasons and diseases? Metabolism. 2022;133:155223. https://doi.org/10.1016/j.metabol.2022.155223.
83. Evans JM, Donnelly LA, Emslie-Smith AM, Alessi DR, Morris AD. Metformin and reduced risk of cancer in diabetic patients. BMJ. 2005;330(7503):1304–5. https://doi.org/10.1136/bmj.38415.708634.F7.
84. Lee M-S, Hsu C-C, Wahlqvist ML, Tsai H-N, Chang Y-H, Huang Y-C. Type 2 diabetes increases and metformin reduces total, colorectal, liver and pancreatic cancer incidences in Taiwanese: a representative population prospective cohort study of 800,000 individuals. BMC Cancer. 2011;11(1):1–10. https://doi.org/10.1186/1471-2407-11-20.
85. Gandini S, Puntoni M, Heckman-Stoddard BM, Dunn BK, Ford L, DeCensi A, et al. Metformin and cancer risk and mortality: a systematic review and meta-analysis taking into account biases and confounders. Cancer Prev Res. 2014;7(9):867–85. https://doi.org/10.1158/1940-6207.CAPR-13-0424.
86. Home P, Kahn S, Jones N, Noronha D, Beck-Nielsen H, Viberti G. Experience of malignancies with oral glucose-lowering drugs in the randomised controlled ADOPT (A Diabetes Outcome Progression Trial) and RECORD (Rosiglitazone Evaluated for Cardiovascular Outcomes and Regulation of Glycaemia in Diabetes) clinical trials. Diabetologia. 2010;53(9):1838–45. https://doi.org/10.1007/s00125-010-1804-y.
87. Stevens R, Ali R, Bankhead C, Bethel M, Cairns B, Camisasca R, et al. Cancer outcomes and all-cause mortality in adults allocated to metformin: systematic review and collaborative meta-analysis of randomised clinical trials. Diabetologia. 2012;55(10):2593–603. https://doi.org/10.1007/s00125-012-2653-7.
88. Ng TP, Feng L, Yap KB, Lee TS, Tan CH, Winblad B. Long-term metformin usage and cognitive function among older adults with diabetes. J Alzheimers Dis. 2014;41(1):61–8. https://doi.org/10.3233/JAD-131901.
89. Koenig AM, Mechanic-Hamilton D, Xie SX, Combs MF, Cappola AR, Xie L, et al. Effects of the insulin sensitizer metformin in Alzheimer's disease: pilot data from a randomized placebo-controlled crossover study. Alzheimer Dis Assoc Disord. 2017;31(2):107–13. https://doi.org/10.1097/WAD.0000000000000202.
90. Zhang Y, Zhang Y, Shi X, Han J, Lin B, Peng W, et al. Metformin and the risk of neurodegenerative diseases in patients with diabetes: a meta-analysis of population-based cohort studies. Diabet Med. 2022;39:e14821. https://doi.org/10.1111/dme.14821.
91. Ping F, Jiang N, Li YX. Association between metformin and neurodegenerative diseases of observational studies: systematic review and meta-analysis. BMJ Open Diabetes Res Care. 2020;8(1):e001370. https://doi.org/10.1136/bmjdrc-2020-001370.
92. Berman AY, Motechin RA, Wiesenfeld MY, Holz MK. The therapeutic potential of resveratrol: a review of clinical trials. npj Precis Oncologia. 2017;1:35. https://doi.org/10.1038/s41698-017-0038-6.
93. Walle T. Bioavailability of resveratrol. Ann N Y Acad Sci. 2011;1215:9–15. https://doi.org/10.1111/j.1749-6632.2010.05842.x.

94. Kane AE, Sinclair DA. Sirtuins and NAD(+) in the development and treatment of metabolic and cardiovascular diseases. Circ Res. 2018;123(7):868–85. https://doi.org/10.1161/CIRCRESAHA.118.312498.
95. Dai H, Sinclair DA, Ellis JL, Steegborn C. Sirtuin activators and inhibitors: promises, achievements, and challenges. Pharmacol Ther. 2018;188:140–54. https://doi.org/10.1016/j.pharmthera.2018.03.004.
96. Campisi J. Senescent cells, tumor suppression, and organismal aging: good citizens, bad neighbors. Cell. 2005;120(4):513–22. https://doi.org/10.1016/j.cell.2005.02.003.
97. Freund A, Orjalo AV, Desprez PY, Campisi J. Inflammatory networks during cellular senescence: causes and consequences. Trends Mol Med. 2010;16(5):238–46. https://doi.org/10.1016/j.molmed.2010.03.003.
98. Laberge RM, Awad P, Campisi J, Desprez PY. Epithelial-mesenchymal transition induced by senescent fibroblasts. Cancer Microenviron. 2012;5(1):39–44. https://doi.org/10.1007/s12307-011-0069-4.
99. Campisi J. Aging, cellular senescence, and cancer. Annu Rev Physiol. 2013;75:685–705. https://doi.org/10.1146/annurev-physiol-030212-183653.
100. Birch J, Gil J. Senescence and the SASP: many therapeutic avenues. Genes Dev. 2020;34(23–24):1565–76. https://doi.org/10.1101/gad.343129.120.
101. Zhang L, Pitcher LE, Prahalad V, Niedernhofer LJ, Robbins PD. Targeting cellular senescence with senotherapeutics: senolytics and senomorphics. FEBS J. 2023;290(5):1362–83. https://doi.org/10.1111/febs.16350.
102. https://www.accessdata.fda.gov/drugsatfda_docs/nda/2006/021986_022072_SprycelTOC.cfm#:~:text=Approval%20Date%3A%2006%2F28%2F2006.
103. Chaib S, Tchkonia T, Kirkland JL. Cellular senescence and senolytics: the path to the clinic. Nat Med. 2022;28(8):1556–68. https://doi.org/10.1038/s41591-022-01923-y.
104. Yousefzadeh MJ, Zhu Y, McGowan SJ, Angelini L, Fuhrmann-Stroissnigg H, Xu M, et al. Fisetin is a senotherapeutic that extends health and lifespan. EBioMedicine. 2018;36:18–28. https://doi.org/10.1016/j.ebiom.2018.09.015.
105. Zhao J, Zhang L, Mu X, Doebelin C, Nguyen W, Wallace C, et al. Development of novel NEMO binding domain mimetics for inhibiting IKK/NF-jB activation. PLoS Biol. 2018;16(6):e2004663. https://doi.org/10.1371/journal.pbio.2004663.
106. Zhang L, Zhao J, Mu X, McGowan SJ, Angelini L, O'Kelly RD, et al. Novel small molecule inhibition of IKK/NF-jB activation reduces markers of senescence and improves healthspan in mouse models of aging. Aging Cell. 2021;20(12):e13486. https://doi.org/10.1111/acel.13486.
107. Cargnello M, Roux PP. Activation and function of the MAPKs and their substrates, the MAPK-activated protein kinases. Microbiol Mol Biol Rev. 2011;75(1):50–83. https://doi.org/10.1128/MMBR.00031-10.
108. Alimbetov D, Davis T, Brook AJ, Cox LS, Faragher RG, Nurgozhin T, et al. Suppression of the senescence-associated secretory phenotype (SASP) in human fibroblasts using small molecule inhibitors of p38 MAP kinase and MK2. Biogerontology. 2016;17(2):305–15. https://doi.org/10.1007/s10522-015-9610-z.
109. Xu M, Tchkonia T, Ding H, Ogrodnik M, Lubbers ER, Pirtskhalava T, et al. JAK inhibition alleviates the cellular senescence-associated secretory phenotype and frailty in old age. Proc Natl Acad Sci USA. 2015;112(46):E6301–10. https://doi.org/10.1073/pnas.1515386112.
110. Bode-Boger SM, Martens-Lobenhoffer J, Teager M, Schreoder H, Scalera F. Aspirin reduces endothelial cell senescence. Biochem Biophys Res Commun. 2005;334(4):1226–32. https://doi.org/10.1016/j.bbrc.2005.07.014.
111. Ota H, Eto M, Kano MR, Kahyo T, Setou M, Ogawa S, et al. Induction of endothelial nitric oxide synthase, SIRT1, and catalase by statins inhibits endothelial senescence through the Akt pathway. Arte4rioscler Thromb Vasc Biol. 2010;30(11):2205–11. https://doi.org/10.1161/ATVBAHA.110.210500.

112. Rolland Y, Sierra F, Ferrucci L, Barzilais N, DeCabo R, Mannick J, et al. Challenges in developing Geroscience trials. Nat Commun. 2023;14(1):5038. https://doi.org/10.1038/s41467-023-39786-7.
113. McCreight LJ, Bailey CJ, Pearson ER. Metformin and the gastrointestinal tract. Diabetologia. 2016;59(3):426–35. https://doi.org/10.1007/s00125-015-3844-9.
114. Infante M, Leoni M, Caprio M, Fabbri A. Long-term metformin therapy and vitamin B12 deficiency: an association to bear in mind. World J Diabetes. 2021;12(7):916–31. https://doi.org/10.4239/wjd.v12.i7.916.
115. Konopka AR, Laurin JL, Schoenberg HM, Reid JJ, Castor WM, Wolff CA, et al. Metformin inhibits mitochondrial adaptations to aerobic exercise training in older adults. Aging Cell. 2019;18(1):e12880. https://doi.org/10.1111/acel.12880.
116. Miller BF, Thyfault JP. Exercise-pharmacology interactions: metformin, statins, and healthspan. Physiology (Bethesda). 2020;35(5):338–47. https://doi.org/10.1152/physiol.00013.2020.
117. Goergen SK, Rumbold G, Compton G, Harris C. Systematic review of current guidelines, and their evidence base, on risk of lactic acidosis after administration of contrast medium for patients receiving metformin. Radiology. 2010;254(1):261–9. https://doi.org/10.1148/radiol.09090690.
118. Qiao H, Li Y, Xu B, Lu Z, Zhang J, Meng E, et al. Metformin can be safely used in patients exposed to contrast media: a systematic review and meta-analysis. Cardiology. 2022;147(5–6):469–78. https://doi.org/10.1159/000527384.
119. Kao TW, Lee KH, Chan WP, Fan KC, Liu CW, Huang Y-C. Continuous use of metformin in patients receiving contrast medium: what is the evidence? A systematic review and meta-analysis. Eur Radiol. 2022;32(5):3045–55. https://doi.org/10.1007/s00330-021-08395-7.
120. Yuan A, Woo SB. Adverse drug events in the oral cavity. Oral Surg Oral Med Oral Pathol Oral Radiol. 2015;119(1):35–47. https://doi.org/10.1016/j.oooo.2014.09.009.
121. Demaria M, Ohtani N, Youssef SA, Rodier F, Toussaint W, Mitchell JR, et al. An essential role for senescent cells in optimal wound healing through secretion of PDGF-AA. Dev Cell. 2014;31(6):722–33. https://doi.org/10.1016/j.devcel.2014.11.012.
122. Calcinotto A, Kohli J, Zagato E, Pellegrini L, Demaria M, Alimonti A. Cellular senescence: aging, cancer, and injury. Physiol Rev. 2019;99(2):1047–78. https://doi.org/10.1152/physrev.00020.2018.

GPSR Compliance

The European Union's (EU) General Product Safety Regulation (GPSR) is a set of rules that requires consumer products to be safe and our obligations to ensure this.

If you have any concerns about our products, you can contact us on ProductSafety@springernature.com

In case Publisher is established outside the EU, the EU authorized representative is:

Springer Nature Customer Service Center GmbH
Europaplatz 3
69115 Heidelberg, Germany

Batch number: 08751879

Printed by Printforce, the Netherlands